T0311797

Nutraceuticals for Aging and Anti-Aging

Nutraceuticals: Basic Research and Clinical Applications

Series Editor:
Yashwant Pathak, PhD

Nutrigenomics and Nutraceuticals
Clinical Relevance and Disease Prevention
Edited by Yashwant Pathak and Ali M. Ardekani

Food By-Product Based Functional Food Powders
Edited by Özlem Tokuşoğlu

Flavors for Nutraceuticals and Functional Foods
M. Selvamuthukumaran and Yashwant Pathak

Antioxidant Nutraceuticals
Preventive and Healthcare Applications
Chuanhai Cao, Sarvadaman Pathak, and Kiran Patil

Advances in Nutraceutical Applications in Cancer
Recent Research Trends and Clinical Applications
Edited by Sheeba Varghese Gupta and Yashwant Pathak

Flavor Development for Functional Foods and Nutraceuticals
M. Selvamuthukumaran and Yashwant Pathak

Nutraceuticals for Prenatal, Maternal and Offspring's Nutritional Health
Priyanka Bhatt, Maryam Sadat Miraghajani, Sarvadaman Pathak, and Yashwant Pathak

Bioactive Peptides
Production, Bioavailability, Health Potential and Regulatory Issues
Edited by John Oloche Onuh, M. Selvamuthukumaran, and Yashwant Pathak

Nutraceuticals for Aging and Anti-Aging
Basic Understanding and Clinical Evidence
Edited by Jayant Lokhande and Yashwant Pathak

For more information about this series, please visit: https://www.crcpress.com/Nutraceuticals/book-series/CRCNUTBASRES

Nutraceuticals for Aging and Anti-Aging

Basic Understanding and Clinical Evidence

Edited by
Jayant N. Lokhande and
Yashwant V. Pathak

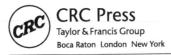

CRC Press
Taylor & Francis Group
Boca Raton London New York

CRC Press is an imprint of the
Taylor & Francis Group, an **informa** business

First edition published 2022
by CRC Press
6000 Broken Sound Parkway NW, Suite 300, Boca Raton, FL 33487-2742

and by CRC Press
2 Park Square, Milton Park, Abingdon, Oxon, OX14 4RN

© 2022 selection and editorial matter, Jayant Nemchand Lokhande, Yashwant Vishnupant Pathak; individual chapters, the contributors

CRC Press is an imprint of Taylor & Francis Group, LLC

Reasonable efforts have been made to publish reliable data and information, but the author and publisher cannot assume responsibility for the validity of all materials or the consequences of their use. The authors and publishers have attempted to trace the copyright holders of all material reproduced in this publication and apologize to copyright holders if permission to publish in this form has not been obtained. If any copyright material has not been acknowledged please write and let us know so we may rectify in any future reprint.

Except as permitted under U.S. Copyright Law, no part of this book may be reprinted, reproduced, transmitted, or utilized in any form by any electronic, mechanical, or other means, now known or hereafter invented, including photocopying, microfilming and recording, or in any information storage or retrieval system, without written permission from the publishers.

For permission to photocopy or use material electronically from this work, access www.copyright.com or contact the Copyright Clearance Center, Inc. (CCC), 222 Rosewood Drive, Danvers, MA 01923, 978-750-8400. For works that are not available on CCC please contact mpkbookspermissions@tandf.co.uk

Trademark notice: Product or corporate names may be trademarks or registered trademarks and are used only for identification and explanation without intent to infringe.

Library of Congress Cataloging-in-Publication Data
Names: Lokhande, Jayant N., editor. | Pathak, Yashwant Vishnupant, editor.
Title: Nutraceuticals for aging and anti-aging : basic understanding and clinical evidence / edited by Jayant Nemchand Lokhande, Yashwant Vishnupant Pathak.
Description: First edition. | Boca Raton : Taylor & Francis, 2022. | Series: Nutraceuticals: basic research/clinical applications | Includes bibliographical references and index.
Identifiers: LCCN 2021026110 (print) | LCCN 2021026111 (ebook) | ISBN 9780367614942 (hardback) | ISBN 9780367628000 (paperback) | ISBN 9781003110866 (ebook)
Subjects: LCSH: Aging—Nutritional aspects. | Functional foods.
Classification: LCC RA776.75 .N88 2022 (print) | LCC RA776.75 (ebook) | DDC 613.2—dc23
LC record available at https://lccn.loc.gov/2021026110
LC ebook record available at https://lccn.loc.gov/2021026111

ISBN: 978-0-367-61494-2 (hbk)
ISBN: 978-0-367-62800-0 (pbk)
ISBN: 978-1-003-11086-6 (ebk)

DOI: 10.1201/9781003110866

Typeset in ITC Garamond
by codeMantra

Contents

Foreword

The advances in biomedical sciences have resulted in improved quality of health care leading to increase in the average life expectancy. Indeed, the world is aging. Aging is a natural, progressive, biological process of changes responsible for increased susceptibility to disease and degeneration, which finally leads to death. This process is common to all living forms, and aging and death are universal. Aging is not a disease, but it can bring on some disabilities and diseases, which can be avoided if one attains healthy aging. Aging process can pose vulnerability as an outcome of several factors, including nutrition, lifestyle and environmental exposure during the earlier stages of development from childhood. The aging process is controlled by genetic and epigenetic factors, which are influenced by environmental conditions. Progressive damage to macromolecules, cells, tissues and organs is responsible for aging. Senescence is the state or process of aging characterized by the declining ability to respond to stress, an increasing homeostatic imbalance and an increased risk of disease. Cellular senescence has been attributed to the shortening of telomeres with each cell cycle. Understanding some of these underlying biological processes is very important to promote healthy aging and longevity.

Anti-aging concept has different connotations but broadly involves a strategy to slow down the process of aging to attain longevity by various means including use of pharmaceuticals, nutraceuticals, antioxidants, and lifestyle and behavior modification. Longevity is living longer, which is the result of healthy aging. Longevity is based on several factors including genetics, lifestyle and environmental factors. Many studies indicate that about one third of the human life span depends on genetics, and the remainder can be attributed to lifestyle and environmental factors, linked to individual choices.

Reasonable scientific consensus is in favor of the free radical theory of aging. The aging process involves reactive oxygen species as free radical reactions responsible for age-related deterioration of the cardiovascular, central nervous and immune systems. It is hypothesized that an effective control of free radical-induced damage may be useful in promoting healthy life span and longevity. Free radical scavenging can be attempted by modifications in diet and lifestyle, including body weight control and diets. Dietary interventions consisting of antioxidants have been shown to reduce free radical reaction damage leading to the increased life span of experimental animals like mice, rats, fruit flies, nematodes and rotifers. Antioxidants have been shown to counter cancers and to enhance humoral and cell-mediated immune responses.

Aging is considered as a natural physiological process starting right from birth. Traditional knowledge systems like Ayurveda and Yoga have much to offer in the attempt to attain healthy aging and longevity. Physical and mental exercise, relaxation, meditation techniques from Yoga and the interventions of Ayurveda through Rasayana and Jara Chikitsa can aid in the prevention of the disabilities of aging. According to Ayurveda, childhood, youth and old age are dominated by Kapha, Pitta and Vata, respectively. Thus, Vata Dosha predominates during old age. Among the three Prakriti types, Kapha Prakriti persons are likely to have longer life spans, while Vata Prakriti persons may have shorter life spans.

Rejuvenation means delaying or reversing aging and is distinctly different from mere extension of the life span. Rejuvenation is a process to prevent or repair such damage. Rejuvenation requires the repair of the aging-related damage and also the replacement of damaged tissue with new tissue. Rejuvenation may result in life extension, but not vice versa. Rejuvenation process is very close to the Ayurveda concept of Rasayana, which actually incorporates both rejuvenation and regeneration. Rasayana drugs have rejuvenation, anti-aging and immunomodulatory properties.

Nutraceuticals for Aging and Anti-Aging: Basic Understanding and Clinical Evidence, edited by Prof Yashwant Pathak and Jayant Lokhande, offers very interesting perspectives on various aspects of aging and anti-aging. This book covers various aspects of science behind the aging process and a positive role of nutraceutical products and health supplements. Prof Pathak brings in rich expertise in pharmaceutical sciences, nutraceuticals and traditional medicine. His understanding of aging and anti-aging from perspectives of Ayurveda, Rasayana, nutrition and modern biology reflects throughout this book. Many eminent authors from different parts of the world have provided state-of-the-art information in well-organized twenty-eight chapters.

I congratulate all the editors and authors and wish the best for the book. I hope this book will offer new insights to those interested in aging, anti-aging and safer solutions with the help of scientifically studied and clinically established nutraceuticals.

Dr. Bhushan Patwardhan, PhD, FNASc, FNAMS
National Research Professor – AYUSH
Interdisciplinary School of Health Sciences
Savitribai Phule Pune University
Pune 411007, India

Preface

Aging can be perceived in two aspects: 'biological and chronological'. Is aging a disease or is it still considered as a 'normal physiological process'? One can have strong argument though! Average human life expectancy has been increasing in the last 200 years globally (from 30 to 80 years), and with all disruptive technological advances entering in human life, there is an estimate that age longevity, shall increase further. The most fundamental contemplation is whether, along with age longevity, age quality has been increased or not. Again, the answer is still not clear; however, that should be the goal in geriatric healthcare. This book puts the spotlight on some of these intricate points and will throw light on how to navigate further research and development in the right context.

The title of this book *Nutraceuticals for Aging and Anti-Aging: Basic Understanding and Clinical Evidence* itself signifies the foundation to be laid down in understanding basic definitions to establish a harmonized thought process and converting the very same into innovations and applications in anti-aging which means maintaining quality of life throughout one's increased biological and/or chronological age. The simplest and easily implementable tool to achieve this objective is nutraceuticals. Nutraceuticals are functionally enhanced and tailor-made dietary molecules. Their clinical evidence can be conducted and practiced in the anti-aging nutraceuticals to offer confidence to the consumer. This book offers what can be the clinical design to validate different anti-aging claims in different physiological systems. The safety, efficacy and quality validation of nutraceuticals are critical, and this book has articulated these aspects in an assured way. At the market level, how regulations are important in different country perspectives and how one can overall incentivize innovation efforts through intellectual property rights claims is also an important addendum of this book. Some proven and recently occurred product developments in this context are elaborated in dedicated chapters of this book like nutraceuticals in neurodegenerative, immunological, endocrinological, cardiovascular and metabolic systems. This book strategically emphasizes in creating a perfect blend of ancient medical wisdom with modern manufacturing technology. This is a key to develop and manufacture affordable anti-aging nutraceuticals. In such context, the most ancient medical treatise like Ayurveda Rasayana bears a prominent and promising place in offering 'sustainably tried and tested' remedies. One of the highlights of this book is to broaden the understanding of aging beyond bodily dimensions like mind, cognizance and consciousness because these dimensions certainly influence aging. How aging can be calibrated at molecular and genetic levels and how epigenetics can play a pivotal role in aging at the next level is one of the hallmarks in this book as well.

We sincerely hope this book can stimulate new thought process and embody a pivotal shift in research and development to explore novel anti-aging nutraceuticals and promise 'quality of life' with 'longevity of life' expectation at consumer end.

Jayant N. Lokhande and Yashwant V. Pathak

Editors

Jayant N. Lokhande, MD (Botanical Drugs), MBA (Biotechnology), is an expert in Botanical Drugs & Biotechnology Business Management. He has successfully strategized and formulated products for several nutraceutical, pharmaceutical and medical food companies in the United States and other developed countries. He has significant clinical experience especially in using botanical drugs and medical foods for complex and chronic diseases. His other professional interests are in biodiversity entrepreneurship, bioprospecting, medical anthropology and disease reversal therapeutics. He is currently working as chief scientific officer and management analyst in Indus Extracts in the United States, and his responsibilities include business analysis, product and technical market development.

Yashwant V. Pathak, PhD, is currently the associate dean for faculty affairs at the newly launched College of Pharmacy, University of South Florida, Tampa, Florida. Pathak earned his MS and PhD degrees in pharmaceutical technology from Nagpur University, Nagpur, India, and EMBA and MS degrees in conflict management from Sullivan University, Louisville, Kentucky. With extensive experience in academia and industry, Pathak has over 120 publications, research papers, abstracts, book chapters and reviews to his credit. He has presented over 150 presentations, posters and lectures worldwide in the field of pharmaceuticals, drug delivery systems and other related topics. He has also coedited six books on nanotechnology and drug delivery systems, two books on nutraceuticals and several books on cultural studies. Dr. Pathak is the holder of two patents. He has travelled extensively to over 75 countries and is actively involved with many pharmacy colleges in different countries.

Contributors

Shima Abdollahi
School of Public Health
North Khorasan University of
    Medical Sciences
Bojnurd, Iran

Niyati Acharya
Institute of Pharmacy
Nirma University
Ahmedabad, India

Ofosua Adi-Dako
Department of Pharmaceutics
    and Microbiology, School of
    Pharmacy
University of Ghana
Accra, Ghana

Ghuncha Ambrin
Biomedical Engineering and
    Biotechnology
University of Massachusetts
    Dartmouth
Dartmouth, Massachusetts

Mary Ann Archer
Centre for Plant Medicine
    Research
Mampong-Akuapem, Ghana

Francis Bentil
Department of Pharmaceutics
    and Microbiology, School of
    Pharmacy
University of Ghana
Accra, Ghana

Pravin Bhat
Sumatibhai Shah Ayurveda
    Mahavidyalaya, Hadapsar
Pune, India

Ramesh Bhonde
Regenerative Medicine Laboratory,
    Dr. D. Y. Patil Vidyapeeth
Pune, India

Vaibhav Changediya
Parul Institute of Pharmacy and
    Research
Parul University
Vadodara, India

Rajiv Dahiya
School of Pharmacy, Faculty of
    Medical Sciences
The University of the West Indies,
    St. Augustine Campus - Madison,
    Wisconsin

Sunita Dahiya
Department of Pharmaceutical
  Sciences, School of Pharmacy,
  Medical Sciences Campus
University of Puerto Rico
San Juan, Puerto Rico

Manoj Dash
College of Ayurvedic Medicine
Banaras Hindu University
Varanasi, India

Shruti Ashok Sawant Desai
M/s Katariya and Associates Pune,
  India

Aaishwarya Deshmukh
Department of Pharmacology
Smt. Kashibai Navale College of
  Pharmacy
Pune, India

Mansa Fredua-Agyeman
Department of Pharmaceutics
  and Microbiology, School of
  Pharmacy
University of Ghana
Accra, Ghana

Swati Gadgil
Department of Rasashastra-
  Bhaishajyakalpana Vigyan,
  College of Ayurveda
Bharati Vidyapeeth (Deemed to be
  University)
Pune, India

Reza Ghiasvand
Food Security Research Center,
  Department of Community
  Nutrition, School of Nutrition
  and Food Science
Isfahan University of Medical
  Sciences
Isfahan, Iran

Benjamin B. Greco
Taneja College of Pharmacy
University of South Florida
Tampa, Florida

Tripti Halder
Institute of Pharmacy
Nirma University
Ahmedabad, India

Keerti Jain
Department of Pharmaceutics
National Institute of
  Pharmaceutical Education and
  Research (NIPER) – Raebareli
Lucknow, India

Rupalben K. Jani
Parul Institute of Pharmacy and
  Research, Faculty of Pharmacy
Parul University
Waghodia, India

Remya Jayakumar
College of Ayurvedic Medicine
Banaras Hindu University
Varanasi, India

Kalpana Joshi
Department of Biotechnology
Sinhgad College of Engineering
  affiliated with Savitribai Phule
  Pune University
Pune, India

Namrata Joshi
College of Ayurvedic Medicine
Banaras Hindu University
Varanasi, India

Vishal Katariya
M/s Katariya and Associates
  Aundh, Pune, India

Archana Kulkarni
Founder and Director of Ayur
  Wellness
Tampa, Florida
Everglades University
Tampa, Florida

Doris Kumadoh
Centre for Plant Medicine
  Research
Mampong-Akuapem, Ghana

Lalit Kumar
Department of Pharmaceutics,
  Manipal College of
  Pharmaceutical Sciences
Manipal Academy of Higher
  Education
Udupi, India

Raj Kumar
Prime Bio, Inc.
Dartmouth, Massachusetts

Jayant N. Lokhande
Indus Extracts
Carson, California

Ankita Mehta
Department of Pharmacology,
  Institute of Pharmacy
Nirma University
Ahmedabad, India

Priti Mehta
Institute of Pharmacy
Nirma University
Ahmedabad, India

Patricia Mendonca
Division of Pharmaceutical
  Sciences, College of
  Pharmacy & Pharmaceutical
  Sciences, Institute of Public
  Health
Florida A&M University
Tallahassee, Florida

Navneet
Department of Pharmaceutics
National Institute of
  Pharmaceutical Education and
  Research (NIPER) – Raebareli
Lucknow, India

Manuela Okaijah
Department of Pharmaceutics
  and Microbiology, School of
  Pharmacy
University of Ghana
Accra, Ghana

Rupali Joshi Panse
Ayurveda
Orlando, Florida

Anita Patel
Faculty of Pharmacy, Nootan
  Pharmacy College
Sankalchand Patel University
Visnagar, India

Bhoomika Patel
Department of Pharmacology,
  Institute of Pharmacy
Nirma University
Ahmedabad, India

Dhavalkumar Patel
Leading Pharma LLC
Fairfield, New Jersey

Gargi Patel
Taneja College of Pharmacy
University of South Florida
Tampa, Florida

Jayvadan Patel
Nootan Pharmacy College, Faculty
   of Pharmacy
Sankalchand Patel University
Visnagar, India

Mayur M. Patel
Department of Pharmaceutics,
   Institute of Pharmacy
Nirma University
Ahmedabad, India

Satish Patel
Prabhu Dental Clinic
Visnagar, India

Yashwant V. Pathak
Taneja College of Pharmacy
University of South Florida
Tampa, Florida
and
Airlangga University
Surabaya, Indonesia

Anagha Ranade
Regional Ayurved Research Center
Pune, India

Shruti U. Rawal
Department of Pharmaceutics,
   Institute of Pharmacy
Nirma University
Ahmedabad, India

Salwa
Department of Pharmaceutics,
   Manipal College of
   Pharmaceutical Sciences
Manipal Academy of Higher
   Education
Udupi, India

Avinash Sanap
Regenerative Medicine Laboratory
   Dr. D. Y. Patil Vidyapeeth
Pune, India

Sahar Saraf-Bank
Food Security Research Center,
   Department of Community
   Nutrition, School of Nutrition
   and Food Science
Isfahan University of Medical
   Sciences
Isfahan, Iran

Shikha Sharma
Institute For Stem Cell Biology
   and Regenerative Medicine,
   Bangalore, India

Bal Ram Singh
Institute of Advanced Sciences
Dartmouth, Massachusetts

Siddhesh Solanke
Department of Technology
Savitribai Phule Pune University
Pune, India

Karam F. A. Soliman
Division of Pharmaceutical
   Sciences, College of Pharmacy
   & Pharmaceutical Sciences,
   Institute of Public Health
Florida A&M University
Tallahassee, Florida

Teeja Suthar
Department of Pharmaceutics
National Institute of
    Pharmaceutical Education and
    Research (NIPER) – Raebareli
Lucknow, India

Kavita Trimal
Department of Technology
Savitribai Phule Pune University
Pune, India

Lei Wang
Biomedical Engineering and
    Biotechnology
University of Massachusetts
    Dartmouth
Dartmouth, Massachusetts

Pankaj Wanjarkhedkar
Ayurveda, Deenanath Mangeshkar
    Hospital, and Research Center
Pune, India

Asmita Wele
Department of Rasashastra-
    Bhaishajyakalpana Vigyan,
    College of Ayurveda
Bharati Vidyapeeth (Deemed to be
    University)
Pune, India

Sajal Yenkar
M/s Katariya and Associates
    Pune, India

Trends in the Functional Food Market and Nutraceutical Product Development

Tripti Halder, Priti Mehta, and Niyati Acharya
Nirma University

Contents

1.1 Introduction

Functional foods (FFs) are foods or part of dietary items which provide nutrients and energy along with health-promoting benefits with some targeting functions like preventing the risk of diseases or enhancing physiological responses. The term was first used by Japan in the 1980s, but there is no satisfactory definition of FFs. However, these are the food items either natural or processed having potentially positive effects on health beyond basic nutrition (Ye et al., 2018). These are generally processed from plant, animal or microbial origin with a potential impact on overall health and physical performance. In recent times, there has been increasing awareness in people about the impact of food on their health as well as the social and environmental consequences (Falguera et al., 2012).

FFs are partially effective with preventive or protective action in various diseases, and self-medication with different FFs as a dietary supplement is in high demand throughout the world. It has been found that 40% of the US and European population consume FFs as a part of their daily diet. So the global market of FFs is highly increasing at a rate of 7% and expected to reach

DOI: 10.1201/9781003110866-1

almost 138 million dollars by 2027 (Supplements, 2020). Phytonutrients like phenolic acids, flavonoids, anthocyanin, stilbenes, coumarins, tannins, etc. provide great health benefits to reduce the risk of developing diseases or help in management or treatment of chronic diseases due to their high antioxidant activity and free radical scavenging activity (Adefegha, 2018). Other natural compounds like terpenoids, carotenoids, alkaloids, etc. have been reported to interact with several enzymes like α-amylase, α-glucosidase, angiotensin-I-converting enzyme, acetyl cholinesterase and arginase and can be helpful to manage some degenerative conditions (Adefegha, 2018). Previously, FFs were categorized as nature's gifted conventional foods including grains, vegetables, fruits, etc., but gradually, other foods like those with provitamins, beta carotene, essential fatty acids like polyunsaturated fatty acids (PUFA), omega 3 fatty acids, dihomo gamma-linoleic acids (DGLA), selenium, coenzyme Q-enriched foods or fortified foods or beverages are also brought under the umbrella of the term FFs. Marine foods like different types of fishes (salmon, tuna, mackerel and steaks), macroalgae and microalgae containing vitamins, micronutrients, omega 3 fatty acids and minerals with antioxidant properties are also forming a part of it. These are extensively consumed by people to help prevent chronic diseases like cardiovascular diseases, cancers, neurodegenerative diseases, diabetes and other inflammatory diseases (Abuajah et al., 2015; Supplements, 2020). In developing countries, intestinal health is a major factor, and some of the gut flora strains show effects on host health due to their nutritional, immunological and physiological functions (Cencic & Chingwaru, 2010). Prebiotics, probiotics and symbiotics are playing a great role in controlling or improving the microbial gut flora with enough scientific evidence. The World Health Organization (WHO) and the Food and Agriculture Organization (FAO) have defined the role of probiotics as the living microorganisms that help to reduce gastrointestinal diseases and improve body resistances. Some non-dairy beverages are also now more attracted items to the consumers with lactose intolerance conditions. Novel technologies have been developed and adopted to deliver FFs and related ingredients in the form of tablet, capsule, powder and coated or encapsulated product. Many FF ingredients from the class of natural bioactive have been developed in the form of nanoformulations to overcome the solubility and stability issues. Nanotechnology helps to deliver nutraceuticals in a proper way with the improvement in bioavailability (Huang et al., 2010). The developed nanocarriers and nanoencapsulated FF ingredients (Zhu & Huang, 2019) are used for different therapeutic and diagnostic purposes (Bano et al., 2020). These delivery systems are more potential to deliver phytochemicals for the treatment of various chronic diseases like cancers (Rizwanullah et al., 2018; Xie et al., 2016), Alzheimer's and cardiovascular diseases, diabetes (Enrico, 2019), obesity and its comorbidities (Goktas et al., 2020) and chemotherapies (Subramanian et al., 2016).

In this chapter, we discuss about different types of functional foods, categories of FF ingredients and their applications in human health. It also addresses new trends in the nutraceutical product development with the use of several new functional foods. Different formulation approaches using nanocarriers for delivery of phytocompounds and different functional foods are also included along with the global market and regulatory scenario for functional food in different countries.

1.2 Classification

Functional foods are classified into three categories on the basis of their available sources. Conventional foods are naturally available foods like vegetables, grains, fishes, dairy products, etc. which are used as a dietary supplement in our daily diet. Modified foods are generally prepared by addition of enhanced or enriched fortified foods like fortified dairy products, fortified beverages like fruit juice with vitamin D and calcium, breads and wraps enriched with folate, etc. These foods have high nutritious value due to the presence of varied types of macro- and micronutrients. Synthetic food, on the other hand, is processed in the laboratory as food or beverages for human health benefits (Domínguez Díaz et al., 2020b; Nwosu & Ubaoji, 2020) (Table 1.1).

1.3 Functional food categories and ingredients

a. **Marine foods:**

Several bioactive compounds like microalgae, seaweeds, different fishes and fish oils are the main sources of marine foods which are called the treasure house of nutrients particularly of protein and peptides. Despite having so much health benefits, marine functional ingredients have been underexploited for food purposes. Nowadays, marine foods are used as a functional ingredient in the bakeries and pasta industries for the development of fortified food with additional nutrients (Kadam & Prabhasankar, 2010). These marine foods not only provide nutritive benefits but also are effective in combating various chronic and degenerative diseases. It has been reported that several

Table 1.1 Classification of Functional Foods (Domínguez Díaz et al., 2020b; Nwosu & Ubaoji, 2020)

Classes	Description	Examples
Conventional food	Naturally occurring and without any modification or fortification	Different veggies, grains, fruits and non-dairy products
Modified foods	Fortified foods (increase nutrient content)	Fruit juice along with vitamin C
	Enhanced foods (modification of nutrient composition)	Fruits with more vitamin and calcium
	Enriched foods (addition of a new nutrient)	Fruit juice with calcium
	Altered foods (altered the present nutrient)	Milk altered with oleic acid
Synthetic food	Processed foods in the laboratory	Probiotic type of foods

marine foods, mainly fish products, are good sources of vitamins, minerals like potassium and omega-3 fatty acids and have proliferative, calcium-binding, ACE-inhibitory and antihypertensive activities (Lordan et al., 2011).

Microalgae are an important marine source for bioactive compounds with high antioxidant properties along with carotenoids, proteins, vitamins, essential amino acids, enzymes and fiber. This promising food is now gaining worldwide attention as using microalgae biomass algae-based novel food can be developed with increased nutritional value. Microalgae have been reported to have potential in preventing cancer, gastric ulcers, diabetes, hypertension, cardiovascular diseases and also as an anti-inflammatory due to their highly antioxidant activity (Matos et al., 2017). Microalgae have been reported to indirectly work as a prebiotic as they contain polysaccharides which degenerate into oligosaccharides in the gastrointestinal tract (GIT) (Camacho et al., 2019). Microalgae-based products are available as powders, tablets, liquid oil, capsules or pastilles with more than 75% of its biomass. Many other items like desserts, dairy products and dietary supplements also contain microalgae as one of the ingredients (Galasso et al., 2019). These are also other sources of taurine, lipids and pigments and also used as a substrate for bioactive peptides (Garcia-Vaquero & Hayes, 2016). Five most important species of microalgae are *Chlorella vulgaris* (in the form of green and carotenogenic properties), *Haematococcus pluvialis* (only carotenogenic), *Spirulina maxima, Diacronema vlkianum* and *Isochrysis galbana*. Last two species, *Diacronema vlkianum* and *Isochrysis galbana*, have high protein (40%) and fat (18%–24%) contents with PUFA, omega 3 fatty acids, etc. Green *Chlorella vulgaris* and *Spirulina maxima* are also very high sources of protein (38% and 44% respectively) and have low fat (5%) content. Carotenogenic *Chlorella vulgaris* and *Haematococcus pluvialis* are known for higher carotenoid content, and *Diacronema vlkianum* is one of the richest sources for mass production of β-carotene (Batista et al., 2013). But the processing technologies of this innovative protein-containing food are not developed fully. It lacks advanced research and investment to improve the technology readiness level (TRL) which will be able to improve the economy of the current situations (Caporgno & Mathys, 2018). Higher production costs, difficult extraction and refining, and sensory and palatability issues are major bottlenecks to formulate novel food products and follow the scale-up technologies (Camacho et al., 2019).

Seaweeds are versatile marine macroalgae, generally found in cold temperatures like in Atlantic Ocean in European countries. Several species of seaweeds are available, but as far as human health benefits are concerned, only three types of seaweeds are considered (Holdt & Kraan, 2011) like red, brown and green macroalgae from marine

Table 1.2 Different Types of Macroalgae (Kılınç et al., 2013)

Algae	Phylum	Classes	No. of Species
Red	Rhodophyta	Rhodophyceae	6,000 species
Brown	Ochrophyta	Phaeophyceae	1,750 species
Green	Chlorophyta	Bryopsidophyceae, Chlorophyceae, Dasycladophyceae, Prasinophyceae and Ulvophyceae	1,200 species
Blue green	Cyanophyta	Cyanophyceae	1500 species

sources. Generally, these algae have different therapeutic activities in various chronic and degenerative diseases like cancer, neurodegenerative, diabetic and various microbial diseases. Most people of the Asian countries like Japan, Korea, Thailand and some South American countries like Brazil, Chile and Peru also take edible seaweeds in their foods for their health benefits (Mohamed et al., 2012). Table 1.2 shows major classes from red, brown, blue and green algae.

Seaweeds contain various macro- and microelements like proteins, lipids, polysaccharides, minerals, vitamins and enzymes. Vitamins like A, E, C and niacin are present in red, brown and green seaweeds. Other bioactive compounds like phlorotannins, carotenoids as fucoxanthin, peptides, ash (21.1%–39.3%) and sulphate (1.3%–5.9%) are also present. They also have omega 3 PUFA and help to increase the concentration of different minerals like potassium, calcium, magnesium and manganese. Generally, seaweeds have been used from the 14th century in Japan followed by China in the 19th century. The hydrocolloids formed with the red and brown algae become the most used product in industries and food applications. Day by day, seaweeds are experiencing increased demand due to the presence of antioxidant compounds and also serve as a good source for alginate, agar and carrageenan. These are highly used in the food industry as food processing agents and in low-calorie food like salad, soups, fermented products and prebiotics. These are also used in thalassotherapy, in which the paste of seaweeds is used in osteoporosis and rheumatism (Cherry et al., 2019; Kılınç et al., 2013). Fucoidan, a natural sulphated polysaccharide extracted from brown seaweed, *Undaria pinnatifida* species, has shown antioxidant, anticoagulant and anticancer activities. Patented products like cookie, beverages, noodles, tea and restructured meat containing fucoidan are reported for their therapeutic claims in arthritis, influenza, malaria, etc. Concomitant administration of fucoidan with letrozole and tamoxifen has proven anticancer therapeutics without the risk of significant pharmacokinetic interactions in breast cancer patients (Tocaciu et al., 2018).

b. **Prebiotics:**

Prebiotics are short-chain carbohydrates like fructooligosaccharides, xylooligosaccharides, cyclodextrins, isomaltulose, palatinose, etc., which maintain the health of probiotics or the beneficial bacteria in our small intestine. Mainly they are non-digestible and fermented in the intestine and produce short-chain fatty acids which are essential for the growth and health of probiotics. Several fruits and vegetables with non-digestible saccharide fibers are able to alter microbiota and help enhance the adhesion of beneficial bacteria by decreasing adhesion of pathogenic bacterial species like *Salmonella typhimurium* and *Staphylococcus aureus* (Al-Sheraji et al., 2013).

A potent prebiotic, disaccharide lactulose was derived from lactose with the rearrangement of glucose to fructose. It helps to induce proliferation in *Lactobacillus* and *Bifidobacterium* flora in gut as it is not able to digest in upper GIT. It is also used in the management of several disorders like hepatic encephalopathy and chronic constipation (Nooshkam et al., 2018). The interaction between gut microbiota and prebiotics manages various chronic conditions like inflammatory bowel diseases (IBD). Flavonoids are good anti-inflammatory agents and help to reduce the inflammation in IBD and colorectal inflammation along with reducing the risk of cancer and other chronic conditions. These are also helpful in obesity and metabolic syndrome and uptake of minerals like calcium and magnesium for improved bone structure. Inulin and oligosaccharides naturally present in onion, asparagus, wheat, artichoke, etc. have great industrial applications in different food products like breakfasts and beverages due to different functional attributes like anti-inflammatory effects, modulation of gut microbiota and bowel habits and alteration on lipid and glucose metabolism (Laparra & Sanz, 2010; Yin et al., 2019).

c. **Probiotics**:

Probiotics are the main beneficial bacteria that help to stimulate or regulate the responses and activities of the host cells and also regulate the hormone release to improve the gut barrier functions. It also improves the gastrointestinal microflora to improve its immune system (Özer & Kirmaci, 2010). Several probiotic genera like *Lactobacillus, Bacillus, Lactococcous, Streptococcus, Bifidobacterium, Saccharomyces*, etc. are useful for a wide range of human health benefits. Probiotics are generally served in modified ways like yogurt fortified with calcium and fibers. Probiotics like *Bifidobacterium* and *Lactobacillus* strains help to prevent irritable bowel-related conditions and improve the immune system (Bimbo et al., 2017). Probiotics and their dietary source help to improve human health by maintaining the gastrointestinal microbial levels, but many processing factors induce stress to the microorganisms resulting in compromised functions and viability (Nagpal et al., 2012; Fiocco et al., 2020). It has been found that commercial fermented milk with *L. helveticus* has antihypertensive

Table 1.3 Plant Sources with Prebiotic Ingredients (George Kerry et al., 2018)

Prebiotics	Plant Sources	Probiotics
Fructo-oligosaccharides	Onion, garlic, asparagus, banana	*Bifidobacterium, Bacteroids*
Xylooligosaccharides	Milk, honey, fruits, vegetables	*Bifidobacterium, Lactobacillus*
Inulin	Onion, garlic, asparagus, banana, wheat, oats	*Bifidobacterium, Lactobacillus*
Lactulose	Skim milk	*Bifidobacterium, Lactobacillus*
Lactosucrose	Milk sugar	*Zymomonas mobilis*
Galacto-oligosaccharides	Lentil, mother milk, green pea, chickpea	*Bifidobacterium*
Isomalto-oligosaccharides	Soya sauce, honey	*Bifidobacterium, Bacteroids*

effects due to the bioactive peptide release after fermentation in GIT (Beltrán-Barrientos et al., 2016). **Sheep milk**-based functional food with high concentrations of protein, fats and minerals has been developed with prebiotic ingredients, or it can be added in the form of probiotic bacterial source (Balthazar et al., 2017) (Table 1.3).

The term postbiotic refers to metabolism by products of the beneficial bacteria like bacteriocins, organic acid, diacetyl, acetaldehyde, etc. These metabolic products can inhibit the pathogenic microbes and have been promoted as an alternative to antibiotics. They help enhance the barrier function in the gut system and also help increase angiogenesis of epithelial cells. They are nontoxic, non-pathogenic compounds, and they cannot be easily hydrolyzed by mammalian enzymes. Symbiotics are defined as combinations of their prebiotics and postbiotics. They show synergistic effects and so are gaining commercial interest for improvement in overall human gut health. Probiotics are used in various functional food products for their anti-pathogenic, anti-obesity, anti-inflammatory and anti-allergic effects (George Kerry et al., 2018). Having increasing benefits of such kind of products, it is a need of time to resolve the problems associated with preservation, storage and sustainability in terms of viability of the probiotics. Several factors affect their viability like the level of oxygen, lactic acid bacterial content and sensitivity of metabolites. So proper development of symbiotic combination with appropriate strain selection and supported prebiotics for sustainable food product development is the area of major research (Terpou et al., 2019).

d. **Non-dairy milk beverage and fermented functional food**:

Dairy probiotics are highly nutritional, but sometimes, consumers prefer milk alternatives due to problems related to lactose intolerance, allergic potential of dairy constituents and hypercholesterolemia (Paul et al., 2020). Several plant-based milk products are available in the market due to the ability of offer varied nutritional ingredients, and it constitutes a major segment in the functional beverages if fortified with essential vitamins and macro/micronutrients. The overall nutritional profile of non-dairy milks is dependent on the source and process used in the formulation development. The sources of these milks are different such as cereal-based like oats and rice, legume-based like soy and pea, seed-based like flax and hemp, nut-based like almond, coconut and cashew and also vegetable-based like potato milk that are available as beverages. These are also highly nutritious for health benefits, contain a high amount of protein and essential fatty acids and are low in calories. Sometimes, these milks are also fortified with different vitamins and minerals to get more benefits (Bridges, 2018). Several fermentation processes have been used to develop fruits, vegetables, cereals, soy and meat-based probiotic beverages, biscuits, breads, cereal breakfast, etc. (Min et al., 2019). Table 1.4 shows variation in the composition of different non-dairy milks and characteristics of most common plant-based milks.

Conventional probiotics face several challenges with respect to the effect of temperature and pH on stability leading to loss of the potency with viability changes of the product. These problems are not associated with plant-based probiotics or non-dairy probiotics (Prado et al., 2008). Non-dairy milk products are prepared by the method of extraction with a suitable solvent followed by separation and starch liquefaction for developing the product base. For the fortification formulation development, various nutrients are added at this stage followed by homogenization to impart stability to the final suspension product. Fermented non-dairy milk products employ the use of lactic acid bacteria for improved sensory and nutritional profile (Mäkinen et al., 2016).

Fruit- and vegetable-based beverages containing probiotics like different strains of *Lactobacillus* species are one of the promising approaches for the functional beverage development. Many fermented/nonfermented beverages with orange juice, pineapple juice,

Table 1.4 Compositional Characteristics of Various Plant-Based Milks (Bridges, 2018; Min et al., 2019)

Plant Based Milk	Compositional Characteristics
Soy milk	Least processed milk with high protein content but high in sugar and fat
Almond milk	Low calorie and high in vitamin E but with relatively low protein content
Oat milk	Fiber, iron, protein, vitamin E, folic acids but has allergenic potential
Coconut milk	Good source of potassium, iron, fiber but relatively with high fat
Hemp milk	3:1 ratio of omega 6: omega 3 fatty acids with good amount of alpha linoleic acids, magnesium, phytosterols, iron, potassium but having earthy flavor
Cashew milk	High vitamin E and relatively less calories but low in protein
Flax milk	Good source of omega 3 fatty acids, low in calorie but very little protein
Pea milk	Good source of protein
Potato milk	High in carbohydrate and low in protein
Rice milk	High carbohydrate, low protein but with less allergic potential compared to other non-dairy milks

litchi juice and pomegranate juice contain probiotic bacterial strains of *Lactobacillus* like *L. casei, L. plantarum,* etc. Fermented vegetable beverages having beet, tomato, carrot, cabbages and green tea are found with *Lactobacillus* and *Bifidobacteria* to improve their potency. This approach also improves storage conditions, stability, and viability of the microorganisms in the fruit and vegetable matrix (Shori, 2016).

e. **Phytochemicals in functional food**:

Several phytochemicals belonging to the class of polyphenols, glycosides, alkaloids, carotenoids, terpenoids and unsaturated fatty acids hold great potential to offer natural blend in nutraceutical formulations. The protective effects of such compounds and polyphenols against oxidative stress and inflammation, two processes associated with the pathogenesis of several common diseases, have been widely evaluated in recent years. Functional foods of plant origin like cruciferous vegetables, oat, flaxseed, tomato, soybean, citrus, berries, tea, grapes, wine and garlic have been already reported for their health benefits. These effects are attributed to the bioactive phytochemicals present in considerable amount, and sufficient scientific evidence supporting such effects has been reported. Table 1.5 covers major classes of different phytochemicals and plant sources with their respective benefits.

Table 1.5 Different Phytocompounds along with Sources and Benefits (Adefegha, 2018; Daliri & Lee, 2015; Nazir et al., 2019)

Phenolics	Active Constituents	Plant Sources	Benefits
	Phenolic acids (gallic acid, chlorogenic acid, caffeic acid, ferulic acid)	Strawberries, bell peepers, brown rice, whole wheat, peanut	Antioxidant activity, potential effects for anticancer, anti-proliferative, immunomodulatory, neuroprotective, antidiabetic, etc.
	Flavonoids: Flavonols (quercetin, myricetin, kaempferol), flavones (luteolin, apigenin), flavanols (catechin epicatechin) Flavanones (naringin, hesperidin) Anthocyanidins Isoflavones (genistein)	Citrus fruits, onion Fruits and vegetables Teas Grapes, citrus fruits Strawberries Soybeans	
Carotenoids	Alpha and beta carotene	Carrots	Antioxidant, anticancer, cataract, anti- carcinogenic specifically help reduce the risk of prostate cancer, etc.
	Lutein	Spinach	
	Lycopene	Tomato, papaya	
Sterols	Phytosterols	Soybean, corn and wheat	Help to reduce blood cholesterol
Glucosinolates	Isothiocyanates	Radish and mustard	Anticancer
	Sulforaphene	Broccoli	Anticancer
	Indoles	Broccoli	Anticancer
	Thiosulfonates	Garlic and onions	Anticancer, antihypertensive, antimicrobial

In addition to their nutritional value as a conventional food, functional foods help in the promotion of optimal health conditions and may reduce the risks of various diseases. They are used enormously in the Indian market based on their nutritional profile and therapeutic claims for the development of foods for special dietary uses (FSDU) and foods for special medical purposes (FSMP). The following are some more plant sources emerging as functional foods evidenced with human health benefits. Regular intake of these functional food-based products can help to reduce the risk of many chronic or degenerative diseases as per their labelling and scientific claims (Table 1.6).

1.4 Formulation approaches

Despite the great health potential of functional food and its ingredients to improve immunity and reduce the risks of several diseases, effective delivery and bioavailability remain the major problems. Novel formulation techniques with cutting-edge principles have been used to overcome solubility- and stability-related problems of functional food ingredients after oral administration. Various delivery approaches like pH-sensitive, carbohydrate-based, protein-based and lipid-based nanoparticles have been developed to get better efficacy and effective delivery at the target site (Xiong et al., 2020). Several photoactive and functional food ingredients like phenolic antioxidants, natural food colorants, antimicrobial agents and essential oils, vitamins, minerals, flavors, fish oils and essential fatty acids have been delivered efficiently with the use of novel nanocarriers and encapsulation-based techniques (Assadpour & Mahdi Jafari, 2019). Phenolic compounds are excellent antioxidants and useful to a great extent in functional food products but associated with poor bioavailability due to their low solubility, instability, passive diffusion and efflux (Li et al., 2015). Nanoformulations like nanoemulsions (Jamali et al., 2019) and lipid nanoformulations (Zhong & Zhang, 2019) including micelles, liposomes (Singh et al., 2019), solid and lipid nanoparticles, nanostructured lipidic carrier (Faridi Esfanjani et al., 2018), niosomes, polymeric nanoparticles, metallic nanoparticles, starch-based nanoparticles (Liu et al., 2016; Qiu et al., 2020), gum-based nanocarriers (Taheri & Jafari, 2019) and different dendrimer-based approaches (Yousefi et al., 2020) have been hugely developed to overcome these hindrances. With the advent and intervention of nanotechnology, it is now possible to deliver stable bioactive compounds (Fahimirad & Hatami, 2019; McClements, 2020) at the target site with enhanced applications in the food industry (Milinčić et al., 2019). Phytochemicals like curcumin, quercetin, paclitaxel and silymarin have been explored with a range of splendid formulations with high entrapment efficiency and bioavailability at the required site (Jadhav et al., 2017). These approaches are not only employed for phenolics but several vegetables, vegetable oils and probiotics (Pandey & Mishra, 2021) are also developed as nano- or microencapsulated products to improve their stability (Delshadi et al., 2020). Besides this green nanotechnology (Lee et al., 2011), ultrasound-based fortification of foods is a highly recommended

Table 1.6 Functional Food Ingredients and Products

Natural Source	Active Compounds	Protective Activity/Benefits	Products	Reference
Chia seeds	Omega 3 fatty acids, dietary fiber, proteins and polyphenolic compounds	Anti-diabetic effects, reduces the risk of cardiovascular diseases	Dairy products, baked items, meat and fish products, used to develop gluten free products	Ikumi et al. (2019); Zettel & Hitzmann (2018)
Drumstick pods/ leaves	Phenolic acids, phytosterols, flavonoids, alkaloids, and vitamins	Anti-cancer, anti-diabetic, anti-inflammatory and antioxidant	Fortification of bakery product, bread, biscuits dairy items like yoghurt, cheese	Ma et al. (2020); Saini et al. (2016)
Barley grass	Gamma-amino butyric acid, flavonoids, saponin, superoxide dismutase (SOD), minerals, vitamins	Antioxidant, antidiabetic, control blood pressure, immunity booster, cardiovascular diseases	Shakes, smoothie, juices, etc.	Zeng et al. (2018)
Bio fortified carrot	Beta-carotene provitamin A, anthocyanin and the nonprovitamin A, lutein, zeaxanthin, lycopene etc.,	Health promoting supplement in vitamin A deficiency	Fortified with increased amounts of carotenoids and lycopene	Arscott and Tanumihardjo (2010)
Quinoa	Protein and peptides, lipids, betaine, saponins phytoedysteroids, phytohormones, antioxidant enzymes	anti-diabetic, immunomodulatory, anti-cancer, anti-microbial, antioxidant	Soups, salad, baby foods, with cereal for malnutrition	Vega-Gálvez et al. (2010); Vilcacundo and Hernández-Ledesma (2017)
Dry beans/pinto beans	Phenols, resistant starch, vitamins, fructo-oligosaccharides, stilbenes	Reduce oxidative stress and cardiovascular disease, diabetes	Protein hydro lysate, canned beans	Cámara et al. (2013)
Green and yellow tea	Polyphenols, fibers, catechins, flavonols	Antioxidant, antimutagenic	Cookies or tea fortified cookies	Gramza-Michałowska et al. (2016)
Turmeric	Polyphenols, curcumin	Antioxidant, anti-inflammatory, anticancer, antiobesity, neurodegenerative, etc.	Nutraceutical, water soluble nanoformulations	Tsuda (2018)

(Continued)

Table 1.6 (Continued) Functional Food Ingredients and Products

Natural Source	Active Compounds	Protective Activity/Benefits	Products	Reference
Pomegranate	Polyphenols like anthocyanin and hydrolysable tannins	Reduce the risk of cancer chemotherapy cardiovascular disease, diabetes, etc.	Juice, functional beverages, fruit extracts	Johanningsmeier & Harris (2011); Wu & Tian (2017)
Oolong tea polyphenols (OTP)	Tea catechins, especially O-methylated derivatives, may have prebiotic-like activity	Reduce the effects of obesity related metabolic problems	As bakery items	Cheng et al. (2018)
Grape pomace	Polyphenol proteins, omega 3 fatty acids, dietary fibers	Antioxidant and antimicrobial	Insoluble fiber-based functional products	Yu & Ahmedna (2013)
Saffron	Crocetin and its glycosidic esters, called crocins, and safranal	Nervous and cardiovascular systems, liver diseases, antidepressant	Cooking as coloring and flavoring agent	José Bagur et al. (2017)
Alliums	Organosulfurs, quercetin, flavonoids, saponins,	Antidiabetic, antioxidants, antimicrobial, neuroprotective and immunological effects	Chutney, pickles, etc.	Zeng et al. (2017)
Acerola cherry	Vitamin C, benzoic acid derivatives, phenylpropanoids, flavonoids, anthocyanin, and carotenoids	Antioxidant, antitumor, antihyperglycemic	As fruits or juices or extract mixed with beverages	Belwal et al. (2018)
Soybeans	Phospholipids, saponins, isoflavones, daidzein, genistein, oligosaccharides and edible fiber	Antioxidant, anticancer, collagen strengthening	Soy milk, soy flour, tofu, okara, fermented products like tempeh and miso	Hu et al. (2020)
Flaxseed	Alpha-linoleic acid, dietary fibers and SDG lignans	Reduce the risks of diabetes, cardiovascular diseases, cancer, arthritis, osteoporosis, etc.	Neat oil, capsules and microencapsulated powder	Goyal et al. (2014)

(Continued)

Table 1.6 (Continued) Functional Food Ingredients and Products

Natural Source	Active Compounds	Protective Activity/Benefits	Products	Reference
Peanut	Proteins, fibers, polyphenols, antioxidants, vitamins and minerals, resveratrol, phenolic acids, flavonoids and phytosterols	Anti-inflammatory, anti-diabetic, cancer prevention	Bakery items, of peanut butter, confections, extenders in meat product formulation, soups and desserts	Arya et al. (2016)
Halophytes	Polyunsaturated fatty acids, carotenoids, vitamins, sterols, essential oils (terpenes), polysaccharides, glycosides, and phenolic compounds	Antioxidant, anti-tumoral, anti-inflammatory, and antimicrobial activities	Novel food products like vinegar, encapsulated oil	Ksouri et al. (2012); Petropoulos et al. (2018)
Whey proteins	High protein, bioactive peptides	Protein hydrolysate is used to promote health benefits in the immune, cardiovascular, nervous and gastrointestinal systems	Whey protein hydrolysate is used in food supplements like tablet, capsules, etc. Also in fermented milk-based products	Dullius et al. (2018)
Mushrooms of genus *Ganoderma Lentinus, Grifola,* etc.	Beta-glucan	Immunomodulatory, anticancer, cardio protective, hepatoprotective, antioxidant and antimicrobial activities	Used as low-calorie and high-fiber substitute for baked products	Khan et al. (2018)
Karela/bitter gourd	Protein, minerals, beta carotene	Anti-diabetic, antioxidant, immunomodulatory	Cooking food, juice, tablet, capsule	Supplements (2020)

technique for formulation development in the food industries (Koshani & Jafari, 2019). Several such approaches used for the functional food or bioactive delivery are mentioned in Table 1.7.

1.5 Functional food market

Functional food market is a very rapidly growing market as reported by the value at $177,770.00 million in 2019 throughout the world and expected to reach up to $267,924.40 million by 2027 as per the CGAR rate reported (TechNavio, 2014), but before 10 years, most of the European countries did not know the details of functional food (Annunziata & Vecchio, 2011). Now people are very cautious about their health, showing their interest in functional food and also gaining knowledge about the beneficial health effects of functional foods. Globally, some of the largest functional food markets are considered as Japan, United States, Europe and the developing countries like Brazil, Peru, China, India, etc. Japan, United States, Europe and Australia's markets are growing at the rate of 38.4%, 31.1%, 28.9% and1.6% of the total global market, respectively (Küster-Boluda & Vidal-Capilla, 2017). Several factors playing a pivotal role in the growth of the FF market are newer trends in FF, collaboration of manufacturers and supplier, increased variety of the functional food products, diverging focus to develop the ecofriendly products, validation and variable dosage delivery forms (Hilton, 2017). Probiotics, mainly the *Lactobacillus* component in the Asian Pacific region, become highly demanding, and the market size was around at 36.6 billion dollars in 2016 and expected to increase to 57.2 billion dollars within 2022 (Diez-Gutiérrez et al., 2020). A wide number of Americans observed increased interest in different functional foods such as Greek yogurt, coconut water, omega 3-enriched foods, gluten, and fat- and lactose-free foods (Daliri & Lee, 2015). The United States is the highest selling market with the reported value of $42 billion dollars, whereas China showed $24.6 billion annual growth rate with a global compound annual growth rate (CAGR) of 8.7% in 2020. Japan and Europe are some other leading countries in the functional food market, and reports stated that Europe accounts for 20.2% of the global market value of functional food, and Brazil market was worth US$ 8.7 billion in 2014 and estimated to reach 12% increase within 2020 (Nazir et al., 2019). Japanese people developed FOSHU or food for specific health issue in 1991, and the market size reached US$ 3.2 billion by 2007. After saturation, a new concept FFC, "food with functional claims", was developed through which the market sales reached US$ 8 billion in 2018 (Iwatani & Yamamoto, 2019). Among the Asian countries, India has also a growing functional food market with the 17.1 % increasing CGAR rate with expected growth up to $4 billion in 2021. In the Indian food market, the highest selling products are from categories like probiotics (9%), omega 3 fatty acids (5%), several vitamins and minerals (36%), etc. Several brands like DSM Nutritional BASF, Merck, Danisco, Chr. Hansen, Yakult, etc. are dominated for their product

Table 1.7 Formulations Developed with Several Functional Foods

Nanoapproach Used	Functional Food/Phytochemical	References
Biogenic silver nanoparticles	*Nigella sativa* extract (NSE)	Kadam et al. (2019)
Nanostructure silver particles	Brown marine algae *Sargassum muticum* aqueous extract	Azizi et al. (2013)
Silver nanoparticles	Peanut red skin	Rehan et al. (2020)
Copper oxide nanoparticles	*Tecoma castanifolia* leaf extract	Sharmila et al. (2016)
Silver, copper and palladium metallic nanoparticles	Mulberry (*Morus alba* L.) fruit	Razavi et al. (2020)
Silver-gold palladium nanoparticles	*Aegle marmelos* leaf and *Syzygium aromaticum* bud extracts	Rao & Paria (2015)
Gold nanoparticles	Aqueous extract of *Elaeis guineensis* leaves	Ahmad et al. (2019)
Gold nanoparticles	Broccoli phytochemicals	Khoobchandani et al. (2013)
Iron oxide nanoparticles	Green biosynthetic method	Mahdavi et al. (2013)
Gold nanoparticles	Cinnamon	Chanda et al. (2011)
Spherical gold nanoparticles	Mangosteen pericarp extract	Park et al. (2017)
Nanoparticles (FA-NPS-PEG and FA-PEG-NPS)	EGCG and FA	Hassani et al. (2020)
Poly(DL-lactide-co-glycolide) (PLGA)	Acerola, guava and passion fruit of by-product extracts	Silva et al. (2014)
PLGA nanoparticle	Thymoquinone	Ganea et al. (2010)
Nanoparticles with 3,4,5-methoxycinnamic acid (3,4,5-TCA) from Chinese herb medicine	Berberine	Han et al. (2020)
Caprolactone and pluronic polymeric nanoparticles	Extracts of red propolis	do Nascimento et al. (2016)
Carbohydrate matrix of gum Arabic and maltodextrin	Green tea polyphenol epigallocatechin-3-gallate (EGCG)	Rocha et al. (2011)
Gum Arabic nanoparticles	Gallic acid	Hassani et al. (2020)
Zein nanoparticles	Curcumin	Zou et al. (2016)
Casein nanoparticles	Encapsulation of curcumin	Pan et al. (2014)
Nanosupramolecular assemblies	Curcumin	Pathak et al. (2015)
Zinc oxide nanoparticles	*Tecoma castanifolia* leaf extract	Sharmila et al. (2019
Methyl cellulose nanoparticles	Gamma oryzanol	Ghaderi et al. (2014)
Nanoparticles	Ginseng	Mathiyalagan and Yang (2017)
Green nanotechnology as gold nanoparticles	Cumin	Katti et al. (2009)
Green nanotechnology as gold nanoparticles	Tea	Nune et al. (2009)
Chitosan nanoparticles/nanofiber	Resveratrol and ferulic acid	Balan et al. (2020)
Bioactive peptide with chitosan nanoparticle	Epigallocatechin-3-gallate (EGCG)	Hu et al. (2013)
Xanthan gum–shellac nanoparticles	Cinnamon bark	Muhammad et al. (2020)
Nanoemulsion	Whey protein	Adjonu et al. (2014)
Water-soluble tomato extract (Fruitflow®)	Platelet inhibition, anti-inflammatory, cardio protective	O'Kennedy et al. (2017)

range with vitamins, minerals, probiotics, etc. The probiotic market (22.6% annual growth) is the most important and shows a positive way for the investment of several industries, and the reflected values are US$ 300 billion within a couple of years (Kaur & Das, 2011; Domínguez Díaz et al., 2020a).

1.6 Regulatory guidelines of functional food in different countries

Functional food science originated from the collaboration of sciences and the public need. It is the melding on food science, nutrition and medicine as it produces substances at the cross section of food and pharmaceuticals. A global perspective offers a comprehensive resource for information on regulatory aspects of the growing and economically important functional food industry. A thorough understanding of laws and regulation within and among key countries with regard to functional foods is critical to the direction of food companies that are developing products for these markets (Hasler, 2007). In the United States, the US Food and Drug Administration (FDA) under the provision of the Federal Food, Drug and Cosmetic Act (FD&C Act) governed the safety and efficacy of the functional food market in 1938. In 1994, the Dietary Supplement Health and Education Act (DSHEA) was developed for dietary supplements, and they defined functional food as a conventional food as helpful for disease prevention and also helpful to maintain the nutrient profile (Wong et al., 2015). They defined dietary supplements as only for ingestion and the ones other than the drug substances like vitamins, minerals and amino acids as dietary substances which cannot be claimed for diagnosis, treatment and prevention for any disease. There is no specific definition for FF, but it can be well described as the extracted or processed food obtained from the original food and used for health benefits beyond its basic nutritional profile. Premarketing approval is not required for marketing functional foods or dietary supplements in the United States (Thakkar et al., 2020). EU regulates herbal medicinal products with the European Medicines Agency (EMA), and the substances for nutrition such as vitamins and minerals or botanical compounds are regulated by following the European Food Safety Authority (EFSA). EC 1925/2006 is based on the precautionary things and high level of consumer protection. Premarketing approval is required for novel food which is produced by several novel technologies, and some additive ingredients to increase nutrient values need to take premarket approval authorization. The EFSA assesses the dossiers to advise the European Commission to give the final decision after taking the dossier from EFSA (Bragazzi et al., 2016; Moors, 2012). In Australia, the Therapeutics Goods Administration (TGA)-governed complementary medicines like different vitamins, herbs, homeopathy, minerals and nutritional supplements were not a conventional part of all health products in the country, and some novel foods which are extracted and processed with new technologies are governed by Food Standards Australia and New Zealand (FSANZ). In Japan, the Ministry of Health, Labour and

Welfare (MHLW) introduced the FOSHU, "Foods for Specified Health Use," in 1991 to regulate the functional food market. After 2009, the food labelling was transferred to the Consumer Affairs Agency. Then, a new health claim termed "foods with function claims" (FFC) was coined to improve the regulations through a better system (Shimizu, 2014). Kampo medicines are developed in Japan with traditional Chinese medicines (TCM). It has been reported that 148 prescriptions and 294 over-the-counter Kampo medicines were approved in Japan (Thakkar et al., 2020). In India, the Food Safety and Standards Authority (FSSA) was developed in 2006 to regulate nutraceutical and food market under the FSSAI act. This act controls the licenses to the local authorities like food manufactures and nutraceutical companies. False product claim enforcements and penalties (Bagchi, 2019; Keservani et al., 2014) have also been applied for noncompliance. In Canada, the Canadian Food Inspection Agency (CFIA) and Health Canada's Food Directorate established Food and Drugs Act and Food and Drug Regulations to regulate and control the food market. Other acts such as Safe Food for Canadians Act and Regulations also help to improve the food safety and quality (Powers et al., 2019). WHO has also developed the guidelines, and according to that, laws for GMPs and marketing of traditional medicines are followed with a proper procedure (Bahorun et al., 2019). In Korea, Health/Functional Food Act (HFF) was established in 2004, and 37 generic products were listed, and the rest are considered as product-specific. As per the new regulation act, the product-specific products should maintain standardization, safety and efficacy and must conform to the international standard of HFF (Kim et al., 2006). In Malaysia, several laws were developed for controlling the functional food like Food Act 1983 and Food Regulation 1985, Control of Drugs and Cosmetics Regulation 1984, and Halal laws and related regulations. Under such newer regulations, the food claims for health benefits like food for reducing cholesterol, improving intestinal health and immune system, etc. can be done (Lau, 2019). The Russian food and functional food markets were controlled by Federal Laws on Technical Regulation, on Food Quality and Safety, on Protection of Consumer Rights, etc. The technical committee created some standards (GOST R) related to functional food. They defined functional food as the diet which helps to reduce the nutrition-related diseases by maintaining balances (Tutelyan et al., 2019). Consumers are increasingly aware of the importance of diet functional food products. The current status of the international regulatory framework is driven by the majority of the health-related claims in functional food products. Specific regulation must control the use of these claims, many a times more than one in the labelling of functional products. Although the European, American and Japanese claims are partly similar in nature, the approval and use procedures and the regulatory framework are quite different. A thorough regulatory landscape focused on consumers' need for making better-informed food decisions and for the food industry in marketing its products with a focus on international trade must be developed.

References

Abuajah, C. I., Ogbonna, A. C., & Osuji, C. M. (2015). Functional components and medicinal properties of food: A review. *Journal of Food Science and Technology.* doi:10.1007/s13197-014-1396-5.

Adefegha, S. A. (2018). Functional foods and nutraceuticals as dietary intervention in chronic diseases; novel perspectives for health promotion and disease prevention. *Journal of Dietary Supplements.* doi:10.1080/19390211.2017.1401573.

Adjonu, R., Doran, G., Torley, P., & Agboola, S. (2014). Whey protein peptides as components of nanoemulsions: A review of emulsifying and biological functionalities. *Journal of Food Engineering.* doi:10.1016/j.jfoodeng.2013.08.034.

Ahmad, T., Bustam, M. A., Irfan, M., Moniruzzaman, M., Asghar, H. M. A., & Bhattacharjee, S. (2019). Mechanistic investigation of phytochemicals involved in green synthesis of gold nanoparticles using aqueous Elaeis guineensis leaves extract: Role of phenolic compounds and flavonoids. *Biotechnology and Applied Biochemistry.* doi:10.1002/bab.1787.

Al-Sheraji, S. H., Ismail, A., Manap, M. Y., Mustafa, S., Yusof, R. M., & Hassan, F. A. (2013). Prebiotics as functional foods: A review. *Journal of Functional Foods.* doi:10.1016/j.jff.2013.08.009.

Annunziata, A., & Vecchio, R. (2011). Functional foods development in the European market: A consumer perspective. *Journal of Functional Foods.* doi:10.1016/j.jff.2011.03.011.

Arscott, S. A., & Tanumihardjo, S. A. (2010). Carrots of many colors provide basic nutrition and bioavailable phytochemicals acting as a functional food. *Comprehensive Reviews in Food Science and Food Safety.* doi:10.1111/j.1541-4337.2009.00103.x.

Arya, S. S., Salve, A. R., & Chauhan, S. (2016). Peanuts as functional food: A review. *Journal of Food Science and Technology.* doi:10.1007/s13197-015-2007-9.

Assadpour, E., & Mahdi Jafari, S. (2019). A systematic review on nanoencapsulation of food bioactive ingredients and nutraceuticals by various nanocarriers. *Critical Reviews in Food Science and Nutrition.* doi:10.1080/10408398.2018.1484687.

Azizi, S., Namvar, F., Mahdavi, M., Ahmad, M. Bin, & Mohamad, R. (2013). Biosynthesis of silver nanoparticles using brown marine macroalga, Sargassum muticum aqueous extract. *Materials.* doi:10.3390/ma6125942.

Bagchi, D. (2019). Nutraceutical and functional food regulations in the United States and around the world. *Nutraceutical and Functional Food Regulations in the United States and around the World.* doi:10.1016/C2018-0-00112-7.

Bahorun, T., Aruoma, O. I., & Neergheen-Bhujun, V. S. (2019). Phytomedicines, nutraceuticals, and functional foods regulatory framework: The African context. *Nutraceutical and Functional Food Regulations in the United States and around the World.* doi:10.1016/B978-0-12-816467-9.00032-0.

Balan, P., Indrakumar, J., Murali, P., & Korrapati, P. S. (2020). Bi-faceted delivery of phytochemicals through chitosan nanoparticles impregnated nanofibers for cancer therapeutics. *International Journal of Biological Macromolecules.* doi:10.1016/j.ijbiomac.2019.09.093.

Balthazar, C. F., Pimentel, T. C., Ferrão, L. L., Almada, C. N., Santillo, A., Albenzio, M., Mollakhalili, N., Mortazavian, A. M., Nascimento, J. S., Silva, M. C., Freitas, M. Q., Sant'Ana, A. S., Granato, D., & Cruz, A. G. (2017). Sheep milk: Physicochemical characteristics and relevance for functional food development. *Comprehensive Reviews in Food Science and Food Safety.* doi:10.1111/1541-4337.12250.

Bano, A., Gupta, A., Sharma, S., & Sharma, R. (2020). Recent developments in nanocarrier-based nutraceuticals for therapeutic purposes. *Biogenic Nano-Particles and their Use in Agro-ecosystems.* doi:10.1007/978-981-15-2985-6_20.

Batista, A. P., Gouveia, L., Bandarra, N. M., Franco, J. M., & Raymundo, A. (2013). Comparison of microalgal biomass profiles as novel functional ingredient for food products. *Algal Research.* doi:10.1016/j.algal.2013.01.004.

Beltrán-Barrientos, L. M., Hernández-Mendoza, A., Torres-Llanez, M. J., González-Córdova, A. F., & Vallejo-Córdoba, B. (2016). Invited review: Fermented milk as antihypertensive functional food. *Journal of Dairy Science*. doi:10.3168/jds.2015-10054.

Belwal, T., Devkota, H. P., Hassan, H. A., Ahluwalia, S., Ramadan, M. F., Mocan, A., & Atanasov, A. G. (2018). Phytopharmacology of Acerola (Malpighia spp.) and its potential as functional food. *Trends in Food Science and Technology*. doi:10.1016/j.tifs.2018.01.014.

Bimbo, F., Bonanno, A., Nocella, G., Viscecchia, R., Nardone, G., De Devitiis, B., & Carlucci, D. (2017). Consumers' acceptance and preferences for nutrition-modified and functional dairy products: A systematic review. *Appetite*. doi:10.1016/j.appet.2017.02.031.

Bragazzi, N. L., Martini, M., Saporita, T. C., Nucci, D., Gianfredi, V., Maddalo, F., Di Capua, A., Tovani, F., & Marensi, L. (2016). Nutraceutical and functional food regulations in the European Union. *Developing New Functional Food and Nutraceutical Products*. doi:10.1016/B9780128027806.000171.

Bridges, M. (2018). "Moo-ove over, cow's milk: The rise of plant-based dairy alternatives. *Practical Gastroenterology* 21. https://practicalgastro.com/wp-content/ uploads/2019/07/ Moo-ove-Over-Cow-Milk-Rise-of-PlantBased-Dairy-Alternatives.pdf. (Accessed 10 August 2020). page no: 20–27.

Camacho, F., Macedo, A., & Malcata, F. (2019). Potential industrial applications and commercialization of microalgae in the functional food and feed industries: A short review. *Marine Drugs*. doi:10.3390/md17060312.

Câmara, C. R. S., Urrea, C. A., & Schlegel, V. (2013). Pinto beans (Phaseolus vulgaris l.) as a functional food: Implications on human health. *Agriculture (Switzerland)*. doi:10.3390/agriculture3010090.

Caporgno, M. P., & Mathys, A. (2018). Trends in microalgae incorporation into innovative food products with potential health benefits. *Frontiers in Nutrition*. doi:10.3389/ fnut.2018.00058.

Cencic, A., & Chingwaru, W. (2010). The role of functional foods, nutraceuticals, and food supplements in intestinal health. *Nutrients*. doi:10.3390/nu2060611.

Chanda, N., Shukla, R., Zambre, A., Mekapothula, S., Kulkarni, R. R., Katti, K., Bhattacharyya, K., Fent, G. M., Casteel, S. W., Boote, E. J., Viator, J. A., Upendran, A., Kannan, R., & Katti, K. V. (2011). An effective strategy for the synthesis of biocompatible gold nanoparticles using cinnamon phytochemicals for phantom CT imaging and photoacoustic detection of cancerous cells. *Pharmaceutical Research*. doi:10.1007/ s11095-010-0276-6.

Cheng, M., Zhang, X., Zhu, J., Cheng, L., Cao, J., Wu, Z., Weng, P., & Zheng, X. (2018). A metagenomics approach to the intestinal microbiome structure and function in high fat diet-induced obesity mice fed with oolong tea polyphenols. *Food and Function*. doi:10.1039/c7fo01570d.

Cherry, P., O'hara, C., Magee, P. J., Mcsorley, E. M., & Allsopp, P. J. (2019). Risks and benefits of consuming edible seaweeds. *Nutrition Reviews*. doi:10.1093/nutrit/nuy066.

Daliri, E. B.-M., & Lee, B. H. (2015). Current Trends and Future Perspectives on Functional Foods and Nutraceuticals. *Beneficial Microorganisms in Food and Nutraceuticals*. doi:10.1007/978-3-319-23177-8_10.

Delshadi, R., Bahrami, A., Tafti, A. G., Barba, F. J., & Williams, L. L. (2020). Micro and nano-encapsulation of vegetable and essential oils to develop functional food products with improved nutritional profiles. *Trends in Food Science and Technology*. doi:10.1016/j.tifs.2020.07.004.

Diez-Gutiérrez, L., San Vicente, L., Luis, L. J., Villarán, M. del C., & Chávarri, M. (2020). Gamma-aminobutyric acid and probiotics: Multiple health benefits and their future in the global functional food and nutraceuticals market. *Journal of Functional Foods*. doi:10.1016/j.jff.2019.103669.

do Nascimento, T. G., da Silva, P. F., Azevedo, L. F., da Rocha, L. G., de Moraes Porto, I. C. C., Lima e Moura, T. F. A., Basílio-Júnior, I. D., Grillo, L. A. M., Dornelas, C. B., Fonseca, E. J. da S., de Jesus Oliveira, E., Zhang, A. T., & Watson, D. G. (2016). Polymeric nanoparticles of brazilian red propolis extract: Preparation, characterization, antioxidant and leishmanicidal activity. *Nanoscale Research Letters.* doi:10.1186/s11671-016-1517-3.

Domínguez Díaz, L., Fernández-Ruiz, V., & Cámara, M. (2020a). An international regulatory review of food health-related claims in functional food products labeling. *Journal of Functional Foods.* doi:10.1016/j.jff.2020.103896.

Domínguez Díaz, L., Fernández-Ruiz, V., & Cámara, M. (2020b). The frontier between nutrition and pharma: The international regulatory framework of functional foods, food supplements and nutraceuticals. *Critical Reviews in Food Science and Nutrition.* doi:10.1080/10408398.2019.1592107.

Dullius, A., Goettert, M. I., & de Souza, C. F. V. (2018). Whey protein hydrolysates as a source of bioactive peptides for functional foods – Biotechnological facilitation of industrial scale-up. *Journal of Functional Foods.* doi:10.1016/j.jff.2017.12.063.

Enrico, C. (2019). Nanotechnology-based drug delivery of natural compounds and phytochemicals for the treatment of cancer and other diseases. *Studies in Natural Products Chemistry.* doi:10.1016/B978-0-444-64185-4.00003-4.

Fahimirad, S., & Hatami, M. (2019). Nanocarrier-based antimicrobial phytochemicals. *Advances in Phytonanotechnology.* doi:10.1016/b978-0-12-815322-2.00013-4.

Falguera, V., Aliguer, N., & Falguera, M. (2012). An integrated approach to current trends in food consumption: Moving toward functional and organic products? *Food Control.* doi:10.1016/j.foodcont.2012.01.051.

Faridi Esfanjani, A., Assadpour, E., & Jafari, S. M. (2018). Improving the bioavailability of phenolic compounds by loading them within lipid-based nanocarriers. *Trends in Food Science and Technology.* doi:10.1016/j.tifs.2018.04.002.

Fiocco, D., Longo, A., Arena, M. P., Russo, P., Spano, G., & Capozzi, V. (2020). How probiotics face food stress: They get by with a little help. *Critical Reviews in Food Science and Nutrition.* doi:10.1080/10408398.2019.1580673.

Galasso, C., Gentile, A., Orefice, I., Ianora, A., Bruno, A., Noonan, D. M., Sansone, C., Albini, A., & Brunet, C. (2019). Microalgal derivatives as potential nutraceutical and food supplements for human health: A focus on cancer prevention and interception. *Nutrients.* doi:10.3390/nu11061226.

Ganea, G. M., Fakayode, S. O., Losso, J. N., Van Nostrum, C. F., Sabliov, C. M., & Warner, I. M. (2010). Delivery of phytochemical thymoquinone using molecular micelle modified poly(D, L lactide-co-glycolide) (PLGA) nanoparticles. *Nanotechnology.* doi:10.1088/0957-4484/21/28/285104.

Garcia-Vaquero, M., & Hayes, M. (2016). Red and green macroalgae for fish and animal feed and human functional food development. *Food Reviews International.* doi:10.1080/87559129.2015.1041184.

George Kerry, R., Patra, J. K., Gouda, S., Park, Y., Shin, H. S., & Das, G. (2018). Benefaction of probiotics for human health: A review. *Journal of Food and Drug Analysis.* doi:10.1016/j.jfda.2018.01.002.

Ghaderi, S., Ghanbarzadeh, S., Mohammadhassani, Z., & Hamishehkar, H. (2014). Formulation of gammaoryzanol-loaded nanoparticles for potential application in fortifying food products. *Advanced Pharmaceutical Bulletin.* doi:10.5681/apb.2014.081.

Goktas, Z., Zu, Y., Abbasi, M., Galyean, S., Wu, D., Fan, Z., & Wang, S. (2020). Recent advances in nanoencapsulation of phytochemicals to combat obesity and its comorbidities. *Journal of Agricultural and Food Chemistry.* doi:10.1021/acs.jafc.0c00131.

Goyal, A., Sharma, V., Upadhyay, N., Gill, S., & Sihag, M. (2014). Flax and flaxseed oil: An ancient medicine & modern functional food. *Journal of Food Science and Technology.* doi:10.1007/s13197-013-1247-9.

Gramza-Michałowska, A., Kobus-Cisowska, J., Kmiecik, D., Korczak, J., Helak, B., Dziedzic, K., & Górecka, D. (2016). Antioxidative potential, nutritional value and sensory profiles of confectionery fortified with green and yellow tea leaves (Camellia sinensis). *Food Chemistry*. doi:10.1016/j.foodchem.2016.05.048.

Han, N., Huang, X., Tian, X., Li, T., Liu, X., Li, W., Huo, S., Wu, Q., Gu, Y., Dai, Z., Xu, B., Wang, P., & Lei, H. (2020). Self-assembled nanoparticles of natural phytochemicals (berberine and 3,4,5-methoxycinnamic acid) originated from traditional Chinese medicine for inhibiting multidrug-resistant Staphylococcus aureus. *Current Drug Delivery*. doi:10.2174/1567201817666201124121918.

Hasler, C. M. (2007). Regulation of functional foods and nutraceuticals: A global perspective. *Regulation of Functional Foods and Nutraceuticals: A Global Perspective*. doi:10.1002/9780470277676.

Hassani, A., Azarian, M. M. S., Ibrahim, W. N., & Hussain, S. A. (2020). Preparation, characterization and therapeutic properties of gum arabic-stabilized gallic acid nanoparticles. *Scientific Reports*. doi:10.1038/s41598-020-71175-8.

Hilton, J. (2017). Growth patterns and emerging opportunities in nutraceutical and functional food categories: Market overview. *Developing New Functional Food and Nutraceutical Products*. doi:10.1016/B978-0-12-802780-6.00001-8.

Holdt, S. L., & Kraan, S. (2011). Bioactive compounds in seaweed: Functional food applications and legislation. *Journal of Applied Phycology*. doi:10.1007/s10811-010-9632-5.

Hu, B., Ting, Y., Zeng, X., & Huang, Q. (2013). Bioactive peptides/chitosan nanoparticles enhance cellular antioxidant activity of (-)-epigallocatechin-3-gallate. *Journal of Agricultural and Food Chemistry*. doi:10.1021/jf304821k.

Hu, C., Wong, W. T., Wu, R., & Lai, W. F. (2020). Biochemistry and use of soybean isoflavones in functional food development. *Critical Reviews in Food Science and Nutrition*. doi:10.1080/10408398.2019.1630598.

Huang, Q., Yu, H., & Ru, Q. (2010). Bioavailability and delivery of nutraceuticals using nanotechnology. *Journal of Food Science*. doi:10.1111/j.1750-3841.2009.01457.x.

Ikumi, P., Mburu, M., & Njoroge, D. (2019). Chia (Salvia hispanica L.) – A potential crop for food and nutrition security in Africa. *Journal of Food Research*. doi:10.5539/jfr.v8n6p104.

Iwatani, S., & Yamamoto, N. (2019). Functional food products in Japan: A review. *Food Science and Human Wellness*. doi:10.1016/j.fshw.2019.03.011.

Jadhav, N. R., Nadaf, S. J., Lohar, D. A., Ghagare, P. S., & Powar, T. A. (2017). Phytochemicals formulated as nanoparticles: Inventions, recent patents and future prospects. *Recent Patents on Drug Delivery & Formulation*. doi:10.2174/1872211311666171120102531.

Jamali, S. N., Assadpour, E., & Jafari, S. M. (2019). Formulation and application of nanoemulsions for nutraceuticals and phytochemicals. *Current Medicinal Chemistry*. doi:10.2174/0929867326666190620102820.

Johanningsmeier, S. D., & Harris, G. K. (2011). Pomegranate as a functional food and nutraceutical source. *Annual Review of Food Science and Technology*. doi:10.1146/annurev-food-030810-153709.

José Bagur, M., Alonso Salinas, G. L., Jiménez-Monreal, A. M., Chaouqi, S., Llorens, S., Martínez-Tomé, M., & Alonso, G. L. (2017). Saffron: An old medicinal plant and a potential novel functional food. *Molecules (Basel, Switzerland)*. doi:10.3390/molecules23010030.

Kadam, D., Momin, B., Palamthodi, S., & Lele, S. S. (2019). Physicochemical and functional properties of chitosan-based nano-composite films incorporated with biogenic silver nanoparticles. *Carbohydrate Polymers*. doi:10.1016/j.carbpol.2019.02.005.

Kadam, S. U., & Prabhasankar, P. (2010). Marine foods as functional ingredients in bakery and pasta products. *Food Research International*. doi:10.1016/j.foodres.2010.06.007.

Katti, K., Chanda, N., Shukla, R., Zambre, A., Suibramanian, T., Kulkarni, R. R., Kannan, R., & Katti, K. V. (2009). Green nanotechnology from cumin phytochemicals: Generation of biocompatible gold nanoparticles. *International Journal of Green Nanotechnology: Biomedicine*. doi:10.1080/19430850902931599.

Kaur, S., & Das, M. (2011). Functional foods: An overview. *Food Science and Biotechnology.* doi:10.1007/s10068-011-0121-7.

Keservani, R. K., Sharma, A. K., Ahmad, F., & Baig, M. E. (2014). Nutraceutical and functional food regulations in India. *Nutraceutical and Functional Food Regulations in the United States and Around the World: Second Edition.* doi:10.1016/B978-0-12-405870-5.00019-0.

Khan, A. A., Gani, A., Khanday, F. A., & Masoodi, F. A. (2018). Biological and pharmaceutical activities of mushroom β-glucan discussed as a potential functional food ingredient. *Bioactive Carbohydrates and Dietary Fibre.* doi:10.1016/j.bcdf.2017.12.002.

Khoobchandani, M., Zambre, A., Katti, K., Lin, C. H., & Katti, K. V. (2013). Green nanotechnology from brassicaceae: Development of broccoli phytochemicals-encapsulated gold nanoparticles and their applications in nanomedicine. *International Journal of Green Nanotechnology.* doi:10.1177/1943089213509474.

Kılınç, B., Cirik, S., & Turan, G. (2013). Seaweeds for food and industrial applications. *Seaweeds for Food and Industrial Applications.* doi:10.5772/53172.

Kim, J. Y., Kim, D. B., & Lee, H. J. (2006). Regulations on health/functional foods in Korea. *Toxicology.* doi:10.1016/j.tox.2006.01.016.

Koshani, R., & Jafari, S. M. (2019). Ultrasound-assisted preparation of different nanocarriers loaded with food bioactive ingredients. *Advances in Colloid and Interface Science.* doi:10.1016/j.cis.2019.06.005.

Ksouri, R., Ksouri, W. M., Jallali, I., Debez, A., Magné, C., Hiroko, I., & Abdelly, C. (2012). Medicinal halophytes: Potent source of health promoting biomolecules with medical, nutraceutical and food applications. *Critical Reviews in Biotechnology.* doi:10.3109/07388551.2011.630647.

Küster-Boluda, I., & Vidal-Capilla, I. (2017). Consumer attitudes in the election of functional foods. *Spanish Journal of Marketing - ESIC.* doi:10.1016/j.sjme.2017.05.002.

Laparra, J. M., & Sanz, Y. (2010). Interactions of gut microbiota with functional food components and nutraceuticals. *Pharmacological Research.* doi:10.1016/j.phrs.2009.11.001.

Lau, T. C. (2019). Regulations, opportunities, and key trends of functional foods in Malaysia. *Nutraceutical and Functional Food Regulations in the United States and around the World.* doi:10.1016/B978-0-12-816467-9.00034-4.

Lee, J., Kim, H. Y., Zhou, H., Hwang, S., Koh, K., Han, D. W., & Lee, J. (2011). Green synthesis of phytochemical-stabilized Au nanoparticles under ambient conditions and their biocompatibility and antioxidative activity. *Journal of Materials Chemistry.* doi:10.1039/c1jm11592h.

Li, Z., Jiang, H., Xu, C., & Gu, L. (2015). A review: Using nanoparticles to enhance absorption and bioavailability of phenolic phytochemicals. *Food Hydrocolloids.* doi:10.1016/j.foodhyd.2014.05.010.

Liu, C., Ge, S., Yang, J., Xu, Y., Zhao, M., Xiong, L., & Sun, Q. (2016). Adsorption mechanism of polyphenols onto starch nanoparticles and enhanced antioxidant activity under adverse conditions. *Journal of Functional Foods.* doi:10.1016/j.jff.2016.08.036.

Lordan, S., Ross, R. P., & Stanton, C. (2011). Marine bioactives as functional food ingredients: Potential to reduce the incidence of chronic diseases. *Marine Drugs.* doi:10.3390/md9061056.

Ma, Z. F., Ahmad, J., Zhang, H., Khan, I., & Muhammad, S. (2020). Evaluation of phytochemical and medicinal properties of Moringa (Moringa oleifera) as a potential functional food. *South African Journal of Botany.* doi:10.1016/j.sajb.2018.12.002.

Mahdavi, M., Namvar, F., Ahmad, M. B., & Mohamad, R. (2013). Green biosynthesis and characterization of magnetic iron oxide (Fe 3O4) nanoparticles using seaweed (Sargassum muticum) aqueous extract. *Molecules.* doi:10.3390/molecules18055954.

Mäkinen, O. E., Wanhalinna, V., Zannini, E., & Arendt, E. K. (2016). Foods for special dietary needs: Non-dairy plant-based milk substitutes and fermented dairy-type products. *Critical Reviews in Food Science and Nutrition.* doi:10.1080/10408398.2012.761950.

Mathiyalagan, R., & Yang, D. C. (2017). Ginseng nanoparticles: A budding tool for cancer treatment. *Nanomedicine*. doi:10.2217/nnm-2017-0070.

Matos, J., Cardoso, C., Bandarra, N. M., & Afonso, C. (2017). Microalgae as healthy ingredients for functional food: A review. *Food and Function*. doi:10.1039/c7fo00409e.

McClements, D. J. (2020). Advances in nanoparticle and microparticle delivery systems for increasing the dispersibility, stability, and bioactivity of phytochemicals. *Biotechnology Advances*. doi:10.1016/j.biotechadv.2018.08.004.

Milinčić, D. D., Popović, D. A., Lević, S. M., Kostić, A., Tešić, Ž. L., Nedović, V. A., & Pešić, M. B. (2019). Application of polyphenol-loaded nanoparticles in food industry. *Nanomaterials*. doi:10.3390/nano9111629.

Min, M., Bunt, C. R., Mason, S. L., & Hussain, M. A. (2019). Non-dairy probiotic food products: An emerging group of functional foods. *Critical Reviews in Food Science and Nutrition*. doi:10.1080/10408398.2018.1462760.

Mohamed, S., Hashim, S. N., & Rahman, H. A. (2012). Seaweeds: A sustainable functional food for complementary and alternative therapy. In *Trends in Food Science and Technology*. https://doi.org/10.1016/j.tifs.2011.09.001

Moors, E. H. M. (2012). Functional foods: Regulation and innovations in the EU. *Innovation*. doi:10.1080/13511610.2012.726407.

Muhammad, D. R. A., Sedaghat Doost, A., Gupta, V., bin Sintang, M. D., Van de Walle, D., Van der Meeren, P., & Dewettinck, K. (2020). Stability and functionality of xanthan gum–shellac nanoparticles for the encapsulation of cinnamon bark extract. *Food Hydrocolloids*. doi:10.1016/j.foodhyd.2019.105377.

Nagpal, R., Kumar, A., Kumar, M., Behare, P. V., Jain, S., & Yadav, H. (2012). Probiotics, their health benefits and applications for developing healthier foods: A review. *FEMS Microbiology Letters*. doi:10.1111/j.1574-6968.2012.02593.x.

Nazir, M., Arif, S., Khan, R. S., Nazir, W., Khalid, N., & Maqsood, S. (2019). Opportunities and challenges for functional and medicinal beverages: Current and future trends. *Trends in Food Science and Technology*. doi:10.1016/j.tifs.2019.04.011.

Nooshkam, M., Babazadeh, A., & Jooyandeh, H. (2018). Lactulose: Properties, techno-functional food applications, and food grade delivery system. *Trends in Food Science and Technology*. doi:10.1016/j.tifs.2018.07.028.

Nune, S. K., Chanda, N., Shukla, R., Katti, K., Kulkarni, R. R., Thilakavathy, S., Mekapothula, S., Kannan, R., & Katti, K. V. (2009). Green nanotechnology from tea: Phytochemicals in tea as building blocks for production of biocompatible gold nanoparticles. *Journal of Materials Chemistry*. doi:10.1039/b822015h.

Nwosu, O. K., & Ubaoji, K. I. (2020). Nutraceuticals: History, classification and market demand. *Functional Foods and Nutraceuticals*. doi:10.1007/978-3-030-42319-3_2.

O'Kennedy, N., Crosbie, L., Song, H. J., Zhang, X., Horgan, G., & Duttaroy, A. K. (2017). A randomised controlled trial comparing a dietary antiplatelet, the water-soluble tomato extract Fruitflow, with 75 mg aspirin in healthy subjects. *European Journal of Clinical Nutrition*. doi:10.1038/ejcn.2016.222.

Özer, B. H., & Kirmaci, H. A. (2010). Functional milks and dairy beverages. *International Journal of Dairy Technology*. doi:10.1111/j.1471-0307.2009.00547.x.

Pan, K., Luo, Y., Gan, Y., Baek, S. J., & Zhong, Q. (2014). PH-driven encapsulation of curcumin in self-assembled casein nanoparticles for enhanced dispersibility and bioactivity. *Soft Matter*. doi:10.1039/c4sm00239c.

Pandey, P., & Mishra, H. N. (2021). Co-microencapsulation of γ-aminobutyric acid (GABA) and probiotic bacteria in thermostable and biocompatible exopolysaccharides matrix. *LWT*. doi:10.1016/j.lwt.2020.110293.

Park, J. S., Ahn, E. Y., & Park, Y. (2017). Asymmetric dumbbell-shaped silver nanoparticles and spherical gold nanoparticles green-synthesized by mangosteen (Garcinia mangostana) pericarp waste extracts. *International Journal of Nanomedicine*. doi:10.2147/IJN.S140190.

Pathak, L., Kanwal, A., & Agrawal, Y. (2015). Curcumin loaded self assembled lipid-bio-polymer nanoparticles for functional food applications. *Journal of Food Science and Technology*. doi:10.1007/s13197-015-1742-2.

Paul, A. A., Kumar, S., Kumar, V., & Sharma, R. (2020). Milk Analog: Plant based alternatives to conventional milk, production, potential and health concerns. *Critical Reviews in Food Science and Nutrition*. doi:10.1080/10408398.2019.1674243.

Petropoulos, S. A., Karkanis, A., Martins, N., & Ferreira, I. C. F. R. (2018). Edible halophytes of the Mediterranean basin: Potential candidates for novel food products. *Trends in Food Science and Technology*. doi:10.1016/j.tifs.2018.02.006.

Powers, J. P., Farrell, M., McMullin, C., Retik, L., & White, J. (2019). Regulation of dietary supplements and functional foods in Canada. *Nutraceutical and Functional Food Regulations in the United States and around the World*. doi:10.1016/B978-0-12-816467-9.00017-4.

Prado, F. C., Parada, J. L., Pandey, A., & Soccol, C. R. (2008). Trends in non-dairy probiotic beverages. *Food Research International*. doi:10.1016/j.foodres.2007.10.010.

Qiu, C., Wang, C., Gong, C., McClements, D. J., Jin, Z., & Wang, J. (2020). Advances in research on preparation, characterization, interaction with proteins, digestion and delivery systems of starch-based nanoparticles. *International Journal of Biological Macromolecules*. doi:10.1016/j.ijbiomac.2020.02.156.

Rao, K. J., & Paria, S. (2015). Mixed phytochemicals mediated synthesis of multifunctional Ag-Au-Pd nanoparticles for glucose oxidation and antimicrobial applications. *ACS Applied Materials and Interfaces*. doi:10.1021/acsami.5b03089.

Razavi, R., Molaei, R., Moradi, M., Tajik, H., Ezati, P., & Shafipour Yordshahi, A. (2020). Biosynthesis of metallic nanoparticles using mulberry fruit (Morus alba L.) extract for the preparation of antimicrobial nanocellulose film. *Applied Nanoscience (Switzerland)*. doi:10.1007/s13204-019-01137-8.

Rehan, M., Elshemy, N. S., Haggag, K., Montaser, A. S., & Ibrahim, G. E. (2020). Phytochemicals and volatile compounds of peanut red skin extract: Simultaneous coloration and in situ synthesis of silver nanoparticles for multifunctional viscose fibers. *Cellulose*. doi:10.1007/s10570-020-03452-8.

Rizwanullah, M., Amin, S., Mir, S. R., Fakhri, K. U., & Rizvi, M. M. A. (2018). Phytochemical based nanomedicines against cancer: Current status and future prospects. *Journal of Drug Targeting*. doi:10.1080/1061186X.2017.1408115.

Rocha, S., Generalov, R., Pereira, M. D. C., Peres, I., Juzenas, P., & Coelho, M. A. N. (2011). Epigallocatechin gallate-loaded polysaccharide nanoparticles for prostate cancer chemoprevention. *Nanomedicine*. doi:10.2217/nnm.10.101.

Saini, R. K., Sivanesan, I., & Keum, Y. S. (2016). Phytochemicals of Moringa oleifera: A review of their nutritional, therapeutic and industrial significance. *3 Biotech*. doi:10.1007/s13205-016-0526-3.

Sharmila, G., Thirumarimurugan, M., & Muthukumaran, C. (2019). Green synthesis of ZnO nanoparticles using Tecoma castanifolia leaf extract: Characterization and evaluation of its antioxidant, bactericidal and anticancer activities. *Microchemical Journal*. doi:10.1016/j.microc.2018.11.022.

Sharmila, G., Thirumarimurugan, M., & Sivakumar, V. M. (2016). Optical, catalytic and antibacterial properties of phytofabricated CuO nanoparticles using Tecoma castanifolia leaf extract. *Optik*. doi:10.1016/j.ijleo.2016.05.142.

Shimizu, M. (2014). History and current status of functional food regulations in Japan. *Nutraceutical and Functional Food Regulations in the United States and Around the World: Second Edition*. doi:10.1016/B978-0-12-405870-5.00015-3.

Shori, A. B. (2016). Influence of food matrix on the viability of probiotic bacteria: A review based on dairy and non-dairy beverages. *Food Bioscience*. doi:10.1016/j.fbio.2015.11.001.

Silva, L. M., Hill, L. E., Figueiredo, E., & Gomes, C. L. (2014). Delivery of phytochemicals of tropical fruit by-products using poly (dl-lactide-co-glycolide) (PLGA) nanoparticles: Synthesis, characterization, and antimicrobial activity. *Food Chemistry*. doi:10.1016/j.foodchem.2014.05.118.

Singh, M., Devi, S., Rana, V. S., Mishra, B. B., Kumar, J., & Ahluwalia, V. (2019). Delivery of phytochemicals by liposome cargos: Recent progress, challenges and opportunities. *Journal of Microencapsulation*. doi:10.1080/02652048.2019.1617361.

Subramanian, A. P., Jaganathan, S. K., Manikandan, A., Pandiaraj, K. N., Gomathi, N., & Supriyanto, E. (2016). Recent trends in nano-based drug delivery systems for efficient delivery of phytochemicals in chemotherapy. *RSC Advances*. doi:10.1039/c6ra07802h.

Supplements, N. (2020). *APTI Women's Forum*. http://aptiindia.org/newsletter/APTI-WF-NL_14_MAY_2_CORR_2020.pdf. May - Jul, 2020

Taheri, A., & Jafari, S. M. (2019). Gum-based nanocarriers for the protection and delivery of food bioactive compounds. *Advances in Colloid and Interface Science*. doi:10.1016/j.cis.2019.04.009.

TechNavio. (2014). *Global Functional Foods and Beverages Market 2014-2018*. 75. https://www.technavio.com/report/functional-foods-and-beverages-market-industry-analysis

Terpou, A., Papadaki, A., Lappa, I. K., Kachrimanidou, V., Bosnea, L. A., & Kopsahelis, N. (2019). Probiotics in food systems: Significance and emerging strategies towards improved viability and delivery of enhanced beneficial value. *Nutrients*. doi:10.3390/nu11071591.

Thakkar, S., Anklam, E., Xu, A., Ulberth, F., Li, J., Li, B., Hugas, M., Sarma, N., Crerar, S., Swift, S., Hakamatsuka, T., Curtui, V., Yan, W., Geng, X., Slikker, W., & Tong, W. (2020). Regulatory landscape of dietary supplements and herbal medicines from a global perspective. *Regulatory Toxicology and Pharmacology*. doi:10.1016/j.yrtph.2020.104647.

Tocaciu, S., Oliver, L. J., Lowenthal, R. M., Peterson, G. M., Patel, R., Shastri, M., Mcguinness, G., Olesen, I., & Fitton, J. H. (2018). The effect of *Undaria pinnatifida* fucoidan on the pharmacokinetics of letrozole and tamoxifen in patients with breast cancer. *Integrative Cancer Therapies*, 17, 99–105.

Tsuda, T. (2018). Curcumin as a functional food-derived factor: Degradation products, metabolites, bioactivity, and future perspectives. *Food and Function*. doi:10.1039/c7fo01242j.

Tutelyan, V. A., Sukhanov, B. P., Kochetkova, A. A., Sheveleva, S. A., & Smirnova, E. A. (2019). Russian regulations on nutraceuticals, functional foods, and foods for special dietary uses. *Nutraceutical and Functional Food Regulations in the United States and around the World*. doi:10.1016/B978-0-12-816467-9.00026-5.

Vega-Gálvez, A., Miranda, M., Vergara, J., Uribe, E., Puente, L., & Martínez, E. A. (2010). Nutrition facts and functional potential of quinoa (Chenopodium quinoa willd.), an ancient Andean grain: A review. *Journal of the Science of Food and Agriculture*. doi:10.1002/jsfa.4158.

Vilcacundo, R., & Hernández-Ledesma, B. (2017). Nutritional and biological value of quinoa (Chenopodium quinoa Willd.). *Current Opinion in Food Science*. doi:10.1016/j.cofs.2016.11.007.

Wong, A. Y. T., Lai, J. M. C., & Chan, A. W. K. (2015). Regulations and protection for functional food products in the United States. *Journal of Functional Foods*. doi:10.1016/j.jff.2015.05.038.

Wu, S., & Tian, L. (2017). Diverse phytochemicals and bioactivities in the ancient fruit and modern functional food pomegranate (punica granatum). *Molecules*. doi:10.3390/molecules22101606.

Xie, J., Yang, Z., Zhou, C., Zhu, J., Lee, R. J., & Teng, L. (2016). Nanotechnology for the delivery of phytochemicals in cancer therapy. *Biotechnology Advances*. doi:10.1016/j.biotechadv.2016.04.002.

Xiong, K., Zhou, L., Wang, J., Ma, A., Fang, D., Xiong, L., & Sun, Q. (2020). Construction of food-grade pH-sensitive nanoparticles for delivering functional food ingredients. *Trends in Food Science and Technology*. doi:10.1016/j.tifs.2019.12.019.

Ye, Q., Georges, N., & Selomulya, C. (2018). Microencapsulation of active ingredients in functional foods: From research stage to commercial food products. *Trends in Food Science & Technology*, 78, 167–179. https://doi.org/10.1016/J.TIFS.2018.05.025

Yin, R., Kuo, H. C., Hudlikar, R., Sargsyan, D., Li, S., Wang, L., Wu, R., & Kong, A. N. (2019). Gut microbiota, dietary phytochemicals, and benefits to human health. *Current Pharmacology Reports*. doi:10.1007/s40495-019-00196-3.

Yousefi, M., Narmani, A., & Jafari, S. M. (2020). Dendrimers as efficient nanocarriers for the protection and delivery of bioactive phytochemicals. *Advances in Colloid and Interface Science*. doi:10.1016/j.cis.2020.102125.

Yu, J., & Ahmedna, M. (2013). Functional components of grape pomace: Their composition, biological properties and potential applications. *International Journal of Food Science and Technology*. doi:10.1111/j.1365-2621.2012.03197.x.

Zeng, Y., Li, Y., Yang, J., Pu, X., Du, J., Yang, X., Yang, T., & Yang, S. (2017). Therapeutic role of functional components in alliums for preventive chronic disease in human being. *Evidence-based Complementary and Alternative Medicine*. doi:10.1155/2017/9402849.

Zeng, Y., Pu, X., Yang, J., Du, J., Yang, X., Li, X., Li, L., Zhou, Y., & Yang, T. (2018). Preventive and therapeutic role of functional ingredients of barley grass for chronic diseases in human beings. *Oxidative Medicine and Cellular Longevity*. doi:10.1155/2018/3232080.

Zettel, V., & Hitzmann, B. (2018). Applications of chia (Salvia hispanica L.) in food products. *Trends in Food Science and Technology*. doi:10.1016/j.tifs.2018.07.011.

Zhong, Q., & Zhang, L. (2019). Nanoparticles fabricated from bulk solid lipids: Preparation, properties, and potential food applications. *Advances in Colloid and Interface Science*. doi:10.1016/j.cis.2019.102033.

Zhu, J., & Huang, Q. (2019). Nanoencapsulation of functional food ingredients. *Advances in Food and Nutrition Research*. doi:10.1016/bs.afnr.2019.03.005.

Zou, L., Zheng, B., Zhang, R., Zhang, Z., Liu, W., Liu, C., Xiao, H., & McClements, D. J. (2016). Enhancing the bioaccessibility of hydrophobic bioactive agents using mixed colloidal dispersions: Curcumin-loaded zein nanoparticles plus digestible lipid nanoparticles. *Food Research International*. doi:10.1016/j.foodres.2015.12.035.

2

Importance of Integrative Health Sciences in Antiaging Nutraceutical Development

Gargi Patel, Jayant N. Lokhande, and Yashwant V. Pathak
University of South Florida

Contents

Nutraceuticals could be defined as substances that provide physiological benefits and protection against severe chronic diseases. One can say that nutraceuticals play an internal part if used to improve health, delay the aging process, increase life expectancy or help in functional support of the body.

In today's modern world, aging is a complex phenomenon, a sum total of changes occurring in living organisms throughout life. Humans decreasing ability to cooperate with stress and increasing ability of functional impairment increase the probability of premature chronological death. Today there is very less awareness and primary data available on nutraceutical products and its efficacy, but nutraceuticals has its potential towards age management.

DOI: 10.1201/9781003110866-2

The studies on nutraceutical products have proven to show promising results through these elements/compounds in various complications. Multiple reviews have been conducted with much effort to present the concepts of effectiveness of nutraceutical products on diseases modifying indications. The prominence have been given to present the various level of effectiveness from the herbal nutraceuticals on hard curative disorders which are associated with oxidative stress like allergy, cardiovascular, cancer, Alzheimer, diabetes, opthalmology, immunity disorders, inflammatory conditions, Parkinson's Disease, and obesity. However, in this chapter, we will focus on aging and its direct association with use of pharmaceutical products [1]. Furthermore, in this chapter, we will introduce various health benefits of integrating nutraceutical products in one's daily life and age-longevity. Their availability is in various parts of the world, with different names, culture and their integration in daily rituals.

2.1 Introduction

The word *nutraceutical* is derived from the term "nutrition" and "pharmaceutics." The word itself differs in its product property by means of isolation from dietary supplements (nutrients), specific diets, herbal products, processed foods such as cereals, soups and beverages in a manner which could be used as a medicine other than just as nutrition. One can say, nutraceuticals play an internal part if used to improve health, delay the aging process and age-longevity by proving to increase life expectancy.

There are multiple theories conducted on aging and skin improvement. Aging is a complex phenomenon, generally defined as a process that results in an age-related increase in health detour or failure rate. However, there are multiple different products used with the sole purpose of delaying the process of aging. For example, it is common in today's modern world for individuals to use different "pharmaceutical drugs", chemical peeling, injectable agents, grafting and surgical procedures to reduce the extrinsic aging process to appear younger. However, the side-effects these products leave behind on human health are not conducive.

In contrast, thanks to our ancient masters and scientists who have managed to discover the "medicine" which has helped in diseases and age modification indications in many individuals who had shown their promise in usage of such natural products. Nowadays, nutraceutical products are receiving considerable interest throughout the globe due to its potential nutritional, safety and therapeutic effects. Some popular nutraceuticals include ginseng, *Echinacea*, green tea, glucosamine, omega-3, lutein, folic acid, and cod liver oil. Majority of the nutraceuticals possess multiple therapeutic properties [2].

2.2 Wisdom of antiaging in ancient health sciences

The quality of life and ability to influence longevity are concepts that are not unexplored. In fact, they have been around the centuries, and ancient text of health sciences are dated back to about 2100 BCE even before the idea of life extension. If one refers to *gotu kola*, *centella asiatica*, *brahmi* or *spade leaf*, all are ancient healing plants that make a profound comeback in the modern science through advancement for preventing aging.

2.3 Contribution of cognition, intelligence, perception, psychology, and emotional intelligence in antiaging

It is comprehensive to say that as time passes, humans are awarded with the titled of "aged". Almost half of the population in the world after 40 would like to find a magical solution to age longevity. However, the stress one faces in today's modern environment is affecting physical, cognitive and emotional health of individuals as years pass. So, the question still remains if the decline in one's health is associated with aging inevitability. According to modern and ancient health science, there is no direct association. Research conducted over the years by doctors and scientists proves that minority of individuals, perhaps 20% or so, whose face ages successfully, have longer health spans and high physical, cognitive, emotional and social functioning if they are more aware [3].

Furthermore, they stay mentally sharp, do not get sick often and are able to avoid chronic disorders such as dementia, depression, heart disease, diabetes and cancer.

What is common is all of these individuals' daily practices or *"Dincharya"* as Ayurveda refers as. The *super agers* practice a healthy lifestyle which leads to a common life of more than 100 years with full functional ability. **The seven longevity lessons are listed below.**

1. **Consume a plant-based diet**: Include intake of more fruits, veggies, whole grains, legumes, and avoid meat, dairy and processed food.
2. **Move naturally**: Practice daily physical exercise
3. **Eat in moderation**: Follow the 80/20 rule, by consuming food until you are 80% full and by cutting 20% of calories out.
4. **Down shift**: Relieve stress by including mediation twice in your daily routine.
5. **Have a purpose**: Determine your life purpose and hold yourself accountable for it.

6. **Enjoy social support**: Make a priority of your social circle; be involved with your friends and family.
7. **Belong**: Be part of spiritual and community practices.

These discoveries of the lessons learned from the *super agers* applied by the Blue Zone communities of Maharishi University of Management in Fairfield, Iowa. It is now up to individuals weather in your 30s, 40s or 70s to allow the effects of such practices to partake in designing of one's aging process [3].

2.4 Impact of time and space elements in antiaging

I need clarity on this on. Are we talking about space elements as away from the Earth or time and space elements in different parts of earth?

2.5 Spiritual science of antiaging

Our eternal life by God is something that promotes and transcends physical longevity. The belief of man in God is the demonstration of man's immortal, spiritual identity and individuality. So, what correlation does God have with the aging process? Well, one of the best antiaging techniques is something that is very simple and can be performed any hour of the day, which is "mediation". Meditations indeed can help in slowing down the process of aging and provide regimentation to stressful mind. Common practices such as yoga and mindfulness are also useful techniques, along with meditation. After all, mediation has originated from yearlong ancient history whose practitioners in Eastern cultures had younger and longer life throughout.

One of the main reasons why meditation slows the aging process is because it reduces stress. Again, most of us have probably seen this anecdotally in our own lives. One can examine the individuals having high stress and traumatic lifestyle. And the question is what makes them still look younger in such pressure. The short answer would be their daily spiritual practices and continuously following self-aware lifestyle. Let's look at some of the common benefits meditation brings in slowing the aging process.

1. It improves individuals' sleep.
2. It makes them more self-aware and gives better understanding of who they are
3. It can help in reduction of blood pressure.
4. It brings clarity of the mind and helps in processing thoughts properly to make useful decisions.
5. It is free and has no side-effects to individuals' body, in contrast significantly to some antiaging treatments that can be considerably expensive.

6. It helps in concentration levels, plus it reduces memory loss and improves your attention span.
7. It can help in reducing the feeling of anxiety and worries and improves overall emotional and mental stage of individuals.
8. It ultimately makes you happier, as happiness has a direct relationship with slowing down the aging process.

In this modern arena, one cannot stop the stress we encounter. But, following some principles or practices can help us deal with stress better, through which our body has an impact in both internal and external level. Thus, it is no harm in understanding the incorporation of spiritual practices for the benefit of age longevity [4].

2.6 Role of Rasayana Ayurveda (Indian System of Medicine) in antiaging nutraceutical development

Ayurveda is considered as one of the oldest healing sciences in the history of mankind. It was discovered by Hindu Indian saints in India more than 5,000 years ago and is often referred to as the "Mother of All Healing." In Sanskrit, Ayurveda means "The Science of Life." The origin of Ayurveda fosters back from the ancient Vedic culture, which was passed on from accomplished masters to their disciples by oral verse teaching. However, as time passes, many of these teachings were set on print a few 1,000 year ago, but most of them had been either lost or still inaccessible. One can refer to many of the natural healing systems which are now available in Western market that has its roots implanted from Ayurveda, including homo-apathy, allopathy and polarity therapy [5]. So one may ask what does Ayurveda have to do with antiaging?

Ayurveda has several formulations for management of aging and related conditions. There are around 200 herbs, minerals and fats stated in the ancient literature to maintain and enhance the health and beauty of the skin [6].

The concept of antiaging is described in Ayurveda as RASAYANA, which aims at maintaining excellent physical and mental health in mature age through a combination of nourishing diet, wholesome activities and gentle herbs. The word Rasayana means clearing the channels for the natural flow of matter and energy. The aim of Rasayana treatments and herbs is to improve the body's own mechanism of repair and detoxification, thereby maintaining better immunity, circulation, musculoskeletal strength and mobility along with balanced cognitive functions. The Rasayana Ayurveda is placed with a higher emphasis on prevention and encouragement of maintenance of health through paying close attention of intake of various food, modest lifestyle, diet and the usage of the herbs [7].

The deep knowledge of Ayurveda helps one to understand how to create balance of mind, body and soul in life and leading one's life in the direction so that one would achieve internal and external homeostasis. There are multiple factors that can disturb this balance and can reflect on individuals' physical, mental and emotional characteristics. Today, modern lifestyle affects individuals at multiple stages leaving an imprint on our emotional state, leading to consequences on work and family relationship and long-lasting physical trauma. Once these factors are understood, one can take appropriate actions to nullify or minimize their effects or eliminate the causes of imbalance and re-establish one's original constitution. *Balance is the natural order; imbalance is disorder.* Health is order; disease is disorder. Many professionals can claim that within one's body, there is constant interaction or battle of order and disorder. If one takes due steps in understanding the nature and the root cause of this disorder, one can guide one's life toward a journey to establish order [5].

Thus, our focus here is to find that one "root cause" or antidote that can help age longevity or stop the aging process. Aging is known as *"Jarā"* in Sanskrit defined as one that has become old by the act of wearing out *"jīryati iti jara"*. Ayurveda divides human life into childhood (up to the age 16 years); youth and middle age [from 16 to 60 years (*charaka*) or 70 years (*sushruta*) and exhibits progressively the traits of growth (*vivardhamana*, 16–20 years of age), youth (*youvana*, 20–30 years), maturity (*sampoornata*, 30–40 years), deterioration (*parihani*, 40 years onwards) which gradually sets in up to 60 years]; old age, wherein after 60–70 years the body elements, sense organs, strength and so forth begin to decay [7].

When describing aging, *Ayurveda* takes into consideration *Prana* (life energy that performs respiration, oxygenation and circulation). It governs two other subtle essence *ojas* and *tejas*. *Ojas* (the essence of the seven *dhatus* or bodily tissues) is responsible for mental intelligence and the auto-immune system. It highly emphasizes that in order to maintain longevity, the *prana, ojas and tejas* should always remain in balance [6].

Furthermore, the imbalance of *tridosh – vatta, pitta and kapha* – can also create a major impact on individuals' health as they play a role in motion, metabolism, structure and bodily wastes [6]. The *vatta* imbalance creates worry, anxiety and oxidative ambulated stress within our minds. To reserve the effected illness, intake of various ancient herbs , which are high in oxygen radical absorbance capacity, can lead to extensive impact. Thus, Rasayana anti-aging treatments with herb-infused oils can help improve circulation, skin health and lubrication in our joints and also include healthy oils within the diet. Ghee (clarified butter), coconut and sesame oil are recommended based on the individual's nature and extent of dryness symptoms. One of the most common Rasayana herbs used in Ayurvedic science is *Triphala*; it is 100 times more powerful in its antioxidant effectiveness compared to any of the berry juices [8].

2.7 Role of Ashtanga Yoga in antiaging nutraceutical development

Humanity is continuously facing significant increase in complexity of diseases such as diabetes mellitus (DM), cardiovascular diseases (CVD), cancer, infertility, etc. due to the tremendous effect of lifestyle changes. Nonetheless, the diseases have a direct impact on cellular aging. However, science has still failed in the areas of expertise in developing a correct gold standard biomarker to identify the cause or monitorization of healthy aging. The knowledge of putative and cardinal biomarkers reading at the cellular level can help depict aging in human life. However, there is still due need of translational research in developing interventions for preventing chronic lifestyle diseases.

A variety of interventions have been studied which helps to determine the influence on preventing lifestyle diseases and promoting health and longevity. They include drugs targeting specific hallmarks of aging, namely, physical exercise, nutrition, caloric restriction and antioxidants. However, there is still no evidence that all these interventions are effective, nor have they been proven to be therapeutic for modern complex lifestyle diseases. Neither has there been any research in benefits for delaying or reversing acceleration of aging. However, ashtanga yoga is an emerging integrative health discipline, which can positively modulate mind, body and soul. It has been shown to improve the clinical profile of patients with various pathologies including depression, obesity, hypertension, asthma, type II diabetes, cancer, etc. The review of yoga suggests that health on this intervention reduces the effects of stress and inflammatory markers in highly diabetic patients. There is evidence further that only practicing yoga for 3–12 weeks could lead to major improvement on biomarker of cellular aging and have a healthy result. Including a combination of yoga, meditation, nutraceutical products, etc. in one's lifestyle apparently led to a positive impact on genomic stability and balance of cellular oxidative stress, well-regulated stress and inflammatory responses, increases neuroplasticity and nutrition sensing and promotes cellular longevity [9].

2.8 Role of traditional Chinese medicine in antiaging nutraceutical development

The Chinese have a tradition of longevity practices that go back to thousands of years and involve a system of diet, exercise and herbal formulas all of which can slow down the aging process and contribute to an active and healthy old age. Even thousands of years ago, the ancient Taoists saw aging in remarkably modern terms. They believed that people are born with a finite amount of "qi" and that this depends on their parents. In modern science, this corresponds to your genes. They then discussed how to supplement this "qi" by eating well, exercising and getting sufficient rest. All this good advice is now part of an emerging field called epigenetics, which is the study of how your environment and your choices can influence your genetic code. Many of the oldest and best-known herbs protect the body from degeneration and fall into the category called *adaptogens*. Adaptogens are called so because they help our body adapt to the strains of daily living and normalize the body's functions in the face of stressors, restoring homeostasis.

The role of traditional Chinese medicine in antiaging is that it regulates cell metabolism and supports the immune system. Chinese soldiers throughout history have used adaptogens before their battle, whereas the Chinese monks used them as a substitute to the food in order to survive in cold. The best herbal apoptogens for antiaging according to the traditional Chinese medicine are *ginseng, cordyceps, rhodiola, turmeric, fo-ti, ginko biloba, royal jelly and green tea* [8].

References

1. Nasri, H., Baradaran, A., Shirzad, H., & Rafieian-Kopaei, M. (2014). New concepts in nutraceuticals as alternative for pharmaceuticals. *International Journal of Preventive Medicine, 5*(12), 1487–1499. https://www.nature.com/articles/d41586-019-02667-5.
2. Bhar G. C. (2016). In search of rationality in human longevity and immortality. *Mens Sana Monographs, 14*(1), 187–213. doi:10.4103/0973-1229.193083.
3. Schneider, R. (2017). Secrets to a longer, healthier life: How modern scientific discoveries and ancient holistic traditions can reverse aging. *Transcendental Meditation.* https://tmhome.com/benefits/secrets-of-longer-healthier-life-reverse-ageing/.
4. Freire, T. (2018). The anti-aging impact of mediation. *Wall Street International.* https://wsimag.com/wellness/35256-the-anti-aging-impact-of-meditation.
5. Lad, V. (2006). Ayurveda: A brief introduction and guide. *The Ayurvedic Institute.* https://www.ayurveda.com/resources/articles/ayurveda-a-brief-introduction-and-guide.
6. Datta, H. S., & Paramesh, R. (2010). Trends in aging and skin care: Ayurvedic concepts. *Journal of Ayurveda and integrative medicine, 1*(2), 110–113. doi:10.4103/0975-9476.65081.
7. Datta, H. S., Mitra, S. K., Paramesh, R., & Patwardhan, B. (2011). Theories and management of aging: Modern and Ayurveda perspectives. *Evidence-Based Complementary and Alternative Medicine, 2011,* Article ID 528527, 6. doi:10.1093/ecam/nep005.
8. Blakeway, J. (2021). Live longer, live stronger: 10 of the best herbal adaptogens for anti-aging. *Yinova.* https://www.yinovacenter.com/blog/live-longer-live-stronger-10-of-the-best-herbal-adaptogens-for-anti-aging/.
9. Tolahunase, M., Sagar, R., & Dada, R. (2017). Impact of yoga and meditation on cellular aging in apparently healthy individuals: A prospective, open-label single-arm exploratory study. *Oxidative Medicine and Cellular Longevity, 2017,* 7928981. doi:10.1155/2017/7928981.

3

Ayurvedic Perspective of Aging and Antiaging with Special Reference to Rasayana

Archana Kulkarni
Everglades University

Yashwant V. Pathak
University of South Florida

Contents

DOI: 10.1201/9781003110866-3

3.1 Introduction

More than 5,000 years ago, Chyavan Rishi, a sage who desired to regain his youthfulness, strength, and vigor, used Chyavanprasha, an ayurvedic nutrient-rich herbo-mineral supplement and restored the strength and vitality. The desire to maintain the vigor, vitality, and longevity of human life has always been the greatest concern of mankind. Over the last century, global life expectancy is continuously increased [1]. The global population aged 60 and older people were just over 1 billion people which is 2.5 times greater than in 1980 (382 million), and it is expected to double by 2050 (nearly 2.1 billion) [2]. It is a remarkable achievement because of research and advancements in biomedical sciences, public health, and technology, but merely increasing the life expectancy also increases age-related morbidities [3]. It is well stated by Dr. Ghebreyesus, Director-General, World Health Organization, "adding more years to life can be a mixed blessing if it is not accompanied by adding more life to years" [2]. Ayurveda, one of the most ancient medical science, has well described various ways to achieve optimal health and longevity.

3.2 Concept of aging in Ayurveda

Aging is a natural phenomenon in every living being. It is a natural biological process accompanied by progressive structural and functional changes, alteration of the body's homeostatic adaptive responses, and increased susceptibility to degeneration, disease, and disability with the time which finally leads to death. The process of aging starts with life. To understand the aging process, it is important to understand the concept of life.

शरीरेन्द्रियसत्त्वात्मसंयोगो धारि जीवितम्।

नित्यगश्चानुबन्धश्च पर्यायैरायुरुच्यते॥४२॥

Ch Su 1/42

Sharirendriya sattvatmsamyogo dhari jeevitam,Nityagashchanubandha shcha paryayaihi ayu uchyate

Ch Su 1/42

According to Ayurveda, life (Ayu) is a four-dimensional entity that conjuncts physical body (Sharir), senses (Indriya), mind (Sattva), and soul or consciousness (Atma). The integrity of individual life is a process of interaction within physical, psychological and spiritual components and with the cosmos [4]. The important principle of Ayurveda is that an individual is a part of the universe as both are made up of five basic elements (panchamahabhutas) ether, air, fire, water, and earth. There is a constant interaction between an individual and the universe to continue the life process. The harmonious interaction and homeostasis within the individual are important for healthy aging and longevity. Disequilibrium of this internal and external environment leads to degeneration and pathogenesis.

Sanskrit term for the body is sharira which is derived from "sheeryate iti shariram" meaning an entity that decays. Natural laws of decaying apply to only the psychophysical component of Ayu and not to the Atma which is immune to the cycle of birth, growth, decay, and death. The aging process in Ayurveda is defined as "Jara – Jiryati iti Jara" which means the act of wearing out. Charak describes degeneration and decay of bodily elements is a natural process [5].

The body (sharira) undergoes the "Jara process" throughout life but its characteristics like loss of strength of body tissues, declination in the power of senses (sensory and motor functions) declination of mental and cognitive functions are remarkably notifiable in the later stage of life termed as Jirna or Vruddhavastha (old age) which synonymously used for Jara.

3.3 Classification of age

Ayurveda describes the human lifespan of 100 years. Charak has divided the lifespan into three stages as Bala (childhood) up to 30 years, Madhya (Youth) 30–60 years, and Jirna (60–100 years). Table 3.1 describes chronological age with respective biological characteristics. It shows aging does not occur at one time or in all tissues together. It is a progressive change that affects different tissues at different periods. People may live shorter or longer life, in that case, three stages should be considered according to person's constitution, quality and functional ability of tissues, physical and mental strength, which denotes the biological age [6]. Jirnavastha can come earlier or later than the expected chronological age duration. This emphasizes multiple factors that influence the natural Jara process, quality, and duration of life.

Table 3.1 Classification of Vaya

Three Stages of Life	Age	Biomarkers	Dosha Predominance
Bala – Childhood	Up to 30 years	Development and growth of body and mind	Kapha (Anabolic phase)
Madhya – Youth	30–60 years	Physical and mental strength, Vigor, stability	Pitta (Metabolic phase)
Jirna – Old age	60–100 years	Degeneration of tissues, declination of physical and mental strength	Vata (Catabolic phase)

3.4 Characteristics of aging

Characteristics of aging which is remarkably noticed at old age because of the dominance of vata in that stage of life, which are described as degeneration changes and diminished functions of body and mind including decay in various tissues, diminished perception power of senses, strength, energy, immunity, neurocognitive impairment, diminished learning ability, memory, intellect, wrinkling of the skin, graying of hair, and baldness [6,7].

3.5 Types of aging

Sushruta describes two types of aging [1]. Kalaj Jara which means natural aging. Signs and symptoms of aging appear corresponding to chronological age. It is healthy aging when one takes care of his health following use of preventive healthcare measures. It is inevitable but can be prolonged. Akalaja Jara means untimely – earlier aging comes when a person does not follow healthy measures [8]. It explains the difference in the rate of aging in different individuals.

3.6 Sequential loss of biological attributes in aging

Aging is a continuous process. Sharangadhar describes a sequential loss of certain biological attributes during life because of the aging process (Figure 3.1). In the first decade, Balya (childhood) will be diminished, in the second decade Vridhhi (growth), in the third decade Chhavi (complexion), in the fourth decade Medha (intellect), in the fifth decade Twak (skin), in the sixth decade Drishti (vision), in the seventh decade Shukra (sexual activity), in the eighth decade Vikrama (physical strength), in the ninth decade Buddhi (wisdom) and in the tenth decade karmendriya (locomotor activity will be diminished [9].

3.7 Key factors affecting aging

दोषधातुमलमूलं हि शरीरं ·

– Su su 15/3

Dosha dhatu mala mulam hi shariram

– Su, su 15/3

Dosha (Biological forces), Dhatu (tissues) and Mala (metabolic waste products) are the building blocks of the body [10]. Undergoing decay is a nature of the

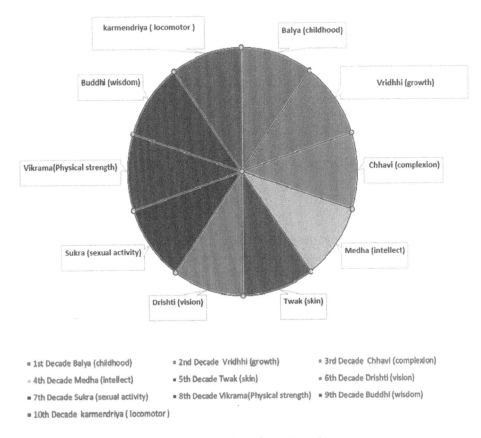

- 1st Decade Balya (childhood)
- 2nd Decade Vridhhi (growth)
- 3rd Decade Chhavi (complexion)
- 4th Decade Medha (intellect)
- 5th Decade Twak (skin)
- 6th Decade Drishti (vision)
- 7th Decade Sukra (sexual activity)
- 8th Decade Vikrama(Physical strength)
- 9th Decade Buddhi (wisdom)
- 10th Decade karmendriya (locomotor)

Figure 3.1 *Sequential loss of biological attributes in aging.*

body but preserving the state of equilibrium, balanced functions of dosha, dhatu, and mala is important for healthy aging. As discussed earlier, Ayu (life) is a 4-dimensional psychophysio-spiritual entity, maintaining a healthy life is multifactorial. Ayurveda explains healthy life is a combination of physical wellbeing in terms of balanced functions of biological energies, healthy functioning tissues, balanced metabolism and proper formation and elimination of metabolic wastes, psychological and spiritual wellbeing. All these factors play a key role in the process of aging.

3.8 Dosha and aging

Tridoshas are the biological energies that govern all physiological and psychological functions of the body and mind from cellular level to systemic level. Vata is responsible for biological movements, pitta for digestion and metabolism, and kapha for growth, development, and strength. These energies show diurnal, seasonal, and chronological variations. Kapha is dominated in early age (Bala), pitta in middle age (Madhya), and vata is in old age (Jirna). Being dry, rough cold and mobile vata energy have more catabolic effects and shows predominant symptoms of aging in old age like degeneration of tissues, declination of physical and mental strength, physical and cognitive disabilities. Pitta represents the fire principle, hot energy. Vitiated pitta leads to inflammatory changes. Research shows chronic inflammation is a biomarker for accelerated aging. High levels of pro-inflammatory markers in cells and tissues, a condition often named inflammaging, is a marker of accelerated aging and age-related diseases [11]. Vitiated, heavy and cold kapha energy slows the metabolism which can hamper tissue nutrition and formation.

3.9 Dhatu and aging

"Dharanat Dhatavah" meaning which sustains the body. Each tissue has a specific role in maintaining a healthy body. Dhatukshaya (tissue emaciation or loss) is a predominant characteristic in aging. It is a gradual depletion of the quality and quantity of tissue with functional disability. Balanced tissue nutrition and metabolism is a prime factor in understanding aging. Ayurveda describes seven tissues form in order. After digestion nutritional fluid (Ahararasa) is carried to the first dhatu for nourishment. With the help of dhatuagni (metabolic fire of each tissue) each tissue nourishes itself, reproduces its new cells, and form sub tissues (updhatu) along with the precursors for the next tissue to potentiate the formation of second tissue. Hypo metabolism or hypermetabolism at the tissue level highly affects tissue formation and quality. During this tissue metabolism along with the formation of qualitatively excellent tissue (Saar tissue), metabolic wastes (Mala) also form which have to be excreted. Disturbance of tissue metabolism or accumulation of malas (metabolic wastes) disturb tissue nutrition and development, which may accelerate the aging process leading to degenerative changes (dhatukshaya). The process of tissue nourishment and metabolism is influenced by many factors like the status of dosha, dhatuagni, diet, lifestyle, environment, etc. These influencing factors influence aging too. According to modern medicine, in all the cells of our body metabolic processes, divisions and multiplications go on from birth to death. In the conjunction and disjunction of cells, the activating factor is vata [12]. In old age, vata is aggravated which can cause metabolic dysfunction. This hampers tissue nutrition leading to Dhatukshaya marked as qualitative and quantitative degradation with impaired tissue functions.

3.10 Mala and aging

Malas are the metabolic wastes in the body. Ayurveda describes any food that undergoes metabolism forms a nutrient part (Saar) and wastes part (Mala). The proper formation of mala in the proper amount and their proper excretion is important to maintain health. Accumulation of malas in the system can block the micro channels and can alter cellular metabolism which contributes to aging. During cellular metabolism molecules are damaged by oxidation, damaged mitochondria, damaged enzyme accumulate in postmitotic cells. The waste product theory of aging shows that intracellular waste accumulation depresses the rate of cellular reproduction and leads to dysfunction, toxicity, aging and cell death [13,14].

3.11 Agni and aging

Aging is strongly related to energy metabolism. Ayurveda describes the concept of "Agni" (biological fire) which are metabolic processes at different levels in the body. Jatharagni, master agni which governs digestion and metabolism at the gastrointestinal tract, dhatvagnis are the metabolic processes at the tissue level, and bhutagnis work at the elemental level (molecular level). The optimum activity of agni maintains vigor and vitality. Bioenergies affect agni. Vata causes irregular metabolism, pitta causes hypermetabolism and Kapha is related to hypometabolism. Hypermetabolism at the dhatu level (excess dhatvagni) causes emaciation of tissues (Dhatukshaya). Hypermetabolism of dhatvagni can be stimulated because of vitiated Pitta leading to the inflammatory response. Research shows inflammation is associated with high resting energy expenditure. The metabolic disorders of the inflammatory response, such as enhanced lipolysis and fat utilization, elevated concentration of catabolic hormones, and extensive protein catabolism results in malnutrition [15]. The Baltimore Longitudinal Study of Aging shows the high metabolic rate is a risk factor for mortality [16]. This can explain that the chronic state of dhatuagni vruddhi (hypermetabolism) can accelerate aging.

Hypofunctioning of agni often leads to the formation of undigested, undesired byproducts called "Ama" in Ayurveda. Ama is sticky in nature, and it can be reactive and toxic. It tends to block the microchannels which can affect the transformation of energy, nutrients, and also the excretion of wastes products. Chronic accumulation of ama can alter metabolism, affects immune function. Ama is not a single entity but is a generalized term, which can be applied to external environmental toxins as well as many malformed substances during the metabolism. Accumulation of amatoxins has a major role in many disease pathogeneses. Ama formed during cellular metabolism can be correlated with free radicles [17,18]. Free radicles formed during metabolism are highly reactive and toxic and major cause of oxidative stress [19]. These reactive oxygen species are mainly responsible for damaging and degenerative conditions responsible for aging and age-related deteriorations [20].

Ayurveda explains at old age, vata increases and kapha decreases, and agni becomes weak leading to a decrease in vigor and vitality and tissue degeneration. This may be due to an age-related decrease in anabolic hormones. Many studies show an age-related decline in basal metabolic rate [21].

3.12 Ojas and aging

The quintessence of all the seven tissues is ojas. It is the final product of tissue nourishment. It is responsible for biological strength, vitality, and immunity. Ojas resides in each cell and protect the body to maintain internal homeostasis. Sushrut describes in absence of ojas body will undergo degeneration [22]. Dhatukshaya (tissue emaciation or loss) is one of the main reasons to initiate pathogenesis in aging. With advancing age inevitable depletion of agni leads to dhatukshaya which ultimately deteriorates immunity. (Ojakshaya). Research shows a progressive decline in immune function as we age leading to immune senescence, a process of senescence of the immune system [23].

3.13 Prakriti and aging

Prakriti is a constitution of an individual which is determined at the time of conception according to the predominance of doshas which are responsible for the physical and mental characteristics of an individual. Prakriti is a uniqueness, genetic makeup of the individual which shows biological variations in terms of physical, physiological, psychological, behavioral characteristics and susceptibility to different diseases. Vata dominating prakriti shows more degenerative changes and has a lesser life span. Pitta dominant people undergo more metabolic changes accelerates the aging process and have a medium life span. Kapha dominant persons having stronger and healthier prakriti undergo delayed aging and has a longer life span [24,25]. A research study on different constitutions and genomics shows significant differences in biochemical and genome-wide expression levels in individuals from three constitution types [26]. The study may show a strong basis for future research on understanding constitutional differences in the aging process. Charak explained the effect of prenatal factors like time of conception and parent's age, the health status of the uterus, maternal diet, and lifestyle, and interaction of five elements (panchamahabhutas) as influencing factors of prakriti [27]. A vast body of research has demonstrated that perinatal factors affect off spring's health and disease susceptibility. Various maternal factors, such as environmental toxicant exposure, diet, stress, exercise, age at conception, and longevity, have the potential to influence age-associated diseases such as cardiovascular disease, obesity, diabetes, and cancer risk in offspring. They can potentially impact offspring's health span and life span-reducing traits as well [28].

3.14 Mind and aging

Ayurveda describes individual life as a physical psychospiritual unit. To maintain health, mental, emotional, and spiritual wellbeing is equally important as physical wellbeing, and they affect each other. Disturbance in mental health brings unwholesome interaction between an individual and his environment. The action of the mind is controlled by three qualities Sattva, Rajas and Tama. Rajas describe the activity and desire, Tama describes inertia, darkness, and Sattva is a state of calmness, a pure mind that keeps the balance between Rajas and Tama activities of the mind. Eight psychological factors described by charak, Mana (emotions, mood), Buddhi (intellect, decision making), Sanjna jnana (orientation and response to external stimuli), Smriti (memory, retention, recall), Bhakti (desire), Shila (habits), Ceshta (psychomotor functions) and Achar (conduct and behavior) are involved in any psychological illnesses in varying orders [29]. These factors are capable to make qualitative and quantitative changes in dosha balance, agni, tissue nutrition and metabolism, ojas and mala functions. These factors that affect your life choices including diet, lifestyle, and behavior can be responsible to accelerate the aging process. As body and mind affect each other, bio-energetic mechanism affects mental health too. Ayurveda describes cognitive and memory impairment as the classical signs of aging in old age, but they start as early as the fourth decade of life [9].

3.15 Diet, lifestyle, and aging

Nutrition and diet are some of the most influential lifestyle factors that contribute to the health as well as development and progression of diseases. "Ahar sambhavam vastu rogaschaharsambhavah" [30] meaning physical body (healthy state) is because of the food same as the diseases. Ayurveda has given extreme importance to diet as preventive and promotive health care. Ayurveda describes wholesome food with all six tastes in diet balances dosha functions and energy metabolism and nourishes body and mind which can delay the aging process. "We are what we eat" is an old phrase that is still relevant and again proven by recent research in diet and epigenetics. Aging is controlled by genetic and epigenetic mechanisms. Diet can influence epigenetic changes, induce epigenetic mechanisms that protect against aging [31]. Along with the quality of food quantity of food is equally important. Research shows a reduction in calories with the maintenance of adequate nutrition to delay aging process through epigenetically mediated changes in gene expressions [32]. Studies on calorie restrictions and aging give light on Charaka's "Matrashisyat" principle – food should be consumed in proper quantity, but it has a more in-depth approach that quantity is not uniformed, it should be varied according to the strength of digestion and metabolism, which again affected by many factors. Ayurveda explains not only quality and quantity of food matter but dietary practices such as the way of eating, way of combining and preparing the food, times of meal along with consideration of prakriti, season, age and super important is the status of agni (metabolic fire) all contribute the process of assimilation, digestion and nourishment of body and mind. Unwholesome diet, wrong dietary practices along with unhealthy life-style (Gramyahar) imbalances dosha functions and energy metabolism, affecting tissue nourishment and immunity.

Dosha shows variations according to day-night schedule, according to the season, and during the stages of the lifespan. Ayurveda recommends following a daily routine (Dinacharya) seasonal routine (Ritucharya) which are basically dietary and lifestyle practices to stay in tune with the natural rhythm of doshas. The diet and lifestyle practices that disturb the doshic rhythm imbalances bioenergetics. This concept correlates with circadian rhythm explained by modern science. It is well understood that circadian rhythms play a vital role in nearly all aspects of physiology and behavior and prolonged disruptions to the clock are associated with aging and morbidities [33].

3.16 Mechanism of aging

Ayurveda considered aging as a natural phenomenon that is influenced by time. Charak has explained in his theory of Swabhavoparamavada that "there is a causative factor for the manifestation of beings but no causative factor as such exists for their deterioration [34]. No exact etiopathology of Jara has been explained in Ayurveda as the process of deterioration occurs naturally with the passage of time. I have tried to explain the possible mechanism of aging and its acceleration (Figure 3.2) based on (i) the factors related to pathophysiology, (ii) signs and symptoms of aging, and (iii) the role of the Rasayana – Ayurvedic management for healthy aging and longevity.

As Ayurveda describes there is a continuous interaction between an individual and the environment. Factors like diet, lifestyle, behavior, psychology, and environment affect the equilibrium of doshas. When these factors help to balance bioenergetics nourishes tissues, form ojas and maintain health and body undergoes healthy aging. With time, natural variations of doshas lead to the dominance of vata energy in old age which is responsible for weakening the agni (metabolic processes), which leads to undernourishment of tissues causing dhatukshaya and finally ojakshaya. The state of Ojakshaya accelerates the degenerative changes leading to multiple aging-associated disorders. This mechanism explains timely aging under balanced interaction within self and his outer environment.

Maintaining a healthy balanced life is not easy in fast-paced modern lives. Inappropriate consumption of these factors (unwholesome diet and wrong dietary practices, unhealthy lifestyle, physical and psychological stress, environmental effects) causes disequilibrium in psychophysiology. Imbalance in bio energies affects the functions of agni at various levels. Deranged metabolism leads to chronic inflammation, disturbed tissue nourishment, and regeneration process, formation, and accumulation of amatoxins (metabolic wastes).

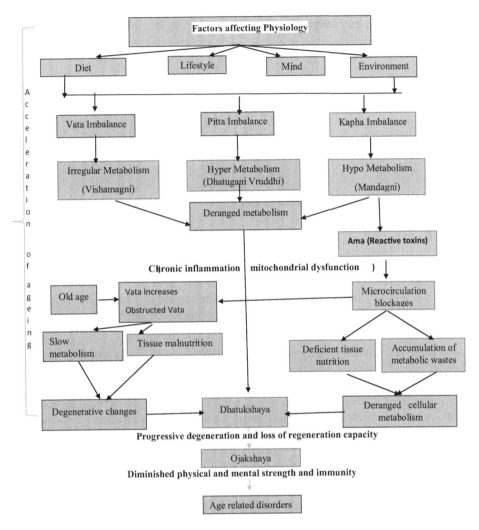

Figure 3.2 *Possible mechanism of aging.*

These amatoxins block the microchannels, vitiate the energies, and deteriorate metabolism. Blockages in microchannels lead to impairment in the flow of nutrients as well as the elimination of toxins. This all leads to progressive degeneration of tissues (dhatukshaya) and diminished strength and immunity (ojakshaya) which may further end up in many age-related disorders and shortening lifespan. This mechanism explains the accelerated aging process causing untimely aging or premature aging (ajkalaj jara).

Other influential factors like prakriti, age, time, quality of tissues, physical and mental strength, satmya (adaptability) contribute to differing the rate of aging in different individuals.

3.17 Antiaging: key to positive health

प्रयोजनं चास्य स्वस्थस्य स्वास्थ्यरक्षणमातुरस्य विकारप्रशमनं च||२६||

-Ch su 30/26

Prayojanam chasya swasthsya swasthya rakshanam aaturasya vikar prashamanam

-Ch su 30/26

Ayurveda has two main objectives [35]:

a. To maintain the health of healthy individuals.
b. To cure the diseases of diseased persons.

Ayurveda gives lots of importance to promotive and preventive health care. Health is a result of the combination and interaction of physical, mental, sensorial, social, and spiritual wellbeing. Maintenance of health plays a key role in preventing diseases, delay aging, and longevity.

Ayurveda recommends general measures of healthy living like the application of Swathavrutta (regimens followed to keep the individual healthy) and following Sadvrutta (good conducts of personal and social behavior) [36] to preserve health and longevity. Swasthvritta practices are self-care practices that include wholesome diet and dietary practices, daily routine (Dinacharya) seasonal routine (Ritucharya) which are recommended to keep the balance and harmonious relation between us and nature. Sadvritta are the ethical and moral principles of life that enforce self-control and choice of right acts. Together, promotes physical, mental, and spiritual health.

In seek of preservation of health and longevity, Ayurveda describes a specialty clinical branch called as Rasayan Tantra which specifically aimed for maintenance of youthfulness, longevity, to increase intelligence, physical and mental strength, and also alleviate the disease [37].

3.18 Concept of antiaging in Ayurveda

Aging is an inevitable progressive process. Ayurveda accepted it as a natural phenomenon with the passage of time. It is the body's nature to decay that won't change. Ayurveda describes the term Vayasthapana meaning, which sustains the youth stage that implies irrespective of chronological aging staying healthy and biologically active. Ayurveda's antiaging approach is to aim for Vayasthapana that to avoid akalaj-jara (premature aging) and to delay kalaj-jara (natural aging) and to sustain a long healthy life. According to Susruta rasayana is vayahsthapana (maintaining youth).

3.19 Rasayana definition

Rasa means juice/fluid, and Ayana means path/movement. Here the meaning of rasa is nutritional fluid. Rasayana means the pathway or movement of nutritional fluid toward all body tissues.

लाभोपायो हि शस्तानां रसादीनां रसायनम्॥८॥

Ch chi 1–8

Labhopayohi shastanam rasadinam rasayanam

Ch chi 1–8

It is a mechanism of nourishment to the formation of optimal qualities of dhatus [38] which leads to optimum physical strength, good memory, intelligence, youthfulness, and excellence of complexion, luster, and increased immunity and attain longevity without the presence of diseases.

रसायनं च तज्ज्ञेयं यज्जराव्याधिनाशनम्

-Sh Pu.4–13

Rasayanm ch tad gyneyam yat jaravyadhi nashanam

-Sh Pu.4–13

Sharangadhar defines Rasayana as the therapy that retards aging and diseases [39].

Rasayana is not a single therapy, but it is a more comprehensive rejuvenation program including pharmacological and nonpharmacological aspects like drugs, diet, and good conduct. It considers the wellbeing of physical, mental, and spiritual components to promote healing and regeneration of tissues. This program is specially described to preserve youthfulness, vigor, vitality, delay aging, and achieve healthy longevity through building the optimal qualities of tissues (Table 3.2).

Table 3.2 Benefits of Rasayana [43]

Health and Longevity	Maintenance of Youth and Retard Aging
Tissue nourishment and prevent degenerative changes	Enhance neurocognitive functions – intelligence, memory improvement
Improves functions of agni (metabolic processes)	Excellence of luster, complexion of skin and beauty
Physical and mental strength and immunity	Enhance strength of Indriyani (senses)

3.20 Classification of Rasayana

Rasayana chikitsa is a comprehensive multi-strategic rejuvenation program that includes pharmacological and nonpharmacological methods. Rasayana has been classified in different ways in different classical texts. Charak has classified Rasayana as per methods of use; according to the aim of chikitsa (treatment), Sushruta and Dalhana elaborated rasayana classification in detail [40].

3.21 Types of Rasayana treatment

A. As per the method of administration
1. Vatatapika rasayana – use of Rasayana in outdoor practice
2. Kutipraveshika rasayana or intensive indoor regimen (inclusive of panchakarma) using a specially designed trigarbha rasayana kuti or therapy chamber
B. As per the objective of the administration
1. Kamya Rasayana – to promote health, vigor, and longevity
2. Naimittika Rasayana – to alleviate the disease
C. Nonpharmacological Rasayana
1. Achara rasayana – good conduct for personal, social, and spiritual wellbeing
2. Ajasrika rasayana – Rejuvenative dietary regimen

Vatatapika Rasayana means the process of using rasayana treatment in the outdoor clinic. The person can do normal work and enjoy outdoor activities while using the rasayana therapy. This form is less restrictive but also less effective compared to Kutipraveshika rasayana in terms of gaining rasayana benefits. **Kutipraveshika Rasayana** is an intensive indoor regimen where a person gets admitted to a specialized build place for rasayana treatment named "Trigarbha Kuti". The person has to undergo biopurification therapies (Panchakarma) before starting the rasayana program and undergoes a strict dietary and lifestyle regimen to maximize the desired effects of rasayana. It seems the method of Kutipraveshika rasayana is more ideal way inclusive physical, behavioral, mental, and spiritual treatments in a controlled environment for complete rejuvenation.

Kamya Rasayana is used to promote health in a healthy person. It is further classified on basis of specific health goals like promoting longevity (Prana kamya), promoting intelligence, retention, and recall (Medha kamya), and promoting luster and beauty (Sri kamya). **Naimittika Rasayana** is a disease-specific rasayana. It is indicated in a diseased person to improve his strength and ability to fight against disease and restore the balance. It can be used as an adjunct therapy along with specific treatment of the diseases for faster and better recovery.

Achar Rasayana is personal and social behavior, based on high ethical and moral principles by which one can acquire the rasayana effect. It includes truthfulness, a calm and relaxed mind devoid of negative emotions like anger, jealousy, greed, nonviolent, loving and compassionate behavior, personal and public cleanliness, having control over mind and senses, and involved in spiritual activities. It increases sattva quality of mind, nourishes ojas, and builds strength and immunity. It has been studied for a long time that psychosocial and behavioral factors can influence health and the chronic course of the disease [41].

Scientific research shows the connection between our emotions and immune states. For instance, emotions like anger, anxiety, mirth, and relaxation can modulate cytokine production and cellular responses to a variety of immune stimuli. Anger has been shown to increase the production of the inflammatory cytokine interleukin-6 (IL-6) and circulating levels of C-reactive protein. Research studying the effects of relaxing interventions shows a significant modulation of the immune response, increasing the number of CD4-positive T cells while buffering the drop in natural killer (NK) and CD8 cells that occurred in human subjects experiencing stress or anxiety [42]. The modern field of psychoneuroimmunology (PNI) research shows similarities with ancient Ayurveda principles.

Ajasrika Rasayana is used in the form of daily consumption of rejuvenative foods like ghrita (clarified butter), ksheer (milk), etc. This diet is sattva nourishing as well as enhancing ojas.

3.22 Mode of action

Rasayana is therapeutic measures that develop the premium qualities of tissues. It promotes the movement of nutritional fluid, provides nourishment to body tissues leading to optimal quality tissues. As mentioned earlier, the process of tissue nourishment starts with absorption and circulation of nutritional fluid (Ahar Rasa) developed at the jatharagni level. Through the microchannels, fluid circulates and nourishes body tissues. Further, dhatuagni (tissue metabolism) processes nutritional rasa for the regeneration of cells, formation of precursor for next tissue, the formation of sub tissues along with metabolic wastes. Considering this process, (i) the best quality of nutritional fluid, (ii) proper metabolism, and (iii) health of microchannels are the important steps during tissue nourishment and development.

The effect of rasayana can be possibly explained through the physiology of "Dhatu Poshana" (tissue nourishment) [40].

1. At the level of Rasa – Rasayana regimen provide excellent nutrients and enrich the quality of nutritional fluid. Examples of nutrient rasayanas like Shatavari (Asparagus racemosus), ksheerkakoli (Lilium polyphyllum), Ghrita (clarified butter), etc.

2. At the level of Agni – Rasayana improves digestive and metabolic processes. Rasayana examples: Pippali (Piper longum), Shunthi (Zingiber officinale), and Bhallataka (Semecarpus anacardium)
3. At the level of Srotasa – Improving the microcirculation, persevering competency of srotasas, cleaning the srotasas, for example, Guggulu (Commiphora wightii).

3.23 Role of Rasayana in healthy aging

The process of human aging is complex and individualized and involves biological, psychological, and social spheres. Nothing can stop the aging process. The multidimensional approach of Rasayana chikitsa including dietary regimen, rasayana drugs, and behavioral, social conduct with spiritual practices makes a perfect model to retard the aging process. Earlier we had discussed factors that influence aging. Consumption of those factors in excessive or less or in a wrong way can accelerate the aging process, affects metabolism, and increase the rate of degeneration leading to dhatukshaya (tissue emaciation) and finally ojakshaya (diminished strength and immunity) which further aggravates the degeneration. Logically it seems suboptimal quality tissues are more prone to premature aging. A qualitative improvement of tissue in terms of structural and functional excellence with rasayana makes them more sustainable to withstand the effects of influencing factors or various stresses. Therefore, "antiaging seems to be a secondary function of the rasayana, subsequent to qualitative up-gradation and stabilization of cells as being its primary function" [44] (Figure 3.3).

Ayurveda recommends a person undergoing rasayana therapy should first do Panchakarma therapy. Panchakarma includes five major bio-purification therapies that cleanse the impurities of the body and mind. Throughout life many toxins, wastes products get accumulated in the body if they are not properly eliminated. They can derange energy metabolism and blocks the microchannels (srotasas) which lead to disturbance inflow of nutrients and further accumulation of metabolic wastes. Rasayana therapy promotes the flow of nutrients and nourishes tissues. Clean and well-functioning srotasas are important for proper utilization of rasayana therapy. Sushruta has clearly described the importance of panchakarma therapy before the administration of Rasayana. It is stated within unpurified body rasayana won't work effectively as expected in the same way as a dirty cloth does not take up due to brightness of color on dyeing [45].

3.24 Decade-wise selection of Rasayana

Rasayana is nutritive care and not only geriatric care. As mentioned earlier, Sharangadhara has described an orderly loss of biological attributes specific to respective decades of life. It shows jara (aging) is an ongoing process and not

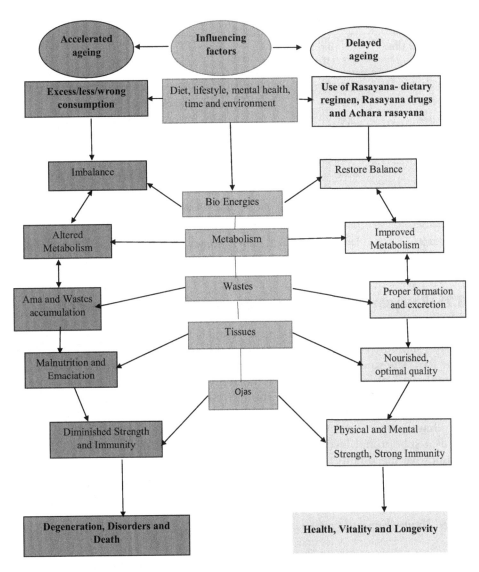

Figure 3.3 Process of accelerated aging vs. delayed aging with application of rasayana.

only affects old age. Sushruta and Vagbhat have described rasayana should be used in the early and middle stages of life to avoid premature aging and to delay aging [46,47]. In early and middle life, tissue strength is good as well as metabolism is strong. The incorporation of rasayana at this time improves the qualities of tissues by nourishing, preventing degeneration and repairing the damaged tissues, and promote regeneration. Table 3.3 shows proposed age-specific rasayana to prevent sequential biological loss [48].

Table 3.3 Age Related Suitable Rasayana Drugs

Decades of Life Span	Bio Value Losses	Suitable Rasayana
First decade	Corpulence	Gambhari (Gmelina arborea) Kshira (milk) Ghrita (clarified butter)
Second decade	Growth	Bala (*Sida cordifolia*), Amalaki (*Emblica officinalis*)
Third decade	Luster	Àmalaki (*Emblica officinalis*), Haridra (*Curcuma longa*)
Fourth decade	Intellect	Brahmi (Bacopa monnieri) Shankhapushpi (*Convolvulus microphyllus*)
Fifth decade	Skin quality	Bhringraja (*Eclipta prostrata*), Haridra (*Curcuma longa*)
Sixth decade	Vision	Triphala (combination of *Emblica officinalis, Terminalia chebula* and *Terminalia bellirica*), Jyotismati (*Celastrus paniculatus*)
Seventh decade	Virility	Ashwagandha (*Withania somnifera*), Kapikacchu (*Mucuna pruriens*)
Eighth decade	Physical strength	Àmalaki (*Emblica officinalis*), Bala (*Sida cordifolia*)
Ninth decade	Thinking	Brahmi (Bacopa monnieri), Shankhapushpi (*Convolvulus microphyllus*)
Tenth decade	Locomotion	Bala (*Sida cordifolia*), Sahachara (Nilgirianthus ciliates)

3.25 Rasayana selection according to seven dhatus (tissue-specific)

Saar is the essence of each dhatu, represents the supreme quality of dhatu comprising supreme constituents and best functional ability. Charak has described Saar Pariksha (qualitative assessment of tissues) to examine the physical and mental strength and immunity of the individual. A person with suboptimal quality of tissues will have less strength and immunity. Achieving supreme qualities of tissues is the desirable effect of rasayana therapy. The person may have only certain tissues with supreme qualities and other tissues may be at a suboptimal level. Dhatu-specific rasayana will be a targeted therapy to improve the quality of that specific tissue and increase disease resistance of that tissue. Table 3.4 describes few examples of dhatu-specific rasayanas.

3.26 Vayasthapana herbs

अमृताऽभयाधात्रीमुक्ताश्वेताजीवन्त्यतिरसामण्डूकपर्णीस्थिरापुनर्नवा इति दशेमानि वयःस्थापनानि भवन्ति (५०),

(Ch Su 4–50)

Charak has described a special group of 10 herbs (Vayasthapan Gana) having age-stabilizing effects, preserve youthfulness, and promote longevity [49].

Vayasthapana herbs being rasayana nourish tissues, improve metabolism, eliminate toxins, promote tissue repair, prevent degeneration, increase physical and mental strength, build immunity, enhance cognitive functions, promote healing, prevent premature aging, and retard the natural aging process. The biological process of aging is a complex phenomenon. Various theories have

Table 3.4 Rasayana Selection According to Tissues

Seven Dhatu	Suitable Rasayana
Rasa dhatu (Plasma)	Shatavari (*Asparagus racemosus*), Guduchi (*Tinospora cardifolia*)
Rakta dhatu (Blood)	Sariva (*Hemidesmus indicus*), Amalaki (*Emblica officinalis*), Lauha bhasma (iron)
Mamsa dhatu (Muscle)	Bala (*Sida cordifolia*), Ashwagandha (*Withania somnifera*)
Meda dhatu (Adipose)	Guggul (*Commiphora mukul*), Shilajit Haritaki (*Terminalia chebula*)
Asthi dhatu (Bones)	Guduchi (*Tinospora cordifolia*), Guggul (*Commiphora mukul*), Asthishrunkhala (*Cissus quadrangularis*)
Majja dhatu (Bone morrow and nervous system)	Ashwagandha (*Withania somnifera*), Brahmi Shankhapushpi (*Convolvulus microphyllus*), Swarna bhasma (Gold bhasma)
Shukra dhatu (Reproductive)	Kapikacchu (*Mucuna pruriens*), Shatvari (*Asparagus racemosus*)

been evaluated to understand the aging process including DNA damage, cellular senescence limiting cell proliferation and resistance to apoptosis, chronic inflammation, immunosenescence is one of the causes of inflammaging, failure in proteostasis leading to accumulation of insoluble proteins in tissues, and oxidative stress by the accumulation of high level of free radicals which is considered an important cause of cellular damage and inflammation [50]. Antioxidant, anti-inflammatory, immunomodulatory, adaptogenic rejuvenation properties can play a potential role in delaying the aging process. We have tried to explain the vayasthapana effect of the ten herbs in the vayasthapana category based on Ayurvedic pharmacology with evidence-based scientific research.

1. Amruta (Guduchi) *Tinospora cardifolia*

Amruta commonly known as guduchi (*Tinospora cardifolia*) is a large deciduous, perennial climber that belongs to the family Menispermaceae. Literally translation of the Sanskrit name "Amrita" is "the root of immortality", has given because of its multiple health benefits including vayasthapana. It is a rejuvenating herb that balances all doshas, restores homeostasis. Being heavy and unctuous in nature and with a sweet post, postdigestive digestive action guduchi proposes nutritive action to the tissues. Bitter and astringent tastes along with heating quality balance metabolism eliminate amatoxins and cleanse microchannels. *T. cardifolia* has been studied extensively for its immunomodulatory [51,52], antioxidant property showing a significant increase in SOD-Super-Oxide Dismutase level and decrease in MDA(Malondialdehyde) level, [53] and also adaptogenic properties [54]. It is described as one of the medhya rasayanas (nootropics to boost cognitive abilities). *T. cardifolia* has reported neuroprotective activity by promoting regeneration, migration, and plasticity of cerebellar neurons and preventing degeneration of neurons induced by glutamate [55]. Neuroprotective action was also studied in *vivo* in *Drosophila* [56]. It has anti-microbial, antipyretic, and anti-inflammatory properties too [57–60]. To assess the longevity effect of *T. cardifolia*, a study was conducted on *D. melanogaster* flies that shows an increase in lifespan of flies which can be attributed to its antioxidant properties [61]. This plant has a wide range of health benefits with a special focus on endocrine and metabolic disorders and as an immune booster aiding for better human life expectancy [62].

2. Abhaya (Haritaki) *Terminalia chebula*

Abhaya is a synonym of Haritaki. It is a medium-sized tree with dark brown bark that belongs to the family Combretaceae. This rejuvenates herb is all dosha balancing. It has been extensively used in vata disorders because of its sweet postdigestive effect and heating quality. Its Rasayana action is mainly because it removes blockages, removes amatoxins, and clears microchannels. With its dry rough qualities and astringent dominating taste, it balances kapha as well as pitta. Long-term use of haritaki is indicated along with different adjuvants at the different seasons to maximize rasayana benefits. Haritaki also acts as a digestive stimulant, amapachan, carminative, anti-inflammatory which aids its Rasayana benefits. *T. chebula* has been studied for multiple pharmacological activities as The plant has been demonstrated to possess multiple pharmacological and medicinal activities, such as antioxidant, antimicrobial, antidiabetic, hepatoprotective, anti-inflammatory, cardioprotective, antiarthritic antimutagenic, antiproliferative, radioprotective, and wound healing [63]. The leaves, bark, and fruit of *T. chebula* showed high antioxidant property [64]. Aqueous extract of *T. chebula* showed inhibition of lipid peroxidation induced by radiation in rat liver microsomes [65].

T. chebula has shown cytoprotective effect and inhibitory effect on cellular aging against UV-induced oxidative damage. *T. chebula* extract showed an inhibitory effect on the age-dependent shortening of the telomere length [66]. Exhibition of development of duodenal ulcer attributed to the cytoprotective effect on the gastric mucosa in vivo [67]. Its adaptogenic [54], immunomodulatory [68], radioprotective [69] and significant hypolipidemic activities [70] have been reported.

3. Dhatri (Amalaki) – *Emblica officianalis*

Emblica officianalis is a deciduous tree that belongs to the family Euphorbiaceae. Amalaki is all doshas balancing especially pitta. Its rejuvenate action is mainly because of balancing pitta with its cooling property and sweet postdigestive effect. It provides tissue nourishment while strengthening the metabolism and eliminating amatoxins. *E. Officinalis* is an abundant source of nutrients like vitamin C, amino acids, and minerals [71]. Pharmacological studies of *E. officinalis* reported broad-spectrum properties like antioxidant, anti-cancer, anti-inflammatory, immunomodulatory, cytoprotective, etc. [72]. Study shows immune stimulant and moderate cytoprotective activity and neuroprotective activity of Amalaki rasayana [73,74]. Since DNA repair gets diminished with aging, a study was conducted on Amalaki rasayana and its effect on UVC-induced DNA strand break repair. After

45 days of administration of Amalaki Rasayana regimen to healthy aged individuals, the study showed stable maintenance of DNA strand break repair without toxic effects [75]. Amalaki Rasayana showed improved oxidative stress tolerance by reducing the accumulation of reactive oxygen species (ROS) and lipid peroxidation while enhancing superoxide dismutase (SOD) activity in aged (35-day-old) wild-type flies [76]. These studies support antiaging activity of Amalaki.

4. Mukta (Rasna) – *Pluchea lanceolate*

   Pluchea lanceolate is a perineal herb that belongs to the family Asteraceae. Charak describes the importance of Rasna as "Rasana vataharanam". It is the best herb for alleviating vata [77], and has been extensively used in Vata-related disorders. Because of its heavy quality and heating energy, it balances vata. Along with Bitter taste and pungent postdigestive effect, it works best as amapachan (detoxify amatoxins) and balances kapha as well. In aging, many degenerative changes are associated with vata aggravation and the presence of reactive amatoxins. Rasna balances vata and detoxify amatoxins, removes the blockages in microchannels leading to better tissue nutrition. *P. lanceolate* has been studied for its antioxidant [78–80] and anti-inflammatory properties. A study shows that *P. lanceolate* extract protects against oxidative stress by significantly lowering MDA levels and measures of lipid peroxidation [81]. Its antioxidant effect is attributed to higher levels of phenolic and ascorbic acid constituents [82]. Flow cytometric studies revealed anti-inflammatory of *P. lanceolate* by the downregulation of pro-inflammatory cytokines. The alcoholic extract of *Pluchea lanceolata* leaves shows immunosuppressive properties by inhibition of the humoral antibody response and cell-mediated immune responses [83]. The neuroprotective effect of *Pluchea lanceolata* was studied in treating ischemic hippocampal injury in Wistar rats. It enhanced the dendritic arborization and reserves oxidative stress through maintaining glutathione peroxidase levels and lipid peroxidation in ischemic conditions [84]. Other studies show its neuroprotective effect by reducing symptoms caused by aluminum chloride, a toxic protein aggregates in many degenerative diseases [85] and reducing neuroinflammation [86].

5. Shweta – *Clitoria ternatea*

   Clitoria ternatea is a perennial climber herb that belongs to the family Fabaceae commonly called as "butterfly". In Ayurveda, it is mainly used as medhya, a drug to improve intelligence and enhance memory. Rasayana effects of this plant are mostly studied for its neurocognitive actions. *C. ternatea* shows improvement in learning and memory by increasing acetylcholine (ACh) content in the rat hippocampus [87]. The root extract of *C. ternatea* restored memory impairment and reduced neural damage induced by chronic cerebral hypoperfusion in male Sprague Dawley rats at doses of 200 and 300 mg/kg [88].

Autophagy is a vital process of cleaning out damaged cells. Neuroprotective effects of *C. ternatea* in stress-induced rat brain shows to improve autophagy by maintaining the selective DNA damage repair pathway and removal of reactive oxygen species [89]. The effect of *C. ternatea* in cognitive impairment was studied on streptozotocin-induced cognitive impairment in Wistar rats. Prevention of impairment was dose-dependent by reducing oxidative stress, cholinesterase activity, and ROCK II expression [90]. Talpate KA, et al. showed C. ternatea's antihyperglycemic and antioxidant properties by significantly increasing SOD and reducing glutathione levels in streptozotocin-induced diabetic rats [91]. The studies show the potential effect of *C. ternatea* as medhya rasayana in neurocognitive impairment.

6. Jivanti – *Leptadenia reticulate*

It is a perennial climber that belongs to the family Asclepiadaceae. The name Jivanti means which gives life. It is a well-known herb for its revitalizing, rejuvenating, and lactogenic properties. Its sweet taste and postdigestive effect, cooling energy and unctuous quality make it a nutritive herb that balances all doshas especially vata and pitta. This rasayana works at the level of rasa, by providing nourishment and helping to build ojas it acts as vayasthapana. A free radical scavenging activity against diphenylpicrylhydrazyl (DPPH), hydroxyl, and nitric oxide radicals has been shown in the study of methanolic extract of *L. reticulate* [92]. *L. reticulate* shows antioxidant property by the significant increase in antioxidant enzymes, superoxide dismutase (SOD), and catalase (CAT) [93]. The aqueous extract of *L. reticulata* showed a significant antipyretic and anti-inflammatory in different animal models at a dose of 200 and 400 mg kg^{-1} body weight, respectively [94]. Immunomodulatory and antioxidant activities were studied using *L. reticulate* extract (100 and 200 mg/kg) in cyclophosphamide-induced immunosuppressed rats showed dose-dependent increase in antibody titer values; increased percentage of neutrophil adhesion to nylon fibers and phagocytosis. A significant improvement in superoxide dismutase (SOD), catalase levels, and decreased lipid peroxidation levels were observed [93]. The hepatoprotective effect was observed in paracetamol–induced hepatotoxicity in rats [95].

7. Atirasa (Shatavari) – *Asparagus racemosus*

Asparagus racemosus is a woody climber that belongs to the family Liliaceae. Atirasa is commonly known as Shatavari and is a best nutritive, cooling rejuvenative plant having special nutritive effects on the female reproductive system. Shatavari with the sweet, bitter taste and cooling energy, balances pitta, and having unctuous, heavy qualities and sweet postdigestive effects it balances vata. Shatavari nourishes tissues, strengthens agni (metabolism), improves learning ability and memory, and has galactagogue activity. Its nourishing and healing effects prevent degenerative changes. *A. racemosus* has been used as an adaptogen to increase the resistance against a variety of stresses [96]. *A. recemosus* is known for its phytoestrogens and has been studied for its use in breast cancer treatment. The extract of *A. recemosus* is studied in vitro T47D cancer cell lines showed excellent antiproliferative activity [97]. The pharmacological studies revealed the potential adaptogenic, anti-inflammatory immunostimulant, phytoestrogenic antioxidant, anti-ulcer, galactagogue, neuroprotective, aphrodisiac, and anti-cancerous activities [98,99]. Tiwari et al. showed that *A. recemosus* significantly inhibited the pro-inflammatory cytokines, generated cellular immune response, and sustained adaptive response with no intrinsic cytotoxicity [100].

8. Mandukparni – *Centella asiatica*

Centella asiatica is a perennial creeper that belongs to the family Umbellifere. Mandukaparni being bitter, astringent in taste, having a sweet postdigestive effect, and cooling energy it pacifies pitta and kapha. Charaka has described it as one of the major medhya Rasayana (cognitive enhancers). It improves strength, metabolism, complexion, and longevity [101]. Mandukaparni increases microcirculation, detoxify toxins. Neuroprotective effect of *C. asiatica* showed it protects monosodium glutamate-induced neurodegeneration [102]. Increased production of reactive oxygen species (ROS) leads to cognitive dysfunction by neuronal synaptic activity and neurotransmission. Study shows an effective increase in SOD and activation of nuclear factor erythroid-2-related factor 2 by *C. asiatica*, and its triterpenoids improve the cognitive impairment in animals [103]. Extract from *C. asiatica* showed improvement in intracellular oxidative stress caused by chemotherapy drugs [104]. Neuroprotective effects of *C. asiatica* appear to be associated with increased mitochondrial activity, inhibition of the pro-inflammatory enzyme, increased dendritic arborization, and synaptogenesis [105]. *C. asiatica* has been studied for its effects on microcirculation. A double-blind study in 87 patients with chronic venous hypertensive microangiopathy showed the efficacy of *C. asiatica* in improving microcirculation parameters [106]. *C. asiatica* has shown connective tissue modulation, improved collagen synthesis, and protecting the venous endothelium in chronic venous hypertension [107].

The wound-healing property of *C. asiatica* has been reported by affecting the proliferation of fibroblasts and collagen synthesis [108,109]. The above studies show *C. asiatica* is vayasthapana drug affects by increasing microcirculation (srotas level action), promoting tissue regeneration and its antioxidant effects (agni level action)

9. Sthira (Shalparani) – *Desmodium gangeticum*

It is a perennial undershrub, belonging to the family Fabaceae, Shalparni with its heavy and unctuous qualities, sweet, bitter taste, and sweet postdigestive effect with heating energy balances all doshas. It is a nourishing, detoxifying rasayana herb. Charak categorized it as "Shwayathu hara" (anti-inflammatory). Pharmacological study shows its immunomodulatory, antioxidant, anti-inflammatory [110,111] antinociceptive, cardioprotective, antiulcer, antiamnesic, and hepatoprotective properties [112]. Flavonoid fraction of *D. gangeticum* showed anti-inflammatory and high antioxidant properties in carrageenan-induced inflamed rats [113]. Cardioprotective effect of *D. gangeticum* was evaluated after ischemia-reperfusion injury in the rat. The aqueous root extract of *D. gangeticum* (L) at a dose of 50 mg/kg body weight was found to be effective in preserving the mitochondrial and sarcoplasmic ATPase in the myocardium [114]. *D. gangeticum* was studied as a nootropic agent. *D. gangeticum* (50, 100, and 200 mg/kg, p.o.) was administered for 7 consecutive days showed significant improvement in learning and memory in mice by reversing scopolamine (0.4 mg/kg, i.p.) induced and natural aging amnesia [115].

10. Punarnava – *Boerhaavia diffusa*

Boerhaavia diffusa is a perennial creeping plant belonging to the family of the Nyctaginaceae. The word punarnava literally means, one which renews the body. Vagabhata has described daily consumption of punarnava with milk for a certain period bring back youthfulness [116]. Rasayan property of punarnava is attributed to its all dosha balancing effect with sweet, bitter, and astringent tastes, sweet postdigestive effect, and heating energy and its effect on the urinary system. It's light, dry heating properties help to detoxify ama, clear the microchannels and improve urinary function, help to eliminate malas (wastes), having cleansing and rejuvenating action. Pharmacological studies show its immunomodulation, hepatoprotection, anticancer activity, antidiabetic activity, anti-inflammation, and diuretic properties [117]. Nephroprotective activity of *B. diffusa* has been studied by various scholars [118]. Treatment of gentamycin-induced nephrotoxicity showed a decrease in BUN, creatinine, kidney malondialdehyde (MDA), and glutathione (GSH) levels and protected against structural and functional damage with *B. diffusa* [119]. The antioxidant property of *B. diffusa* was studied in hyperoxaluric oxidative stress and renal cell injury. Aqueous extract of *B. diffusa* roots at the dose of 100 and 200 mg/kg was given to nephrolithiasis treated rats for 28 days. *B. diffusa* treatment significantly reduced the level of MDA, BUN, and creatinine and also inhibited renal damage. The results attributed to the antioxidant property of *B. diffusa* [120]. A comparative analysis of bioactivities of *B. diffusa* extracts showed the most notable antioxidant property along with thrombolytic and anti-bacterial properties [121]. Wound-healing property was studied with methanol extract of *B. diffusa* showed enhanced viability and migration of human keratinocyte cells. Topical application of B. diffusa extract showed a significant decrease in wound area by the 14th day in the excision wound rat model [122].

These studies show that rasayana herbs used for the purpose of vayasthapana have qualities to promote cellular repair and regeneration, to prevent the damages from oxidative stress, to eliminate toxins, to balance energy metabolism, and provide the richest qualities nutrients which explain their potential as "Vayasthapana".

3.27 Summary

"Antavanta ime deha", a phrase from Bhagavat Gita, describes the perishable nature of the human body. Though aging is an inevitable process longevity has been always a cherished desire of mankind. Healthy aging with longevity is more important than just merely adding years to life. WHO defines healthy aging as "the process of developing and maintaining the functional ability that enables well-being in older age" [2]. Functional ability comprises an individual's interaction within himself and with his environment. Ayurveda describes healthy aging and longevity depends on a person's physical, mental, sensorial, and spiritual balanced interactions. Aging is natural and that comes over time. Intrinsic key factors like dosha (bio-energies), dhatu (tissue), mala (wastes), functions of agni (metabolic processes), mental health, prakriti (constitution), and extrinsic factors like diet, lifestyle, and environment affect the aging process. Their interaction with each other leads to either early aging (akalaj jara) or chronological aging (kalaj jara).

Rasayana therapy is the process of developing and maintaining functional ability. The purpose of rasayana therapy is to form optimal quality tissues which lead to the effects of rasayana such as longevity, vitality, preserving youthfulness, delayed aging, better immunity, physical and mental strength, intellectual competence, and prevention of diseases. Rasayana therapy has a comprehensive approach including rasayana drugs, nutrient-rich dietary regimen, and personal-social behavioral modifications for a positive rejuvenating lifestyle. Bio-purification of body and mind with panchakarma therapy is an essential element before starting rasayana therapy. Rasayana herbs, minerals, or compounds are bioactive micromolecules that provide tissue nourishment and promote repair, regeneration, and development of tissue by promoting cellular metabolism, detoxifying, and eliminating metabolic wastes which are the important factors in the aging mechanism.

In recent years, studies about epigenetics and aging mechanisms show a broad range of diets that mediate epigenetic processes have been identified as "epigenetic diets". Long-term consumption of these bioactive dietary compounds is highly associated with a low incidence of various aging-related degenerative diseases such as cancer and cardiovascular disease, suggesting that these bioactive diets may affect aging processes [32]. These studies may open a new avenue for nutrigenomic research on ancient traditional rasayana as a promising candidate for healthy and delayed aging.

Rasayana effect of ten important herbs categorized by Charak as Vayasthapana herbs (herbs to maintain youthfulness) has been described on basis of ayurvedic pharmacology and scientific research evidence. Most of the herbs possess common properties like antioxidant, immunomodulatory, adaptogenic, and neuroprotective, which may explain their valuable role in delaying the aging process. Obviously, these studies are not adequate, and they evaluated the pharmacological aspect of rasayana studying the effects of herbs or minerals and did not include prerasayana panchakarma, dietary rasayana, and behavioral rasayana therapy as advocated by Ayurveda. Also, the application of rasayana therapy including drug selection, dosages, time, and adjuvant drug/diet highly varies according to the individual's prakriti, strength, metabolism, season, etc. Further strategic research studies considering the whole rasayana approach will provide beneficial insights into aging and degenerative conditions.

References

1. Beltrán-Sánchez H, Soneji S, Crimmins EM. Past, present, and future of healthy life expectancy. *Cold Spring Harbor Perspectives in Medicine.* 2015 November 2;5(11):a025957.
2. Decade of healthy ageing: baseline report. Geneva: World Health Organization; 2020. Licence: CC BY-NC-SA 3.0 IGO.
3. Brown GC. Living too long: The current focus of medical research on increasing the quantity, rather than the quality, of life is damaging our health and harming the economy. *EMBO Reports.* 2015 February;16(2):137–41.
4. Agnivesha, CharakSamhita with AyurvedaDipika Commentary Of Chakrapani Datta, Acharya Y.D ed.Varanasi, India: Chaukhambha Surbharti Prakashan, 2000; Sutrasthan Chapter 1, verse 42;8.
5. Agnivesha, CharakSamhita with AyurvedaDipika Commentary Of Chakrapani Datta, Acharya Y.D ed.Varanasi, India: Chaukhambha Surbharti Prakashan, 2000; Sutrasthan Chapter 16, verse 27;97.
6. Agnivesha, CharakSamhita with AyurvedaDipika Commentary Of Chakrapani Datta, Acharya Y.D ed.Varanasi, India: Chaukhambha Surbharti Prakashan, 2000; Vimansthan Chapter 8, verse 122; 280.
7. Sushrut, Sushrut Samhita with Ayurvedatattva Sandipika, Shastri A. ed. Edition12th, Varanasi, Choukhanba Sanskrit Sansthan, 2001; Sutrasthan Chapter 35, verse 36;135.
8. Sushrut, Sushrut Samhita with Ayurvedatattva Sandipika, Shastri A. ed. Edition12th, Varanasi, Choukhanba Sanskrit Sansthan, 2001; Sutrasthan Chapter 24, verse 8;101.
9. Sharangadhara, Sharangadhara Samhita, commentary by Vidyasagar P, 5th ed, Chaukhambha Orientalia; 2002 Pratham khand, Chapter 6, verse 20;72.
10. Sushrut, Sushrut Samhita with Ayurvedatattva Sandipika, Shastri A. ed. Edition12th, Varanasi, Choukhanba Sanskrit Sansthan, 2001; Sutrasthan Chapter 15, verse 3;56.
11. Ferrucci L, Fabbri E. Inflammageing: Chronic inflammation in ageing, cardiovascular disease, and frailty. *Nature Reviews Cardiology.* 2018 September;15(9):505–522.
12. Sharma V, Chaudhary AK. Concepts of Dhatu Siddhanta (theory of tissues formation and differentiation) and Rasayana;probable predecessor of stem cell therapy. *Ayu.* 2014;35:231–236.
13. Hirsch HR, Coomes JA, Witten M. The waste-product theory of aging: Transformation to unlimited growth in cell cultures. *Experimental Gerontology.* 1989;24(2):97–112.
14. Diggs J. Accumulative waste theory of aging. In: Loue S.J., Sajatovic M. (eds) *Encyclopedia of Aging and Public Health.* Boston, MA, Springer, 2008. doi:10.1007/978-0-387-33754-8_6.

15. Utaka S, Avesani CM, Draibe SA, Kamimura MA, Andreoni S, Cuppari L. Inflammation is associated with increased energy expenditure in patients with chronic kidney disease. *The American Journal of Clinical Nutrition.* 2005 October;82(4):801–805.
16. Ruggiero C, Metter EJ, Melenovsky V, Cherubini A, Najjar SS, Ble A, Senin U, Longo DL, Ferrucci L. High basal metabolic rate is a risk factor for mortality: the Baltimore Longitudinal Study of Aging. J Gerontol A Biol Sci Med Sci. 2008 Jul;63(7):698–706.
17. Tripathi JS, Singh RH. Possible correlates of free radicals and free radical mediated disorders in Ayurveda with special reference to Bhutagni Vyapara and Ama at molecular level. *Ancient Science of Life.* 1999 July;19(1–2):17–20.
18. Ranjan R, Srivastava S. Correlation of concept of ama and free radical theory. *International Journal of Ayurveda and Pharma Research.* 2014;2(2):9–13.
19. Liochev SI. Reactive oxygen species and the free radical theory of aging. *Free Radical Biology and Medicine.* 2013 July;60:1–4.
20. Giorgi C, Marchi S, Simoes ICM, et al. Mitochondria and reactive oxygen species in aging and age-related diseases. *International Review of Cell and Molecular Biology.* 2018;340:209–344.
21. Bartke A, Brannan S, Hascup E, Hascup K, Darcy J. Energy metabolism and aging. *World Journal of Men's Health.* 2021 Apr;39(2):222–232
22. Sushrut, Sushrut Samhita with Ayurvedatattva Sandipika, Shastri A. ed. Edition12th, Varanasi, Choukhanba Sanskrit Sansthan, 2001; Sutrasthan Chapter 15, verse 27;61.
23. Deleidi M, Jäggle M, Rubino G. Immune aging, dysmetabolism, and inflammation in neurological diseases. *Frontiers in Neuroscience.* 2015 June 3;9:172.
24. Agnivesha, CharakSamhita with AyurvedaDipika Commentary Of Chakrapani Datta, Acharya Y.D ed.Varanasi, India: Chaukhambha Surbharti Prakashan, 2000; Vimansthan Chapter 8, verse 96–98;277.
25. Purvya MC, Meena MS. A review on role of prakriti in aging. *Ayu,* 2011;32(1):20–24.
26. Prasher B, Negi S, Aggarwal S, et al. Whole genome expression and biochemical correlates of extreme constitutional types defined in Ayurveda. *Journal of Translational Medicine.* 2008;6:48.
27. Agnivesha, CharakSamhita with AyurvedaDipika Commentary Of Chakrapani Datta, Acharya Y.D ed.Varanasi, India: Chaukhambha Surbharti Prakashan, 2000; Vimansthan Chapter 8, verse 95; 277.
28. Preston JD, Reynolds LJ, Pearson KJ. Developmental origins of health span and life span: A mini-review. *Gerontology,* 2018;64(3):237–245.
29. Singh RH, The Holistic Principles of Ayurvedic Medicine 1st ed. Varanasi, Chaukhambha Surbharti Prakashan, 1998;197–198.
30. Agnivesha, CharakSamhita with AyurvedaDipika Commentary Of Chakrapani Datta, Acharya Y.D ed.Varanasi, India: Chaukhambha Surbharti Prakashan, 2000; Sutrasthan Chapter 28, verse 45; 181.
31. Daniel M, Tollefsbol TO. Epigenetic linkage of aging, cancer, and nutrition. *Journal of Experimental Biology.* 2015;218(Pt 1):59–70.
32. Li Y, Daniel M, Tollefsbol TO. Epigenetic regulation of caloric restriction in aging. *BMC Medicine.* 2011;9:98. Published 2011 August 25.
33. Brown SA, Schmitt K, Eckert A. Aging and circadian disruption: causes and effects. *Aging,* 2011;3(8):813–817.
34. Agnivesha, CharakSamhita with AyurvedaDipika Commentary Of Chakrapani Datta, Acharya Y.D ed.Varanasi, India: Chaukhambha Surbharti Prakashan, 2000; Sutrasthan Chapter 16, verse 27; 97.
35. Agnivesha, CharakSamhita with AyurvedaDipika Commentary Of Chakrapani Datta, Acharya Y.D ed.Varanasi, India: Chaukhambha Surbharti Prakashan, 2000; Sutrasthan Chapter 30, verse 6; 187.
36. Agnivesha, CharakSamhita with AyurvedaDipika Commentary Of Chakrapani Datta, Acharya Y.D ed.Varanasi, India: Chaukhambha Surbharti Prakashan, 2000; Sutrasthan Chapter 5–8; 36–61.

37. Sushrut, Sushrut Samhita with Ayurvedatattva Sandipika, Shastri A. ed. Edition12th, Varanasi, Choukhanba Sanskrit Sansthan, 2001; Sutrasthan Chapter 1, verse 15; 4.

38. Agnivesha, CharakSamhita with AyurvedaDipika Commentary Of Chakrapani Datta, Acharya Y.D ed. Varanasi, India: Chaukhambha Surbharti Prakashan, 2000; Chikitsasthan Chapter 1, verse 8; 376.

39. Sharangadhara, Sharangadhara Samhita, commentary by Vidyasagar P, Edition 1st, Chaukhambha Orientalia; Pratham khand, Chapter 4, verse 13; 37.

40. Singh RH, The Holistic Principles of Ayurvedic Medicine 1st ed. Varanasi, Chaukhambha Surbharti Prakashan, 1998; 120–121.

41. Institute of Medicine (US) Committee on Health and Behavior: Research, Practice, and Policy. *Health and Behavior: The Interplay of Biological, Behavioral, and Societal Influences*. Washington, DC: National Academies Press (US); 2001. 2, Biobehavioral Factors in Health and Disease. Available from: https://www.ncbi.nlm.nih.gov/books/NBK43737/.

42. Brod S, Rattazzi L, Piras G, D'Acquisto F. 'As above, so below' examining the interplay between emotion and the immune system. *Immunology*. 2014;143(3):311–318. doi:10.1111/imm.12341.

43. Agnivesha, CharakSamhita with AyurvedaDipika Commentary Of Chakrapani Datta, Acharya Y.D ed. Varanasi, India: Chaukhambha Surbharti Prakashan, 2000; Chikitsasthan Chapter 1, verse 7–8; 376.

44. Rastogi S. Building bridges between Ayurveda and modern science. *International Journal of Ayurveda Research*. 2010 January;1(1):41–46.

45. Sushrut, Sushrut Samhita with Ayurvedatattva Sandipika, Shastri A. ed. Edition12th, Varanasi, Choukhanba Sanskrit Sansthan, 2001; Chikitsasthan Chapter 27, verse 4;120.

46. Sushrut, Sushrut Samhita with Ayurvedatattva Sandipika, Shastri A. ed. Edition12th, Varanasi, Choukhanba Sanskrit Sansthan, 2001; Chikitsasthan Chapter 27, verse 3;120.

47. Vagbhat, Ashtang Hriday, Garde GK Marathi translation –Sarth Vagbhat,4{{sup}}th Edition, Pune, India: Anamol Prakashan 2001;Uttartantra, Chapter 39, Verse 3;475

48. Patel V, Wilson P, Singh RH. Nutraceuticals of antiquity. In Pathak Y, ed. *Handbook of Nutraceuticals Vol I Ingradients, Formulltations, and Applications*. CRC Press Boca Raton, FL:2010;10.

49. Agnivesha, CharakSamhita with AyurvedaDipika Commentary Of Chakrapani Datta, Acharya Y.D ed.Varanasi, India: Chaukhambha Surbharti Prakashan, 2000; Sutrasthan Chapter 4, Verse 50;34.

50. Campisi J, Kapahi P, Lithgow GJ, Melov S, Newman JC, Verdin E. From discoveries in ageing research to therapeutics for healthy ageing. *Nature*. 2019;571 (7764):183–192.

51. Manjrekar PN, Jolly CI, Narayanan S. Comparative studies of the immunomodulatory activity of Tinospora cordifolia and Tinospora sinensis. *Fitoterapia*. 2000;71:254–257.

52. Aranha I, Clement F, Venkatesh YP. Immunostimulatory properties of the major protein from the stem of the Ayurvedic medicinal herb, guduchi (Tinospora cordifolia). *Journal of Ethnopharmacology*. 2012 January 31;139(2):366–372.

53. Kuchewar VV, Borkar MA, Nisargandha MA. Evaluation of antioxidant potential of Rasayana drugs in healthy human volunteers. *Ayu*. 2014 January;35(1):46–49.

54. Rege NN, Thatte UM, Dahanukar SA. Adaptogenic properties of six rasayana herbs used in Ayurvedic medicine. *Phytotherapy Research*. 1999 June;13(4):275–291.

55. Sharma A, Kaur G. Tinospora cordifolia as a potential neuroregenerative candidate against glutamate induced excitotoxicity: an in vitro perspective. *BMC Complementary and Alternative Medicine*. 2018 October 1;18(1):268.

56. Ramakrishna MK, Ramesh SR, Darshan CG, Sarojini BK. Neuroprotective activity of phytochemical combination of Quercetin and Curcumin against paraquat induced oxidative stress markers in Drosophila melanogaster. Vol. 93. Oklahoma: Drosophila Information Service; 2010:147–148.

57. Mistry KS, Sanghvi Z, Parmar G, Shah S. The antimicrobial activity of Azadirachta indica, Mimusops elengi, Tinospora cardifolia, Ocimum sanctum and 2% chlorhexidine gluconate on common endodontic pathogens: An in vitro study. *European Journal of Dentistry.* 2014 April;8(2):172–177.

58. Ashok BK, Ravishankar B, Prajapati PK, Bhat SD. Antipyretic activity of Guduchi Ghrita formulations in albino rats. *Ayu.* 2010 July;31(3):367–370.

59. Patgiri B, Umretia BL, Vaishnav PU, Prajapati PK, Shukla VJ, Ravishankar B. Anti-inflammatory activity of Guduchi Ghana (aqueous extract of Tinospora Cordifolia Miers.). *Ayu.* 2014 Jan;35(1): 108–10.

60. Hussain L, Akash MS, Ain NU, Rehman K, Ibrahim M. The analgesic, anti-inflammatory and anti-pyretic activities of Tinospora cordifolia. *Advances in Clinical and Experimental Medicine.* 2015 November-December;24(6):957–964.

61. Pathak P, Vyas M, Vyas H, Naria M. Rasayana effect of Guduchi Churna on the life span of Drosophila melanogaster. *Ayu.* 2016;37(1):67–70.

62. Dhama K, Sachan S, Khandia R, et al. Medicinal and beneficial health applications of Tinospora cordifolia (Guduchi): A miraculous herb countering various diseases/ disorders and its immunomodulatory effects. *Recent Patents on Endocrine, Metabolic & Immune Drug Discovery.* 2017;10(2):96–111.

63. Bag A, Bhattacharyya SK, Chattopadhyay RR. The development of Terminalia chebula Retz. (Combretaceae) in clinical research. *Asian Pacific Journal of Tropical Biomedicine.* 2013;3(3):244–252.

64. Chang CL, Lin CS. Development of antioxidant activity and pattern recognition of Terminalia chebula Retzius extracts and its fermented products. *HungKuang Journal.* 2010;61:115–129.

65. Lee HS, Won NH, Kim KH, Lee H, Jun W, Lee KW. Antioxidant effects of aqueous extract of Terminalia chebula in vitvo and *in vitro. Biological and Pharmaceutical Bulletin.* 2005;28(9):1639–1644.

66. Minkyun NA, Wan BAE, Kang SS, Min BS, Yoo JK, Yuk OK, et al. Cytoprotective effect on oxidative stress and inhibitory effect on cellular aging of Terminialia chebula fruit. *Phytotherapy Research.* 2004;18:737–741.

67. Lee HS, Koo YC, Suh HJ, Kim KY, Lee KW. Preventive effects of chebulic acid isolated from Terminalia chebula on advanced glycation endproduct-induced endothelial cell dysfunction. *Journal of Ethnopharmacology.* 2010 October 5;131(3):567–574.

68. Aher VD. Immunomodulatory effect of alcoholic extract of Terminalia chebula ripe fruits. *Journal of Pharmaceutical Sciences and Research.* 2010;2(9):539–544.

69. Gandhi NM, Nayar CKK. Radiation protection by Terminalia chebula some mechanistic aspects. *Molecular and Cellular Biochemistry.* 2005;277(1–2):43–48.

70. Maruthappan V, Shree KS. Hypolipidemic activity of haritaki (terminalia chebula) in atherogenic diet induced hyperlipidemic rats. *Journal of Advanced Pharmaceutical Technology and Research.* 2010 April;1(2):229–235.

71. Gantait S, Mahanta M, Bera S, Verma SK. Advances in biotechnology of Emblica officinalis Gaertn. syn. Phyllanthus emblica L.: A nutraceuticals-rich fruit tree with multifaceted ethnomedicinal uses. *3 Biotech.* 2021;11(2):62.

72. Yadav SS, Singh MK, Singh PK, Kumar V. Traditional knowledge to clinical trials: A review on therapeutic actions of Emblica officinalis. *Biomedicine & Pharmacotherapy.* 2017 September;93:1292–1302.

73. Rajani J, Ashok BK, Galib BJ, Prajapati PK, Ravishankar B. Immunomodulatory activity of Āmalaki Rasāyana: An experimental evaluation. *Ancient Science of Life.* 2012 October;32(2):93–98.

74. Tiwari V, Saba K, Veeraiah P, Jose J, Lakhotia SC, Patel AB. Amalaki Rasayana improved memory and neuronal metabolic activity in AbPP-PS1 mouse model of Alzheimer's disease. *Journal of Biosciences.* 2017 September;42(3):363–371.

75. Vishwanatha U, Guruprasad KP, Gopinath PM, Acharya RV, Prasanna BV, Nayak J, Ganesh R, Rao J, Shree R, Anchan S, Raghu KS, Joshi MB, Paladhi P, Varier PM, Muraleedharan K, Muraleedharan TS, Satyamoorthy K. Effect of Amalaki rasayana on DNA damage and repair in randomized aged human individuals. *Journal of Ethnopharmacology.* 2016 September 15;191:387–397. doi:10.1016/j. jep.2016.06.062.

76. Dwivedi V, Lakhotia SC. Ayurvedic Amalaki Rasayana promotes improved stress tolerance and thus has anti-aging effects in Drosophila melanogaster. *Journal of Biosciences.* 2016 December;41(4):697–711. doi:10.1007/s12038-016-9641-x.

77. Agnivesha, CharakSamhita with AyurvedaDipika Commentary Of Chakrapani Datta, Acharya Y.D ed.Varanasi, India: Chaukhambha Surbharti Prakashan, 2000; Sutrasthan Chapter 25, verse 40; 131.

78. Sharma SK, Goyal N, In vitro antioxidant activity of root extract of Pluchea lanceolata. *Journal of Pharmaceutical and Biomedical Sciences.* 2011;10:1–3.

79. Jahangir T, Safhi MM, Sultana S, Ahmad S. Pluchea lanceolata protects against Benzo(a) pyrene induced renal toxicity and loss of DNA integrity. *Interdisciplinary Toxicology.* 2013 March;6(1):47–54.

80. Sruthi CV, Sindhu A. A comparison of the antioxidant property of five Ayurvedic formulations commonly used in the management of vata vyadhis. *Journal of Ayurveda and Integrative Medicine.* 2012 January;3(1):29–32.

81. Talluri M, Yathapu SR, Bharatraj DK. Evaluation of Rasna panchaka (indigenous drug) as oxidative stress down-regulator using serum-free explant culture system. *Indian Journal of Pharmacology.* 2018;50(6):326–331.

82. Arya D, Patni V, Nair P, Kale RD. In vivo and in vitro determination of total phenolics, ascorbic acid content and antioxidant activity of Pluchea lanceolata (Oliver & Hiern). *International Journal of Pharmaceutical Sciences and Research.* 2015;6:875–879.

83. Bhagwat DP, Kharya MD, Bani S, Kaul A, Kaur K, Chauhan PS, Suri KA, Setti NK. Immunosuppressive properties of Pluchea lanceolata leaves. *Indian Journal of Pharmacology.* 2010;42:21–26.

84. Mundugaru R, Sivanesan S, Popa-Wagner A, Udaykumar P, Kirubagaran R, Kp G, Vidyadhara DJ. Pluchea lanceolata protects hippocampal neurons from endothelin-1 induced ischemic injury to ameliorate cognitive deficits. *Journal of Chemical Neuroanatomy.* 2018 December;94:75–85.

85. Mundugaru R, Sivanesan S, Udaykumar P, Rao N, Chandra N. Protective effect of Pluchea lanceolata against aluminum chloride-induced neurotoxicity in Swiss Albino Mice. *Pharmacognosy Magazine.* 2017 October;13(Suppl 3):S567–S572.

86. Srivastava P, Mohanti S, Bawankule DU, Khan F, Shanker K. Effect of Pluchea lanceolata bioactives on LPS-induced neuroinflammation in C6 rat glial cells. *Naunyn-Schmiedeberg's Archives of Pharmacology.* 2014 February;387(2):119–127.

87. Rai KS, Murthy KD, Karanth KS, Nalini K, Rao MS, Srinivasan KK. Clitoria ternatea root extract enhances acetylcholine content in rat hippocampus. *Fitoterapia.* 2002 December;73(7–8):685–689.

88. Damodaran T, Cheah PS, Murugaiyah V, Hassan Z. The nootropic and anticholinesterase activities of Clitoria ternatea Linn. root extract: Potential treatment for cognitive decline. *Neurochemistry International.* 2020 October;139:104785.

89. Raghu KS, Shamprasad BR, Kabekkodu SP, Paladhi P, Joshi MB, Valiathan MS, Guruprasad KP, Satyamoorthy K. Age dependent neuroprotective effects of medhya rasayana prepared from Clitoria ternatea Linn. in stress induced rat brain. *Journal of Ethnopharmacology.* 2017 February 2;197:173–183.

90. Mehla J, Pahuja M, Gupta P, Dethe S, Agarwal A, Gupta YK. Clitoria ternatea ameliorated the intracerebroventricularly injected streptozotocin induced cognitive impairment in rats: Behavioral and biochemical evidence. *Psychopharmacology (Berl).* 2013 December;230(4):589–605.

91. Talpate KA, Bhosale UA, Zambare MR, Somani R. Antihyperglycemic and antioxidant activity of Clitorea ternatea Linn. on streptozotocin-induced diabetic rats. *Ayu.* 2013 October;34(4):433–439.

92. Wakade AS, Juvekar AR, Hole RC, Nachankar RS, Kulkarni MP. Antioxidant and cardioprotective effect of Leptadenia reticulata against adriamycin–induced myocardial oxidative damage in rat experiments. *Planta Medica.* 2007;73:443.

93. Pravansha S, Thippeswamy BS, Veerapur VP. Immunomodulatory and antioxidant effect of Leptadenia reticulata leaf extract in rodents: Possible modulation of cell and humoral immune response. *Immunopharmacology and Immunotoxicology.* 2012;34:1010–1019.

94. Bherji S., M. Ganga R., Namile D. Evaluation of antipyretic and anti–inflammatory activity of aqueous Extract of Leptadenia reticulata in animal models. *Journal of Natural Remedies.* 2016 April;16(2):40–44.

95. Nema A.K., Agarwal A., Kashaw V. Screening of hepatoprotective potential of Leptadenia reticulata stems against paracetamol–induced hepatotoxicty in rats. *International Journal of Research in Pharmaceutical and Biomedical Sciences.* 2011;2:666–671.

96. Bopana N, Saxena S. Asparagus racemosus – Ethnopharmacological evaluation and conservation needs. *Journal of Ethnopharmacology.* 2007 March 1;110(1):1–15.

97. Sharma R, Jaitak V. Asparagus racemosus (Shatavari) targeting estrogen receptor α: An in-vitro and in-silico mechanistic study. *Natural Product Research.* 2020 June;34(11):1571–1574.

98. Chikhale RV, Sinha SK, Patil RB, et al. In-silico investigation of phytochemicals from Asparagus racemosus as plausible antiviral agent in COVID-19. *Journal of Biomolecular Structure and Dynamics.* 2020;1–15.

99. Alok S, Jain SK, Verma A, Kumar M, Mahor A, Sabharwal M. Plant profile, phytochemistry and pharmacology of Asparagus racemosus (Shatavari): A review. *Asian Pacific Journal of Tropical Disease.* 2013;3(3):242–251. doi:10.1016/S2222.

100. Tiwari N, Gupta VK, Pandey P, Patel DK, Banerjee S, Darokar MP, Pal A. Adjuvant effect of Asparagus racemosus Willd. derived saponins in antibody production, allergic response and pro-inflammatory cytokine modulation. *Biomedicine & Pharmacotherapy.* 2017 February;86:555–561.

101. Agnivesha, CharakSamhita with AyurvedaDipika Commentary Of Chakrapani Datta, Acharya Y.D ed. Varanasi, India: Chaukhambha Surbharti Prakashan, 2000; Chikitsasthan Chapter 1, Pad 4 verse 30–31; 386.

102. Ramanathan M, Sivakumar S, Anandvijayakumar PR, Saravanababu C, Pandian PR. Neuroprotective evaluation of standardized extract of Centella asciatica in monosodium glutamate treated rats. *Indian Journal of Experimental Biology.* 2007 May;45(5):425–431.

103. Gray NE, Zweig JA, Matthews DG, Caruso M, Quinn JF, Soumyanath A. Centella asiatica attenuates mitochondrial dysfunction and oxidative stress in Aβ-exposed hippocampal neurons. *Oxidative Medicine and Cellular Longevity.* 2017;2017:7023091.

104. Welbat JU, Chaisawang P, Pannangrong W, Wigmore P. Neuroprotective properties of asiatic acid against 5-fluorouracil chemotherapy in the hippocampus in an adult rat model. *Nutrients.* 2018 August 9;10(8):1053.

105. Gray NE, Alcazar Magana A, Lak P, et al. Soumyanath A. Centella asiatica - Phytochemistry and mechanisms of neuroprotection and cognitive enhancement. *Phytochemistry Reviews.* 2018 February;17(1):161–194.

106. Cesarone MR, Laurora G, De Sanctis MT, et al. Attività microcircolatoria della Centella asiatica nell'insufficienza venosa. Studio in doppio cieco [The microcirculatory activity of Centella asiatica in venous insufficiency. A double-blind study]. *Minerva Cardioangiologica.* 1994 June;42(6):299–304.

107. Incandela L, Cesarone MR, Cacchio M, et al. Total triterpenic fraction of Centella asiatica in chronic venous insufficiency and in high-perfusion microangiopathy. *Angiology.* 2001 October;52(Suppl 2):S9–S13.

108. Yao CH, Yeh JY, Chen YS, Li MH, Huang CH. Wound-healing effect of electrospun gelatin nanofibres containing Centella asiatica extract in a rat model. *Journal of Tissue Engineering and Regenerative Medicine.* 2017 March;11(3):905–915.

109. Sh Ahmed A, Taher M, Mandal UK, et al. Pharmacological properties of Centella asiatica hydrogel in accelerating wound healing in rabbits. *BMC Complementary and Alternative Medicine.* 2019 August 14;19(1):213.

110. K Yadav A, Agrawal J, Pal A, Gupta MM. Novel anti-inflammatory phytoconstituents from Desmodium gangeticum. *Natural Product Research.* 2013;27(18):1639–1645.

111. Rathi A, Rao ChV, Ravishankar B, De S, Mehrotra S. Anti-inflammatory and antinociceptive activity of the water decoction Desmodium gangeticum. *Journal of Ethnopharmacology.* 2004 December;95(2–3):259–263.

112. Rastogi S, Pandey MM, Rawat AK. An ethnomedicinal, phytochemical and pharmacological profile of Desmodium gangeticum (L.) DC. and Desmodium adscendens (Sw.) DC. *Journal of Ethnopharmacology.* 2011 June 22;136(2):283–296.

113. Govindarajan R, Vijayakumar M, Rao CV, Shirwaikar A, Kumar S, Rawat AK, Pushpangadan P. Antiinflammatory and antioxidant activities of Desmodium gangeticum fractions in carrageenan-induced inflamed rats. *Phytotherapy Research.* 2007 October;21(10):975–979.

114. Kurian GA, Paddikkala J. Role of mitochondrial enzymes and sarcoplasmic ATPase in cardioprotection mediated by aqueous extract of desmodium gangeticum (L) DC root on ischemic reperfusion injury. *Indian Journal of Pharmaceutical Sciences.* 2010 November;72(6):745–752.

115. Joshi H, Parle M. Antiamnesic effects of Desmodium gangeticum in mice. *Yakugaku Zasshi.* 2006 September;126(9):795–804.

116. Vagbhat, Ashtang Hriday, Garde GK Marathi translation –Sarth Vagbhat,4{{sup}}th Edition, Pune, India: Anamol Prakashan 2001;Uttartantra, Chapter 39, verse 155; 485.

117. Mishra S, Aeri V, Gaur PK, Jachak SM. Phytochemical, therapeutic, and ethnopharmacological overview for a traditionally important herb: Boerhavia diffusa Linn. *BioMed Research International.* 2014;2014:808302. doi:10.1155/2014/808302.

118. Sharma S, Baboota S, Amin S, Mir SR. Ameliorative effect of a standardized polyherbal combination in methotrexate-induced nephrotoxicity in the rat. *Pharmaceutical Biology.* 2020;58(1):184–199. doi:10.1080/13880209.2020.1717549.

119. Sawardekar SB, Patel TC. Evaluation of the effect of Boerhavia diffusa on gentamicin-induced nephrotoxicity in rats. *Journal of Ayurveda and Integrative Medicine.* 2015 April-June;6(2):95–103.

120. Pareta SK, Patra KC, Mazumder PM, Sasmal D. Aqueous extract of Boerhaavia diffusa root ameliorates ethylene glycol-induced hyperoxaluric oxidative stress and renal injury in rat kidney. *Pharmaceutical Biology.* 2011 December;49(12):1224–1233.

121. Apu AS, Liza MS, Jamaluddin AT, Howlader MA, Saha RK, Rizwan F, Nasrin N. Phytochemical screening and in vitro bioactivities of the extracts of aerial part of Boerhavia diffusa Linn. *Asian Pacific Journal of Tropical Biomedicine.* 2012 September;2(9):673–678.

122. Juneja K, Mishra R, Chauhan S, Gupta S, Roy P, Sircar D. Metabolite profiling and wound-healing activity of Boerhavia diffusa leaf extracts using in vitro and in vivo models. *Journal of Traditional and Complementary Medicine.* 2019 February 19;10(1):52–59.

Changes in the Regulation of Energy Metabolism with Aging Nutraceutical Applications

Rupalben K. Jani
Parul University

Contents

DOI: 10.1201/9781003110866-4

4.1 Introduction

4.1.1 The metabolism of energy

4.1.1.1 Basic terms of the metabolism of energy

Metabolism can be a chain of all chemical reactions within the organism. They mean a change in nutrients, catalyzed and constrained in certain circumstances.

Indeed metabolic reactions are paired with each other to design metabolism pathways where one compound is converted into another via a sequence of chemical reactions. This method gives rise to countless intercedes supporting different metabolic pathways as an initial substrate [1].

Pyruvate, for example, can be converted to lactate in the process of gluconeogenesis, or it may potentially convert into an amino acid called alanine, takes part in the development of glucose, or can be converted into acetyl-CoA to constitute a source of energy.

This nutrient interconversion is what we call an intermediate (or intermediate) metabolism with completely different intermediate products.

In general, metabolic reactions are indeed separated into anabolic and catabolic forms.

1. **Anabolic reactions**:
   Anabolic reactions are artificial, with simpler compounds making complex compounds. These require energy expended during the response, which is why they belong to an endergonic reaction group.
   Gluconeogenesis, glycogen synthesis, fatty acids, amino acids, proteins, ketones, urea, or other compounds consist of anabolic reactions in the human body [1].
2. **Catabolic reactions**:
   Catabolic reactions include cleavage, deprivation, or putrefaction into simpler ones of composite substances. During this process, the energy is released and could be used to promote macroergic molecules.

Our body has essential catabolic reactions such as glycolysis, glycogenolysis, lipolysis, and beta-oxidation, which are the deprivation of ketone bodies, proteins, or amino acids.

Anabolic and catabolic reactions are characteristics of metabolic pathways called amphibolic reactions (gr. amfi- both).

A citric acid cycle finishes the oxidation of a carbon skeleton of entire nutrients (catabolic pathway). Its intermediate function substrates for anabolic pathways could be a good example (alpha-ketoglutarate converting to glutamate fatty acid synthesis uses succinyl-CoA to hem or citrate).

Anaplerotic reactions are a group of responses that manage to integrate the transitional products with other metabolic pathways. This reaction completes the Citric acid cycle with some certain Oxalacetate (by glucose, glucogenic amino acids, or lactate) and Alpha-ketoglutarate (from glutamate).

Constant regeneration of macroergic compounds, serving as a free energy source for endergonic reactions, can be the energy metabolism essential to sustaining life.

Their development begins with high molecular catabolism. The fragments obtained by this method getting converted into core intercedes (such as acetyl-CoA), which are further oxygenized in the citric acid cycle (in the case of aerobic metabolism), and the resulting coenzymes (NADH+H+−NADH2) are used to produce energy (ATP) in the electron transport chain.

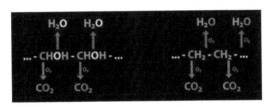

4.2 ATP

The most substantial and universal macroergic substance is ATP. It serves partly as an energy stock but principally provides free energy (G) to transfer to cells. Although macroergic compounds are capable of releasing more energy than ATP, they are not widely used. The details for this are the absolute constancy of the anhydride bond, which is immune (unlike other anhydrides) to spontaneous hydrolysis and will be the only split in the existence of enzymes.

Additional negative values are constituents with free energy. In ATP progression, rejuvenation (e.g., phosphoenolpyruvate, phosphocreatine, and 1,3-bisphosphoglycerate) is considered.

4.2.1 The role of organs in the metabolism of energy
4.2.1.1 Liver

In intermediate metabolism, liver cells (hepatocytes) have an inimitable function. They play a dynamic role in so long as homeostasis, synthesis of different molecules, intermediate metabolism, and control of storing and proclaiming energy. In the breakdown of all nutrients, the liver takes part.

1. **Liver and saccharide metabolism**:
   The liver plays a vital role in glycemic control in the short term (in hours) and, in a long time (in the span of days to weeks) known as the liver's glucostatic purpose. The liver began the glycogen synthesis

process, which uses blood glucose when the volume of glucose in *Vena portae* peaks afterward the suppertime. During fasting, the opposite mechanism takes place as the level of blood sugar decreases.

In the bloodstream, glucose gets absorbed by glycogenolysis, which means disintegration of stored glycogen, and gluconeogenesis, which means glycogen source reduces. Galactose and fructose breakdown also takes place in the liver [2].

2. **Liver-lipid metabolism**:

Many mechanisms of lipid metabolisms (such as ketone body synthesis) are inimitable to the liver. However, most occur in other things (though the liver is always the essential organ in quantitative terms).

Fatty acid oxidation occurs here and accelerates to the point that such energy is released more than the liver requires during fasting and offers surplus acetyl-CoA that forms ketone bodies.

Ketone bodies cannot be used by the liver and are released into the blood where they act as an alternate source of energy.

The liver acts as a critical role in the formation of lipoproteins as well. VLDL units, some of which are HDL, are synthesized, IDL is converted into LDL, and fragments of chylomicrons, HDL, and a component of LDL are degraded. Cholesterol synthesis takes place here also.

3. **Metabolism of protein in the liver as well as amino acids**:

Protein and amino acid metabolism reactions occur almost entirely in the liver (urea synthesis). Others may also occur in other tissues (amino acid deamination and transamination, nonessential AA synthesis). The liver synthesizes, except for immunoglobulins, all proteins from plasma (e.g., coagulation factors or albumin).

4.2.2 Further organs

4.2.2.1 Kidneys

Vast amounts of energy use in the urine concentration and transportation processes of substances originate in the kidneys. That is the reason ATP utilization, explicitly in the renal cortex, is high. ATP creates· by the oxidative digestion of glucose, lactate, unsaturated fats, and amino acids.

The kidneys are the second most crucial site of gluconeogenesis after the Liver (mostly throughout fasting). The carbon skeleton of amino acids is its primary substrate (particularly glutamine). Ammonia, the outcome of these reactions, is metabolized right into the urine, which acts as a buffer.

4.2.2.2 Skeletal muscles

Vital muscles of the skeletons consume a considerable amount of energy. ATP regeneration occurs via aerobic and anaerobic glycolysis, fatty acid degradation, and creatine phosphate [3].

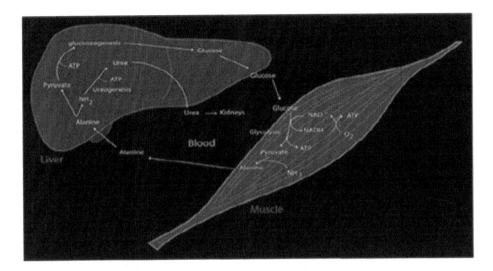

Figure 4.1 *The alanine cycle.*

The skeletal muscle plays a significant part in amino acid metabolism, mostly a chain of amino acids (leucine, isoleucine, valine). The carbon skeletons gained in this procedure produce energy and the amino group's aid as a substratum to form glutamine, glutamate, and alanine. These amino acids ultimately release into the arteries moderately in large amounts. The liver can use the alanine produced by skeletal muscles in the glucose regeneration (the alanine cycle) (Figure 4.1).

4.2.2.3 Adipose tissue

The storage location for TAG postprandially is adipose tissue (where insulin predominates after appetite). It stores food-derived lipids and those synthesized in the liver as well. During fasting times, lipolysis occurs due to glucagon's influence, the deprivation of lipid into fatty acids, and glycerol.

4.2.2.4 Brain

Glucose is the primary energy font for the brain. Its daily intake is about 100–120 g. However, the brain can cover up to 50% of its energy needs by oxidizing ketone bodies throughout altered fasting (which occurs roughly after 3 weeks without ample energy stream).

As shown in Figure 4.2, during workouts, the interaction of our organs discloses.

4.2.3 Human metabolism of nutrients

The primary components of foods are carbohydrates, lipids, and proteins, which act as fuel molecules for the humanoid body. The breakdown in the

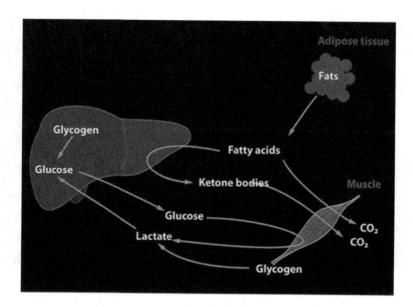

Figure 4.2 *Our organs' interaction during physical activity.*

food tract of these nutrients and the following absorption (entry into the bloodstream) of the digestive system's end products makes it possible for tissues and cells to turn the latent chemical energy of food into practical work.

Monosaccharides, mostly monoacylglycerol glucose (from carbohydrates), long-chain fatty acids (from lipids), small peptides, and amino acids are the major consumed end products of food digestion (out of protein). Various cells can metabolize these nutrients once they are in the bloodstream. It has known that carbohydrates, lipids, and protein groups of molecules are energy sources for metabolism in humans. However, it is a common misconception (especially among undergraduates) that human cells only use glucose as an energy source [2]. This misrepresentation can arise from the definition of energy metabolism in most textbooks, highlighting glycolysis (the metabolic pathway for glucose degradation) and failing fatty acid or amino acid oxidation.

4.2.4 Energy metabolism historical review

The early studies, initiated by Joseph Priestley, Joseph Black, Antoine Lavoisier, and Carl Wilhelm Scheele, played a distinct part during the 18th century, distinguishing gases, oxygen, and carbon dioxide, are essential for the generation of energy. The air we inhale is sort by the nobleman of French who holds the designation of "father of modern chemistry" is Lavoisier. The primary studies perform on energy conservation and changes in the body.

Scientist Lavoisier disclosed that the breath-out air confined carbon dioxide, which forms Lavoisier, also discovered that heat is incessantly produced by the body while breathing. Justus Liebig then performed animal experiments in the mid of the 19th century and comprehended carbohydrates, proteins, and fats oxidize in the body. Finally, the studies of Max Rubner made revolutionary contributions to metabolism and nutrition. Voit disclosed that O_2 utilization is the creation of metabolism in the cell. In contrast, Rubner described caloric standards, which are still used today by calculating the main energy content of some foods like Sugars and proteins to produce around 4–5 kcal/g of energy, while lipids can produce up to 9–10 kcal/g. Rubner's findings show that heat productivity was equal to heat elimination for a resting animal, suggesting the law of energy conservation, as described in the early experiments of Lavoisier, applied to living organisms. Therefore, converting the potential chemical energy of molecules hooked on different forms of powers like chemical, motion, kinetic, and thermal energy from a sequence of oxygen-enabled reactions inside a cell is what makes life possible [4].

4.3 What is the regulation of energy metabolism?

Energy is a type of fuel separated from the food we consume by the body's metabolic processes. This energy generates numerous catabolic pathways and stores the elevated energy phosphate bonds of the body's energy loading fragment of Adenosine Triphosphate (ATP).

The process by which energy transforms into ATP recognizes as cellular inhalation. Often known as the powerhouse of the cell, mitochondria are the main component of this cellular respiration.

Glucose is the ideal energy basis for the production of ATP in the body. However, it is also possible to metabolize other carbohydrates, fats, and proteins into acetyl coenzyme A (CoA), entry of the citric acid cycle (Krebs), and, if necessary, oxidize into carbon dioxide and water (Figure 4.3).

A. **Changes in the regulation of energy intake**:
   One literature review studied whether elder age correlates with transformed energy consumption responses to forced overfeeding and underfeeding, which was the first study of this subject. Since day-to-day energy intake variability is usually 20%–25% while day-to-day energy outlays variability is stereotypically only 10%, significant daily energy balance fluctuations are inevitably present.
   Overfeeding and underfeeding proprieties are typically an effort to investigate the effects of inconsistency in energy consumption magnitudes and energy equilibrium during everyday life. The same result obtains under contrary investigational circumstances (overfeeding and underfeeding) revealed a fundamental alteration slightly than an experimental artifact between age groups and indicates that aging correlates with a diminished capability to precisely control energy balance through energy intake changes [5].

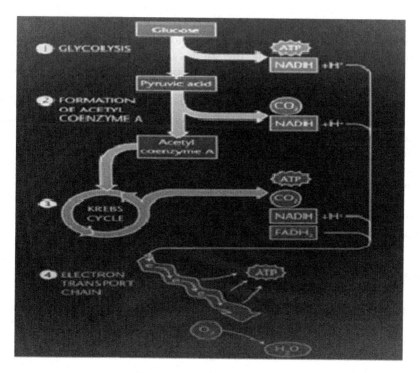

Figure 4.3 *Cycle of energy metabolism regulation.*

B. How does the body regulate energy metabolism?

A dynamic mechanism involving various biological substances and chemical processes is the regulation of energy absorption. The body entails vitamins and minerals to generate energy, mostly because vitamins and minerals do not encompass calories. They thus do not generate energy directly, but without them, the body itself does not create energy as of macronutrients [3].

Thiamin, riboflavin, vitamin B6, vitamin B3, vitamin B9, vitamin B12, pantothenic acid, and biotin are especially essential in enhancing energy metabolism. It is necessary to consume these water-soluble vitamins every day, except for vitamin B12, as the body does not have a storage point. Contrariwise, these vitamins' excess limits get wash out in the urine, either from diet or supplementation. The primary function of B-vitamins is to turn as coenzymes in many metabolic processes.

The coenzyme is a molecule that helps it do its job to activate it and combines it with an enzyme. Six coenzymes such as biotin, pantothenic acid, vitamin B6, niacin, thiamine, and riboflavin are mainly involved in the metabolism of energy, whereas the other two (vitamin B9 and vitamin B12) effort principally in the renewal of cells and red

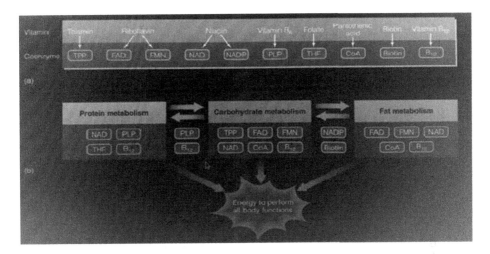

Figure 4.4 Role of vitamins B to promote the metabolism of energy.

blood cell synthesis, as shown in (Figure 4.4). However, vitamin B9 and vitamin B12 have minor roles in energy metabolism [5].

As we have said, except folate and B12, B-vitamins' primary role is to promote energy production in the body. The other nutrients in energy metabolism include a vitamin-like substance called choline, and the minerals iodine, sulfur, chromium, and manganese [2].

C. **Roles of micronutrients in energy metabolism**:

Several micronutrients are needed to turn dietary sources of energy in the ATP form, like carbohydrates, fats, and proteins, through cell energy, such as coenzymes and enzyme reaction cofactors, structural enzymes, and mitochondrial cytochrome components, and active electron and proton carriers in the breathing chain producing ATP.

The part of vitamins in the breakdown of energy continues to attract interest in science. The literature review revealed the critical role of vitamins B6, B9, and B12 in managing one-carbon mitochondrial exchange sequences via mitochondrial enzymes' control.

In their research paper, some authors stressed the B vitamin family's essential function in sustaining mitochondrial power breakdown and how mitochondria are affected by a lack of B vitamins in their process as the cellular organs responsible for energy metabolism. There is a growing interest in certain minerals in energy metabolism [1].

A trace element like copper is a critical cytochrome C-oxidase cofactor, a part of the mitochondrial breathing chain, intricate in iron metabolism. Chromium potentiates the action of insulin, hence endorsing glucose agreement by the cells. Manganese is a cofactor of many enzymes complex in gluconeogenesis and carbohydrate breakdown. Zinc is an integral component of over 100 enzymes, some of which are complex in energy breakdown. Reviews of substantially active entities reveal magnesium consumption in some athletes' classes does not comply with adult guidelines. A few studies have shown that supplements of magnesium increase strength and enhance exercise efficiency [1].

4.4 How energy metabolism gets affected during aging processes?

Age is one of the most significant reasons behind improvements in the metabolism of energy. Skeletal musculature volume decreases, and with age, the percentage of adipose tissue increases. The reduction in muscle physique relative to the entire body shows to be principally responsible for the age-related deterioration in the basal metabolic rate.

A. Some more factors were studied and discussed by various scientists, directly affected during aging processes and change energy metabolism regulation. Here, this chapter explained all the aspects in detail.
   I. **Basal Metabolic Rate (BMR)**:
      Basal metabolic rate (BMR) reflects sufficiently to add up energy needed at full rest for the body's cellular metabolism (postabsorptive, thermally neutral, lying relaxed in bed). AH BMR tables show a gradual decline from birth to old age, and accurate quantitative parameters sometimes are given, perhaps "a 23% fall during adulthood." The decrease probably reduces the relative function of most of the body's organs, tissues, and an actual reduction in the mass of organs and tissues. There are especially evident examples of the skeleton and skeletal muscle. In the decrease in BMR, however, there must be a lot of individual variabilities. The data available, which almost entirely consists of cross-sectional studies, does not allow us to be reliable whether we are concerned with individuals with particular groups. The drop in BMR is more likely than any perceived age-related metabolism switch to interpret a change in body structure with age (more fat and less muscle, for example). Elderly folks have denied these changes in the body, at least up to somewhat advanced age (70–75 years or so). A slight decrease in BMR could well demonstrate the composition [6].
   II. **Physical activity**:
      Same as BMR, physical activity also plays a significant role in energy metabolism with aging processes. The mutable likely to emphasize differences in energy metabolism among older people is regular exercise. For the elderly, physical activity has several degrees of significance. In simple nutritional terms, energy expenditure elevates when physical activity increases and the energy necessary to reduce the spending is similarly enhanced. Hunger increases, then the volume of nutrition consumed is consistently

higher. A secondary issue of increased food consumption is that the intake of protein, minerals, and other vitamins might also be more extensive. The physical activity itself results in more significant muscle tone, increased strength of the muscles and joints, an enhancement of social interactions, and a gradual improvement in "well-being" feeling. There is a great deal of personal and indirect information that predicts that, on average, perception from young adulthood onwards could drop substantially [7].

The line of work has an insignificant correlation to leisure activities. However, generally, it is probably of little implications. In contrast, most work situations in industrialized countries' energy metabolism do not require a level of physical activity that would be strenuous for an average healthy older person. Consequently, the significant impact of occupation might be whether or not the degree of physical activity on withdrawal augmented.

The enhanced tendency to suffer from one or more degenerative diseases of the circulatory and respiratory systems, mainly bones and joints, which may hinder physical activity, is another aspect of aging. Due to old age, many seniors involve because getting around is inconvenient, uncomfortable, or even painful. The proportion of older people who suffer from joint disabilities sufficient to incapacitate or inhibit movement is unknown and probably varies considerably for different countries, climates, occupations, and so forth. The general conclusion may be that, whereas there is a negative relationship of aging to physical activity, up to 70 age or so, the trend will often be relatively gradual. It will be affected by the standard of health and the amount of activity in the earlier régime.

III. **Body weight and composition**:

Modifications in body mass through aging are not well predictable. The majority of cross-sectional data shows a decreased height, which for those between 30 and 70 years of age can be as much as 5–7 cm. With the socio-economic group, it tends to differ significantly. More substantial variations in height in industrial areas arise with aging compared to rural populations with the occupation. Professional groups from the more affluent social classes, on the other hand, seem to be showing no shift. Weight changes seem more complicated and vary between sexes so that at 65–70 years of age, men tend to have a small bodyweight than at 40 years of age, while women also display an increase in body weight over this time.

In general, data show that weight rises with age and height decrease in both the United States and the United Kingdom, with weight stabilizing in men around the age of about 70 years and then steadily decreasing due to the liberal loss of skeletal muscle and potentially also fat. In general, this refers to the average population of both males and females in each country. Most of these body composition data were collected from cross-sectional studies, although the accurate longitudinal information is limited. Redistribution of fat was also defined by Brozik, with substantially less fat in the subcutaneous than the truncal sites in older individuals, which we have also reported. The remaining outcome of a progressive rise in body weight up to a certain age is that the elderly would expend additional energy to a younger group of adults for every given amount and type of exercise [8].

IV. **Temperature of body**:

Logically, it is probable that a fundamental decrease in core temperature could impact metabolic activity that could occur in advanced age due to decreased metabolism of tissue, but this was not on record [9].

V. **Sympathetic nervous system**:

The probability that the nervous system's sympathetic activity rises with the aging process and can affect diet and exercise has studied. However, the proof is uncertain and hard to examine (for many reasons, including methodological problems). There is little practical significance to its exact relationship with energy metabolism in the elderly [10].

VI. **Muscle fiber type**:

In the elderly body, there tends to be a selective loss of type II fibers, which may decrease the muscle glycogen stores and result in a moderated compression power, but this may be more perception than an actual aging effect with lower sports participation. Amidst this shift in the context of the failing function, however, muscle strength is still capable of developing from a reasonable exercise plan to a significantly older age [10].

VII. **Absorption of nutrients and digestion**:

One of the other changes in activity generally considered to occur in the aged, of absolute possible nutritional value, is the relative metabolic derangement of foods. Decent scientific proof in courtesy of this is difficult to corner. Southgate and Durnin discussed this as a by-product of measuring the energy values of protein, fat, and carbohydrates calculated by chemical methods. Bomb calorimetry absorbs the entire meal, and groups of young and older males and females excrete the urine and faces. The outcomes disclosed no mark of declined proficiency of digestion and absorption with aging [10].

VIII. **Metabolism of carbohydrate and fat**:

The ratios of carbohydrates and fats that provide energy to the body could have caloric significance and may differ with aging, even though there is no strong evidence for this [11].

IX. **Altered energy intake because of dietary fiber**:
In the elderly, it is probable but doubtful that someone will have a significant intake of fiber and limited overall dietary nutritional consumption. The ingestion and absorption of the nutrients have hindered. These can sometimes be severe enough to result in malnutrition. The accessibility of carbohydrates, fat, and protein in the food diminishes to the range that the total net energy is insufficient [5].

X. **Low energy intake disturbing with protein metabolism**:
The ratio of protein compared to the whole energy in the régime may be within usual limitations. However, assume the entire diet is insufficient in providing the energy necessities. In that scenario, the protein will be used as an energy source and, thus, be inadequate for protein metabolism's daily needs. Because this situation in senior citizens is presumably not scarce, probably living independently, with an inadequate diet and little desire to prepare good meals, small degrees of nutritional deficiencies, particularly in older sets of old patients, maybe predictable. The potentially strong research in the United Kingdom and the United States that would have revealed these cases if they occurred did not seem to indicate much evidence of malnutrition is complicated, but restricted protein scantiness is distinctive. The complaint may therefore be more common than is appearing [12].

XI. **Actual energy disbursements**:
While published statistics suggest that some older men have high energy expenditure levels, the proportion of older people is more than 3,000 kcal/d, which is of more immediate concern. Their energy intake is so inadequate that it will lead to insignificant nutrient intake by consuming energy to supply the amount. There must be dissatisfaction with the nutrient intake levels, often in the younger elderly population [13].

B. **Potential mediators of impaired regulation such as glucose and insulin**:
- Theoretically, a reduced gastric emptying rate may justify consistently higher postprandial glucose and insulin levels in later life because gastric emptying will boost the quality of gastric emptying in old age when nutrients occur in the flow due to prolonged intake.
- Simultaneously, this is not the only conceivable reason for high circulating glucose after meal intake in older people (delay uptake of glucose by the muscle and liver can explain). Most studies investigative gastric emptying concerning age have reported a decreased rate in the elderly. In general, delayed gastric emptying has been associated with reduced starvation and improved engorgement and can potentially lead to increased satiety and satiation or decreased elderly appetite [14].

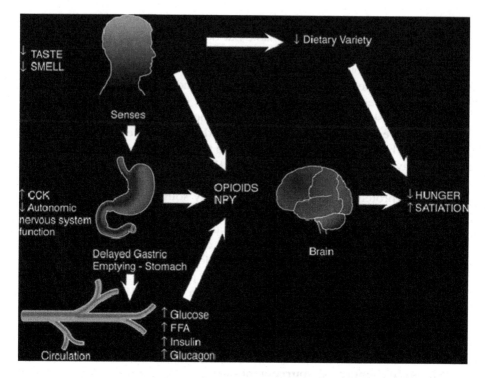

Figure 4.5 *Nutrients metabolism through various internal organs.*

- The period during which glucose and other energy substrates consume extend by potential delays in gastric emptying. Modifications in gastric emptying in the old phase will likely also result in an extended period of stomach swelling and affect appetite over the period of postprandial nutritional availability. It could also directly extend repletion through afferent pneumogastric signals. Morley also indicated that reducing stomach production of nitric oxide in older adults can increase repletion by dropping fundus relaxation and speeding up food movement to the antrum [5,15] (Figure 4.5).

4.5 What are the outcomes of the loss of such activity?

It states that many disease states prevalent in old age, such as cancer, are associated with body weight and fat loss. However, until recently, there was no clarity about whether healthy aging is associated with weight loss mediated by a reduced capacity to manage energy intake [16].

A. **Variations in the regulation of energy intake**:
 1. The causes of apparent deregulation of old-age food consumption are not well known, primarily because they do not fully

understand the mechanisms of original effective energy control at any age.

2. As illustrated in some recent studies, there are several entrants for age-related modifications that might lead to aging anorexia. It is vital to note that severance in energy management mechanisms is possibly due to preserving the energy equilibrium within parameters. That does not impact during reproduction in young adult life and species survival generally. Before a measurable deficiency in energy control, observations in many mechanisms need to fail in old age [17]. Therefore, for impaired control of energy intake to be seen, quite many candidate mechanisms can potentially be impaired in old age, and work is required to define which agents are quantitatively appropriate [18].

3. Sturm and colleagues proposed that both decreased premeal starvation and increased postmeal repletion are autonomous contributors to diminished old-age energy control. Increased satiation after meal intake correlates with the increased antral region (and possibly distension).

B. **Changes in taste and smell with aging processes become potential contributors to energy metabolism**:

This assumption is also congruent with animal reports claiming short energy intake foremost to weight loss in aging rats caused by the information of shorter suppertimes at a reduced pace rather than portioned meals [19]. In combination, these findings indicate that a decreased sense of starvation or increased satiety precedes and leads to weight loss in old age [20]. Changes in taste and smell with aging processes become potential contributors to energy metabolism

1. There are well-predictable age-associated declines in taste and smell compassion.

2. In particular, most studies suggest that exposure and acknowledgment thresholds for salt and other specific tastes increase with age because of suppositories that impact taste and a loss of functional taste bud number and structure, and a diminished sense of smell.

3. Suppose the losses in taste and smell related to aging have a corresponding effect (i.e., making diet seem blander, as commonly testified). The anticipated reduction in gastric emptying and possibly delayed absorption of nutrients could explain the recorded increase in repletion and decrease in starvation in old age [20].

C. **Reduced dietary variety as a mediator of diminished regulation of food intake**:

Experiments in lab mice, cats, and guinea pigs have shown that most foods give higher energy intake. Energy consumption is higher than when only a single food provides. Several single-meal studies in humans also indicate this effect. While two longer-term studies have exposed that lab rats have more significant body fat and body fat benefit when fed a range of foods than when only a single food provides. Until recently, long-term studies have been lacking in humans. The long-term suggestion between dietary variability and body obesity in healthy adult men and women has been recently documented [21]. Dietary type from a combined category of candy, snacks, condiments, entrees, and carbohydrates was positively associated with body fatness in multiple regression studies adjusted for age and sex. Body fat was negatively associated with dietary variety from vegetables of the same model. In other words, people who ate a wide range of higher-energy foods combined with a common type of vegetables were comparatively fatter [22].

1. **Social factors and medical**:
   - Many aging-related social and medical changes indicate weight loss, such as poverty, homelessness, social alienation, weak dentition, chronic illness, and the use of multiple medications.
   - Furthermore, depression causes a significant reason of weight loss among the aging, a finding that supports a cohort data review.
   - However, it is fascinating to write that the study disclosed that depression was linked with weight loss only in entities aged 55 years or older and was associated with weight gain in younger adults. One potential description for this verdict is that psychosocial aspects are potential catalysts for weight loss only when a primary impairment in the food intake parameter allows impediments to bother to be stated [17].
   - Regarding social seclusion, the literature review stated that less energy, requires at meals taken alone than meals eaten in the company, with the difference in energy intake between the two situations being a considerable 30%. While some reports conclude that social eating is disadvantageous because it encourages overeating and obesity, the reverse is an equally correct interpretation that eating alone contributes to undereating and weight loss [18]. It is particularly true as it considers that humans are a gregarious species of animals and naturally eat in social groups. It is directly related to low energy consumption in the older population since social interaction can constrain bereavement and functional disabilities.
   - Thus, one of the factors leading to short energy consumption in older adults could be the increased frequency of eating alone. Besides, there is a confident relationship between the rate of eating restaurant food and body fat, and older adults may eat out less often for reasons of social seclusion and practical infirmities [18].

- In support of this suggestion, adults younger than 45 years of age stated suppertimes almost twice as much as individuals older than 65 in the newly recorded NHANES 1999–2000 study [19]. The synthesis of these various observations and results indicates that limiting social meals and consuming out has a potentially significant role in the short energy consumption and body weight loss of older grownups, which is autonomous of any age-related genetic impairment [21] (Table 4.1).

Table 4.1 Strength of Worldwide Available Nutritional Constituents

Sr. No.	Nutritional Constituent	Digestive Component	Physical Advantages	Test Parameters	Daily Intake Limit
1	Margarine	Esters of sterol and stanol	Reduce cholesterol	All stages of clinical trials	1.3 g/d for sterols 1.7 g/d for stanols
2	Psyllium	Soluble fiber	Lessen cholesterol	All stages of clinical trials	1 g/d
3	Soy	Protein	Diminish cholesterol	All stages of clinical trials	25 g/d
4	Whole oat products	Glucan	Decrease cholesterol	All stages of clinical trials	3 g/d
5	Cranberry juice	Proanthocyanidin	Reduce frequency of UTI	A small number of clinical trials	300 mL/d
6	Fatty fish	(n-3) Fatty acids	Reduce TG, reduce heart disease, cardiac deaths, and fatal and nonfatal myocardial infarction	All stages of clinical trials	2/wk
7	Garlic	Organosulfur components	Decrease cholesterol	All stages of clinical trials	600–900 mg/d
8	Green tea	Catechins	Decrease chances of different types of cancer	Study of epidemiology	
9	Spinach, kale, collard greens	Lutein/ zeaxanthin	Decrease the chances of age-related Degeneration	Study of epidemiology	6 mg/d
10	Tomatoes and Processed Tomato products	Lycopene	Decrease the frequency of prostate cancer	Study of epidemiology	Daily
11	Cruciferous, Vegetables	Glucosinolates, indoles	Decrease chances of different types of cancer	Study of epidemiology	Three or more servings/wk
12	Fermented dairy Products	Probiotics	Improve immunity	Release study data of *in-vivo* and *in-vitro* studies	Daily

4.6 Other materials used in recovery?

Aging is associated with reduced immunity, increased infectious agent mortality, morbidity, and low nutritional status. Widespread are deficiencies in vitamin E, vitamin B6, folate, zinc, and selenium, and defects in these micronutrients report to hinder immunity. Therefore, if nutraceutical products may improve micronutrient status, elderly population's everyday use of nutraceuticals can provide an opportunity to enhance resistance at-risk populations [23].

4.6.1 Functional food

The idea was first introduced in Japan in the 1980s when the Ministry of Health and Welfare implemented a regulatory system in the face of rising health care costs to permit such foods with reported health benefits to improve the aging population's health. Foods for Specified Health Use recognizes as foods that are eligible to tolerate a distinct seal [24].

Functional foods have no such regulatory identity in the United States. However, for this modern type of food, many groups have suggested definitions.

Food and Nutrition Board (FNB) of the National Academies of Sciences specified functional foods in 1994 as any altered food or food ingredient that may provide a health advantage beyond the traditional nutrients it contains [25].

The International Life Sciences Institute describes them as "diets that provide a health advantage beyond basic nutrition in the presence of physiologically active components." The American Dietetic Association defined functional foods in a 1999 position paper as foods that are whole, fortified, enriched, or developed but more importantly, states that such foods must be ingested [24].

For customers to enjoy their possible health benefits, part of a diverse diet regularly, at appropriate levels'.

Foods with an FDA-approved health claim (sterol or stanol esters, oats, psyllium, soy) are usually backed by two dozen or more reported clinical trials that are well-designed [26].

For example, 40 clinical trials have been included in the soy health claim petition, although there are only a few experimental trials on cranberry juice and urinary tract infections.

4.6.2 Medical foods

A holistic approach to the medicinal food concept derives from the research that foods do not mean to fulfill hunger, provide the body with only necessary macronutrients and micronutrients, and offer bioactive ingredients. They help minimize diseases linked to diet and ensure physical and mental well-being [27]. On the other hand, nutraceutical food means "food or part of food that provides medical or health benefits, including disease prevention and treatment." The critical difference is that nutraceuticals may take as pills, capsules, or tablets in a nonfood matrix form. In contrast, functional or therapeutic foods are considered part of a typical food pattern [28].

For dietary purposes, the consumption and type of medicinal food should limit the usually expected.

4.6.3 Dietary supplements

All of these foods come from old-style health and healing classifications. For this reason, we must differentiate between how nations regulate the practice of medicine and how they control marketed products used in a therapeutic way or as foods, as shown in Figure 4.6. The US method is governed by the states, while the federal government monitors advertised diet and medicinal products in regional trade [27].

4.7 How can nutraceuticals help in recovery?

Nutraceuticals are oral nutritional components naturally found in diets and held to have therapeutic or health benefits. Nutraceuticals derive from pharmaceuticals and nutrition. The name applies to products that are isolated from herbal products, dietary supplements (nutrients), specific diets, and processed foods in addition to nutritional, which also uses for medicinal purposes [5].

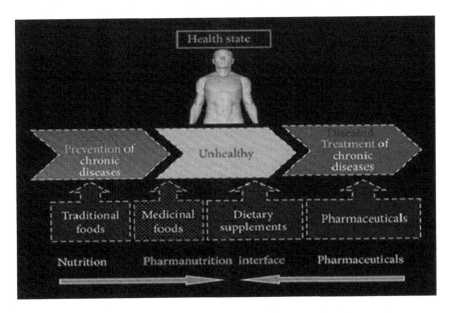

Figure 4.6 Role of nutrition and pharmaceuticals in the health state.

A. **Nutraceuticals can help in recovery or improve energy metabolism with aging**:

Essential (EAAs) or branched-chain amino acids (BCAAs) dietary supplementation controls breakdown and the balance of energy [29].

Many micronutrients have an essential function in energy metabolism, which has various vitamins [thiamine (B1), riboflavin (B2), nicotinic acid, and niacin (B3), pyridoxine (B6), vitamin B12], folic acid, minerals (calcium, phosphorus, magnesium, and trace elements like copper, chromium, iron, manganese, zinc [30]).

Macronutrients can catalyze the released energy (carbohydrates, lipids, and proteins). Vitamins and minerals play a decisive role in energy metabolism; they are vital as functional components of enzymes involved in the release and stored energy [6].

1. **Thiamine (B1)**:

It is vital in glucose breakdown, RNA, DNA, and ATP formation. For energy production, it serves as a cofactor for enzymes that break down glucose [1].

2. **Riboflavin (B2)**:

Flavoproteins are an essential component of riboflavin (B2) in many metabolic pathways and coenzymes intricate in the breakdown of carbohydrates, lipids, and proteins. Reach sources are whole grains, enriched flour products, milk, eggs, plain yogurt, and green leafy vegetables [1].

3. **Niacin (B3)**:

It is present in the form of nicotinamide or nicotinic acid (niacinamide). It is a part of the nicotinamide adenine dinucleotide (NAD) coenzyme. Its phosphorylated form (NADP) is intricate in carbohydrate catabolism or metabolism and produces energy.

Safe sources include whole grains, fortified flour, beef, eggs, peanuts, legumes, and protein-containing tryptophan, such as meat and poultry [1].

4. **Pantothenic acid (B5)**:

Coenzyme A, which is active in lipid, cholesterol, and acetylcholine synthesis, forms pantothenic acid. Pantothenic acid present in all foods, but whole grains, oats, tomatoes, broccoli, meat, particularly chicken, milk, egg yolks, and sunflower seeds are better sources [1].

5. **Pyridoxine (B6)**:

It plays a role in the synthesis and catabolism of amino acids. It also releases glucose from glycogen in glycogenolysis's catabolic process and is essential by enzymes for synthesizing multiple neurotransmitters and hemoglobin. A good source includes poultry such as chicken or turkey, peanuts, soya beans, wheat gram, oats, meats, potatoes, and bananas [1].

6. **Biotin (B7)**:
   This vitamin assists in glucose, fat and protein metabolism, and amino acid synthesis. Excellent dietary sources: meat, fish, milk, egg yolks, and peanut. Biotin is also present in many foods, but only at deficient levels [1].

7. **Folate**:
   Folate is an essential coenzyme for the amino acid methionine synthesis and the development of RNA and DNA. Rapidly dividing cells are, thus, most exaggerated by folate deficit. WBC, RBC, and platelets incessantly produce in the bone marrow from distributing stem cells. The excellent sources include broccoli, brussels sprouts, green leafy vegetables, cabbage, kale, spring greens and spinach, peas, sunflower seeds, and orange juice [1].

8. **Cobalamin (B12)**:
   Cobalamin contains cobalt and is also the only vitamin encompassing a metal ion. Cobalamin is a vital coenzyme element. Catabolism of fats and proteins, the activity of folate coenzymes, and synthesis of hemoglobin require it. Malabsorption of vitamin B12 is most common in older individuals who may have weakened the digestive organ's function, a natural compound of old age. Good sources of nutraceuticals are animal-derived foods and fortified breakfast cereals [1].

B. **Nutraceuticals can give the body the extra push needed to increase energy metabolism**:
   Metabolism is the capacity of the body to break food down into energy. The energy used to keep all organs working and metabolism may impair inadequate nutrition that works appropriately [5].

   Nutraceuticals supplements (minerals) that increase the metabolism are given below.

1. **Iron**:
   Iron transforms energy too nutrients and helps transport oxygen to the body's cells. The more oxygen the cell has, the more fat that cells can burn [3].

   Familiar sources of iron include spinach, shellfish, lean meats, and beans.

2. **Magnesium**:
   Magnesium is essential for the production of energy and encompasses a broad range of enzyme reactions. Common sources of magnesium include nuts, green leafy vegetables, and seeds [3].

3. **Acetyl L-carnitine**:
   Acetyl L-carnitine affects mitochondrial function and energy metabolism. Familiar sources of acetyl L-carnitine include meat and fish [1].

   Nutrition can be enhanced, and energy metabolism is increased by supplements such as iron and acetyl L-carnitine [31].

4. **Micronutrients with multiple phenol groups are polyphenols**:
   The polyphenol present in red cabbage, spinach, fruit, red grapes, wine, and peanuts is resveratrol adding to its influence on sirtuins and the breakdown of carbohydrates lipids. On the gut microbiome, resveratrol may have beneficial effects. It can improve the intestine function, activate metabolites in the intestinal tract, and arbitrate microflora's biotransformation in the gut [31].
5. Many other natural plant-derived polyphenols, with thyme, chime, and chrysin, have been shown to boost lipolysis magnolol and honokiol components of bark extract in Asian trees. It's been used for therapeutic purposes and includes sources of dietary polyphenols that may offer a possible safe treatment option for having lipolysis in overweight patients by provoking the SNS and starting the WAT [31].
6. Green tea extraction contains epigallocatechin gallate can provoke thermogenesis to facilitate weight control. This outcome is most assumed due to the inhibition of norepinephrine degradation and the substantial increase in BAT sympathetic stimulation [32].

4.8 Conclusion

The effects of fruit or plant extract nutraceuticals on minimizing oxidative damage and encouraging safe aging in invertebrate models demonstrate numerous studies. In nutraceuticals, the active ingredients that plants generally produce as secondary composites seem to support plants withstand traumatic circumstances. Numerous phytochemicals, for example, flavonoids, anthocyanin glycosides, triterpenoids, and proanthocyanidin oligomers, partner nutraceutical valuable properties.

Nutraceuticals do not have an official legal definition, but conventional foods, nutritional supplements, and medicinal diets may be generally defined. There is no authorized aspect of nutraceuticals and functional foods, but they are identifiable as conventional food items and are different from other nutraceuticals. On the other hand, dietary supplements are legally specified, precisely specifying, amid other criteria, that a substance classified as a dietary supplement must not signify traditional food.

Medical foods, the final category, can be differentiated from functional foods and dietary supplements by requiring that medicinal foods fulfill an illness or disease's specific nutritional criteria. Medicinal foods must be food for oral or tube feeding. They must be labeled for the healthy management of a particular medical disorder, disease, or state for recognized dietary criteria and projected for medically controlled practice.

References

1. E. Huskisson, S. Maggini, M. Ruf, The role of vitamins and minerals in energy metabolism and well-being, *J. Int. Med. Res.* 35 (2007) 277–289. doi:10.1177/147323000703500301.

2. JTLVM Manore, *The Science of Nutrition*, 4th ed., Pearson, 2017. https://www.vitalsource.com/educators/products/the-science-of-nutrition-janice-thompson-linda-v9780135351123?term=9780135351123.

3. Byerley, Apus : An introduction to nutrition, libretexts-medicine. (2020) 244–278.

4. B. Lindshield, New prairie press Kansas State University Human Nutrition (FNDH 400) flexbook, 2018. https://newprairiepress.org/ebooks/19/.

5. S.B. Roberts, I. Rosenberg, Nutrition and aging: Changes in the regulation of energy metabolism with aging, *Physiol. Rev.* 86 (2006) 651–667. doi:10.1152/physrev.00019.2005.

6. A. Bartke, S. Brannan, E. Hascup, K. Hascup, J. Darcy, Energy metabolism, and aging, *World J. Men's. Health.* 38 (2020) 1–11. doi:10.5534/wjmh.200112.

7. S.B. Roberts, G.E. Dallal, Energy requirements and aging, *Public Health Nutr.* 8 (2005) 1028–1036. doi:10.1079/PHN2005794.

8. I. Bratic, A. Trifunovic, Mitochondrial energy metabolism and aging, *Biochim. Biophys. Acta - Bioenerg.* 1797 (2010) 961–967. doi:10.1016/j.bbabio.2010.01.004.

9. R. Starling, E. Poehlman, Assessment of energy requirements in elderly populations, *Eur. J. Clin. Nutr.* 54 (2000) S104–S111. doi:10.1038/sj.ejcn.1601031.

10. JVGA Durnin, Energy Metabolism in the Elderly, *Nature.* 29 (1992) 51–63.

11. Z. Feng, R.W. Hanson, N.A. Berger, A. Trubitsyn, Reprogramming of energy metabolism as a driver of aging, *Oncotarget.* 7 (2016) 15410–15420. doi:10.18632/oncotarget.7645.

12. P. Ritz, Factors affecting energy and macronutrient requirements in elderly people, *Public Health Nutr.* 4 (2001) 561–568. doi:10.1079/PHN2001141.

13. T.P.J. Solomon, C.M. Marchetti, R.K. Krishnan, F. Gonzalez, J.P. Kirwan, Effects of aging on basal fat oxidation in obese humans, *Metabolism.* 57 (2008) 1141–1147. doi:10.1016/j.metabol.2008.03.021.

14. C. López-Otín, L. Galluzzi, J.M.P. Freije, F. Madeo, G. Kroemer, Metabolic control of longevity, *Cell.* 166 (2016) 802–821. doi:10.1016/j.cell.2016.07.031.

15. V. Azzu, T.G. Valencak, Energy metabolism and ageing in the mouse: A mini-review, *Gerontology.* 63 (2017) 327–336. doi:10.1159/000454924.

16. A.K. Kant, B.I. Graubard, Eating out in America, 1987-2000: Trends and nutritional correlates, *Prev. Med. (Baltim).* 38 (2004) 243–249. doi:10.1016/j.ypmed.2003.10.004.

17. T. Kaneda, S. Makino, M. Nishiyama, K. Asaba, K. Hashimoto, Differential neuropeptide responses to starvation with aging, *J. Neuroendocrinol.* 13 (2001) 1066–1075. doi:10.1046/j.1365-2826.2001.00730.x.

18. S.B. Roberts, High-glycemic index foods, hunger, and obesity: Is there a connection? *Nutr. Rev.* 58 (2000) 163–169. doi:10.1111/j.1753-4887.2000.tb01855.x.

19. S. Boghossian, C. Veyrat-Durebex, J. Alliot, Age-related changes in adaptive macronutrient intake in swimming male and female Lou rats, *Physiol. Behav.* 69 (2000) 231–238. doi:10.1016/S0031-9384(99)00233-4.

20. BA. Horwitz, C.A. Blanton, R.B. McDonald, Physiologic determinants of the anorexia of aging: Insights from animal studies, *Annu. Rev. Nutr.* 22 (2002) 417–438. doi:10.1146/annurev.nutr.22.120301.071049.

21. R. Ren, A. Ocampo, G.-H. Liu, J.C. Izpisua Belmonte, Regulation of stem cell aging by metabolism and epigenetics, *Cell Metab.* 26 (2017) 460–474. doi:10.1016/j.cmet.2017.07.019.

22. P.J. Scarpace, M. Matheny, Y. Zhang, N. Tümer, C.D. Frase, E.W. Shek, B. Hong, V. Prima, S. Zolotukhin, Central Leptin gene delivery evokes persistent Leptin signal transduction in young and aged-obese rats, but physiological responses become attenuated over time in aged-obese rats, *Neuropharmacology.* 42 (2002) 548–561. doi:10.1016/s0028-3908(02)00003-5.

23. J. Dwyer, P. Coates, M. Smith, Dietary supplements: Regulatory challenges and research resources, *Nutrients.* 10 (2018) 41. doi:10.3390/nu10010041.

24. A. Cencic, W. Chingwaru, The role of functional foods, nutraceuticals, and food supplements in intestinal health, *Nutrients.* 2 (2010) 611–625. doi:10.3390/nu2060611.

25. S. Roberts, Regulation of energy intake in relation to metabolic state and nutritional status, *Eur. J. Clin. Nutr.* 54 (2000) S64–S69. doi:10.1038/sj.ejcn.1601027.

26. C.M. Hasler, Functional foods: Benefits, concerns, and challenges—A position paper from the American Council on Science and Health, *J. Nutr.* 132 (2002) 3772–3781. doi:10.1093/jn/132.12.3772.

27. N. Ramalingam, M.F. Mahomoodally, The therapeutic potential of medicinal foods, *Adv. Pharmacol. Sci.* 2014 (2014) 1–18. doi:10.1155/2014/354264.

28. C. Gupta, D. Prakash, Nutraceuticals for geriatrics, *J. Tradit. Complement. Med.* 5 (2015) 5–14. doi:10.1016/j.jtcme.2014.10.004.

29. B. Chelluboina, R. Vemuganti, Therapeutic potential of nutraceuticals to protect the brain after stroke, *Neurochem. Int.* 142 (2021) 104908. doi:10.1016/j.neuint.2020.104908.

30. H.H.V. Michael, J. Gibney, S.A. Lanham-New, A. Cassidy, *Introduction to Human Nutrition*, Wiley-Blackwell, 2013. https://www.wiley.com/en-in/9781118684702.

31. F. Bifari, C. Ruocco, I. Decimo, G. Fumagalli, A. Valerio, E. Nisoli, Amino acid supplements, and metabolic health: a potential interplay between intestinal microbiota and systems control, *Genes Nutr.* 12 (2017) 27. doi:10.1186/s12263-017-0582-2.

32. KK. Karna, Y.S. Shin, B.R. Choi, H.K. Kim, J.K. Park, The role of endoplasmic reticulum stress response in male reproductive physiology and pathology: A review, *World J. Men's. Health.* 37 (2019) 484. doi:10.5534/WJMH.190038.

5

Neurodegenerative and Cognition Losses during Aging (Memory) and Nutraceuticals

Reza Ghiasvand
Isfahan University of Medical Sciences

Shima Abdollahi
North Khorasan University of Medical Sciences

Sahar Saraf-Bank
Isfahan University of Medical Sciences

Contents

5.1 What are the neurodegenerative and cognition losses during aging?

Life expectancy for men and women has increased over the past century, and it is estimated that the US population over the age of 65 rose to ~120% between 2010 and 2050 [1]. As the population ages, age-related health complications and the need for effective prevention and treatment strategies will increase. Although cardiovascular diseases are still the leading cause of death in the elderly [2], age-related neurodegenerative disorders are among the top causes of death, with no definitive treatment [3].

DOI: 10.1201/9781003110866-5

Aging affects the nervous system, as well as all organs, including neuronal structure alterations, dismantling of synapses, impairment in connectivity of neuronal networks, and cognitive decline corresponding to disability and dependency in older people [4]. Although the exact reason is not yet fully understood, there are several factors contributing to cumulative brain damage. Possible factors include trauma, inflammation, cerebrovascular ischemia [5], heavy alcohol drink, hormonal changes [6,7], oxidative stress, cardiovascular disease risk factors such as hypertension, diabetes and obesity, and genetic (for instance, *APOE4* genotype) and neurodegenerative disorders such as Alzheimer's disease (AD). Increasing accumulation of two abnormal proteins called beta-amyloid plaques and tau tangles in neurons are also associated with neuron loss and brain shrink [8,9].

It is not well-known whether the neurodegeneration accelerates aging or aging leads to this process; however, studies showed that the prevalence of Alzheimer's and Parkinson's diseases – the most common neurodegenerative diseases – continues to rise with increasing age [10,11]. Brain size and function gradually decrease with increasing age, and it intensifies after 50 years [12]. At the 60-year threshold, most people become increasingly susceptible to neurological disorder disease [13–15]. In 2020, it is reported that 5.8 million Americans suffered from AD, of which 17% are in the age group of 65–74, and 47% are in the age group of 75–84 years [3].

Some cognitive abilities related to skills, historical memories, procedural memories, vocabulary and general information are not affected by normal aging and even may improve through the life. In contrast, some other abilities steadily decline with age [16], including retrieval of new information, process speed, language, numerical ability, visuospatial judgment [17] and executive functions [18] involving problem-solving, attention and focus on multitasks. There are also age-related declines in aspects of concept formation and mental flexibility, especially in subjects over 70 years [17]. These changes are usually mild and undetectable in onset but gradually develop and get revealed to family members and close friends. As the disease progresses, walking, swallowing and everyday activities are affected, and full-blown dementia may accrue [19]. However, severe memory loss is not considered as a consequence of the normal aging process.

Patients with dementia are exposed to several behavioral and psychological complications, including delirium, falls, accidents, fractures and infections. They may also forget to take medication, which may lead to worsen comorbidities. They are at the risk of malnutrition due to forgetting to eat and inability to prepare foods. Loneliness and social isolation also put these people at the risk of depression. The complicated condition of demented patients affects also the health of their family caregivers, and they may experience increased anxiety, depression, chronic fatigue and sleep disorders [20]. The quality of life for both patients and caregivers is decrease by dementia. Caring for these patients is costly and may expose them to abandonment. The global burden of neurodegenerative diseases has outpaced that of cancer and cardiovascular disease [21,22]. Therefore, appropriate medical, psychological and social services are necessary for both.

The age-related neurodegeneration has currently no cure. However, there is emerging evidence that healthy lifestyle may slow down late-life neurodegeneration, including healthy food choices, exercise, stress management, cognitive activation, management of weight and comorbidities [23]. Any approach that could delay the onset of age-related cognition impairment would increase the quality of life and reduce the cost of treatment of millions of older adults worldwide. In particular, the neuroprotection effects of nutraceuticals have been the subject of considerable attention, recently. Several of these are discussed below.

5.2 Omega-3 fatty acids

Long-chain polyunsaturated fatty acids (LC-PUFAs), notably EPA (eicosapentaenoic acid, 20:5n-3), and DHA (docosahexaenoic acid, 22:6n-3)-essential nutrients in human are being increasingly investigated because of their role in the stability of neuron cell membranes and their antioxidant properties [24,25]. There are growing evidence suggesting inverse association between n-3 LC-PUFAs levels and brain shrink or cognitive impairment [26], and protective effects on depression [27], AD [28] and lower atrophy of cerebral cortex [29]. A healthy brain is high in fatty acids, and DHA – a key component of brain cell membranes [30] – plays a critical role in brain metabolism. *In vitro* studies suggested that lower levels of DHA may affect cortical and hippocampal neural networks, and areas related to memory [31,32]. Studies have shown that n-3 LC-PUFAs exhibit beneficial effects on memory and learning through improvement in neuronal cell membranes, synaptic consolidation processes, neurogenesis and neurotransmission and modulate expression of glutamate receptors [33]. It is also showed DHA increases brain-derived neurotrophic factor (BDNF) and grows hippocampal volume [34]. Moreover, DHA may reduce the production of the β-amyloid peptide and modulate tau phosphorylation by inhibiting glycogen synthase kinase 3, leading to lower aggregation of the abnormal proteins in the brain [35]. EPA also has been shown to be effective in modulating proinflammatory cytokines in neuronal tissue of patients with Alzheimer's [36]. Devassy et al. concluded that EPA may have beneficial effects on mood disorders, while DHA appears more efficient in integrity of brain structures [37]. Plant-based n-3 LC-PUFAs such as alpha-linolenic acid (ALA) have also been investigated and revealed to have significant neuroprotection by anti-apoptotic properties [38], cerebrovascular flow improvement [39], inhibition of microglia activation [40] and increased learning ability [41] and functional outcomes [42].

However, some others showed no effectiveness of n-3 LC-PUFAs on cognition and make it difficult to draw a conclusion [43,44]. A meta-analysis of clinical trials concluded that n-3 LC-PUFAs may significantly improve cognitive development in infants but do not appear to benefit cognitive performance or prevent neurodegeneration disorders during the remaining lifespan [45]. Although there is insufficient evidence to recommend the use of omega-3 supplements to prevent or treat age-related neurodegenerative disorders, a meta-analysis of cohort studies resulted that each one serving/week increment of fish intake was associated with 5% and 7% lower risk of dementia and Alzheimer's diseases, respectively [46]. The 2013 International Conference on Nutrition and the Brain also recommends modifying dietary fat intake to increase omega-3 PUFAs to prevent AD [47].

5.3 Polyphenols

Polyphenols are plant-derived compounds that protect them against reactive oxygen species (ROS), pathogens and other damages [48]. Studies are describing the beneficial effects of polyphenols on age-related cognitive decline and synaptic plasticity and promote neurogenesis [49,50] by antioxidant activities [51] and inhibiting neural death [52]. Higher consumption of oxygen by brain tissue makes it more vulnerable to oxidative damage [53], and polyphenols with high antioxidant properties can protect against brain damage and the neurodegenerative process. Accumulation of oxidative stress damages over time, and the simultaneous reduction of antioxidant mechanisms is one of the accepted theories in the process of brain aging [54,55]. ROS also can increase β-amyloid production and contribute to the progression of AD [56]. Polyphenols due to the presence of aromatic rings bound to hydroxyl groups in their biochemical structure can directly scavenger active species by donating hydrogen atom or electrons [51]. Moreover, polyphenolic compounds can reduce ROS by inhibiting enzymes involved in their production, including monoamine oxidase [57]. Some of these phytochemicals also can make pro-oxidant metals inaccessible by chelating these ions, such as cooper, zinc and iron, partially responsible for oxidative damage and neurotoxicity, etc. [58].

5.4 Flavonoids

Flavonoids are the most abundant polyphenols found naturally in plants [59]. There are six subclasses of flavonoids, including flavonols, flavones, flavanols, isoflavones, anthocyanidins and flavanones. More than 4,000 flavonoids have been found in various plant species [60]. There is enormous evidence supporting cognitive benefits of flavonoids. Higher flavonoid intake is associated with better memory and cognitive performance in middle and older adults [61,62], and it may also slower cognitive decline [62]. Moreover, it seems that higher intake of flavonoids also delays the onset of Alzheimer, in *APOE4* carriers [63]. Animal studies showed beneficial effects of blueberry as a rich source of flavonoids on spatial memory [64], recognition memory

[65], learning [66], long-term memory and short-term memory [64,67]. A long-term prospective human study also revealed that higher intake of berries was associated with slower rate of cognitive decline and may delay cognitive aging for 2.5 years [68].

It is reported that the incidence of neurodegenerative diseases in people who drink wine 3–4 glasses a day is 80% lower than in people who drink less [69]. Resveratrol (3,4′,5-trihydroxystilbene; $C_{14}H_{12}O_3$), a natural polyphenol, seems to be responsible for the antioxidant properties of red wine. It is also found in peanuts, grapes, berries and dark chocolate [70]. There are several trials supporting the beneficial effects of resveratrol in neurodegenerative diseases [71,72]. It seems that resveratrol induces its metabolic effects through a variety of pathways. It has been shown that silent informationregulator-1 (SIRT1) is one of the targets of resveratrol [73]. This protein plays an essential role in neural cell growth, synaptic plasticity, learning and memory and prevents neural death [74,75] by its nicotinamide adenine dinucleotide (NAD)-dependent deacetylation activities [76]. It is also reported that β-amyloid production elevates when SIRT1 expression decreases [76], and overexpression of SIRT1 can suppress β-amyloid production [77]. SIRT1 exerts this effect by upregulating secretase gene, an enzyme that breaks down the amyloid precursor protein [78]. Peroxisome proliferator-activated receptor gamma coactivator 1-alpha (PGC-1α), p53 and forkhead box O (FOXO) also are deacetylated by SIRT1, resulting in mitochondrial function improvement, inhibition β-amyloid aggregation [79], reduction in inflammation and neuronal apoptosis [80,81]. The anti-inflammatory effects of resveratrol are also mediated by inhibiting signaling pathways including nuclear factor-κB (NF-κB), extracellular signal-regulated kinase-1 and kinase-2, and mitogen-activated protein kinase (MAPK) [82].

Another subgroup of flavonoids is anthocyanins, which are responsible for the red, purple and blue color of fruits [83]. Studies have demonstrated that dietary anthocyanins can reduce age-related learning decline [84,85], improve cognition performance [86,87], protect stress-induced cerebral damage [88] and increase activity in brain regions associated with cognition [89]. These studies indicated that neuroprotective effects of anthocyanins are mainly related to their antioxidant properties. Anthocyanins have been shown to directly increase glutathione peroxidase activity and indirectly increase detoxification enzymes, such as superoxide dismutase by modulating nuclear factor erythroid 2-related factor 2 (Nrf2) activity, a master regulator of antioxidant genes [90,91]. Besides, pro-inflammatory pathways including c-Jun-N-terminal kinase (JNK), p38-mitogen activated protein kinase (p38-MAPK), extracellular signal-regulated kinase 1/2 (ERK1/2) and Akt also attenuate by anthocyanin treatment, contributing to NF-κB downregulation and pro-inflammatory genes consequently [92,93].

Quercetin, myricetin, catechins, etc. are other most common flavonoids. Recently, quercetin – found in onions, broccoli and leeks – has been reported to exert preventive effects against neuronal loss [94], improve memory, learning

[95], mitochondrial function, AMP-activated protein kinase activity and ATP production and ameliorate cognitive defect when administered in mice with AD [96]. These studies indicated that the beneficial effects of quercetin may be attributed to decreased malondialdehyde [97], nitrite [98], lipid peroxidation [98], acetylcholinesterase activity [99] and enhanced expression of BDNF [100], cerebral blood flow [97] and glutathione [97] in brain. However, results from human studies are controversial [101].

Myricetin, another lipophilic flavonoid in fruits and vegetables, also has shown neuronal protective effects through its antioxidant activities, anti-apoptotic properties and iron-chelating capability [102]. It may also promote neuronal recovery, hippocampal neurogenesis, learning, memory and cognition [103].

Catechins such as epicatechin, epigallocatechin gallate, epigallocatechin and others are natural flavonoids found mostly in tea leaves, one of the most consumed beverages [104]. Meta-analysis studies found that higher intake of tea was associated with 35% reduction in risk of cognitive disorders [105] and 26% reduction in Parkinson's disease [106]. It is reported that catechins may produce favorable effects on cognition performance by inactivating inflammatory signaling pathways and preventing neuronal apoptosis [107]. Moreover, in a trial, epigallocatechin gallate increased cerebral blood flow and cerebral activity [108]. Since loss of dopaminergic neurons is known as a suspected cause of the cognitive impairment, catechins may have a protection role by increasing catecholamine levels [109]. Moreover, it is suggested that catechins may exhibit anxiolytic, relaxation and mindfulness properties through binding to the gamma-aminobutyric acid (GABA) receptors [110]. Other potential mechanisms are related to enhancing endothelial functions [111] and inhibiting copper or iron-β amyloid complex formation as a chelator of redox-active metals [112].

5.5 Carotenoids

The neural tissue is one of the tissues that are particularly exposed to oxidative stress. This happens because of the high oxygen demand in the nervous system. The brain, which contains only 2% of an adult's body weight, consumes nearly 20% of the oxygen received by the system. In addition, intensive oxygen metabolism leads to increased production of ROS, which is formed as a by-product of cellular respiration [113].

The cell membranes of neurons are rich in polyunsaturated fatty acids, so they are sensitive to oxidation. Moreover, the neural tissue in the central nervous system has a poor ability to repair, which prevents its normal regeneration and function after damage caused by ROS [114].

High metabolic activity combined with the PUFA-rich structure makes the brain very vulnerable to oxidative stress. In addition, an increase in DHA oxidation has been observed in patients with dementia and cognitive impairment [115]. Age-related cognitive functions might be affected by dietary patterns and eating habits [116].

Carotenoids are a broad group of natural pigments, usually red, orange or yellow, of which more than 750 compounds have been identified. Carotenoids that have 9–11 conjugated double bonds exhibit strong antioxidant effects on singlet oxygen. Although humans are not able to synthesize carotenoids, they need them for various functions [117].

There are two classification methods for carotenoids: (i) oxygen-based: carotenes (oxygen-free) and xanthophylls (oxygen-containing) [118], and (ii) based on provitamin A: provitamin A (β-carotene and β-cryptoxanthin) and non-provitamin A carotenoids (lycopene and lutein). Provitamin A group of carotenoids can convert to retinal [119].

AD is one of the most serious neurodegenerative disorders characterized by an increase in amyloid-β (Aβ), which is formed by the breakdown of amyloid precursor proteins by β- and γ-secretase [120]. Carotenoids such as lutein, lycopene, astaxanthin, β-cryptoxanthin and fucoxanthin have been shown to prevent Aβ42 aggregation. In this context, lutein has the highest activity in inhibiting accumulation of Aβ42 rather than zeaxanthin, β-cryptoxanthin and β-carotene. This result hypothesized that the number of hydroxyl groups may play an important role in inhibiting Aβ aggregation [121]. Lakey-Beitia et al. have shown that lutein is the most potent carotenoid against Aβ accumulation [122].

Cognitive functions are mental processes that consist of memory, attention, processing speed and executive function [123]. Lutein/zeaxanthin supplementation improves cognition in young adults. Lieblin-Buff et al. have suggested that lutein is associated with major neurotransmitters (such as glutamate and γ-aminobutyric acid) that are well known to affect cognition [124]. Unlike nonpolar carotenoids (β-carotene and lycopene), lutein has polar groups at the end of the molecule that probably causes the molecule to be placed perpendicular or semi-perpendicular to the surface of the membrane [125,126]. This is in line with the evidence that lutein is located in the PUFA-rich membrane domain (including DHA) and specifies that the presence of lutein in membranes is to prevent the oxidation of these brain fats [127,128]. This accumulation in the brain is thought to be due to the presence of a specific lutein-binding protein [129]. Lutein is one of the major carotenoids in human brain tissue [130]. It is selectively distributed in the frontal cortex, visual cortex and hippocampus [124]. Lutein, found in dark green leafy vegetables, corn, eggs and avocados, as well as its isomer, zeaxanthin, can cross the blood-retina barrier and blood-brain barrier (BBB). Therefore, they have antioxidant and anti-inflammatory functions directly in the eyes and the brain [131]. A recent study reported that lutein consumption for 6 months elevated total antioxidant capacity and BDNF in young adults [132]. Since inflammation affects BDNF expression, BDNF levels are considered an anti-inflammatory biomarker [133]. A review article showed that the effective doses of lutein and astaxanthin to affect cognitive function are very different from the average daily intake of the diet. The amount of lutein in the diet is about 2 mg/day, while in the trial studies 12 mg of lutein per day has been shown to be effective [133]. Astaxanthin is a ketocarotenoid found in crustacean shells. Its function as a free radical scavenger is to protect neurons from apoptosis by reducing caspase-3 activity and enhancement of neurogenesis by affecting mitogen-activated kinases [134,135]. Lee et al. found that astaxanthin could prevent nitric oxide production both in vitro and in vivo [136].

Lycopene with its acyclic and highly conjugated structure can inhibit Aβ42 formation. Wang et al. showed that lycopene with its antioxidant properties and suppressing the activation of microglia can reduce the Aβ aggregation and inhibit the inflammatory response. In addition, lycopene has been shown to improve cognitive deficits by reducing the inflammation in the intestinal-liver-brain axis as well as improving glycolipid metabolism [137]. Other mechanisms of lycopene include inhibition of neural apoptosis and restoration of mitochondrial function, which provides neurocognitive protection [138]. Research carried out by Rahman and Rhim has shown that apart from ensuring that ROS is reduced by lycopene, this carotenoid has a reducing effect on the risk of b-amyloid, tau protein and a-synuclein deposit [139]. It is worth noting that these misfolded proteins have a crucial role in AD and Parkinson's disease [140].

However, the precise mechanisms by which carotenoids may affect neural health across the lifespan remain unclear. Moreover, associations by race/ethnicity and other personal characteristics are not well-evaluated, but given the sum of evidence so far and low dietary intake, it is necessary to try to establish the recommended intake for this group of nutrients.

5.6 Probiotics

A normal aging process is associated with physiologic changes in the central nervous system. In this life cycle, reduced cognition and memory and mood disorders are common among the elderly [141,142]. Change of gut microbiota composition and function (proteolytic bacteria elevation and saccharolytic bacteria reduction) can affect the health status of subjects during aging [143,144]. Based on the gut-brain-axis concept, any intestinal dysbiosis influences cognition, learning and memory status [145]. Therefore, keeping the intestinal microbiota balance is an important strategy for a healthy late life [146,147]. Several factors can affect gut microbiota [148]. Manipulation of dietary factors is considered as a potential approach to increase brain health and function particularly cognition and memory through gut-brain-axis modification [149].

It is shown that supplementation of probiotics – live microorganisms – can improve CNS (central nervous system) function and exert an influence on

CNS-related disorders (such as cognitive impairment) through its anti-inflammatory and immunomodulatory properties [150,151]. Several previous studies have evaluated the potential effects of probiotic consumption either from the supplement or enriched foods on cognition loss [148,151–154].

It is proposed that probiotic supplementation can improve cognitive function and mood status through neurotransmitters and neurochemical production [155]. Neurotransmitters like serotonin [156] and dopamine [157] and neurochemicals like BDNF [158] are attributed to cognitive deficit prevention. Chronic low-grade inflammation is a feature of normal aging and may be an important factor in neuroinflammation and progression of neurodegenerative disorders, particularly cognitive impairment [155,159]. Probiotics with their anti-inflammatory effect can eliminate the activation of brain resident macrophage known as microglia, which has an important role in inflammatory cytokine increment in the brain [160]. Also, probiotic supplementation can be considered an efficient approach to control severe anxiety and depression (a prevalent problem among this population) that has a linear association with cognitive deficits [161,162].

It must be kept in mind that the number of available clinical trials is limited, and drawing a net conclusion needs performing several clinical trials in healthy older adults and patients who suffered from cognition loss and other neurodegenerative disorders.

5.7 Ginseng

Ginseng is the root of plants of the *Panax* family and one of the most popular herbal remedies. Ginseng has long been used for therapeutic purposes, especially in Asian regions. There are several active agents in ginseng, including ginsenosides, polysaccharides, peptides, vitamins, saponins and enzymes [163]. Ginsenosides are the main active component and responsible for most of the therapeutic effects of ginseng. Growing *in vivo* studies indicated a cognition-enhancing effect of ginseng in animals; however, long-term human evidence is limited. Animal studies found that ginsenosides may enhance cholinergic system's function by increasing choline acetyltransferase activity and inhibition of acetylcholinesterase activity [164], which is contributed to cognition and memory. Early studies found that ginsenoside administration in mice significantly improved the thickness of cortex, synapse density [165] and proliferation in the hippocampal region [166], the region related to the short-term and long-term memory. Furthermore, there is some evidence suggesting that ginseng may be a cognitive enhancer by reducing amyloid plaque deposition [167]. It is also reported that ginseng can increase neurotransmitters such as dopamine and serotonin in the brain, associated with its anti-depressant effects [168]. Human trials also reported the beneficial effect of ginseng on cognitive function and memory [169]. Moreover, other neuroprotective mechanisms including inhibition of the expression of NADPH oxidase, cyclooxygenase-2, TNF-α, IL-1β and IL-6 and improvement in Nrf2 and HO-1 antioxidant enzyme activity in brain tissue have also been reported [170,171].

5.8 Garlic

Garlic (*Allium sativum*) belongs to the Allium family and has been widely used in folk medicine, especially for improving immune function and adjuvant treatment of bacterial or fungal infections [172]. Recently, it has been considered for its positive effects on AD. Garlic is a source of various useful biochemicals, including sulfur-containing compounds, allyl thiosulfinates and polyphenols. It is reported that repeated administration of garlic increases brain serotonin and enhances cognitive performance in rats [173]. Garlic is also found to inhibit caspase-3 activation, an enzyme involved in the formation of β-amyloid [174]. Sulfur compounds extracted from garlic also showed anti-inflammatory effects [175]. Investigators indicated that garlic extract can increase a number of antioxidant activities, such as superoxide dismutase (SOD), catalase, glutathione peroxidase and glutathione and also protect β-amyloid-induced neuronal toxicity [176]. Allicin, another active agent in garlic, responsible for the pungent smell, is known to have antioxidative, anticancerous and antibacterial properties [177,178]. It is also shown that Allicin is effective in boosting antioxidant detoxification enzyme activity and amelioration of neuron cell death [179,180]. Moreover, acetylcholinesterase and butyrylcholinesterase are also inhibited by Allicin, leading to increased acetylcholine levels, learning and memory capacity [181]. However, there are limited human studies, and it is not yet clear how much garlic consumption can show its beneficial effects.

5.9 Vitamins

There is growing evidence supporting the protective role of a number of micronutrients in age-related cognition decline [182]. Most of the observed beneficial effects seem to be related to antioxidant properties of nutrients, such as vitamin E, vitamin C, lipoic acid, and coenzyme Q10. Homocysteine levels have been shown to increase with vitamin B deficiency (vitamin B2, vitamin B6, vitamin B12 and folate), which accelerates amyloid and tau protein aggregation and neuronal death, with a direct effect on cognition impairment. It is thought that vitamin B supplementation can improve memory, sensorimotor speed and information processing speed in older adults, partly due to the reduction in homocysteine levels [183–185]. Homocysteine also can induce neurotoxicity through activation of N-methyl-D-aspartate subtype of glutamate receptor, contributed to brain damage [186]. There is also some evidence indicating that vitamin B supplementation can slow down the rate of brain atrophy and cognitive decline in adults with mild cognitive impairment [187–189].

Recently, studies suggested a pivotal role of vitamin D in the etiology of cognitive dysfunction and all-cause dementia [190]. *In vitro* studies showed that vitamin D increases the clearance of the β-amyloid plaques, by stimulating macrophages [191], and vitamin D deficiency is linked to brain atrophy [192]. Additionally, vitamin D may act as a neuroprotection agent, by regulating nerve growth factor neurotrophin, glial cell-derived neurotrophic factor and choline acetyl transferase production. The EPIDOS cohort study also found that vitamin D deficiency predicted the onset of non-Alzheimer dementias in older women [193]. A meta-analysis also showed that patients with AD have lower concentration of vitamin D, compared to control group [194].

As one of the most popular mechanisms proposed for aging is oxidative pathways, antioxidants can mediate several beneficial effects on redox oxidative pathways. Rotterdam study showed an association between higher vitamin C intake and lower risk of AD [195]. A meta-analysis study also found that higher intake of dietary vitamin C, E and β-carotene is associated with lower risk of AD, with the most protective effects of vitamin E [196]. However, a large 6-year trial found no significant effect of vitamin E, selenium supplementation on AD prevention [197]. These antioxidants are involved in the biosynthesis of catecholamines, myelin formation, synaptic function, scavenging activity against ROS, suppressing inflammatory mediators by inhibiting MAPK and NF-κB signaling pathways, reduction of glutamate toxicity and cytotoxicity of β-amyloid by chelating metals [198–203].

Neurodegenerative diseases are one of the late-life diseases, whose prevalence continues to increase with increasing age. However, there is no definitive treatment for it, and interventions are being done to improve the quality of life. Among different approaches, the role of diet and nutrients as a preventive tool for cognitive decline has been an object of intensive research in the last years. However, most of the studies conducted in vitro were trial in design. Obviously, the dose of the nutrients was much higher than the amounts in foods, and their bioavailability has not been considered in these studies. However, since oxidative damage is one of the proposed mechanisms of age-related neurodegeneration, it seems that diets rich in antioxidants can have beneficial effects in improvement or delaying the onset of the diseases.

References

1. Vincent GK, Velkoff VA. The next four decades: The older population in the United States: 2010 to 2050: US Department of Commerce, Economics and Statistics Administration, US; 2010.
2. Cross SH, Warraich HJ. Changes in the place of death in the United States. *New England Journal of Medicine.* 2019;381(24):2369–70.
3. 2020 Alzheimer's disease facts and figures. ALZHEIMER'S ASSOCIATION REPORT. 2020;16(3):391–460.
4. Bishop NA, Lu T, Yankner BA. Neural mechanisms of ageing and cognitive decline. *Nature.* 2010;464(7288):529–35.

5. Pluta R, Ulamek-Koziol M, awomir Januszewski SÂÂÂ, Czuczwar SJ. From brain ischemia to Alzheimer-like neurodegeneration. 2018.
6. Compton J, Van Amelsvoort T, Murphy D. HRT and its effect on normal ageing of the brain and dementia. *British Journal of Clinical Pharmacology.* 2001; 52(6):647–53.
7. van Dam PS, Aleman A. Insulin-like growth factor-I, cognition and brain aging. *European Journal of Pharmacology.* 2004;490(1–3):87–95.
8. Hanseeuw BJ, Betensky RA, Jacobs HI, Schultz AP, Sepulcre J, Becker JA, et al. Association of amyloid and tau with cognition in preclinical Alzheimer disease: A longitudinal study. *JAMA Neurology.* 2019;76(8):915–24.
9. Sato C, Barthélemy NR, Mawuenyega KG, Patterson BW, Gordon BA, Jockel-Balsarotti J, et al. Tau kinetics in neurons and the human central nervous system. *Neuron.* 2018;97(6):1284–98. e7.
10. Mayeux R, Stern Y. Epidemiology of Alzheimer disease. *Cold Spring Harbor Perspectives in Medicine.* 2012;2(8):a006239.
11. Reeve A, Simcox E, Turnbull D. Ageing and Parkinson's disease: Why is advancing age the biggest risk factor? *Ageing Research Reviews.* 2014;14:19–30.
12. Mendonca GV, Pezarat-Correia P, Vaz JR, Silva L, Heffernan KS. Impact of aging on endurance and neuromuscular physical performance: The role of vascular senescence. *Sports Medicine.* 2017;47(4):583–98.
13. Aarsland D, Creese B, Politis M, Chaudhuri KR, Weintraub D, Ballard C. Cognitive decline in Parkinson disease. *Nature Reviews Neurology.* 2017;13(4):217–31.
14. Kalia L, Lang A. Parkinson's disease. *Lancet* [Internet]. 2015;386(9996):896–912.
15. Mattson MP. Addendum: Pathways towards and away from Alzheimer's disease. *Nature.* 2004;431(7004):107.
16. Murman DL. The impact of age on cognition. *Semin Hear.* 2015;36(3):111–121. doi:10.1055/s-0035-1555115
17. Lezak MD, Howieson DB, Loring DW, Hannay H, Fischer JS. *Neuropsychological Assessment (4th edn.).* New York: Oxford University Press. 2004.
18. Salthouse TA. Selective review of cognitive aging. *Journal of the International Neuropsychological Society: JINS.* 2010;16(5):754.
19. Peters R. Ageing and the brain. *Postgraduate Medical Journal.* 2006;82(964):84–8.
20. Guerriero Austrom M, Damush TM, West Hartwell C, Perkins T, Unverzagt F, Boustani M, et al. Development and implementation of nonpharmacologic protocols for the management of patients with Alzheimer's disease and their families in a multiracial primary care setting. *The Gerontologist.* 2004;44(4):548–53.
21. Collins PY, Patel V, Joestl SS, March D, Insel TR, Daar AS, et al. Grand challenges in global mental health. *Nature.* 2011;475(7354):27–30.
22. Luchtman DW, Song C. Cognitive enhancement by omega-3 fatty acids from childhood to old age: Findings from animal and clinical studies. *Neuropharmacology.* 2013;64:550–65.
23. Fotuhi M, Do D, Jack C. Modifiable factors that alter the size of the hippocampus with ageing. *Nature Reviews Neurology.* 2012;8(4):189–202.
24. Dangour AD, Andreeva VA, Sydenham E, Uauy R. Omega 3 fatty acids and cognitive health in older people. *British Journal of Nutrition.* 2012;107(S2):S152–S8.
25. Jiao J, Zhang Y. Transgenic biosynthesis of polyunsaturated fatty acids: a sustainable biochemical engineering approach for making essential fatty acids in plants and animals. *Chemical Reviews.* 2013;113(5):3799–814.
26. Tan Z, Harris W, Beiser A, Au R, Himali J, Debette S, et al. Red blood cell omega-3 fatty acid levels and markers of accelerated brain aging. *Neurology.* 2012;78(9): 658–64.
27. Mocking R, Harmsen I, Assies J, Koeter M, Ruhé H, Schene A. Meta-analysis and meta-regression of omega-3 polyunsaturated fatty acid supplementation for major depressive disorder. *Translational Psychiatry.* 2016;6(3):e756.

28. Eriksdotter M, Vedin I, Falahati F, Freund-Levi Y, Hjorth E, Faxen-Irving G, et al. Plasma fatty acid profiles in relation to cognition and gender in Alzheimer's disease patients during oral omega-3 fatty acid supplementation: The omegad study. *Journal of Alzheimer's Disease*. 2015;48(3):805–12.

29. Daiello LA, Gongvatana A, Dunsiger S, Cohen RA, Ott BR, Initiative AsDN. Association of fish oil supplement use with preservation of brain volume and cognitive function. *Alzheimer's & Dementia*. 2015;11(2):226–35.

30. Arterburn LM, Hall EB, Oken H. Distribution, interconversion, and dose response of n− 3 fatty acids in humans. *The American Journal of Clinical Nutrition*. 2006; 83(6):1467S–76S.

31. Hashimoto M, Hossain S. Neuroprotective and ameliorative actions of polyunsaturated fatty acids against neuronal diseases: beneficial effect of docosahexaenoic acid on cognitive decline in Alzheimer's disease. *Journal of Pharmacological Sciences*. 2011;116(2):150–62.

32. Tanabe Y, Hashimoto M, Sugioka K, Maruyama M, Fujii Y, Hagiwara R, et al. Improvement of spatial cognition with dietary docosahexaenoic acid is associated with an increase in Fos expression in rat CA1 hippocampus. *Clinical and Experimental Pharmacology and Physiology*. 2004;31(10):700–3.

33. Lee LK, Shahar S, Chin A-V, Yusoff NAM. Docosahexaenoic acid-concentrated fish oil supplementation in subjects with mild cognitive impairment (MCI): A 12-month randomised, double-blind, placebo-controlled trial. *Psychopharmacology*. 2013; 225(3):605–12.

34. Fujita S, Ikegaya Y, Nishikawa M, Nishiyama N, Matsuki N. Docosahexaenoic acid improves long-term potentiation attenuated by phospholipase A2 inhibitor in rat hippocampal slices. *British Journal of Pharmacology*. 2001;132(7):1417.

35. Cole GM, Frautschy SA. DHA may prevent age-related dementia. *The Journal of Nutrition*. 2010;140(4):869–74.

36. Serini S, Bizzarro A, Piccioni E, Fasano E, Rossi C, Lauria A, et al. EPA and DHA differentially affect in vitro inflammatory cytokine release by peripheral blood mononuclear cells from Alzheimer's patients. *Current Alzheimer Research*. 2012;9(8):913–23.

37. Devassy JG, Leng S, Gabbs M, Monirujjaman M, Aukema HM. Omega-3 polyunsaturated fatty acids and oxylipins in neuroinflammation and management of Alzheimer disease. *Advances in Nutrition*. 2016;7(5):905–16.

38. Lang-Lazdunski L, Blondeau N, Jarretou G, Lazdunski M, Heurteaux C. Linolenic acid prevents neuronal cell death and paraplegia after transient spinal cord ischemia in rats. *Journal of Vascular Surgery*. 2003;38(3):564–75.

39. Blondeau N, Pétrault O, Manta S, Giordanengo V, Gounon P, Bordet R, et al. Polyunsaturated fatty acids are cerebral vasodilators via the TREK-1 potassium channel. *Circulation Research*. 2007;101(2):176–84.

40. Liu Y, Sun Q, Chen X, Jing L, Wang W, Yu Z, et al. Linolenic acid provides multi-cellular protective effects after photothrombotic cerebral ischemia in rats. *Neurochemical Research*. 2014;39(9):1797–808.

41. Yamamoto N, Saitoh M, Moriuchi A, Nomura M, Okuyama H. Effect of dietary alpha-linolenate/linoleate balance on brain lipid compositions and learning ability of rats. *Journal of Lipid Research*. 1987;28(2):144–51.

42. King VR, Huang WL, Dyall SC, Curran OE, Priestley JV, Michael-Titus AT. Omega-3 fatty acids improve recovery, whereas omega-6 fatty acids worsen outcome, after spinal cord injury in the adult rat. *Journal of Neuroscience*. 2006;26(17):4672–80.

43. Forbes SC, Holroyd-Leduc JM, Poulin MJ, Hogan DB. Effect of nutrients, dietary supplements and vitamins on cognition: a systematic review and meta-analysis of randomized controlled trials. *Canadian Geriatrics Journal*. 2015;18(4):231.

44. Wu S, Ding Y, Wu F, Li R, Hou J, Mao P. Omega-3 fatty acids intake and risks of dementia and Alzheimer's disease: A meta-analysis. *Neuroscience & Biobehavioral Reviews*. 2015;48:1–9.

45. Jiao J, Li Q, Chu J, Zeng W, Yang M, Zhu S. Effect of n– 3 PUFA supplementation on cognitive function throughout the life span from infancy to old age: A systematic review and meta-analysis of randomized controlled trials. *The American Journal of Clinical Nutrition*. 2014;100(6):1422–36.

46. Zhang Y, Chen J, Qiu J, Li Y, Wang J, Jiao J. Intakes of fish and polyunsaturated fatty acids and mild-to-severe cognitive impairment risks: A dose-response meta-analysis of 21 cohort studies–3. *The American Journal of Clinical Nutrition*. 2015;103(2):330–40.

47. Barnard ND, Bush AI, Ceccarelli A, Cooper J, de Jager CA, Erickson KI, et al. Dietary and lifestyle guidelines for the prevention of Alzheimer's disease. *Neurobiology of Aging*. 2014;35:S74–S8.

48. Pandey KB, Rizvi SI. Plant polyphenols as dietary antioxidants in human health and disease. *Oxidative Medicine and Cellular Longevity*. 2009;2:270–8.

49. Fernández-Fernández L, Comes G, Bolea I, Valente T, Ruiz J, Murtra P, et al. LMN diet, rich in polyphenols and polyunsaturated fatty acids, improves mouse cognitive decline associated with aging and Alzheimer's disease. *Behavioural Brain Research*. 2012;228(2):261–71.

50. Liu P, Kemper LJ, Wang J, Zahs KR, Ashe KH, Pasinetti GM. Grape seed polyphenolic extract specifically decreases aβ* 56 in the brains of Tg2576 mice. *Journal of Alzheimer's Disease*. 2011;26(4):657–66.

51. Sandoval-Acuña C, Ferreira J, Speisky H. Polyphenols and mitochondria: An update on their increasingly emerging ROS-scavenging independent actions. *Archives of Biochemistry and Biophysics*. 2014;559:75–90.

52. Smolensky D, Rhodes D, McVey DS, Fawver Z, Perumal R, Herald T, et al. High-polyphenol sorghum bran extract inhibits cancer cell growth through ROS induction, cell cycle arrest, and apoptosis. *Journal of Medicinal Food*. 2018;21(10):990–8.

53. Foley TD. Reductive reprogramming: A not-so-radical hypothesis of neurodegeneration linking redox perturbations to neuroinflammation and excitotoxicity. *Cellular and Molecular Neurobiology*. 2019:1–14.

54. Rizvi SI, Maurya PK. Alterations in antioxidant enzymes during aging in humans. *Molecular Biotechnology*. 2007;37(1):58–61.

55. Rizvi SI, Maurya PK. Markers of oxidative stress in erythrocytes during aging in humans. *Annals of the New York Academy of Sciences*. 2007;1100(1):373–82.

56. Palacino JJ, Sagi D, Goldberg MS, Krauss S, Motz C, Wacker M, et al. Mitochondrial dysfunction and oxidative damage in parkin-deficient mice. *Journal of Biological Chemistry*. 2004;279(18):18614–22.

57. Hollman PC, Cassidy A, Comte B, Heinonen M, Richelle M, Richling E, et al. The biological relevance of direct antioxidant effects of polyphenols for cardiovascular health in humans is not established. *The Journal of Nutrition*. 2011;141(5):989S–1009S.

58. Pandey K, Rizvi S. Plant polyphenols as dietary antioxidants in human health and disease. *Oxidative Medicine and Cellular Longevity*. 2009;2:270–278.

59. Manach C, Scalbert A, Morand C, Rémésy C, Jiménez L. Polyphenols: food sources and bioavailability. *The American Journal of Clinical Nutrition*. 2004;79(5):727–47.

60. Petri G, Krawczyk U, Kery A. Spectrophotometric and chromatographic investigation of bilberry anthocyanins for quantification purposes. *Microchemical Journal*. 1997;55(1):12–23.

61. Kesse-Guyot E, Fezeu L, Andreeva VA, Touvier M, Scalbert A, Hercberg S, et al. Total and specific polyphenol intakes in midlife are associated with cognitive function measured 13 years later. *The Journal of Nutrition*. 2012;142(1):76–83.

62. Letenneur L, Proust-Lima C, Le Gouge A, Dartigues J-F, Barberger-Gateau P. Flavonoid intake and cognitive decline over a 10-year period. *American Journal of Epidemiology*. 2007;165(12):1364–71.

63. Dai Q, Borenstein AR, Wu Y, Jackson JC, Larson EB. Fruit and vegetable juices and Alzheimer's disease: The Kame Project. *The American Journal of Medicine*. 2006;119(9):751–9.

64. Williams CM, Abd El Mohsen M, Vauzour D, Rendeiro C, Butler LT, Ellis JA, et al. Blueberry-induced changes in spatial working memory correlate with changes in hippocampal CREB phosphorylation and brain-derived neurotrophic factor (BDNF) levels. *Free Radical Biology and Medicine*. 2008;45(3):295–305.

65. Goyarzu P, Malin DH, Lau FC, Taglialatela G, Moon WD, Jennings R, et al. Blueberry supplemented diet: effects on object recognition memory and nuclear factor-kappa B levels in aged rats. *Nutritional Neuroscience*. 2004;7(2):75–83.

66. Barros D, Amaral OB, Izquierdo I, Geracitano L, Raseira MdCB, Henriques AT, et al. Behavioral and genoprotective effects of vaccinium berries intake in mice. *Pharmacology Biochemistry and Behavior*. 2006;84(2):229–34.

67. Ramirez MR, Izquierdo I, Raseira MdCB, Zuanazzi JÂ, Barros D, Henriques AT. Effect of lyophilised Vaccinium berries on memory, anxiety and locomotion in adult rats. *Pharmacological Research*. 2005;52(6):457–62.

68. Devore EE, Kang JH, Breteler MM, Grodstein F. Dietary intakes of berries and flavonoids in relation to cognitive decline. *Annals of Neurology*. 2012;72(1):135–43.

69. Scarmeas N, Luchsinger JA, Mayeux R, Stern Y. Mediterranean diet and Alzheimer disease mortality. *Neurology*. 2007;69(11):1084–93.

70. Jardim FR, de Rossi FT, Nascimento MX, da Silva Barros RG, Borges PA, Prescilio IC, et al. Resveratrol and brain mitochondria: a review. *Molecular Neurobiology*. 2018;55(3):2085–101.

71. Moussa C, Hebron M, Huang X, Ahn J, Rissman RA, Aisen PS, et al. Resveratrol regulates neuro-inflammation and induces adaptive immunity in Alzheimer's disease. *Journal of Neuroinflammation*. 2017;14(1):1.

72. Thordardottir S, Ståhlbom AK, Almkvist O, Thonberg H, Eriksdotter M, Zetterberg H, et al. The effects of different familial Alzheimer's disease mutations on APP processing in vivo. *Alzheimer's Research & Therapy*. 2017;9(1):9.

73. Markus MA, Morris BJ. Resveratrol in prevention and treatment of common clinical conditions of aging. *Clinical Interventions in Aging*. 2008;3(2):331.

74. Gao J, Wang W-Y, Mao Y-W, Gräff J, Guan J-S, Pan L, et al. A novel pathway regulates memory and plasticity via SIRT1 and miR-134. *Nature*. 2010;466(7310):1105–9.

75. Michán S, Li Y, Chou MM-H, Parrella E, Ge H, Long JM, et al. SIRT1 is essential for normal cognitive function and synaptic plasticity. *Journal of Neuroscience*. 2010;30(29):9695–707.

76. Kumar R, Nigam L, Singh AP, Singh K, Subbarao N, Dey S. Design, synthesis of allosteric peptide activator for human SIRT1 and its biological evaluation in cellular model of Alzheimer's disease. *European Journal of Medicinal Chemistry*. 2017;127:909–16.

77. Gomes BAQ, Silva JPB, Romeiro CFR, Dos Santos SM, Rodrigues CA, Gonçalves PR, et al. Neuroprotective mechanisms of resveratrol in Alzheimer's disease: role of SIRT1. *Oxidative Medicine and Cellular Longevity*. 2018;2018. Article ID 8152373.

78. Pallàs M, Casadesús G, Smith MA, Coto-Montes A, Pelegri C, Vilaplana J, et al. Resveratrol and neurodegenerative diseases: activation of SIRT1 as the potential pathway towards neuroprotection. *Current Neurovascular Research*. 2009;6(1):70–81.

79. Sweeney G, Song J. The association between PGC-1α and Alzheimer's disease. *Anatomy & Cell Biology*. 2016;49(1):1–6.

80. Bernier M, Paul RK, Martin-Montalvo A, Scheibye-Knudsen M, Song S, He H-J, et al. Negative regulation of STAT3 protein-mediated cellular respiration by SIRT1 protein. *Journal of Biological Chemistry*. 2011;286(22):19270–9.

81. Ramis MR, Esteban S, Miralles A, Tan D-X, Reiter RJ. Caloric restriction, resveratrol and melatonin: Role of SIRT1 and implications for aging and related-diseases. *Mechanisms of Ageing and Development*. 2015;146:28–41.

82. Zhang Q, Yuan L, Zhang Q, Gao Y, Liu G, Xiu M, et al. Resveratrol attenuates hypoxia-induced neurotoxicity through inhibiting microglial activation. *International Immunopharmacology*. 2015;28(1):578–87.

83. Milbury PE, Kalt W. Xenobiotic metabolism and berry flavonoid transport across the blood– brain barrier. *Journal of Agricultural and Food Chemistry*. 2010; 58(7):3950–6.

84. Casadesus G, Shukitt-Hale B, Stellwagen HM, Zhu X, Lee H-G, Smith MA, et al. Modulation of hippocampal plasticity and cognitive behavior by short-term blueberry supplementation in aged rats. *Nutritional Neuroscience*. 2004;7(5-6):309–16.

85. Joseph JA, Shukitt-Hale B, Denisova NA, Bielinski D, Martin A, McEwen JJ, et al. Reversals of age-related declines in neuronal signal transduction, cognitive, and motor behavioral deficits with blueberry, spinach, or strawberry dietary supplementation. *Journal of Neuroscience*. 1999;19(18):8114–21.

86. Albert MS, DeKosky ST, Dickson D, Dubois B, Feldman HH, Fox NC, et al. The diagnosis of mild cognitive impairment due to Alzheimer's disease: recommendations from the National Institute on Aging-Alzheimer's Association workgroups on diagnostic guidelines for Alzheimer's disease. *Alzheimer's & Dementia*. 2011;7(3):270–9.

87. Petersen RC. Mild cognitive impairment as a diagnostic entity. *Journal of Internal Medicine*. 2004;256(3):183–94.

88. Rahman MM, Ichiyanagi T, Komiyama T, Sato S, Konishi T. Effects of anthocyanins on psychological stress-induced oxidative stress and neurotransmitter status. *Journal of Agricultural and Food Chemistry*. 2008;56(16):7545–50.

89. Boespflug EL, Eliassen JC, Dudley JA, Shidler MD, Kalt W, Summer SS, et al. Enhanced neural activation with blueberry supplementation in mild cognitive impairment. *Nutritional Neuroscience*. 2018;21(4):297–305.

90. Curti V, Capelli E, Boschi F, Nabavi SF, Bongiorno AI, Habtemariam S, et al. Modulation of human miR-17-3p expression by methyl 3-O-methyl gallate as explanation of its in vivo protective activities. *Molecular Nutrition & Food Research*. 2014;58(9):1776–84.

91. Tsuji PA, Stephenson KK, Wade KL, Liu H, Fahey JW. Structure-activity analysis of flavonoids: direct and indirect antioxidant, and antiinflammatory potencies and toxicities. *Nutrition and Cancer*. 2013;65(7):1014–25.

92. Ye J, Meng X, Yan C, Wang C. Effect of purple sweet potato anthocyanins on β-amyloid-mediated PC-12 cells death by inhibition of oxidative stress. *Neurochemical Research*. 2010;35(3):357–65.

93. Poulose SM, Fisher DR, Larson J, Bielinski DF, Rimando AM, Carey AN, et al. Anthocyanin-rich açai (Euterpe oleracea Mart.) fruit pulp fractions attenuate inflammatory stress signaling in mouse brain BV-2 microglial cells. *Journal of Agricultural and Food Chemistry*. 2012;60(4):1084–93.

94. Jembrek MJ, Vuković L, Puhović J, Erhardt J, Oršolić N. Neuroprotective effect of quercetin against hydrogen peroxide-induced oxidative injury in P19 neurons. *Journal of Molecular Neuroscience*. 2012;47(2):286–99.

95. Priprem A, Watanatorn J, Sutthiparinyanont S, Phachonpai W, Muchimapura S. Anxiety and cognitive effects of quercetin liposomes in rats. *Nanomedicine: Nanotechnology, Biology and Medicine*. 2008;4(1):70–8.

96. Wang D-M, Li S-Q, Wu W-L, Zhu X-Y, Wang Y, Yuan H-Y. Effects of long-term treatment with quercetin on cognition and mitochondrial function in a mouse model of Alzheimer's disease. *Neurochemical Research*. 2014;39(8):1533–43.

97. Tota S, Awasthi H, Kamat PK, Nath C, Hanif K. Protective effect of quercetin against intracerebral streptozotocin induced reduction in cerebral blood flow and impairment of memory in mice. *Behavioural Brain Research*. 2010;209(1):73–9.

98. Kim JH, Lee J, Lee S, Cho EJ. Quercetin and quercetin-3-β-d-glucoside improve cognitive and memory function in Alzheimer's disease mouse. *Applied Biological Chemistry*. 2016;59(5):721–8.

99. Maciel RM, Carvalho FB, Olabiyi AA, Schmatz R, Gutierres JM, Stefanello N, et al. Neuroprotective effects of quercetin on memory and anxiogenic-like behavior in diabetic rats: Role of ectonucleotidases and acetylcholinesterase activities. *Biomedicine & Pharmacotherapy*. 2016;84:559–68.

100. Liu R, Zhang T-t, Zhou D, Bai X-y, Zhou W-l, Huang C, et al. Quercetin protects against the Aβ25–35-induced amnesic injury: Involvement of inactivation of RAGE-mediated pathway and conservation of the NVU. *Neuropharmacology*. 2013;67:419–31.

101. Broman-Fulks JJ, Canu WH, Trout KL, Nieman DC. The effects of quercetin supplementation on cognitive functioning in a community sample: A randomized, placebo-controlled trial. *Therapeutic Advances in Psychopharmacology*. 2012;2(4):131–8.

102. Yao Y, Lin G, Xie Y, Ma P, Li G, Meng Q, et al. Preformulation studies of myricetin: A natural antioxidant flavonoid. *Die Pharmazie-An International Journal of Pharmaceutical Sciences*. 2014;69(1):19–26.

103. Ramezani M, Darbandi N, Khodagholi F, Hashemi A. Myricetin protects hippocampal CA3 pyramidal neurons and improves learning and memory impairments in rats with Alzheimer's disease. *Neural Regeneration Research*. 2016;11(12):1976.

104. Higdon JV, Frei B. Tea catechins and polyphenols: health effects, metabolism, and antioxidant functions. 2003.

105. Ma Q-P, Huang C, Cui Q-Y, Yang D-J, Sun K, Chen X, et al. Meta-analysis of the association between tea intake and the risk of cognitive disorders. *PLoS One*. 2016;11(11):e0165861.

106. Qi H, Li S. Dose–response meta-analysis on coffee, tea and caffeine consumption with risk of Parkinson's disease. *Geriatrics & Gerontology International*. 2014;14(2):430–9.

107. Koh S-H, Kwon H, Kim KS, Kim J, Kim M-H, Yu H-J, et al. Epigallocatechin gallate prevents oxidative-stress-induced death of mutant Cu/Zn-superoxide dismutase (G93A) motoneuron cells by alteration of cell survival and death signals. *Toxicology*. 2004;202(3):213–25.

108. Wightman EL, Haskell CF, Forster JS, Veasey RC, Kennedy DO. Epigallocatechin gallate, cerebral blood flow parameters, cognitive performance and mood in healthy humans: A double-blind, placebo-controlled, crossover investigation. *Human Psychopharmacology: Clinical and Experimental*. 2012;27(2):177–86.

109. Chen W-Q, Zhao X-L, Wang D-L, Li S-T, Hou Y, Hong Y, et al. Effects of epigallocatechin-3-gallate on behavioral impairments induced by psychological stress in rats. *Experimental Biology and Medicine*. 2010;235(5):577–83.

110. Brown AL, Lane J, Coverly J, Stocks J, Jackson S, Stephen A, et al. Effects of dietary supplementation with the green tea polyphenol epigallocatechin-3-gallate on insulin resistance and associated metabolic risk factors: Randomized controlled trial. *British Journal of Nutrition*. 2008;101(6):886–94.

111. Wang M-H, Chang W-J, Soung H-S, Chang K-C. (–)-Epigallocatechin-3-gallate decreases the impairment in learning and memory in spontaneous hypertension rats. *Behavioural Pharmacology*. 2012;23(8):771–80.

112. Kim JS, Kim J-M, Jeong-Ja O, Jeon BS. Inhibition of inducible nitric oxide synthase expression and cell death by (–)-epigallocatechin-3-gallate, a green tea catechin, in the 1-methyl-4-phenyl-1, 2, 3, 6-tetrahydropyridine mouse model of Parkinson's disease. *Journal of Clinical Neuroscience*. 2010;17(9):1165–8.

113. Chong ZZ, Li F, Maiese K. Oxidative stress in the brain: Novel cellular targets that govern survival during neurodegenerative disease. *Progress in Neurobiology*. 2005;75(3):207–46.

114. Barnham KJ, Masters CL, Bush AI. Neurodegenerative diseases and oxidative stress. *Nature Reviews Drug Discovery*. 2004;3(3):205–14.

115. Friedman J. *Why is the Nervous System Vulnerable to Oxidative Stress? Oxidative Stress and Free Radical Damage in Neurology*. Springer's Humana Press, New Jersey; 2011. p. 19–27.

116. Grodzicki W, Dziendzikowska K. The role of selected bioactive compounds in the prevention of Alzheimer's disease. *Antioxidants*. 2020;9(3):229.

117. Vershinin A. Biological functions of carotenoids-diversity and evolution. *Biofactors*. 1999;10(2-3):99–104.

118. Britton G. *Carotenoids. Natural Food Colorants.* Springer, Boston, MA; 1996. p. 197–243.
119. Waris G, Ahsan H. Reactive oxygen species: role in the development of cancer and various chronic conditions. *Journal of Carcinogenesis.* 2006;5:14.
120. Lozupone M, Solfrizzi V, D'Urso F, Di Gioia I, Sardone R, Dibello V, et al. Anti-Amyloid-β Protein agents for the treatment of Alzheimer's Disease: An update on emerging drugs. *Expert Opinion on Emerging Drugs.* 2020;25(3):319–35.
121. Katayama S, Ogawa H, Nakamura S. Apricot carotenoids possess potent anti-amyloido-genic activity in vitro. *Journal of Agricultural and Food Chemistry.* 2011;59(23):12691–6.
122. Lakey-Beitia J, Kumar D J, Hegde ML, Rao K. Carotenoids as novel therapeutic mol-ecules against neurodegenerative disorders: Chemistry and molecular docking analy-sis. *International Journal of Molecular Sciences.* 2019;20(22):5553.
123. Baudouin A, Isingrini M, Vanneste S. Executive functioning and processing speed in age-related differences in time estimation: a comparison of young, old, and very old adults. *Aging, Neuropsychology, and Cognition.* 2019;26(2):264–81.
124. Lieblein-Boff JC, Johnson EJ, Kennedy AD, Lai C-S, Kuchan MJ. Exploratory metab-olomic analyses reveal compounds correlated with lutein concentration in fron-tal cortex, hippocampus, and occipital cortex of human infant brain. *PLoS One.* 2015;10(8):e0136904.
125. Krinsky NI, Mayne ST, Sies H. *Carotenoids in Health and Disease.* CRC Press, Boca Raton; 2004.
126. Gruszecki WI, Sujak A, Strzalka K, Radunz A, Schmid GH. Organisation of xanthophyll-lipid membranes studied by means of specific pigment antisera, spectro-photometry and monomolecular layer technique lutein versus zeaxanthin. *Zeitschrift Für Naturforschung C.* 1999;54(7–8):517–25.
127. Wisniewska A, Subczynski WK. Accumulation of macular xanthophylls in unsatu-rated membrane domains. *Free Radical Biology and Medicine.* 2006;40(10):1820–6.
128. Rapp LM, Maple SS, Choi JH. Lutein and zeaxanthin concentrations in rod outer segment membranes from perifoveal and peripheral human retina. *Investigative Ophthalmology & Visual Science.* 2000;41(5):1200–9.
129. Tanprasertsuk J, Li B, Bernstein PS, Vishwanathan R, Johnson MA, Poon L, et al. Relationship between concentrations of lutein and StARD3 among pediatric and geri-atric human brain tissue. *PLoS One.* 2016;11(5):e0155488.
130. Vishwanathan R, Kuchan MJ, Sen S, Johnson EJ. Lutein and preterm infants with decreased concentrations of brain carotenoids. *Journal of Pediatric Gastroenterology and Nutrition.* 2014;59(5):659–65.
131. Stringham JM, Johnson EJ, Hammond BR. Lutein across the lifespan: From child-hood cognitive performance to the aging eye and brain. *Current Developments in Nutrition.* 2019;3(7):nzz066.
132. Stringham NT, Holmes PV, Stringham JM. Effects of macular xanthophyll supplemen-tation on brain-derived neurotrophic factor, pro-inflammatory cytokines, and cogni-tive performance. *Physiology & Behavior.* 2019;211:112650.
133. Nouchi R, Suiko T, Kimura E, Takenaka H, Murakoshi M, Uchiyama A, et al. Effects of lutein and astaxanthin intake on the improvement of cognitive functions among healthy adults: A systematic review of randomized controlled trials. *Nutrients.* 2020;12(3):617.
134. Che H, Li Q, Zhang T, Wang D, Yang L, Xu J, et al. Effects of astaxanthin and docosahexaenoic-acid-acylated astaxanthin on Alzheimer's disease in APP/PS1 dou-ble-transgenic mice. *Journal of Agricultural and Food Chemistry.* 2018;66(19):4948–57.
135. Grimmig B, Kim S-H, Nash K, Bickford PC, Shytle RD. Neuroprotective mechanisms of astaxanthin: A potential therapeutic role in preserving cognitive function in age and neurodegeneration. *Geroscience.* 2017;39(1):19–32.
136. Lee D-H, Lee YJ, Kwon KH. Neuroprotective effects of astaxanthin in oxygen-glucose deprivation in SH-SY5Y cells and global cerebral ischemia in rat. *Journal of Clinical Biochemistry and Nutrition.* 2010;47(2):121–9.

137. Wang J, Wang Z, Li B, Qiang Y, Yuan T, Tan X, et al. Lycopene attenuates Western-diet-induced cognitive deficits via improving glycolipid metabolism dysfunction and inflammatory responses in gut–liver–brain axis. *International Journal of Obesity*. 2019;43(9):1735–46.

138. Chen D, Huang C, Chen Z. A review for the pharmacological effect of lycopene in central nervous system disorders. *Biomedicine & Pharmacotherapy*. 2019;111:791–801.

139. Rahman MA, Rhim H. Therapeutic implication of autophagy in neurodegenerative diseases. *BMB Reports*. 2017;50(7):345.

140. Przybylska S. Lycopene–a bioactive carotenoid offering multiple health benefits: A review. *International Journal of Food Science & Technology*. 2020;55(1):11–32.

141. Mattson MP, Arumugam TV. Hallmarks of brain aging: Adaptive and pathological modification by metabolic states. *Cell Metabolism*. 2018;27(6):1176–99.

142. Nilsson LG. Memory function in normal aging. *Acta Neurologica Scandinavica*. 2003;107:7–13.

143. O'Toole PW, Jeffery IB. Gut microbiota and aging. *Science*. 2015;350(6265):1214–5.

144. Bischoff SC. Microbiota and aging. *Current Opinion in Clinical Nutrition & Metabolic Care*. 2016;19(1):26–30.

145. Gareau MG. *Microbiota-Gut-Brain Axis and Cognitive Function. Microbial Endocrinology: The Microbiota-Gut-Brain Axis in Health and Disease*. Springer-Verlag, New York; 2014. p. 357–71.

146. Clark RI, Walker DW. Role of gut microbiota in aging-related health decline: insights from invertebrate models. *Cellular and Molecular Life Sciences*. 2018;75(1):93–101.

147. Claesson MJ, Jeffery IB, Conde S, Power SE, O'connor EM, Cusack S, et al. Gut microbiota composition correlates with diet and health in the elderly. *Nature*. 2012;488(7410):178–84.

148. Akbari E, Asemi Z, Daneshvar Kakhaki R, Bahmani F, Kouchaki E, Tamtaji OR, et al. Effect of probiotic supplementation on cognitive function and metabolic status in Alzheimer's disease: A randomized, double-blind and controlled trial. *Frontiers in Aging Neuroscience*. 2016;8:256.

149. Proctor C, Thiennimitr P, Chattipakorn N, Chattipakorn SC. Diet, gut microbiota and cognition. *Metabolic Brain Disease*. 2017;32(1):1–17.

150. Wraith DC, Nicholson LB. The adaptive immune system in diseases of the central nervous system. *The Journal of Clinical Investigation*. 2012;122(4):1172–9.

151. Xiao J, Katsumata N, Bernier F, Ohno K, Yamauchi Y, Odamaki T, et al. Probiotic bifidobacterium breve in improving cognitive functions of older adults with suspected mild cognitive impairment: A randomized, double-blind, placebo-controlled trial. *Journal of Alzheimer's Disease*. 2020(Preprint):1–9.

152. Benton D, Williams C, Brown A. Impact of consuming a milk drink containing a probiotic on mood and cognition. *European Journal of Clinical Nutrition*. 2007;61(3):355–61.

153. Kim C-S, Cha L, Sim M, Jung S, Chun WY, Baik HW, et al. Probiotic supplementation improves cognitive function and mood with changes in gut microbiota in community-dwelling elderly: A randomized, double-blind, placebo-controlled, multicenter trial. *The Journals of Gerontology: Series A*. 2020;76:32–40.

154. Chung Y-C, Jin H-M, Cui Y, Jung JM, Park J-I, Jung E-S, et al. Fermented milk of Lactobacillus helveticus IDCC3801 improves cognitive functioning during cognitive fatigue tests in healthy older adults. *Journal of Functional Foods*. 2014;10:465–74.

155. Di Benedetto S, Müller L, Wenger E, Düzel S, Pawelec G. Contribution of neuroinflammation and immunity to brain aging and the mitigating effects of physical and cognitive interventions. *Neuroscience & Biobehavioral Reviews*. 2017;75:114–28.

156. Jenkins TA, Nguyen JC, Polglaze KE, Bertrand PP. Influence of tryptophan and serotonin on mood and cognition with a possible role of the gut-brain axis. *Nutrients*. 2016;8(1):56.

157. Backman L, Nyberg L, Lindenberger U, Li SC, Farde L. The correlative triad among aging, dopamine, and cognition: current status and future prospects. *Neuroscience & Biobehavioral Reviews*. 2006;30(6):791–807.

158. Komulainen P, Pedersen M, Hänninen T, Bruunsgaard H, Lakka TA, Kivipelto M, et al. BDNF is a novel marker of cognitive function in ageing women: the DR's EXTRA Study. *Neurobiology of Learning and Memory*. 2008;90(4):596–603.

159. Capuron L, Schroecksnadel S, Féart C, Aubert A, Higueret D, Barberger-Gateau P, et al. Chronic low-grade inflammation in elderly persons is associated with altered tryptophan and tyrosine metabolism: Role in neuropsychiatric symptoms. *Biological Psychiatry*. 2011;70(2):175–82.

160. Chunchai T, Thunapong W, Yasom S, Wanchai K, Eaimworawuthikul S, Metzler G, et al. Decreased microglial activation through gut-brain axis by prebiotics, probiotics, or synbiotics effectively restored cognitive function in obese-insulin resistant rats. *Journal of Neuroinflammation*. 2018;15(1):11.

161. Liu RT, Walsh RFL, Sheehan AE. Prebiotics and probiotics for depression and anxiety: A systematic review and meta-analysis of controlled clinical trials. *Neuroscience & Biobehavioral Reviews*. 2019;102:13–23.

162. Bierman E, Comijs H, Jonker C, Beekman A. Effects of anxiety versus depression on cognition in later life. *The American Journal of Geriatric Psychiatry*. 2005;13(8):686–93.

163. Xiang YZ, Shang HC, Gao XM, Zhang BL. A comparison of the ancient use of ginseng in traditional Chinese medicine with modern pharmacological experiments and clinical trials. *Phytotherapy Research*. 2008;22(7):851–8.

164. Su C-F, Cheng J-T, Liu I-M. Increase of acetylcholine release by Panax ginseng root enhances insulin secretion in Wistar rats. *Neuroscience Letters*. 2007;412(2):101–4.

165. Ying Y, Zhang J, Shi C, Qu Z, Liu Y. Study on the nootropic mechanism of ginsenoside Rb1 and Rg1--influence on mouse brain development. *Yao xue xue bao= Acta Pharmaceutica Sinica*. 1994;29(4):241–5.

166. Shen L-h, Zhang J-t. Ginsenoside Rg1 promotes proliferation of hippocampal progenitor cells. *Neurological Research*. 2004;26(4):422–8.

167. Hwang SH, Shin E-J, Shin T-J, Lee B-H, Choi S-H, Kang J, et al. Gintonin, a ginseng-derived lysophosphatidic acid receptor ligand, attenuates Alzheimer's disease-related neuropathies: Involvement of non-amyloidogenic processing. *Journal of Alzheimer's Disease*. 2012;31(1):207–23.

168. Jin Y, Cui R, Zhao L, Fan J, Li B. Mechanisms of Panax ginseng action as an antidepressant. *Cell Proliferation*. 2019;52(6):e12696.

169. Wesnes K, Ward T, McGinty A, Petrini O. The memory enhancing effects of a Ginkgo biloba/Panax ginseng combination in healthy middle-aged volunteers. *Psychopharmacology*. 2000;152(4):353–61.

170. Lee Y, Oh S. Administration of red ginseng ameliorates memory decline in aged mice. *Journal of Ginseng Research*. 2015;39(3):250–6.

171. Jung JS, Shin JA, Park EM, Lee JE, Kang YS, Min SW, et al. Anti-inflammatory mechanism of ginsenoside Rh1 in lipopolysaccharide-stimulated microglia: critical role of the protein kinase A pathway and hemeoxygenase-1 expression. *Journal of Neurochemistry*. 2010;115(6):1668–80.

172. HERMAN-ANTOSIEWICZ A, Powolny AA, Singh SV. Molecular targets of cancer chemoprevention by garlic-derived organosulfides 1. *Acta Pharmacologica Sinica*. 2007;28(9):1355–64.

173. Haider S, Naz N, Khaliq S, Perveen T, Haleem DJ. Repeated administration of fresh garlic increases memory retention in rats. *Journal of Medicinal Food*. 2008;11(4):675–9.

174. Peng Q, Buz'Zard AR, Lau BH. Neuroprotective effect of garlic compounds in amyloid-β peptide-induced apoptosis in vitro. *Medical Science Monitor*. 2002;8(8):BR328–BR37.

175. Lin GH, Lee Y-J, Choi D-Y, Han SB, Jung JK, Hwang BY, et al. Anti-amyloidogenic effect of thiacremonone through anti-inflammation in vitro and in vivo models. *Journal of Alzheimer's Disease.* 2012;29(3):659–76.

176. Borek C. Garlic reduces dementia and heart-disease risk. *Journal of Nutrition.* 2006;136(3 Suppl):810s–2s.

177. Wu X, Santos RR, Fink-Gremmels J. Analyzing the antibacterial effects of food ingredients: model experiments with allicin and garlic extracts on biofilm formation and viability of Staphylococcus epidermidis. *Food Science & Nutrition.* 2015;3(2):158–68.

178. Zhu X, Zhang F, Zhou L, Kong D, Chen L, Lu Y, et al. Diallyl trisulfide attenuates carbon tetrachloride-caused liver injury and fibrogenesis and reduces hepatic oxidative stress in rats. *Naunyn-Schmiedeberg's Archives of Pharmacology.* 2014;387(5):445–55.

179. Xu XH, Li GL, Wang BA, Qin Y, Bai SR, Rong J, et al. Diallyl trisufide protects against oxygen glucose deprivation-induced apoptosis by scavenging free radicals via the PI3K/Akt-mediated Nrf2/HO-1 signaling pathway in B35 neural cells. *Brain Research.* 2015;1614:38–50.

180. Li X-H, Li C-Y, Xiang Z-G, Zhong F, Chen Z-Y, Lu J-M. Allicin can reduce neuronal death and ameliorate the spatial memory impairment in Alzheimer's disease models. *Neurosciences (Riyadh, Saudi Arabia).* 2010;15(4):237–43.

181. Hasselmo ME. The role of acetylcholine in learning and memory. *Current Opinion in Neurobiology.* 2006;16(6):710–5.

182. Gillette-Guyonnet S, Van Kan GA, Andrieu S, Barberger-Gateau P, Berr C, Bonnefoy M, et al. IANA task force on nutrition and cognitive decline with aging. *Journal of Nutrition Health and Aging.* 2007;11(2):132.

183. Durga J, van Boxtel MP, Schouten EG, Kok FJ, Jolles J, Katan MB, et al. Effect of 3-year folic acid supplementation on cognitive function in older adults in the FACIT trial: A randomised, double blind, controlled trial. *The Lancet.* 2007;369(9557):208–16.

184. Walker JG, Batterham PJ, Mackinnon AJ, Jorm AF, Hickie I, Fenech M, et al. Oral folic acid and vitamin B-12 supplementation to prevent cognitive decline in community-dwelling older adults with depressive symptoms—the Beyond Ageing Project: a randomized controlled trial. *The American Journal of Clinical Nutrition.* 2012;95(1):194–203.

185. Kwok T, Lee J, Law C, Pan P, Yung C, Choi K, et al. A randomized placebo controlled trial of homocysteine lowering to reduce cognitive decline in older demented people. *Clinical Nutrition.* 2011;30(3):297–302.

186. Garcia A, Zanibbi K. Homocysteine and cognitive function in elderly people. *Cmaj.* 2004;171(8):897–904.

187. Smith AD, Smith SM, De Jager CA, Whitbread P, Johnston C, Agacinski G, et al. Homocysteine-lowering by B vitamins slows the rate of accelerated brain atrophy in mild cognitive impairment: a randomized controlled trial. *PLoS One.* 2010;5(9):e12244.

188. de Jager CA, Oulhaj A, Jacoby R, Refsum H, Smith AD. Cognitive and clinical outcomes of homocysteine-lowering B-vitamin treatment in mild cognitive impairment: a randomized controlled trial. *International Journal of Geriatric Psychiatry.* 2012;27(6):592–600.

189. Littlejohns TJ, Henley WE, Lang IA, Annweiler C, Beauchet O, Chaves PH, et al. Vitamin D and the risk of dementia and Alzheimer disease. *Neurology.* 2014;83(10):920–8.

190. Dickens AP, Lang IA, Langa KM, Kos K, Llewellyn DJ. Vitamin D, cognitive dysfunction and dementia in older adults. *CNS Drugs.* 2011;25(8):629–39.

191. Mizwicki MT, Menegaz D, Zhang J, Barrientos-Durán A, Tse S, Cashman JR, et al. Genomic and nongenomic signaling induced by 1α, 25 (OH) 2-vitamin D 3 promotes the recovery of amyloid-β phagocytosis by Alzheimer's disease macrophages. *Journal of Alzheimer's Disease.* 2012;29(1):51–62.

192. Annweiler C, Montero-Odasso M, Hachinski V, Seshadri S, Bartha R, Beauchet O. Vitamin D concentration and lateral cerebral ventricle volume in older adults. *Molecular Nutrition & Food Research.* 2013;57(2):267–76.

193. Annweiler C, Rolland Y, Schott A-M, Blain H, Vellas B, Beauchet O. Serum vitamin D deficiency as a predictor of incident non-Alzheimer dementias: a 7-year longitudinal study. *Dementia and Geriatric Cognitive Disorders*. 2011;32(4):273–8.

194. Balion C, Griffith LE, Strifler L, Henderson M, Patterson C, Heckman G, et al. Vitamin D, cognition, and dementia: a systematic review and meta-analysis. *Neurology*. 2012;79(13):1397–405.

195. Engelhart MJ, Geerlings MI, Ruitenberg A, van Swieten JC, Hofman A, Witteman JC, et al. Dietary intake of antioxidants and risk of Alzheimer disease. *Jama*. 2002;287(24):3223–9.

196. Li F-J, Shen L, Ji H-F. Dietary intakes of vitamin E, vitamin C, and β-carotene and risk of Alzheimer's disease: a meta-analysis. *Journal of Alzheimer's Disease*. 2012;31(2):253–8.

197. Kryscio RJ, Abner EL, Caban-Holt A, Lovell M, Goodman P, Darke AK, et al. Association of antioxidant supplement use and dementia in the prevention of Alzheimer's disease by vitamin E and selenium trial (PREADViSE). *JAMA Neurology*. 2017;74(5):567–73.

198. Nualart F, Mack L, García A, Cisternas P, Bongarzone ER, Heitzer M, et al. Vitamin C transporters, recycling and the bystander effect in the nervous system: SVCT2 versus gluts. *Journal of Stem Cell Research & Therapy*. 2014;4(5):209.

199. Harrison FE, Bowman GL, Polidori MC. Ascorbic acid and the brain: Rationale for the use against cognitive decline. *Nutrients*. 2014;6(4):1752–81.

200. Maczurek A, Hager K, Kenklies M, Sharman M, Martins R, Engel J, et al. Lipoic acid as an anti-inflammatory and neuroprotective treatment for Alzheimer's disease. *Advanced Drug Delivery Reviews*. 2008;60(13-14):1463–70.

201. Ono K, Hirohata M, Yamada M. α-Lipoic acid exhibits anti-amyloidogenicity for β-amyloid fibrils in vitro. *Biochemical and Biophysical Research Communications*. 2006;341(4):1046–52.

202. Juan YS, Chuang SM, Mannikarottu A, Huang CH, Li S, Schuler C, et al. Coenzyme Q10 diminishes ischemia–reperfusion induced apoptosis and nerve injury in rabbit urinary bladder. *Neurourology and Urodynamics: Official Journal of the International Continence Society*. 2009;28(4):339–42.

203. Yang X, Zhang Y, Xu H, Luo X, Yu J, Liu J, et al. Neuroprotection of coenzyme Q10 in neurodegenerative diseases. *Current Topics in Medicinal Chemistry*. 2016;16(8):858–66.

6

Nutraceutical Activation of the Transcription Factor Nrf2 as a Potential Approach for Modulation of Aging

Patricia Mendonca and Karam F. A. Soliman
Florida A&M University

Contents

6.1 Introduction

The aging process is induced by numerous exogenous and endogenous stressors that can cause genetic modifications, epigenetic changes, and alteration in protein homeostasis, speeding up the aging process. Another critical factor that also plays a significant role during cellular senescence is the production of reactive oxygen species (ROS), showing benefits at optimal levels, but harmful effects when in excess [1]. In organisms that use oxygen in their respiratory

DOI: 10.1201/9781003110866-6

chain, the mitochondria generate oxygen radicals, and efficient electron transport decreases over time [2]. The malfunction of mitochondria increases ROS production and induces cell damage and aging [3]. ROS production can alter proteins, lipids, carbohydrates, and nucleic acids, changing cellular function [4]. ROS accumulation activates inflammation and oxidative stress, and the chronic production of ROS leads to the induction of age-related diseases [5]. Increased oxidative stress levels increase the susceptibility to pathologies associated with age due to damages in essential intracellular components that alter the cell's overall redox, metabolic, and protein homeostasis [4]. Oxidative stress has been reported as associated with the aging process and numerous chronic-aged diseases such as neurodegeneration and cancer [6].

Besides oxidative stress, ROS accumulation may cause electrophile stress, damage of membranes, the formation of DNA adducts, and mutations, ultimately leading to tissue degeneration and early aging, apoptosis, and the transformation of normal cells and cancer [7]. Oxidative stress seems to be the crucial factor that drives premature aging; therefore, modulatory mechanisms that can delay the increase of cell oxidation products can induce longevity [8].

6.2 The role of Nrf2 in reducing oxidative stress

Accumulation of oxidative damage plays a key role in the aging process; hence, prooxidants' use or increased antioxidant levels may extend the lifespan [9]. In a protective mechanism against oxidative stress, cells can activate antioxidant defenses, including the transcription factor nuclear factor (erythroid-derived 2)-like 2 (Nrf2), which is considered as a master regulator of antioxidation and the aging process [10]. Nrf2 belongs to the leucine-zipper transcription factor family. It controls the expression of more than 200 cytoprotective and antioxidant genes that encode proteins to neutralize and detoxify toxins, eliminate ROS, and help maintain high-quality proteome assist in the regulation of cell cycle and growth [11,12].

The Kelch-like ECH-associated protein 1 (Keap1)-Nrf2 is a critical cell antioxidant response and protection against oxidative damage. Nrf2 is a potent transcription factor, and Keap1 works as an Nrf2 negative regulator during homeostasis. Keap1 is also in charge of the inducible activation of Nrf2 against oxidative and electrophilic stress [13–16]. Under homeostatic conditions, with low oxidative stress levels, Nrf2 is maintained in its inactivated form in the cytoplasm, bound to Keap1. In this state, Nrf2 is targeted by Keap1 and by ubiquitination and degradation, resulting in lower levels of expression [17]. Conversely, high levels of oxidative stress exposure change in Keap1 cysteine residues leading to conformational alterations, protecting Nrf2 from ubiquitination and degradation [18], consequently causing Nrf2 accumulation and activation [6]. Free Nrf2 then translocates to the nucleus, dimerizes with musculoaponeurotic fibrosarcoma (Maf) proteins, and binds to the antioxidant response element (ARE) in the promoter region of downstream genes. These genes encode cytoprotective, antioxidant, and phase II detoxifying enzymes or proteins, such as NAD(P)H: quinone reductase-1 (NQO1), heme oxygenase-1 (HO-1), and glutathione synthetase (GSS) [19]. The Nrf2/Keap1/ARE signaling pathway can be activated by various exogenous and endogenous small molecules [20,21] and controls the expression of genes involved in regulating cell proliferation and survival [22].

6.3 The role of Nrf2 in aging

It was described that old organisms present a compromised nucleophilic tone that leads to chronic oxidative stress [23,24]. The exacerbated age-associated oxidative state diminishes the organism's antioxidant capacity, which will present an inefficient proteasome action and a decreased mitochondrial Lon protease activity. These alterations lead to the accumulation of intra-mitochondrial and intracellular masses of oxidized and cross-linked aggregation of protein [25–27]. Evidence indicates that a decrease in antioxidants' adaptive response to an oxidative stimulus has an essential function in the buildup of age-related oxidative stress. It may be associated with a decline in the efficiency of the Nrf2 signaling [28–30].

As we age, there is a gradual decline in cell signaling, higher protein dysfunction levels, and an increased possibility of cell death. The gradual decline observed in Nrf2 expression has been associated with an upregulation of its negative regulators and a downregulation of Nrf2 protein expression and pathway responsiveness [31].

The role of Nrf2 in gene regulation was explored in an Nrf2 knockout mice model. The results showed that Nrf2 knockout aged mice presented elevated sensitivity to electrophiles and oxidants [32–34], higher susceptibility to cancer [35–37], and other environmental insult diseases [38] and were more susceptible to skin aging due to ultraviolet B [39]. Moreover, the hearing capacity of Nrf2 null mice was shown to be impaired compared to age-matched wild-type animals [40]. Therefore, these studies indicated that a decrease in Nrf2 activity might lead to some of the age-associated phenotypes.

Furthermore, studies have also reported that PI3K and PCK activity may be involved in the nuclear translocation and export of Nrf2 protein. Shih and Yen described that an age-dependent decline of Nrf2 protein and Nrf2-dependent genes was linked with a decreased activation of mitogen-activated protein kinase (MAPK) cascade in the liver of aged rats [41]. An age-related decrease in PI3K/AKT signaling was observed in the skeletal muscle of old mice [42], hepatocytes of old rats [43], brains [44] and hippocampus of old mice [45], and elderly individuals' macrophages [46].

Numerous factors are involved in Nrf2 downregulation, including the promoter's silencing by epigenetic factors, higher degradation of Nrf2 in mRNA and protein levels, and competition with other transcription factors [47]. These

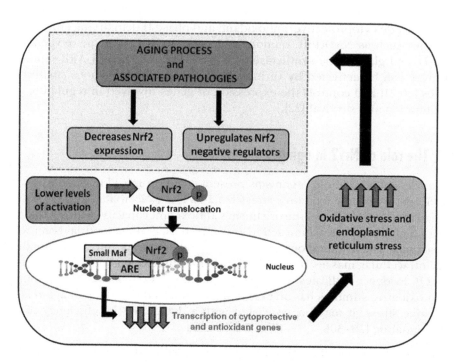

Figure 6.1 *The association of oxidative stress, Nrf2 downregulation, and the aging process. The figure describes how the decline in Nrf2 activation leads to increased oxidative and endoplasmic reticulum stress levels, resulting in the progression of the aging process and the development of age-related pathologies.*

factors can eventually reduce the transcription of cytoprotective genes mediated by Nrf2, leaving the cells more susceptible to oxidative stress and endoplasmic reticulum stress, contributing to the aging process [4]. A reduction in Nrf2 expression allows cells to shift to a pathogenic state due to superoxide accumulation, hydroxyl radicals, and hydrogen peroxide. Nrf2 level is a crucial component of the aging process, and lower levels result in increased oxidative stress. Since decreased Nrf2 expression may lead to protease loss, instability of genome, epigenetic changes, dysfunction of mitochondria, nutrient sensing deregulation, cellular senescence, exhaustion of stem cell, and distorted intercellular communications, it is crucial to develop Nrf2-based therapeutics to lessen aging and its associated pathologies [4] (Figure 6.1).

6.4 The beneficial properties of flavonoids

Recent studies using nutraceuticals have indicated that these compounds present a potential approach for slowing down the aging process in humans by reducing oxidative stress and the risk of diseases associated with age, improving health, and lifespan.

Plants are important sources of natural compounds and phytochemicals and have been investigated for their antiaging properties and improving cells' ability to keep the ROS-antioxidant balance. Phenolic compounds such as quercetin, resveratrol, and cyanidin are natural antioxidants due to the presence of free hydroxyl groups that can donate hydrogen atoms to protect cells against lipid peroxidation [48] and have the ability to potentiate antioxidant enzymes endogenously, including superoxide dismutase (SOD) and catalase [49].

Polyphenols are naturally occurring compounds classified according to the number of phenol rings and the structures that hold them together [50]. The main groups of polyphenols are flavonoids divided into flavones, flavonols, anthocyanidins, flavanones, catechins, and isoflavones [51]. Their structure is based on the 15-carbon skeleton (C6-C3-C6 fashion or two phenyl rings (A and B) associated with a three-carbon bridge). Their differentiation can be noticed based on the B ring attachment position, by the oxygenation degree and pattern, by the occurrence or not of the C-ring and C2-C3 double bond, and other variations [52]. As the secondary metabolites of plants, polyphenols are implicated in the defense against ultraviolet radiation or pathogens, but in the food, they provide bitterness, astringency, color, flavor, odor, and oxidative stability [53]. They are part of the human diet and are found in vegetables, fruits, cereal, chocolate, and beverages, including red wine, tea, and coffee [54,55] (Table 6.1).

Table 6.1 Flavonoid Structure and Classification

Flavonoids	Basic Structure		
Subclasses	Chemical Structure	Examples	Natural Sources
Flavones		Luteolin Apigenin Vitexin Orientin	Parsley, celery seed, oregano
Flavonols		Quercetin Kaempferol Myricetin Isorhamnetin Rutin Silymarin	Onions, apples, tea, berries

(Continued)

Table 6.1 (*Continued*) Flavonoid Structure and Classification

Flavonoids	Basic Structure		
Flavonones		Hesperetin Naringenin Eriodictyol Naringin	Citrus fruits and juices
Flavon-3-ols		Epicatechin Epigallocatechin Epicatechin 3-gallate Theaflavin Thearubigins	Green tea, chocolate, tree fruits, grapes, red wine
Anthocyanins		Cyanidin Delphinidin Malvidin Pelargonidin Peonidin Petunidin	Most berries, stone fruits
Isoflavones		Genistein Daidzein Glycitein	Soybeans, soy-based foods, legumes

The table shows flavonoid's chemical structure classified according to molecular configuration, examples of flavonoid compounds, and natural sources.

The beneficial effect of dietary polyphenols has been studied mainly due to their pharmacological properties, including antioxidant, anti-inflammatory, and anticancer effects. They have been linked to lower chances of developing cancer [56–60]. Meta-analyses indicated that long-term diets rich in polyphenols reduced the incidence of cancers, cardiovascular diseases, diabetes, osteoporosis, neurodegenerative diseases, and others [61,62] (Figure 6.2).

Even under normal conditions, oxidative stress and consequent damages occur in the cells; however, with aging, the rate of this damage speeds up because of deficient antioxidant mechanisms and a decrease in repair mechanisms [63,64]. A dietary intake of antioxidants may increase plasma antioxidant capacity and be reported as a significant factor to lessen the harmful effects of aging. Several studies have suggested that polyphenols may provide efficacy as antiaging compounds due to their antioxidant and anti-inflammatory properties [65,66].

Flavonoids are also found in high levels in fruits and vegetable extracts with a high total antioxidant activity. It was described that spinach, strawberry,

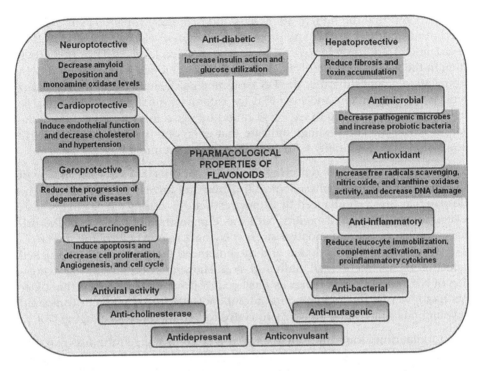

Figure 6.2 *Pharmacological properties of flavonoids. The figure shows the numerous pharmacological effects of flavonoids already described in the literature.*

or blueberry extracts used as dietary supplementation for 8 weeks were successful in counteracting age-related deficits in brain and behavioral function in aged rats [67]. The anthocyanins, found in berry fruits, concord grapes, and grape seeds, provided the color of the fruits and were described as having potent antioxidant and anti-inflammatory activities and inhibitory effects in lipid peroxidation and the cyclo-oxygenase (COX)-1 and -2 [68]. Tea catechins were also described as having potent activity against aging, and their consumption may delay the onset of aging [69]. Resveratrol from grapes has also been described as an antiaging compound. This compound targets sirtuin-1 (SIRT-1), which belongs to a class of nicotinamide adenine dinucleotide (NAD)-dependent deacetylases and seems to mediate the beneficial effects on health and longevity of both caloric restriction and resveratrol [70].

6.5 The effect of flavonoids on Nrf2 expression

Oxidative damage of proteins, lipids, and DNA has been described as one of the major causes of many aging disorders, including cataracts. Age-related cataracts are formed with the contribution of high levels of oxidative stress and antioxidants' protection failure. Nrf2 plays a crucial role in lens epithelial cells maintaining the redox balance through ROS elimination. Palsamy et al.

demonstrated that the human aging lens and diabetic cataractous lenses present diminished Nrf2 mRNA and protein expression levels, augmented levels of Keap1 mRNA and protein expression, and enhanced levels of DNA demethylation in the Keap1 promoter [71]. Conversely, clear human lens presented DNA methylation, suggesting that the DNA promoter's demethylation in the *Keap1* gene is age-dependent and essential for cataract formation [72] through the activation of Keap1 protein expression and increase in proteasomal degradation of Nrf2 [71]. The findings indicate that compounds that can induce Nrf2 expression may potentially help treat age-related cataracts.

During the aging process, removing the senescent cells that lost the capacity of dividing would improve physiological function and increase longevity [73]. The lifespan may also be enhanced by caloric restriction, causing a delay in diseases related to age [74]. In this regard, Nrf2 was demonstrated to be one of the primary regulators against oxidative stress, playing a role in controlling the favorable effects of calorie restriction and the enhanced autophagy and diminished induction of senescence cell. Shih and Yean showed a decrease in the expression of Nrf2 and its target genes as rats aged [75]. Suh et al. observed that older rats had lower levels of expression of total and nuclear Nrf2 protein compared to young rats, suggesting an Nrf2 protective role in the process of aging [76].

Using tomatidine, found in tomatoes, Gang et al. prolonged the lifespan and health span in *Caenorhabditis elegans*, which is considered an animal aging model that shares vital longevity associated with mammals' pathways via the Nrf2 pathway [77]. Protandim was demonstrated to be an Nrf2 activator from botanical extracts, increasing mice longevity, and its oral intake increased the levels of SOD and catalase in healthy humans' erythrocytes [78–80]. These studies suggest that activation of Nrf2 may prolong the lifespan and they may lead to the delay of the aging process.

Natural compounds, mostly polyphenols, from medicinal plants or dietary supplements containing polyphenols are known for their ability to eliminate free radicals by scavenging effects or inhibition of ROS production via chelation with metal ions to exhibit antioxidant defenses boosting [52]. By far, flavonoids are the most diverse group of phenolic secondary metabolites that present numerous biochemical activities [52]. The most studied and potent effect of flavonoids is their ability to work as antioxidants, depending on their functional groups' arrangement about the nuclear structure. The number of hydroxyl groups may also influence their antioxidant activity mechanism, radical scavenging, and metal ion chelation [81,82]. Flavonoids' phenolic structure with the more prominent activity associated with the diorthohydroxyl (catechol) functional moiety provides their direct ROS scavenging effect [83–85]. The antioxidant effects of flavonoids may involve inhibition of ROS production, ROS scavenging, and increased protection by antioxidant defenses [86,87]. They are known for their ability to work as free radical scavengers, and their benefits are, in part, attributed to a direct antioxidant activity through the modulation of signaling processes [88].

Polyphenols may also prevent oxidative damage by stimulating the transcription factor Nrf2, which is redox-sensitive. Nrf2 expression regulates genes that help to counteract oxidative stress and detoxify xenobiotics [89,90], controls cell survival and metabolic genes, and also plays a role in adipocyte differentiation [91]. The therapeutic potential of numerous polyphenols on Nrf2 expression and aging has been explored as described below.

6.6 Quercetin

Numerous studies have indicated the crucial role of oxidative stress in age-related macular degeneration (AMD), to cause irreversible blindness in older adults [92]. Quercetin, a naturally occurring flavonoid, was described as having antioxidant, ROS-scavenging, anti-inflammatory, and antitumor effects [93]. *In vivo* studies showed that quercetin effects showed potent protective effects on retina oxidative damage by activating Nrf2 expression and increasing antioxidant enzyme levels [94]. These studies showed that quercetin exerted its antioxidative and anti-inflammatory effects through the upregulation of the Nrf-2 signaling pathway, suggesting that this polyphenol may have a potential to be used as an antiaging compound.

6.7 Tangeretin

Tangeretin, a Chinese herb and the main phytochemical in tangerine peels, presented many pharmacological properties, including antioxidative and anti-inflammatory activities [95] by upregulating the Nrf2 signaling together with a reduction in the enzymatic and nonenzymatic antioxidant levels and inflammatory cytokines [96,97]. Li et al. described that tangeretin decreases oxidative stress damage in arthritic rats and controls the expression of inflammatory cytokines, decreasing the expression of pro-inflammatory cytokines (IL-1β, TNF-α, IFN-γ, and PGE2), increasing the expression of the anti-inflammatory cytokine IL-10, and enhancing the activity of antioxidant enzymes. The study showed that tangeretin exerted its antioxidative and anti-inflammatory effects through the upregulation of the Nrf-2 signaling pathway, suggesting that this polyphenol may have potential as a therapeutic agent in the treatment of arthritic and aging [98].

6.8 Resveratrol

Resveratrol, found in many foods, particularly in grapes, has been studied mainly for its antioxidant properties. In diabetic rats, resveratrol normalized renal Nrf2/Keap1 expression and the levels of its downstream regulatory proteins, providing kidney protection against hyperglycemia-mediated oxidative damage [99]. In testicular apoptotic cells, resveratrol attenuated type 1 diabetes-induced apoptosis, mostly related to Akt's Nrf2 activation via p62-dependent Keap1 degradation [100].

6.9 Caffeic acid

Caffeic acid, a coffee polyphenol, was shown to stimulate Nrf2 expression, and its electrophilic moiety was crucial for Keap1 protein oxidation [101]. Pang et al.'s studies showed that caffeic acid could inhibit Keap1 binding to Nrf2 through a decrease in Keap1 expression. This decrease leads to the activation of Nrf2 and consequent upregulation in the expression of antioxidants such as HO-1 and NQO1, which prevented hepatotoxicity caused by acetaminophen [102]. Moreover, Shen et al. demonstrated that caffeic acid also decreased Keap1 expression by p62/Sequestosome1-mediated autophagy, building up Nrf2 levels [103]. Kimet et al. also demonstrated that caffeic acid phenethyl ester, an analog of caffeic acid, had the ability to precipitate Keap1 and enhance the Nrf2 antioxidant pathway. The compound's effect was only completely activated in pathological conditions presenting oxidative stress, suggesting that caffeic acid phenethyl ester can be an Nrf2 activator [104].

6.10 Epigallocatechin gallate

Another well-known Nrf2 activator is *Epigallocatechin gallate* (EGCG), found in green tea. EGCG was reported to elevate the antioxidant activity and phase II enzymes in pulmonary fibrosis rat models treated with bleomycin but did no modify Keap1 levels considerably [105]. Thangapandiyan et al. reported that EGCG preadministration normalized Nrf2/Keap1 expression in the kidney of rats treated with fluoride [106]. Moreover, the activation of Nrf2 was significantly increased in the animal testis, showing enhanced expression of the target genes HO-1, NQO1, and γ-GCS, together with an inhibition of Keap1 [107]. EGCG also abolished oxidative stress induced by fluoride in lung injury through the activation of Nrf2/Keap1 signaling [108]. All these studies show evidence of the potential of EGCG as an Nrf2 activator to be used in the prevention and treatment of diseases associated with oxidative stress and inflammation. Phase I clinical studies using EGCG oral administration combined with radiotherapy were safe and effective, and phase II studies recommended a concentration of 440 µmol/L [109].

6.11 Gallic acid

A natural polyphenol, gallic acid, was described as having an inhibitory effect in hepatotoxicity induced by tertbutyl hydroperoxide by stimulating extracellular regulated kinase (ERK)/Nrf2-mediated antioxidant signaling. Gallic acid enhanced the nuclear translocations of Nrf2 and increased Nrf2 target proteins HO-1, glutamate-cysteine ligase catalytic (GCLC), and glutathione (GSH) [110]. Chandrasekhar et al. reported that pretreatment with gallic acid reversed Keap1 upregulation and Nrf2 downregulation caused by 6-OHDA and protected nerve cells from 6-OHDA-induced injury [111].

6.12 Luteolin

Luteolin, a flavone present in numerous fruits, vegetables, and herbs, has been reported to inhibit carcinogenesis and colon cancer through a high antioxidant effect [112–114]. It reduced ROS levels in colon cancer cells and enhanced the Nrf2 levels by an increased Nrf2 transcription mediated by DNA demethylation of its promoter. Furthermore, luteolin stimulated the association of Nrf2 and p53, inducing the expression of antioxidant enzymes and proteins associated with apoptosis. The studies indicated luteolin's therapeutic potential in cancer prevention and treatment through Nrf2 modulation [115].

6.13 7-O-methylbiochanin A

Li et al. analyzed the association of flavonoids' structure-activity and their effect on Nrf2 activation and oxidative stress prevention. The results demonstrated that the isoflavone 7-O-methylbiochanin A (7-MBA) activated the Nrf2 signaling pathway and provided protection to human lung epithelial cells against cell death induced by sodium arsenite in an Nrf2-dependent way [116]. By increasing Nrf2 stabilization, blocking its ubiquitination, and regulating its phosphorylation, 7-MBA induced the Nrf2-dependent antioxidant system's upregulation. Considering that kinases play an essential role in Nrf2 phosphorylation and activation, the authors also reported that the 7-MBA mechanism to activate Nrf2 involves PI3K, MAPK, PKC, and PERK pathways. The findings suggest that 7-MBA may have a potential in the prevention of oxidative stress through Nrf2 activation [116].

6.14 Conclusion

The aging process leads to a decline in the Nrf2 activation and induces oxidative stress and associated diseases. Therefore, nutraceuticals can activate Nrf2 signaling, which induces the transcription of cytoprotective and antioxidant genes, maybe a potential approach for modulation of aging. Although several natural flavonoids have been described as Nrf2 activators, only a few of them are commercially available or easily obtained. Thus, more investigations are needed to discover novel flavonoids that may work as Nrf2 activators. More clinical studies are necessary to confirm their beneficial therapeutic effects against aging and age-associated diseases (Figure 6.3).

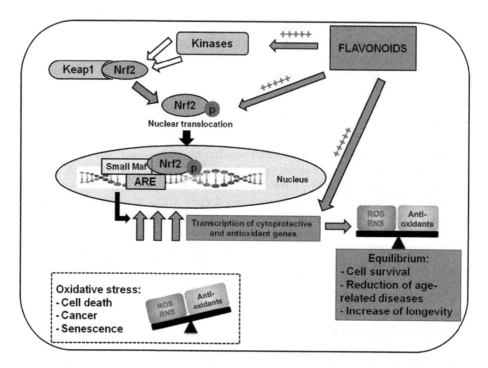

Figure 6.3 *The beneficial role of flavonoids in Nrf2 modulation. The diagram shows the effect of flavonoids in Nrf2 activation and transcription of cytoprotective genes essential to maintain cell survival, reduce age-associated disease, decrease oxidative stress levels, and increase lifespan.*

References

1. López-Otín, C.; Blasco, M.A.; Partridge, L.; Serrano, M.; Kroemer, G. The hallmarks of aging. *Cell* **2013**, *153*, 1194–1217, doi:10.1016/j.cell.2013.05.039.
2. Lenaz, G. Role of mitochondria in oxidative stress and aging. *Biochimica et Biophysica Acta (BBA)-Bioenergetics* **1998**, *1366*, 53–67.
3. Harman, D. The free radical theory of aging affects age on serum copper levels. *J. Gerontol.* **1965**, *20*, 151–153.
4. Schmidlin, C.J.; Dodson, M.B.; Madhavan, L.; Zhang, D.D. Redox regulation by NRF2 in aging and disease. *Free Radic. Biol. Med.* **2019**, *134*, 702–707, doi:10.1016/j.freeradbiomed.2019.01.016.
5. Green, DR; Galluzzi, L.; Kroemer, G. Mitochondria and the autophagy–inflammation–cell death axis in organismal aging. *Science* **2011**, *333*, 1109–1112.
6. Bruns, D.R.; Drake, J.C.; Biela, L.M.; Peelor, F.F.; Miller, B.F.; Hamilton, K.L. Nrf2 Signaling and the Slowed Aging Phenotype: Evidence from Long-Lived Models. *Oxid. Med. Cell. Longev.* **2015**, *2015*, 732596, doi:10.1155/2015/732596.
7. Kaspar, J.W.; Niture, S.K.; Jaiswal, A.K. Nrf2:INrf2 (Keap1) signaling in oxidative stress. *Free Radic. Biol. Med.* **2009**, *47*, 1304–1309, doi:10.1016/j.freeradbiomed.2009.07.035.
8. Harman, D. Free radical theory of aging: An update: increasing the functional life span. *Ann. N. Y. Acad. Sci.* **2006**, *1067*, 10–21, doi:10.1196/annals.1354.003.
9. Salmon, A.B.; Richardson, A.; Pérez, V.I. Update on the oxidative stress theory of aging: does oxidative stress play a role in aging or healthy aging? *Free Radic. Biol. Med.* **2010**, *48*, 642–655, doi:10.1016/j.freeradbiomed.2009.12.015.

10. Lewis, K.N.; Mele, J.; Hayes, J.D.; Buffenstein, R. Nrf2, a guardian of healthspan and gatekeeper of species longevity. *Integr. Comp. Biol.* **2010**, *50*, 829–843, doi:10.1093/icb/icq034.

11. Lee, J.M.; Calkins, M.J.; Chan, K.; Kan, Y.W.; Johnson, J.A. Identification of the NF-E2-related factor-2-dependent genes conferring protection against oxidative stress in primary cortical astrocytes using oligonucleotide microarray analysis. *J. Biol. Chem.* **2003**, *278*, 12029–12038, doi:10.1074/jbc.M211558200.

12. Liu, X.M.; Peyton, K.J.; Ensenat, D.; Wang, H.; Hannink, M.; Alam, J.; Durante, W. Nitric oxide stimulates heme oxygenase-1 gene transcription via the Nrf2/ARE complex to promote vascular smooth muscle cell survival. *Cardiovasc. Res.* **2007**, *75*, 381–389, doi:10.1016/j.cardiores.2007.03.004.

13. Leiser, S.F.; Miller, R.A. Nrf2 Signaling, a mechanism for cellular stress resistance in long-lived mice. *Mol. Cell. Biol.* **2010**, *30*, 871–884, doi:10.1128/mcb.01145-09.

14. Uruno, A.; Motohashi, H. The Keap1-Nrf2 system as an in vivo sensor for electrophiles. *Nitric Oxide* **2011**, *25*, 153–160, doi:10.1016/j.niox.2011.02.007.

15. Ahmed, S.M.; Luo, L.; Namani, A.; Wang, X.J.; Tang, X. Nrf2 signaling pathway: Pivotal roles in inflammation. *Biochimica et Biophysica Acta. Mol. Basis Dis.* **2017**, *1863*, 585–597, doi:10.1016/j.bbadis.2016.11.005.

16. Bellezza, I. Oxidative stress in age-related macular degeneration: Nrf2 as therapeutic target. *Front. Pharmacol.* **2018**, *9*, 1280-1280, doi:10.3389/fphar.2018.01280.

17. Itoh, K.; Wakabayashi, N.; Katoh, Y.; Ishii, T.; Igarashi, K.; Engel, J.D.; Yamamoto, M. Keap1 represses nuclear activation of antioxidant responsive elements by Nrf2 through binding to the amino-terminal Neh2 domain. *Genes Dev.* **1999**, *13*, 76–86.

18. Tong, K.I.; Kobayashi, A.; Katsuoka, F.; Yamamoto, M. Two-site substrate recognition model for the Keap1-Nrf2 system: A hinge and latch mechanism. *Biol. Chem.* **2006**, *387*, 1311–1320.

19. Tebay, L.E.; Robertson, H.; Durant, S.T.; Vitale, S.R.; Penning, T.M.; Dinkova-Kostova, A.T.; Hayes, J.D. Mechanisms of activation of the transcription factor Nrf2 by redox stressors, nutrient cues, and energy status and the pathways through which it attenuates degenerative disease. *Free Radic. Biol. Med.* **2015**, *88*, 108–146.

20. Baird, L.; Dinkova-Kostova, A.T. The cytoprotective role of the Keap1-Nrf2 pathway. *Arch. Toxicol.* **2011**, *85*, 241–272, doi:10.1007/s00204-011-0674-5.

21. Paunkov, A.; Chartoumpekis, D.V.; Ziros, P.G.; Sykiotis, G.P. A bibliometric review of the Keap1/Nrf2 pathway and its related antioxidant compounds. *Antioxidants* **2019**, *8*, 353.

22. Malhotra, D.; Portales-Casamar, E.; Singh, A.; Srivastava, S.; Arenillas, D.; Happel, C.; Shyr, C.; Wakabayashi, N.; Kensler, T.W.; Wasserman, W.W. Global mapping of binding sites for Nrf2 identifies novel targets in cell survival response through ChIP-Seq profiling and network analysis. *Nucleic Acids Res.* **2010**, *38*, 5718–5734.

23. Sykiotis, G.P.; Bohmann, D. Stress-activated cap'n'collar transcription factors in aging and human disease. *Sci. Signal* **2010**, *3*, re3, doi:10.1126/scisignal.3112re3.

24. Miura, Y.; Endo, T. Survival responses to oxidative stress and aging. *Geriatrics Gerontol. Int.* **2010**, *10 Suppl 1*, S1–9, doi:10.1111/j.1447-0594.2010.00597.x.

25. Bota, D.A.; Davies, K.J.A. Lon protease preferentially degrades oxidized mitochondrial aconitase by an ATP-stimulated mechanism. *Nat. Cell Biol.* **2002**, *4*, 674–680, doi:10.1038/ncb836.

26. Bota, D.A.; Van Remmen, H.; Davies, K.J. Modulation of Lon protease activity and aconitase turnover during aging and oxidative stress. *FEBS Lett.* **2002**, *532*, 103–106, doi:10.1016/s0014-5793(02)03638-4.

27. Ngo, J.K.; Pomatto, L.C.; Davies, K.J. Upregulation of the mitochondrial Lon Protease allows adaptation to acute oxidative stress dysregulation is associated with chronic stress, disease, and aging. *Redox Biol* **2013**, *1*, 258–264, doi:10.1016/j.redox.2013.01.015.

28. El Assar, M.; Angulo, J.; Rodríguez-Mañas, L. Oxidative stress and vascular inflammation in aging. *Free Radic. Biol. Med.* **2013**, *65*, 380–401, doi:10.1016/j.freeradbiomed.2013.07.003.

29. Volonte, D.; Liu, Z.; Musille, P.M.; Stoppani, E.; Wakabayashi, N.; Di, YP; Lisanti, M.P.; Kensler, T.W.; Galbiati, F. Inhibition of nuclear factor-erythroid 2-related factor (Nrf2) by caveolin-1 promotes stress-induced premature senescence. *Mol. Biol. Cell* **2013**, *24*, 1852–1862, doi:10.1091/mbc.E12-09-0666.

30. Gounder, SS; Kannan, S.; Devadoss, D.; Miller, C.J.; Whitehead, K.J.; Odelberg, S.J.; Firpo, M.A.; Paine, R., 3rd; Hoidal, J.R.; Abel, E.D., et al. Impaired transcriptional activity of Nrf2 in age-related myocardial oxidative stress is reversible by moderate exercise training. *PLoS One* **2012**, *7*, e45697, doi:10.1371/journal.pone.0045697.

31. Zhang, H.; Davies, K.J.A.; Forman, H.J. Oxidative stress response and Nrf2 signaling in aging. *Free Radic. Biol. Med.* **2015**, *88*, 314–336, doi:10.1016/j.freeradbiomed.2015.05.036.

32. Chan, K.; Kan, Y.W. Nrf2 is essential for protection against acute pulmonary injury in mice. *Proc. Natl. Acad. Sci. U. S. A.* **1999**, *96*, 12731–12736, doi:10.1073/pnas.96.22.12731.

33. Enomoto, A.; Itoh, K.; Nagayoshi, E.; Haruta, J.; Kimura, T.; O'Connor, T.; Harada, T.; Yamamoto, M. High sensitivity of Nrf2 knockout mice to acetaminophen hepatotoxicity associated with decreased expression of ARE-regulated drug-metabolizing enzymes and antioxidant genes. *Toxicol. Sci.* **2001**, *59*, 169–177, doi:10.1093/toxsci/59.1.169.

34. Kojima, T.; Dogru, M.; Higuchi, A.; Nagata, T.; Ibrahim, O.M.; Inaba, T.; Tsubota, K. The effect of Nrf2 knockout on ocular surface protection from acute tobacco smoke exposure: Evidence from Nrf2 knockout mice. *Am. J. Pathol.* **2015**, *185*, 776–785, doi:10.1016/j.ajpath.2014.11.014.

35. Ramos-Gomez, M.; Kwak, M.K.; Dolan, P.M.; Itoh, K.; Yamamoto, M.; Talalay, P.; Kensler, T.W. Sensitivity to carcinogenesis is increased, and chemoprotective efficacy of enzyme inducers is lost in nrf2 transcription factor-deficient mice. *Proc. Natl. Acad. Sci. U. S. A.* **2001**, *98*, 3410–3415, doi:10.1073/pnas.051618798.

36. Khor, To; Huang, M.T.; Prawan, A.; Liu, Y.; Hao, X.; Yu, S.; Cheung, W.K.; Chan, J.Y.; Reddy, B.S.; Yang, C.S., et al. Increased susceptibility of Nrf2 knockout mice to colitis-associated colorectal cancer. *Cancer Prev. Res. (Phila.)* **2008**, *1*, 187–191, doi:10.1158/1940-6207.capr-08-0028.

37. Cheung, K.L.; Lee, J.H.; Khor, TO; Wu, T.Y.; Li, GX; Chan, J.; Yang, C.S.; Kong, A.N. Nrf2 knockout enhances intestinal tumorigenesis in Apc(min/+) mice due to attenuation of antioxidative stress pathway while potentiates inflammation. *Mol. Carcinog.* **2014**, *53*, 77–84, doi:10.1002/mc.21950.

38. Meakin, P.J.; Chowdhry, S.; Sharma, R.S.; Ashford, F.B.; Walsh, S.V.; McCrimmon, R.J.; Dinkova-Kostova, A.T.; Dillon, J.F.; Hayes, J.D.; Ashford, M.L. Susceptibility of Nrf2-null mice to steatohepatitis and cirrhosis upon consumption of a high-fat diet is associated with oxidative stress, perturbation of the unfolded protein response, and disturbance in the expression of metabolic enzymes but not with insulin resistance. *Mol. Cell. Biol.* **2014**, *34*, 3305–3320, doi:10.1128/mcb.00677-14.

39. Mitsuishi, Y.; Motohashi, H.; Yamamoto, M. The Keap1-Nrf2 system in cancers: stress response and anabolic metabolism. *Front. Oncol.* **2012**, *2*, 200, doi:10.3389/fonc.2012.00200.

40. Hoshino, T.; Tabuchi, K.; Nishimura, B.; Tanaka, S.; Nakayama, M.; Ishii, T.; Warabi, E.; Yanagawa, T.; Shimizu, R.; Yamamoto, M. et al. Protective role of Nrf2 in age-related hearing loss and gentamicin ototoxicity. *Biochem. Biophys. Res. Commun.* **2011**, *415*, 94–98, doi:10.1016/j.bbrc.2011.10.019.

41. Shih, P.H.; Yen, G.C. Differential expressions of antioxidant status in aging rats: the role of transcriptional factor Nrf2 and MAPK signaling pathway. *Biogerontology* **2007**, *8*, 71–80, doi:10.1007/s10522-006-9033-y.

42. Li, M.; Li, C.; Parkhouse, W.S. Age-related differences in the des IGF-I-mediated activation of Akt-1 and p70 S6K in mouse skeletal muscle. *Mech. Ageing Dev.* **2003**, *124*, 771–778, doi:10.1016/s0047-6374(03)00124-6.

43. Shay, K.P.; Hagen, T.M. Age-associated impairment of Akt phosphorylation in primary rat hepatocytes is remediated by alpha-lipoic acid through PI3 kinase, PTEN, and PP2A. *Biogerontology* **2009**, *10*, 443–456, doi:10.1007/s10522-008-9187-x.
44. Jiang, T.; Yin, F.; Yao, J.; Brinton, R.D.; Cadenas, E. Lipoic acid restores age-associated impairment of brain energy metabolism modulation of Akt/JNK signaling and PGC1α transcriptional pathway. *Aging Cell* **2013**, *12*, 1021–1031, doi:10.1111/acel.12127.
45. Yang, F.; Chu, X.; Yin, M.; Liu, X.; Yuan, H.; Niu, Y.; Fu, L. mTOR, and autophagy in normal brain aging and caloric restriction ameliorate age-related cognition deficits. *Behav. Brain Res.* **2014**, *264*, 82–90, doi:10.1016/j.bbr.2014.02.005.
46. Verschoor, C.P.; Johnstone, J.; Loeb, M.; Bramson, J.L.; Bowdish, D.M. Antipneumococcal deficits of monocyte-derived macrophages from the advanced-age, frail elderly and related impairments in PI3K-AKT signaling. *Hum. Immunol.* **2014**, *75*, 1192–1196, doi:10.1016/j.humimm.2014.10.004.
47. Silva-Palacios, A.; Ostolga-Chavarria, M.; Zazueta, C.; Konigsberg, M. Nrf2: Molecular and epigenetic regulation during aging. *Ageing Res Rev* **2018**, *47*, 31–40, doi:10.1016/j.arr.2018.06.003.
48. Moran, J.F.; Klucas, R.V.; Grayer, R.J.; Abian, J.; Becana, M. Complexes of iron with phenolic compounds from soybean nodules and other legume tissues: Prooxidant and antioxidant properties. *Free Radic. Biol. Med.* **1997**, *22*, 861–870, doi:10.1016/s0891-5849(96)00426-1.
49. Si, H.; Liu, D. Dietary antiaging phytochemicals and mechanisms associated with prolonged survival. *J Nutr Biochem* **2014**, *25*, 581–591, doi:10.1016/j.jnutbio.2014.02.001.
50. Stevenson, D.E.; Hurst, R.D. Polyphenolic phytochemicals – Just antioxidants or much more? *Cell. Mol. Life Sci.* **2007**, *64*, 2900–2916, doi:10.1007/s00018-007-7237-1.
51. Lotito, SB; Frei, B. Consumption of flavonoid-rich foods and increased plasma antioxidant capacity in humans: Cause, consequence, or epiphenomenon? *Free Radic. Biol. Med.* **2006**, *41*, 1727–1746, doi:10.1016/j.freeradbiomed.2006.04.033.
52. Habtemariam, S. The Nrf2/HO-1 axis as targets for flavanones: Neuroprotection by pinocembrin, naringenin, and eriodictyol. *Oxid. Med. Cell. Longev.* **2019**, *2019*, 4724920, doi:10.1155/2019/4724920.
53. Beckman, C.H. Phenolic-storing cells: keys to programmed cell death and periderm formation in wilt disease resistance and general defense responses in plants? *Physiol. Mol. Plant Pathol.* **2000**, *57*, 101–110, doi:10.1006/pmpp.2000.0287.
54. Scalbert, A.; Manach, C.; Morand, C.; Rémésy, C.; Jiménez, L. Dietary polyphenols and the prevention of diseases. *Crit. Rev. Food Sci. Nutr.* **2005**, *45*, 287–306, doi:10.1080/1040869059096.
55. Spencer, J.P.; Abd El Mohsen, MM; Minihane, A.M.; Mathers, J.C. Biomarkers of the intake of dietary polyphenols: strengths, limitations, and application in nutrition research. *Br. J. Nutr.* **2008**, *99*, 12–22, doi:10.1017/s0007114507798938.
56. Knekt, P.; Järvinen, R.; Seppänen, R.; Hellövaara, M.; Teppo, L.; Pukkala, E.; Aromaa, A. Dietary flavonoids and the risk of lung cancer and other malignant neoplasms. *Am. J. Epidemiol.* **1997**, *146*, 223–230, doi:10.1093/oxfordjournals.aje.a009257.
57. Cao, G.; Russell, R.M.; Lischner, N.; Prior, RL Serum antioxidant capacity is increased by consumption of strawberries, spinach, red wine, or vitamin C in elderly women. *J. Nutr.* **1998**, *128*, 2383–2390, doi:10.1093/jn/128.12.2383.
58. Garcia-Closas, R.; Gonzalez, C.A.; Agudo, A.; Riboli, E. Intake of specific carotenoids and flavonoids and the risk of gastric cancer in Spain. *Cancer Causes Control* **1999**, *10*, 71–75, doi:10.1023/a:1008867108960.
59. Levi, F. Cancer prevention: epidemiology and perspectives. *Eur. J. Cancer* **1999**, *35*, 1912–1924, doi:10.1016/s0959-8049(99)00294-4.
60. Knekt, P.; Kumpulainen, J.; Järvinen, R.; Rissanen, H.; Heliövaara, M.; Reunanen, A.; Hakulinen, T.; Aromaa, A. Flavonoid intake and risk of chronic diseases. *Am. J. Clin. Nutr.* **2002**, *76*, 560–568, doi:10.1093/ajcn/76.3.560.

61. Graf, B.A.; Milbury, P.E.; Blumberg, J.B. Flavonols, flavones, flavanones, and human health: epidemiological evidence. *J. Med. Food* **2005**, *8*, 281–290, doi:10.1089/jmf.2005.8.281.
62. Arts, IC; Hollman, P.C. Polyphenols, and disease risk in epidemiologic studies. *Am. J. Clin. Nutr.* **2005**, *81*, 317s-325s, doi:10.1093/ajcn/81.1.317S.
63. Rizvi, S.I.; Maurya, PK Alterations in antioxidant enzymes during aging in humans. *Mol. Biotechnol.* **2007**, *37*, 58–61, doi:10.1007/s12033-007-0048-7.
64. Pandey, K.B.; Rizvi, S.I. Markers of oxidative stress in erythrocytes and plasma during aging in humans. *Oxid. Med. Cell. Longev.* **2010**, *3*, 2–12, doi:10.4161/oxim.3.1.10476.
65. Cao, G.; Booth, S.L.; Sadowski, J.A.; Prior, RL Increases in human plasma antioxidant capacity after consumption of controlled diets high in fruit and vegetables. *Am. J. Clin. Nutr.* **1998**, *68*, 1081–1087, doi:10.1093/ajcn/68.5.1081.
66. Joseph, J.A.; Shukitt-Hale, B.; Casadesus, G. Reversing the deleterious effects of aging on neuronal communication and behavior: Beneficial properties of fruit polyphenolic compounds. *Am. J. Clin. Nutr.* **2005**, *81*, 313s-316s, doi:10.1093/ajcn/81.1.313S.
67. Shukitt-Hale, B.; Lau, F.C.; Joseph, J.A. Berry fruit supplementation and the aging brain. *J. Agric. Food Chem.* **2008**, *56*, 636–641, doi:10.1021/jf072505f.
68. Seeram, N.P.; Cichewicz, R.H.; Chandra, A.; Nair, M.G. Cyclooxygenase inhibitory and antioxidant compounds from crabapple fruits. *J. Agric. Food Chem.* **2003**, *51*, 1948–1951, doi:10.1021/jf025993u.
69. Maurya, PK; Rizvi, S.I. Protective role of tea catechins on erythrocytes subjected to oxidative stress during human aging. *Natural product research* **2009**, *23*, 1072–1079, doi:10.1080/14786410802267643.
70. Markus, M.A.; Morris, B.J. Resveratrol in prevention and treatment of common clinical conditions of aging. *Clin. Interv. Aging,* **2008**, *3*, 331–339.
71. Palsamy, P.; Ayaki, M.; Elanchezhian, R.; Shinohara, T. Promoter demethylation of Keap1 gene in human diabetic cataractous lenses. *Biochem. Biophys. Res. Commun.* **2012**, *423*, 542–548.
72. Gao, Y.; Yan, Y.; Huang, T. Human age-related cataracts: Epigenetic suppression of the nuclear factor erythroid 2-related factor 2-mediated antioxidant system. *Mol. Med. Report.* **2015**, *11*, 1442–1447.
73. Naylor, R.; Baker, DJ; Van Deursen, J. Senescent cells: A novel therapeutic target for aging and age-related diseases. *Clin. Pharmacol. Ther.* **2013**, *93*, 105–116.
74. Bishop, N.A.; Guarente, L. Two neurons mediate diet-restriction-induced longevity in C. elegans. *Nature* **2007**, *447*, 545–549.
75. Shih, P.-H.; Yen, G.-C. Differential expressions of antioxidant status in aging rats: the role of transcriptional factor Nrf2 and MAPK signaling pathway. *Biogerontology* **2007**, *8*, 71–80.
76. Suh, J.H.; Shenvi, S.V.; Dixon, B.M.; Liu, H.; Jaiswal, AK; Liu, R.-M.; Hagen, T.M. Decline in transcriptional activity of Nrf2 causes age-related loss of glutathione synthesis, which is reversible with lipoic acid. *Proc. Nat. Acad. Sci.* **2004**, *101*, 3381–3386.
77. Fang, E.F.; Waltz, T.B.; Kassahun, H.; Lu, Q.; Kerr, J.S.; Morevati, M.; Fivenson, E.M.; Wollman, B.N.; Marosi, K.; Wilson, M.A. Tomatidine enhances lifespan and healthspan in C. elegans through mitophagy induction via the SKN-1/Nrf2 pathway. *Sci. Rep.* **2017**, *7*, 46208.
78. Velmurugan, K.; Alam, J.; McCord, J.M.; Pugazhenthi, S. Synergistic induction of heme oxygenase-1 by the components of the antioxidant supplement Protandim. *Free Radic. Biol. Med.* **2009**, *46*, 430–440.
79. Strong, R.; Miller, R.A.; Antebi, A.; Astle, C.M.; Bogue, M.; Denzel, M.S.; Fernandez, E.; Flurkey, K.; Hamilton, K.L.; Lamming, DW Longer lifespan in male mice treated with a weakly estrogenic agonist, an antioxidant, an α-glucosidase inhibitor or an Nrf2-inducer. *Aging cell* **2016**, *15*, 872–884.

80. Nelson, S.K.; Bose, S.K.; Grunwald, G.K.; Myhill, P.; McCord, J.M. The induction of human superoxide dismutase and catalase in vivo: a fundamentally new approach to antioxidant therapy. *Free Radic. Biol. Med.* **2006**, *40*, 341–347.

81. Heim, K.E.; Tagliaferro, A.R.; Bobilya, D.J. Flavonoid antioxidants: chemistry, metabolism, and structure-activity relationships. *J Nutr Biochem* **2002**, *13*, 572–584.

82. Pandey, A.; Mishra, A.; Mishra, A. Antifungal and antioxidative potential of oil and extracts derived from leaves of Indian spice plant Cinnamomum tamala. *Cell. Mol. Biol.* **2012**, *58*, 142–147.

83. De Martino, L.; Mencherini, T.; Mancini, E.; Aquino, R.P.; De Almeida, L.F.; De Feo, V. In vitro phytotoxicity and antioxidant activity of selected flavonoids. *Int. J. Mol. Sci.* **2012**, *13*, 5406–5419, doi:10.3390/ijms13055406.

84. Pallauf, K.; Duckstein, N.; Hasler, M.; Klotz, L.-O.; Rimbach, G. Flavonoids as putative inducers of the transcription factors Nrf2, FoxO, and PPARγ. *Oxid. Med. Cell. Longev.* **2017**, *2017*, 4397340, doi:10.1155/2017/4397340.

85. Kumar, S.; Pandey, A.K. Chemistry, and biological activities of flavonoids: An overview. *Sci. World J.* **2013**, *2013*, 162750, doi:10.1155/2013/162750.

86. Mishra, A.; Kumar, S.; Pandey, A.K. Scientific validation of the medicinal efficacy of *Tinospora cordifolia*. *Sci. World J.* **2013**, *2013*, 292934, doi:10.1155/2013/292934.

87. Halliwell, B.; Gutteridge, J.M.C. *Free Radicals in Biology and Medicine*, 5th ed.; Oxford University Press: Oxford, 2015; pp. 944, doi:10.1093/acprof:oso/9780198717478.001.0001.

88. Williams, R.J.; Spencer, J.P.; Rice-Evans, C. Flavonoids: Antioxidants or signalling molecules? *Free Radic. Biol. Med.* **2004**, *36*, 838–849, doi:10.1016/j.freeradbiomed.2004.01.001.

89. Alam, J.; Stewart, D.; Touchard, C.; Boinapally, S.; Choi, A.M.; Cook, J.L. Nrf2, a Cap'n'Collar transcription factor, regulates induction of the heme oxygenase-1 gene. *J. Biol. Chem.* **1999**, *274*, 26071–26078, doi:10.1074/jbc.274.37.26071.

90. Venugopal, R.; Jaiswal, A.K. Nrf1 and Nrf2 positively and c-Fos and Fra1 negatively regulate the human antioxidant response element-mediated expression of NAD(P)H: Quinone oxidoreductase1 gene. *Proc. Natl. Acad. Sci. U. S. A.* **1996**, *93*, 14960–14965, doi:10.1073/pnas.93.25.14960.

91. Chorley, B.N.; Campbell, M.R.; Wang, X.; Karaca, M.; Sambandan, D.; Bangura, F.; Xue, P.; Pi, J.; Kleeberger, S.R.; Bell, DA Identification of novel NRF2-regulated genes by ChIP-Seq: Influence on retinoid X receptor-alpha. *Nucleic Acids Res.* **2012**, *40*, 7416–7429, doi:10.1093/nar/gks409.

92. Chiras, D.; Kitsos, G.; Petersen, M.B.; Skalidakis, I.; Kroupis, C. Oxidative stress in dry age-related macular degeneration and exfoliation syndrome. *Crit. Rev. Clin. Lab. Sci.* **2015**, *52*, 12–27, doi:10.3109/10408363.2014.968703.

93. Russo, M.; Spagnuolo, C.; Tedesco, I.; Bilotto, S.; Russo, G.L. The flavonoid quercetin in disease prevention and therapy: facts and fancies. *Biochem. Pharmacol.* **2012**, *83*, 6–15, doi:10.1016/j.bcp.2011.08.010.

94. Shao, Y.; Yu, H.; Yang, Y.; Li, M.; Hang, L.; Xu, X. A solid dispersion of quercetin shows enhanced Nrf2 activation and protective effects against oxidative injury in a mouse model of dry age-related macular degeneration. *Oxidat. Med. Cell. Long.* **2019**, *2019*, 1479571, doi:10.1155/2019/1479571.

95. Campo, G.M.; Avenoso, A.; Campo, S.; Ferlazzo, A.M.; Altavilla, D.; Calatroni, A. Efficacy of treatment with glycosaminoglycans on experimental collagen-induced arthritis in rats. *Arthritis Res. Ther.* **2003**, *5*, R122–R131, doi:10.1186/ar748.

96. Lakshmi, P., Bhanu, PK, Venkata, SK and Josthna, P. Herbal and medicinal plants molecules towards treatment of cancer: A mini-review. *Am. J. Ethnomed.* **2015**, *2*(2), 136–142.

97. Liang, F.; Fang, Y.; Cao, W.; Zhang, Z.; Pan, S.; Xu, X. Attenuation of tert-Butyl Hydroperoxide (t-BHP)-induced oxidative damage in HepG2 Cells by Tangeretin: Relevance of the Nrf2–ARE and MAPK signaling pathways. *J. Agric. Food Chem.* **2018**, *66*, 6317–6325, doi:10.1021/acs.jafc.8b01875.

98. Li, X.; Xie, P.; Hou, Y.; Chen, S.; He, P.; Xiao, Z.; Zhan, J.; Luo, D.; Gu, M.; Lin, D. Tangeretin Inhibits oxidative stress and inflammation via upregulating Nrf-2 signaling pathway in collagen-induced arthritic rats. *Pharmacology* **2019**, *104*, 187–195, doi:10.1159/000501163.

99. Palsamy, P.; Subramanian, S. Resveratrol protects diabetic kidneys by attenuating hyperglycemia mediated-oxidative stress and renal inflammatory cytokines via Nrf2-Keap1 signaling. *Biochimica et Biophysica Acta – Mol. Basis Dis.* **2011**, *1812*, 719–731, doi:10.1016/j.bbadis.2011.03.008.

100. Zhao, Y.; Song, W.; Wang, Z.; Wang, Z.; Jin, X.; Xu, J.; Bai, L.; Li, Y.; Cui, J.; Cai, L. Resveratrol attenuates testicular apoptosis in type 1 diabetic mice: Role of Akt-mediated Nrf2 activation and p62-dependent Keap1 degradation. *Redox Biol.* **2018**, *14*, 609–617, doi:10.1016/j.redox.2017.11.007.

101. Sirota, R.; Gibson, D.; Kohen, R. The role of the catecholic and the electrophilic moieties of caffeic acid in Nrf2/Keap1 pathway activation in ovarian carcinoma cell lines. *Redox Biol.* **2015**, *4*, 48–59, doi:10.1016/j.redox.2014.11.012.

102. Pang, C.; Zheng, Z.; Shi, L.; Sheng, Y.; Wei, H.; Wang, Z.; Ji, L. Caffeic acid prevents acetaminophen-induced liver injury by activating the Keap1-Nrf2 antioxidative defense system. *Free Radic. Biol. Med.* **2016**, *91*, 236–246, doi:10.1016/j.freeradbiomed.2015.12.024.

103. Shen, J.; Wang, G.; Zuo, J. Caffeic acid inhibits HCV replication via induction of IFNα antiviral response through p62-mediated Keap1/Nrf2 signaling pathway. *Antiviral Res.* **2018**, *154*, 166–173, doi:10.1016/j.antiviral.2018.04.008.

104. Kim, H.; Kim, W.; Yum, S.; Hong, S.; Oh, J.E.; Lee, J.W.; Kwak, M.K.; Park, E.J.; Na, DH; Jung, Y. Caffeic acid phenethyl ester activation of Nrf2 pathway is enhanced under oxidative state: Structural analysis and potential as a pathologically targeted therapeutic agent in the treatment of colonic inflammation. *Free Radic. Biol. Med.* **2013**, *65*, 552–562, doi:10.1016/j.freeradbiomed.2013.07.015.

105. Sriram, N.; Kalayarasan, S.; Sudhandiran, G. Epigallocatechin-3-gallate augments antioxidant activities and inhibits inflammation bleomycin-induced experimental pulmonary fibrosis through Nrf2-Keap1 signaling. *Pulm. Pharmacol. Ther.* **2009**, *22*, 221–236, doi:10.1016/j.pupt.2008.12.010.

106. Thangapandiyan, S.; Miltonprabu, S. Epigallocatechin gallate supplementation protects against renal injury induced by fluoride intoxication in rats: Role of Nrf2/HO-1 signaling. *Toxicol. Rep.* **2014**, *1*, 12–30, doi:10.1016/j.toxrep.2014.01.002.

107. Thangapandiyan, S.; Miltonprabu, S. Epigallocatechin gallate exacerbates fluoride-induced oxidative stress-mediated testicular toxicity in rats through the activation of Nrf2 signaling pathway. *Asian Pac. J. Reprod.* **2015**, *4*, 272–287, doi:10.1016/j.apjr.2015.07.005.

108. Shanmugam, T.; Selvaraj, M.; Poomalai, S. Epigallocatechin gallate potentially abrogates fluoride-induced lung oxidative stress, inflammation via Nrf2/Keap1 signaling pathway in rats: An in-vivo and in-silico study. *Int. Immunopharmacol.* **2016**, *39*, 128–139, doi:10.1016/j.intimp.2016.07.022.

109. Zhao, H.; Zhu, W.; Xie, P.; Li, H.; Zhang, X.; Sun, X.; Yu, J.; Xing, L. A phase I study of concurrent chemotherapy and thoracic radiotherapy with oral epigallocatechin-3-gallate protection in patients with locally advanced stage III non-small-cell lung cancer. *Radiother. Oncol.* **2014**, *110*, 132–136, doi:10.1016/j.radonc.2013.10.014.

110. Feng, R.B.; Wang, Y.; He, C.; Yang, Y.; Wan, J.B. Gallic acid, a natural polyphenol, protects against tert-butyl hydroperoxide- induced hepatotoxicity by activating ERK-Nrf2-Keap1-mediated antioxidative response. *Food Chem. Toxicol.* **2018**, *119*, 479–488, doi:10.1016/j.fct.2017.10.033.

111. Chandrasekhar, Y.; Phani Kumar, G. Gallic acid protects 6-OHDA induced neurotoxicity by attenuating oxidative stress in human dopaminergic cell line. **2018**, *43*, 1150–1160, doi:10.1007/s11064-018-2530-y.

112. Pandurangan, A.K.; Dharmalingam, P.; Sadagopan, S.K.A.; Ramar, M.; Munusamy, A. Luteolin induces growth arrest in colon cancer cells through the involvement of Wnt/β-catenin/GSK-3β signaling. *J. Environ. Pathol. Toxicol. Oncol.* **2013**, *32*.
113. Kang, K.A.; Hyun, J.W. Oxidative stress, Nrf2, and epigenetic modification contribute to anticancer drug resistance. *Toxicol. Res.* **2017**, *33*, 1–5.
114. Pandurangan, A.K.; Sadagopan, S.K.A.; Dharmalingam, P.; Ganapasam, S. Luteolin, a bioflavonoid, attenuates azoxymethane-induced effects on mitochondrial enzymes in BALB/c mice. *Asian Pac. J. Cancer, Prev.* **2013**, *14*, 6669–6672.
115. Kang, K.A.; Piao, MJ; Hyun, Y.J.; Zhen, A.X.; Cho, S.J.; Ahn, MJ; Yi, J.M.; Hyun, J.W. Luteolin promotes apoptotic cell death via upregulation of Nrf2 expression by DNA demethylase and the interaction of Nrf2 with p53 in human colon cancer cells. *Exp. Mol. Med.* **2019**, *51*, 1–14, doi:10.1038/s12276-019-0238-y.
116. Li, Y.-R.; Li, G.-H.; Zhou, M.-X.; Xiang, L.; Ren, D.-M.; Lou, H.-X.; Wang, X.-N.; Shen, T. Discovery of natural flavonoids as activators of Nrf2-mediated defense system: Structure-activity relationship and inhibition of intracellular oxidative insults. *Bioorg. Med. Chem.* **2018**, *26*, 5140–5150, doi:10.1016/j.bmc.2018.09.010.

7

Nutraceuticals Against Neurodegeneration
Understanding the Mechanistic Pathways

Teeja Suthar, Navneet, and Keerti Jain
*National Institute of Pharmaceutical Education
and Research (NIPER) – Raebareli*

Contents

DOI: 10.1201/9781003110866-7

Acronyms

6-OHDA: 6-hydroxy dopamine

8-OHG: 8-hydroxyguanine

AD: Alzheimer's disease

ALS: Amyotrophic lateral sclerosis

APP: Amyloid precursor protein

Aβ: Amyloid beta

BBB: Blood-brain barrier

C9orf72: Chromosome 9 open reading frame 72

CAG: Cytosine, adenine and guanine

CNS: Central nervous system

CoQ10: Coenzyme Q10

COX: Cyclooxygenase

CSE: Cystathionine-λ-lyase

DHA: Docosahexaenoic acid

DSB: Double-strand breaks

EGCG: Epigallocatechin-gallate

EPOX: Epoxygenase

ER: Endoplasmic reticulum

ETC: Electron transport chain

FUS: Fused in sarcoma

GDNF: Glial cell-derived neurotrophic factor

GSH: Glutathione

HD: Huntington's disease

HTT: Huntingtin

IL-1: Interlukin-1

LOX: Lipoxygenase

LPS: Lipopolysaccharides

MAPK: Mitogen-activated protein kinase

mHTT: Mutant huntingtin

MND:	Motor neuron disease
MPP⁺:	1-methyl-4-phenylpyridinium
MPTP:	1-methyl-4-phenyl-1, 2, 5, 6-tetrahydropyridine
mPTP:	Mitochondrial permeability transition pore
mtDNA:	Mitochondrial DNA
NDDs:	Neurodegenerative diseases
nDNA:	Nuclear DNA
NF-κB:	Nuclear factor kappa B
NO:	Nitric oxide
PD:	Parkinson's disease
PGE-2:	Prostaglandin E2
PINK1:	PTEN-induced kinase 1
PNS:	Peripheral nervous system
PUFAs:	Polyunsaturated fatty acids
ROS:	Reactive oxygen species
SN:	Substantia nigra
SOD1:	Superoxide dismutase 1
SSB:	Single-strand breaks
TDP43:	Transactive DNA-binding protein 43
TLRs:	Toll-like receptors
TNF-α:	Tumor necrosis factor-α

7.1 Introduction

Neurodegenerative diseases (NDDs) are a diverse group of disorders affecting nerve cells and causing neuronal death. They are characterized by progressive degeneration of the structure and function of the central nervous system (CNS) and/or peripheral nervous system (PNS) [1]. Most of the NDDs are genetic, but few may be caused due to exposure to various toxins and chemicals [2]. Major symptoms accompanying these disorders are slowness of movement, motor impairment, tremor, rigidity, dysphagia, dementia and cognitive impairments [3–5]. NDDs have a very high morbidity and mortality rate, which possess an enormous socioeconomic burden and are majorly associated with aging, and hence the occurrence rate is higher in the elderly population than young adults owing to reduced or altered hormone secretions, increased oxidative stress, and neuronal inflammation [6–8]. The number of people living with dementia worldwide is currently estimated at 50 million, and the total number of people with dementia is projected to reach 82 million in 2030 and about 152 million by the year 2050 [9,10].

The major NDDs include Alzheimer's disease (AD), Parkinson's disease (PD), amyotrophic lateral sclerosis (ALS), Huntington's disease (HD), prion disease, motor neuron disease (MND), spinocerebellar ataxia, spinal muscular atrophy, etc. [11,12]. These NDDs mainly occur due to decreased neuronal counts (decreased neural progenitor cells) or loss of neuronal integrity (protein aggregation/tangles) as well as lack of communication (decreased number of neurotransmitters), eventually resulting in the loss of cognitive, motor and sensory functions [13]. The clinical treatment recommended for these disorders provides only symptomatic relief to the patient by increasing the lifespan to a few years. A lot of research still needs to be carried out to identify the therapeutic markers associated with these diseases [14]. In the following subsections, we will discuss the major NDDs including AD, PD, ALS and HD, particularly in detail along with highlight on their pathogenic mechanisms.

7.1.1 Alzheimer's disease

AD is a progressive and irreversible NDD with a complex pathological phenotype characterized by abnormal deposition of amyloid beta (Aβ) plaques and accumulation of neurofibrillary tangles of hyperphosphorylated Tau protein. It is associated with various cognitive impairments and is the leading cause of dementia [4,15–19]. To date, several hypotheses, such as (i) the amyloid cascade hypothesis, (ii) the cholinergic hypothesis, (iii) the Tau hypothesis and (iv) the oxidative stress hypothesis have been proposed for the pathogenesis of AD [20,21]. Therapeutic strategies aimed at the pathological aspect of this disease have given promising results in preclinical models but failed to produce the same in clinical practice. The multifaceted, progressive degenerative phenotype of AD suggests that successful treatment strategies must be equally multifaceted and disease-stage specific [22,23].

Neurotoxic oligomeric peptide Aβ, which is the main neuropathological diagnostic criteria, and the protein Tau are mediators of neurodegeneration that is among the main causal factors associated with AD [24,25]. However, these processes are enhanced mainly by the presence of oxidative stress. The oxidative stress can occur as a result of an increase in the number of free radicals or a decrease in antioxidant defense. Free radicals are mainly formed by the reduction of molecular oxygen in water, which on addition of an electron produces the superoxide radical followed by hydrogen peroxide. The reduction of hydrogen peroxide produces reactive oxygen species (ROS) that reacts with lipids, nucleic acids, proteins and other molecules and alters their structure and functions. The brain is the most vulnerable organ which is affected by ROS since it is made up of easily oxidizable lipids. ROS production can have a deleterious effect on the body and lead to various diseases and aging. However, antioxidant treatments have shown some success in the treatment of AD, which suggests that AD is associated with oxidative stress [15,17,19,22,26,27].

7.1.2 Parkinson's disease

PD is the second most common degenerative disorder of the CNS. Prevalence of PD increases with age, and PD affects about 1% of the population above 60 years. The onset of the disease is usually at the age of 65–70 years [28–31]. PD is a progressive disorder with motor behavioral abnormalities occurring due to a loss of dopaminergic neurons in the substantia nigra (SN) and intraneuronal α-synuclein inclusion [29,30,32]. PD was originally described by James Parkinson in 1817 in his "Essay on the shaking palsy", outlining the major symptoms of the disease that are still considered as the hallmarks of PD: bradykinesia, rigidity, tremor and loss of postural reflexes [28,33].

Pathophysiology of PD includes, but is not limited to, mitochondrial dysfunctions, oxidative stress and neuroinflammation [34,35]. Characterization of PD can be done by the presence of the major neuropathological findings such as α-synuclein-containing Lewy bodies and loss of dopaminergic neurons in the SN region of the brain, leading to reduced facilitation of voluntary movements. As the PD progresses, α-synuclein accumulation becomes more widespread with Lewy bodies spreading to cortical and neocortical regions [36–38]. The main mechanisms of neurodegeneration in PD are mitochondrial dysfunction due to increased ROS species and an increase in the misfolded proteins, collectively which have a role in dopaminergic neurodegeneration [34,35,39,40].

7.1.3 Amyotrophic lateral sclerosis

ALS was first described in the year 1869 by the French neurologist Jean-Martin Charcot. In the United States, the disease is often referred to as Lou Gehrig's disease after the name of an American baseball player who was diagnosed as having ALS in the year 1939 [41,42]. ALS has a prevalence of about 5 in 100,000 individuals, with an incidence of 1.9 per 100,000 individuals, and a median survival time of 3–5 years. The average age of onset is between 55 and 65 years [43]. ALS, the most common subtype of MND, is marked by progressive degeneration of both upper and lower motor neurons and other neuronal cells, resulting in muscle atrophy, gradual paralysis, severe disability and death, usually resulting from respiratory failure [44,45]. Various symptoms of ALS include difficulty in walking, weakness, and deterioration of muscles in the arms, leg, trunk, and bulbar region, difficulty with speech and swallowing, and breathlessness. Common terminal events occurring in ALS patients are bronchial pneumonia and respiratory failure, resulting in the death of the patient [46]. Pathogenic mechanisms underlying the MND include RNA toxicity, glutamate excitotoxicity, disturbance in proteostasis, defects in axonal transport, oxidative stress, and mitochondrial dysfunction [47–49]. Neuroinflammation is another common pathological process observed in ALS which is distinguished by various inflammatory responses involving CNS microglia and astroglia, infiltrating proinflammatory peripheral monocytes, lymphocytes, and macrophages [50].

ALS is classified as sporadic ALS or familial ALS. Most of the cases of ALS are sporadic, but very few cases, *i.e.*, around 10% are classified as familial ALS. More than 30 different genes have been linked to the familial form of ALS [51–53]. The most common genetic cause of ALS is hexanucleotide repeat expansions in chromosome 9 open reading frame 72 gene (C9orf72) observed in about 40% of the familial ALS patients and 10% of sporadic ALS patients [51,54,55]. Mutations in various other genes such as superoxide dismutase 1 (SOD1), TAR DNA-binding protein 43 (TDP-43), and fused in sarcoma (FUS) are also responsible for enhancing the neuroinflammation and immune dysregulations in ALS patients [48]. These mutations lead to impaired degradation of aggregated proteins and compromised glial protective responses and contribute to proinflammatory-mediated motoneuron injury and thus, the progression of the disease [50,56].

Specific diagnostic tests are not available for ALS, and diagnosis is usually performed on the basis of clinical findings such as progressive weakness and upper and lower motor dysfunctions, electromyography results and genetic tests [57]. Treatment of ALS is best provided by a multidisciplinary team by using a combination of disease-modifying treatments and management of symptoms. The Food and Drug Administration has approved two disease-modifying treatments for ALS *viz.* glutamate receptor antagonist, riluzole, and recently in 2017, a free radical scavenger, edaravone. Other treatment strategies that can be exploited are stem cell therapy and antisense oligonucleotide gene therapy [58,59].

7.1.4 Huntington's disease

HD is a prototypical NDD initially described by George Huntington in the year 1872. He wrote an account of hereditary chorea, where he mentioned the hereditary nature of the disease, accompanying psychiatric and cognitive symptoms. He described the progressive nature of the disease by stating, "once it begins, it clings to the bitter end" [60–62]. HD is a fully penetrant autosomal-dominant inherited NDD of genetic origin characterized by a triad of the motor, cognitive, and psychiatric features. It is a movement disorder with a heterogeneous phenotype illustrated by neuronal loss in striatum, involuntary dance-like gait, motor impairment, bioenergetic deficits, emotional, cognitive and psychiatric deficits [63–65]. HD typically shows a late onset of appearance in mid-life with development of symptoms over 10–15 years, and the manifestation of the disease usually occurs in adult life between 30 and 40 years of age [63,66].

HD is caused by an abnormal expansion of cytosine, adenine, and guanine (CAG) trinucleotide repeats in the N-terminal of the huntingtin (HTT) gene, which results in the production of mutant huntingtin (mHTT) protein with abnormally long polyglutamine repeats on translation [67–69]. The number of pathogenic CAG repeats is associated with the severity and age of onset of the disease. HD exhibits a late-onset appearance in people carrying 39–60 repeats and an early or juvenile onset in people with more than 60 CAG repeats [64]. HTT, the protein mutated in HD, is essential for development, and it is reported to be involved in chemical signaling, binding to various proteins, transporting materials, and protecting the cells from apoptotic death [70]. The genetic mutations in HTT protein were first identified in the year 1993. Intensive efforts of researchers from all over the globe have led to the discovery of various cellular pathological mechanisms underlying disease development. Most of the mechanisms involve the presence of the mHTT protein, which is universally expressed and is thought to be the major cause of the disease [68,69].

Neuropathologically, HD is predominantly characterized by the loss of medium-sized spiny neurons in the neostriatum, but as the disease progresses, neuropathology is also observed in other brain regions including the cerebral cortex, globus pallidus, subthalamic nucleus, nucleus accumbens, SN, thalamus, and cerebellum [71,72]. Currently, no disease-modifying treatments are available for the management of HD; the available treatments only provide symptomatic relief. There has been a large growth in understanding the potential therapeutic targets and clinical trials since the last decade [73,74].

A general description of various NDDs discussed in this chapter is given in Table 7.1. The next section of the chapter deals with various mechanisms associated with NDDs such as mitotoxicity-mediated neurodegeneration, oxidative damage, inflammation, calcium overload and DNA damage.

7.2 Mechanisms underlying neurodegeneration

Various mechanisms namely mitochondrial dysfunction, calcium overload, oxidative stress, inflammation and DNA damage have been found to be majorly associated with neurodegeneration which are diagrammatically presented in Figure 7.1.

7.2.1 Mitochondrial dysfunction-mediated neuronal damage

Mitochondria are ATP-generating organelles that play an important role in the pathogenesis of various NDDs such as AD, PD, ALS and HD. Mitochondria are involved in many functions such as energy production, calcium regulation, free-radical scavenging, alteration of the redox potential of cells and activation of apoptotic cell death [75,76]. The functions of mitochondria are regulated by

Table 7.1 General Description of the Neurodegenerative Diseases Discussed in this Chapter

S. No.	Disease	Symptoms	Age of Onset	Affected Neurons	Associated Proteins	Genetic Factors	Drugs	Mechanism of Action or Targets	Ref.
1.	AD	Behavioral and cognitive impairments	60–65 years	Loss of cortical and hippocampal neurons	Amyloid β plaques and neurofibrillary tangles of protein Tau.	APP, Presenlin 1 (PSEN1), Presenilin 2 (PSEN2) and APOE	Memantine Tacrine, Rivastigmine, Galantamine, Donepezil	Blocks NMDA receptors, reduces excitotoxicity Acetylcholinesterase inhibitors – increase the concentration of acetylcholine in the brain	[4,14,16,23]
2.	PD	Tremor, bradykinesia, rigidity and impaired posture	60 years or older	Dopaminergic neurons in substantia nigra pars compacta	Lewy bodies formed by aggregation of α-synuclein	Synuclein, Parkin, PINK1, DJ-1 and LRRK2	Levodopa	Increased amount of dopamine in substantia nigra neurons	[30,32,38,209]
3.	ALS	Fasciculations (muscle twitches), muscle cramps, spasticity, muscle weakness and eventually paralysis.	55–65 years	Motor neurons of the spinal cord, cortex and brain stem.	SOD1, FUS, TDP-43, OPTN, UBQLN2	SOD1, C90RF72, TDP-43, and FUS	Riluzole, Edaravone	Antiglutamatergic, inhibits NMDA receptors, blocks Na$^+$ channels.	[41–43,210,211]
4.	HD	Chorea, dystonia and cognitive impairments.	30–40 years	Loss of striatal medium spiny neurons, mainly in the striatum and also the frontal and temporal cortex.	Mutant huntingtin	HTT	Tetrabenazine, Deutetrabenazine	Antidopamine (VMAT2 inhibitor, reduces the amount of released dopamine and inhibits monoamine uptake)	[62,64,66,212]

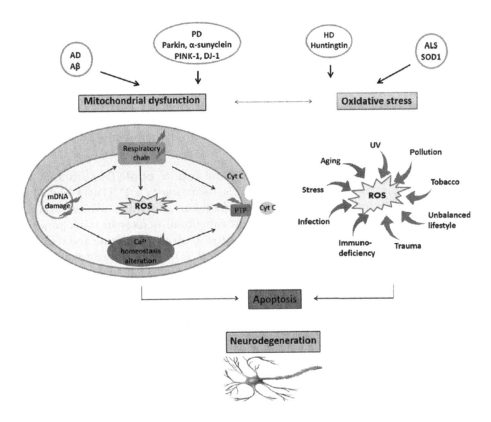

Figure 7.1 *Mechanisms underlying neurodegeneration in various neurodegenerative disorders [214].*

two genomes namely nuclear DNA (nDNA) and mitochondrial DNA (mtDNA). Mutations in these two genomes can lead to mitochondrial toxicity and thus, neurodegeneration [77–80]. Several antioxidants such as glutathione peroxidase, peroxiredoxin and catalase neutralize the ROS species and establish an equilibrium between ROS production and antioxidants. Mitochondrial dysfunction leads to an increase in ROS production, thus disturbing the equilibrium and causing oxidative stress [81,82].

Aβ peptide, an important component of AD pathogenesis, can negatively affect mitochondrial functions. It affects homeostasis, contributes to ROS production and affects the function of the electron transport chain (ETC) [83]. Another pathologic attribute associated with AD is hyperphosphorylation of protein Tau. Accumulation of hyperphosphorylated Tau in the neurons blocks mitochondrial transport, decreases ATP production and increases ROS production [84]. 1-Methyl-4-phenylpyridinium (MPP+), formed from the neurotoxic precursor, 1-methyl-4-phenyl-1,2,3,6-tetrahydropyridine (MPTP), concentrates in the mitochondria of dopaminergic neurons [85]. It contributes to the progression of PD, by inhibiting complex 1 of the respiratory ETC. Defects in complex 1 of ETC in the SN region is considered as a major causative factor of the sporadic PD [86]. Mutations in various genes encoding PARKIN, PTEN-induced kinase 1 (PINK1) and α-synuclein also contribute to the progression of mitochondrial dysfunction-induced PD. Mutations in genes encoding α-synuclein mediate the autosomal dominant form of PD, and mutations in genes encoding PARKIN and PINK1 cause autosomal recessive PD [87–90]. Mutated α-synuclein accumulates in the mitochondrial membrane and leads to defects in complex I of ETC and an increase in the number of ROS species and thus, neuronal cell death [38].

Mitochondrial dysfunction is also a prevalent feature of MNDs such as ALS. Several proteins have been linked to ALS, including SOD1, TDP43 and FUS interacting with mitochondria. Human patients and mice overexpressing mutant SOD1 have shown structural and functional defects in mitochondria [48,91]. Mutant SOD1 accumulates in the mitochondrial membrane and reduces the activity of ETC complexes [92,93]. Mutated TDP-43 accumulates in mitochondria and binds the mRNA of the mtDNA and causes impairments in complex I [94,95]. Overexpression of FUS or mutations in FUS leads to enhanced ROS production and reduced mitochondrial ATP production [96]. mHTT, the gene responsible for the progression of HD, interacts with the mitochondrial outer membrane and triggers Ca^{2+} release. mHTT is also known to impair the structure and functions of mitochondria. HD patients show an altered mitochondrial membrane potential, impaired mitochondrial complexes and defects in mitochondrial calcium handling [97]. The role of oxidative stress, calcium overload, inflammation and DNA damage in the progression of neurodegeneration has been discussed below.

7.2.2 Intracellular calcium overload-mediated neuronal damage

The role of calcium in various NDDs was discovered in the early 1970s. The concentration of Ca^{2+} ions is higher in extracellular space than that inside the cells under normal physiological conditions. This difference is mainly due to the selective permeability of plasma membrane, presence of ATP-dependent Ca^{2+}-ATPase pump and Na^+/Ca^{2+} exchangers that pumps Ca^{2+} outside the cells [98]. Ca^{2+} accumulation in the cells can occur as a result of various Ca^{2+} ion channels. The rise in intracellular Ca^{2+} ions causes disturbance in Ca^{2+} homeostasis in the mitochondria and endoplasmic reticulum (ER), which is associated with the pathogenesis of various NDDs. The sharp rise in Ca^{2+} levels in the cells becomes a threat to the neurons. It can lead to mitotoxicity, reduced ATP synthesis, and eventually leads to impaired neuronal functions and cell death. Thus, the maintenance of Ca^{2+} levels in the cells is important for the proper functioning of nerve cells [99,100].

Dysregulation in Ca^{2+} homeostasis is one of the major contributing factors for neurodegeneration in AD. Higher Ca^{2+} levels in the ER results in altered neuronal Ca^{2+} signaling and enhanced ROS production and thus, causing cognitive impairments and neurodegeneration [101,102]. Moreover, disturbance in Ca^{2+} homeostasis leads to the destruction of dopaminergic neurons in the PD. Continuous Ca^{2+} influx makes the neurons vulnerable by causing mitochondrial oxidative stress. Mutations in the PINK1 gene leads to decreased Ca^{2+} efflux in the dopaminergic neurons and favors mitochondrial depolarization induced cell death. Expression of α-synuclein and its accumulation in Lewy bodies also affects ER mitochondrial coupling and leads to an impairment in Ca^{2+} regulation, and thus, enhances neurodegeneration [103,104].

High levels of Ca^{2+} are observed in the motor neurons of ALS patients. Disturbances in Ca^{2+} homeostasis could lead to the death of motor neurons due to excitotoxicity in ALS patients. In a study performed in Cu/Zn SOD1 mutant mice model, an increased mitochondrial Ca^{2+} level was observed. SOD mutations make the neurons vulnerable to oxidative stress and excitotoxicity. Calbindin-D28K and parvalbumin are Ca^{2+} binding proteins that protect the motor neurons and delay the onset of disease. These proteins were not found in the motor neurons of ALS patients [105–109]. In HD, repeat expansions of CAG in the HTT gene cause mitochondrial dysfunction, changes in membrane potential, and thus, imbalances in the Ca^{2+} levels. In the cells of HD patients, expressing mHTT, the role of disturbed Ca^{2+} homeostasis in neuronal degeneration can be observed. Mitochondrial Ca^{2+} overload leads to the opening of mitochondrial permeability transition pore (mPTP) and thus, leads to the release of Ca^{2+} ions from the ER due to the presence of mHTT. Moreover, mHTT binds to IP3 receptors and enhances their opening to release Ca^{2+} from the ER [110–112]. The next subsection of the chapter deals with the oxidative stress-mediated neurodegeneration mechanism in detail.

7.2.3 Oxidative stress-mediated neuronal damage

Imbalances in various biochemical processes result in an excessive generation of ROS species and lead to a condition called oxidative stress. Oxidative stress caused due to ROS and reactive nitrogen species (RNS) forms the basis for the pathogenesis of various NDDs. Oxidative stress may be caused due to higher oxygen consumption, lower antioxidant reserves, the presence of redox-active transition metals and the presence of polyunsaturated fatty acids (PUFAs) [113].

In AD patients, oxidative damage to DNA, lipids and proteins leads to Aβ accumulation and neuronal degeneration. Aβ accumulation and neurofibrillary tangles bind mitochondrial proteins and lead to impairments in mitochondrial function, ETC activity and increased production of ROS [114–116]. In PD, MPP+ exposure leads to inhibition of complex I in ETC and subsequently, oxidative stress. Oxidative damage to DNA and proteins in the SN region can be seen in the brain of PD patients. Another mechanism for the development of PD is the oxidation of dopamine to 6-hydroxy dopamine (6-OHDA). α-synuclein accumulation in the brain of PD patients reduces the complex I activity and increases ROS generation in SN neurons. Various genes such as PINK1 and PINK2 maintain the mitochondrial and ROS homeostasis. Mutations in PINK1 inhibits complex I and leads to impairment in the ROS production [34,38,40,117].

In ALS patients, oxidative stress can induce mutations in Cu/Zn SOD1 and can cause damage to the proteins, lipids and DNA. SOD1 is a ubiquitous enzyme that scavenges free radicals. Mutation in SOD1 leads to familial ALS. Mutations in this gene lead to protein misfolding in mitochondrial membrane space and produce ROS, which leads to cell death. Mutant SOD1 also causes impairments in the biosynthesis of amino acids [118,119]. In HD, abnormal CAG expansions in HTT lead to the formation of ROS and neuronal damage. mHTT interacts with mitochondrial proteins and disrupts mitochondrial proteostasis, enhances ROS production and affects the expression of cystathionine-ƛ-lyase (CSE). A low level of CSE decreases cysteine in the cell and subsequently leads to enhanced ROS production [69,97].

The studies stated above indicates a definite relationship between oxidative stress and neurodegeneration. This infers that treatment with antioxidants or agents that boosts endogenous antioxidant reserves could prove an important therapeutic strategy for the amelioration of NDDs. Other mechanisms underlying neurodegeneration will be discussed in the subsequent subsections.

7.2.4 Inflammation-mediated neuronal damage

Emerging research has highlighted the role of inflammation in the pathogenesis of various NDDs. Neuronal inflammation occurs as a result of interaction between glial cells, immune cells and neurons. Glial cells, *i.e.*, astroglia and microglia play a key role in neuroinflammation and neuronal cell death. Microglia are the resident immune cells present in the CNS. They can be activated by various signals released from the neighboring cells. On activation, microglial cells release proinflammatory cytokines and other factors such as IL-1, tumor necrosis factor-α (TNFα), NO, PGE2 and superoxide that are toxic to neurons. These microglia-based phagocytic and cytotoxic processes are responsible for neuronal damage. Toll-like receptors (TLRs) also play a crucial role in innate immunity. TLRs contribute to inflammation by augmenting the release of proinflammatory cytokines and chemokines [120–124].

In AD patients, inflammatory responses lead to changes in the morphology of microglial cells from ramified to amoeboid. Astrogliosis can also be observed around senile plaques in AD. Accumulation of Aβ plaques results in inflammatory responses and oxidative damage by the generation of ROS. The AD brain shows an increased level of proinflammatory cytokines, such as PGE2 and γ-secretase, which act as stimulators of neuroinflammation. Various proinflammatory mediators include major histocompatibility complex (MHC) class II, cyclooxygenase (COX)-2, TNF-α, IL-1β and IL-6. Moreover, higher levels of cytokines and chemokines like IL-1α, CXCR2, CCR3, CCR5 and TGF-β, have been recorded in the postmortem of AD patient's brain. Inflammation in the neuronal cells can lead to a significant cognitive decline [125,126]. The exact cause of PD is not properly understood yet. The disease was earlier thought to be caused due to loss of dopaminergic neurons, but it is now recognized that PD is also associated with inflammation. Microglial cells expressing human leukocyte antigen-DR and CD11b, and Lewy bodies, are found in the SN region of PD patients. Inflammation occurs *via* lipid peroxidation, SOD activity and formation of ROS in the SN region. Higher levels of cytokines are also reported in the blood of PD patients. PD is also associated with alterations in lipoxygenase (LOX), COX and epoxygenase (EPOX) pathways. Other pathogenic mechanisms involve the decreased function of ETC complexes, which leads to oxidative stress and generation of isofurans *via* nonenzymatic oxidation of docosahexaenoic acid (DHA) [35,90,127].

Neuroinflammation is also observed in the CNS and spinal cord of both human ALS patients and mouse models of the disease. Inflammation in ALS can be explained by gliosis and the accumulation of glial cells. Glial cells get activated due to increased production of ROS, COX-2, IL-1β, IL-6 and TNF-α. Mutations in TDP-43 also lead to activation of microglia from the surface of the CD14 receptors [50,128]. Proinflammatory cytokines like IL-1β, IL-6 and TNF-α were also found in the brain of HD patients. Kynurenine monooxygenase is an enzyme of the kynurenine pathway, which is the major catabolic route of tryptophan. kynurenine 3-monooxygenase is predominantly overexpressed in the microglial cells of HD patients. Various studies reported the presence of 3-hydroxykynurenine in Huntington mouse possibly due to the increased KMO activity [67,69,97,129,130].

7.2.5 DNA damage-mediated neuronal damage

As seen in many NDDs, the question of whether DNA damage is the cause or consequence of neurodegeneration still exists, and probably, both are true. DNA damage refers to any modifications in the basic structure of DNA that change the normal function of transcription or replication. DNA damage can occur in many different forms such as apurinic/apyrimidinic sites, adducts, single-strand breaks (SSBs), double-strand breaks (DSBs), DNA-protein cross-links, and chemical addition/ disruption. DNA damage disrupts the transcription and replication processes, thereby triggering cell death and aging. More attention is given to oxidative DNA damage since the brain has a high metabolic rate, generates more ROS and a smaller ratio of antioxidant to prooxidant enzymes. Oxidative DNA damage in nDNA results in the build-up of DNA adducts and triggers neuronal death, whereas in mtDNA, it results in base substitutions and deletions leading to errors in gene transcription in

ETC with mitochondrial dysfunction, augmented oxidative stress and neuronal death [77,131–134].

AD patients show elevated levels of DNA strand breaks, reduced levels of DSB repair proteins such as DNA-PKcs and MRN complex proteins. The base excision repair (BER) pathway is mainly involved in the repair of oxidative damage. A reduction in the DNA BER activity was reported in postmortem brain regions of AD patients. Excessive ROS production leads to oxidative attack to DNA bases and leads to the formation of 8-hydroxyguanine (8-OHG), an oxidized base adduct. Elevated levels of 8-OHG can be observed in the brain of AD patients [18,115]. DNA damage activates various response signaling pathways in toxicant models of PD. Following MPP+ exposure, ataxia telangiectasia mutated, and its downstream effector p53 gets activated and induces apoptosis. 6-OHDA also leads to an increase in polyADP-ribosylation, causing cell death. α-synuclein accumulates in Lewy bodies and leads to familial PD. Nuclear α-synuclein binds DNA, and overexpression of α-synuclein causes DNA SSBs and DSBs, particularly under oxidative stress [135].

Neuroinflammation is one of the main pathogenic features of ALS caused due to stimulation of microglia, astrocytes and inflammatory T cells. The microglial cells secrete proinflammatory cytokines such as IL-1β, TNF-α and interferon-γ. Mutant human TDP43 and FUS lead to DNA damage in ALS. Similarly, enhanced levels of oxidative damage and SSBs have been recorded in the neurons of ALS patients [136,137]. Increased incidences of oxidative DNA strand breaks are reported to be associated with HD. A significant increase in the levels of 8-OHdG in nDNA has been found in the postmortem tissue of HD patients [138].

The mechanisms involved in neurodegeneration in various NDDs are depicted in Figure 7.1. The multifaceted nature of these NDDs requires intervention with natural phytochemicals having strong antioxidant, anti-inflammatory and neuroprotective activities. The natural phytochemicals or nutraceuticals may prove to be safer and more efficient alternatives to reduce the progression of such debilitating NDDs.

7.3 Nutraceuticals against neurodegeneration

Around 2,000 years ago, Hippocrates correctly quoted that "let thy food be thy medicine and thy medicine be thy food". According to various epidemiological studies, it has been hypothesized that appropriate nutrition and caloric restriction could largely reduce the risk of many debilitating NDDs. The term "Nutraceutical" was coined by Dr. Stephen L DeFelice, from the words "nutrition" and "pharmaceuticals" in the year 1989 [139,140]. Nutraceuticals is a broad umbrella term that includes any substance that is a food or part of a food and provides medical or health benefits, including the prevention and/or treatment of a disease and/or disorder [139,141]. Nutraceuticals act on multiple cellular

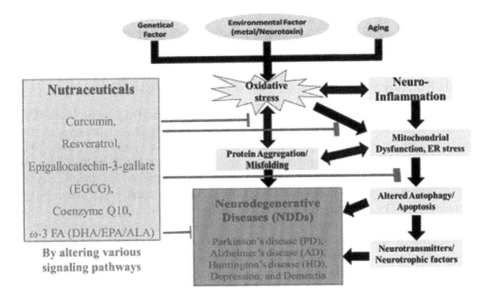

Figure 7.2 *General neuroprotective mechanisms of emerging nutraceuticals in various neurodegenerative disorders [144].*

pathways to support their beneficial role in the treatment and/or prevention of persistent ailments such as NDDs, and they are anticipated to improve overall neuronal health [142,143]. Various pathways associated with neuronal damage and nutraceutical-mediated neuroprotection are represented in Figure 7.2.

Nutraceuticals such as curcumin, coenzyme Q10 (CoQ10), resveratrol, epigallocatechin-3-gallate (EGCG), hesperidin, vitamin C, vitamin D, vitamin E, ginseng and ω-3 fatty acids are some of the antioxidants having therapeutic effects against various NDDs. They typically act by counteracting the oxidative damage, augmenting the endogenous antioxidant levels and stabilizing mitochondrial functions. Nutraceuticals can act as a neuroprotective by virtue of their ability to directly scavenge the free radicals, upsurge the antioxidant reserves, enhancing in anti-inflammatory activities and thus, increasing the antioxidative defenses. They regulate various signaling pathways such as Nrf2/ARE signaling pathway, protein kinase C (PKC), mitogen-activated protein kinase (MAPK), Janus kinase/signal transducer and activator of transcription (JAK-STAT), etc. which have essential roles in cell growth, cell survival and stress responses [143,144].

Several studies have insinuated the advantageous effects of a vast number of nutraceuticals in the management of various NDDs; however, we will discuss only the nutraceuticals for which mechanistic shreds of evidence with special reference to clinical trials (including *in vitro* and animal studies) for neuroprotection are available. The nutraceuticals selected for this book chapter were obtained from various search engines including Google Scholar, ScienceDirect,

PubMed and Publons. Using a combination of various keywords such as "neuroprotection, nutraceuticals, neuroprotective, NDDs and alternate medicine" in clinical trials as well as *in vitro* and animal studies were also included.

7.3.1 Curcumin

Curcumin ((1E,6E)-1,7-bis (4-hydroxy-3-methoxyphenyl)-1,6-heptadiene-3,5-dione), a polyphenolic flavonoid, is a major phytoconstituent present in the rhizomes of *Curcuma longa Linn.* It is widely used as a spice in Indian and Asian cuisine. Curcumin easily crosses the blood-brain barrier (BBB), and it has an outstanding safety profile. Several studies conducted on different cells of the nervous system presented the neuroprotective activity of curcumin by scavenging ROS and neutralizing nitric oxide free radicals. It alleviates the cytotoxicity, oxidative stress and apoptotic cell death in various NDDs. The therapeutic effects of curcumin are linked to its anti-inflammatory, antioxidant, anticancer and anti-protein aggregation activities. Various research studies have been conducted to prove the beneficial effects of curcumin in several medical conditions including cancer, arthritis, gastric ulcers, cystic fibrosis and liver diseases [145,146].

Several studies have reported that curcumin can inhibit inflammation-associated AD. It binds Aβ, enhances its cellular uptake and thus, prevents the deposition of Aβ plaques. *In vivo* experiments have shown the ability of curcumin to reduce the activation of microglial cells, decrease the astrocyte proliferation and improve myelinogenesis. It can modulate Tau protein processing and phosphorylation [142,147]. It also reduces proinflammatory cytokine production and inhibits the nuclear factor kappa B (NF-κB)-associated signaling pathway [148]. Liu et al. (2016) has reported that curcumin activates the peroxisome proliferator-activator receptor gamma (PPARγ) in rats with AD and reduces the neuroinflammation induced by Aβ [149].

Curcumin is also researched to be effective in reducing the disease progression in PD restoring the glutathione (GSH) levels, thus reducing oxidative stress and preserving the neurons against protein oxidation and restoring mitochondrial functional activities. Curcumin administration has been proven to be effective in protecting the dopaminergic neurons and suppressing apoptosis, inducing microglial activation *via* MAPK signaling pathways and improving locomotion. It was also found to prevent the aggregation of α-synuclein, disrupt the preformed α-synuclein aggregates and decrease the overexpression of α-synuclein in the cells. It prevents α-synuclein and MPTP/MPP+-induced neurotoxicity in SHSY-5Y cells by targeting various signaling pathways including JNK, Bcl-2 mitochondria and ROS–iNOS pathways [150,151].

Some studies suggest the potential of curcumin to reduce the aggregation of HTT protein, thus providing symptomatic relief in HD by suppressing neuronal cell death. It has also been demonstrated to be beneficial in altering the biomarkers of depression and uplifting the mood of the patients suffering from depression [152]. However, curcumin possesses various issues such as low bioavailability, internal metabolization and a lack of clinical studies proving its therapeutic potential in various NDDs such as AD, PD and HD. Clinical studies are required to explore the complete therapeutic potential of curcumin in treating NDDs [153].

7.3.2 Resveratrol

Resveratrol (3,5,4′-trihydroxystilbene) is a polyphenolic phytoalexin found in grapes, red cherries, peanuts, pomegranate, pine, blueberries, raspberries and mulberries. It is one of the most popular nutraceuticals that is known to promote health by virtue of its antioxidant, anti-inflammatory, antiaging, anti-cancer, antiviral, antidiabetic, antihyperlipidemic activity as well as cardioprotective and neuroprotective properties. It can easily cross the BBB. It is safe and well-tolerated by almost all types of population. Few disadvantages with resveratrol are low bioavailability, high metabolism and poor lipophilicity. It can be formulated by liposomal-encapsulation to overcome these disadvantages [144,154–156].

Resveratrol has been extensively explored for its potential applications in the treatment of AD. In a Tau transgenic mouse model, hyperphosphorylated Tau protein binds resveratrol and gets stabilized, thus preventing Tau protein from aggregating into tangles [157]. When resveratrol is administered in a PS19 mouse model tauopathy, the treatment resulted in reduced cognitive deficits, reduced levels of phosphorylated Tau and reduced neuroinflammation in the brain of the mouse [158]. In a study, Zhao et al. (2015) studied the effect of resveratrol in the AD rat model. They reported that it inhibits $A\beta_{1-42}$-mediated neuroinflammation by downregulating the expression of NF-κB and protects the integrity of the BBB [159]. In the potential treatment of PD, resveratrol is known to protect dopaminergic neurons against MPTP⁻, MPP⁺, 6-OHDA⁻ and lipopolysaccharides (LPS)-induced toxicity in rodent models. It prevents the aggregation of the α-synuclein protein and thus the formation of Lewy bodies. Furthermore, it acts as a neuroprotective agent by reducing oxidative damage and conserving dopamine in the 6-OHDA rat model of PD [160]. Resveratrol is also proven to be beneficial in the treatment of HD. In the 3-nitropropionic acid-induced mouse model of HD, it inhibits COX activity leading to significant improvement in motor and cognitive impairments. Moreover, it reduces the neurotoxicity caused due to mHTT through SIRT1 activation [161]. Resveratrol is also known to have beneficial effects in the treatment of ALS.

7.3.3 Epigallocatechin-3-gallate (EGCG)

Epigallocatechin-gallate ((2R,3R-5,7-dihydroxy-2-(3,4,5-trihydroxyphenyl) chroman-3-yl) 3,4,5-trihydroxybenzoate) is a polyphenolic flavonoid obtained from leaves of Camellia sinensis. It is the main antioxidant compound found in green tea. It can easily cross the BBB. EGCG is shown to possess antioxidant, antitumoral, antibacterial, and neuroprotective activities. It scavenges the free radicals and reduces neuroinflammation, oxidative stress and autophagy and thus, acts as a neuroprotective agent. It enhances the mitochondrial restoration *via* various signaling pathways by blocking the expression of iNOS, COX-2 and other enzymes which leads to the generation of pro-inflammatory mediators [144,154–156].

In AD, EGCG inhibits the formation of amyloid fibrils and binds amyloid precursor protein (APP) and Tau protein and inhibits aggregation. It enhances the α-secretase activity [162]. In the treatment of PD, EGCG acts as an antagonist for NF-κB and reduces the α-synuclein accumulation. It improves the motor functions in PD patients and reduces neuronal toxicity by restoring dopamine levels. The catechol group of EGCG has free radical scavenging and iron-chelating activities. It is shown to protect against 6-OHDA⁻ and MPTP⁻-induced parkinsonism in mice models [163,164]. EGCG can also be used for the treatment of HD, as it is known to modulate the HTT misfolding and reduce neurodegeneration [165].

7.3.4 Coenzyme Q10 (ubiquinone)

Coenzyme Q10 (CoQ10) also known as ubiquinone is a fat-soluble vitamin-like quinone found in almost all organs but abundantly in the heart, liver, kidney and brain. CoQ10 is an important component of the mitochondrial ETC, and it plays a role in mitochondrial ATP synthesis. It has been exploited for its use as an antioxidant in the treatment of NDDs. It has very few side effects and is usually well tolerated by almost all people. It is found to be effective against rotenone-induced mitochondrial dysfunction by preventing apoptosis and maintaining the mitochondrial membrane potential [166–170].

CoQ10 has been found to inhibit the formation of Aβ and α-synuclein fibrils and destabilize the preformed fibrils [171]. In PD rodent models, CoQ10 reduces MPTP-induced neurotoxicity, due to the transfer of electrons between mitochondrial complex 1 and other complexes of the ETC. It is demonstrated to protect against MPP⁺/MPTP⁻-mediated mitochondrial damage, neurotoxicity and locomotor deficits. It is found to restore the dopamine levels and functions of dopaminergic neurons in the MPTP-induced PD model [172]. CoQ10 improves the mitochondrial deficits in an HD mice model [168].

7.3.5 Quercetin

Quercetin (2-(3,4-dihydroxy phenyl)-3,5,7-trihydroxy-4H-chromen-4-one) is a polyphenolic flavonoid usually found in foods such as apples, onion, broccoli and capers. It is a widely explored nutraceutical for its antioxidant, anti-inflammatory, anticancer and neuroprotective properties. It has the ability to cross the BBB easily. Quercetin alleviates neurodegeneration by reducing cognitive impairments [154,173]. It has been proven to inhibit several aggregation proteins, including Tau protein, Aβ and α-synuclein *in vitro*. It interacts with misfolded proteins and inhibits fibril growth. In various *in vivo* studies, it has been demonstrated to be effective in reducing the number of ROS species, enhancing the levels of GSH and antioxidant enzyme function. Quercetin also inhibits the activation of NF-κB and thus inhibits the activation of proinflammatory cytokines like interleukins [174].

AD is associated with elevated levels of $A\beta_{(1-42)}$. Quercetin modulates oxidative stress and reduces neuronal toxicity caused by Aβ. Quercetin is known to protect the human brain microvascular endothelial cells from fibrillar $A\beta_{(1-40)}$ by enhancing the cell viability. It improves the pathology of AD by reducing the cognitive impairments in the triple transgenic AD mouse model [175]. In PD patients, quercetin is known to reverse dopaminergic depletion and neuronal damage. In *in vivo* studies in rat PD models, quercetin has shown neuroprotective activity by restoring the dopaminergic neurons against 6-OHDA. Quercetin treatment significantly attenuates MPP+-induced toxicity [176,177].

7.3.6 Hesperidin

Hesperidin, ((2S)-5-hydroxy-2-(3-hydroxy-4-methoxyphenyl)-7-[(2S,3R,4S,5S,6R)-3,4,5-trihydroxy-6-{[(2R,3R,4R,5R,6S)-3,4,5-trihydroxy-6-methyloxan-2-yl]oxy-methyl}oxan-2-yl]oxy-2,3-dihydrochromen-4-one), a flavanone glycoside, is a natural phenolic compound usually present in citrus fruits such as oranges, grapes and lemons. It is known to possess a wide range of biological effects including antioxidant, anti-inflammatory, antihypertensive, antiviral, anticarcinogenic and neuroprotective effects. It also has vitamin-like activities, and it decreases capillary permeability (vitamin P), leakiness and fragility. Hesperidin has the ability to cross the BBB, and it can act as a neuroprotective agent against various NDDs, including AD, PD, ALS and HD [178,179].

Hesperidin is found to reduce the Nrf2-mediated oxidative stress, neuroinflammation and Aβ-mediated neurodegeneration in animal models of AD. It also improved the memory and cognitive impairments in various mice and rat models of AD as analyzed by the Morris Water Maze test and Y-maze test. In the aluminium chloride ($AlCl_3$)-induced rat model of AD, hesperidin, inhibited the memory and cognitive impairments by its ability to act as an AChE inhibitor. It also inhibited the APP expression *via* the NF-κB pathway. It also attenuated the LPS-induced neurodegeneration and cognitive impairments in the mouse model of AD [180,181]. In PD, hesperidin remarkably reduces the motor dysfunction in the 6-OHDA-induced rat model of PD. It potentially inhibits the depletion of dopamine, restores GSH levels and attenuates ROS production. It restores the mitochondrial enzyme complex activities by enhancing the activities of mitochondrial complexes I–IV [182]. Hesperidin has also shown promising outcomes in the treatment of HD. It suppresses the NO synthase levels in cortical, striatal and hippocampal regions [183].

Hesperidin can reverse various inducers of NDDs, including protein aggregation, oxidative damage, inflammation and apoptosis, making it a promising alternative for the amelioration of various NDDs.

7.3.7 Vitamin C

Vitamin C or ascorbic acid is a water-soluble vital antioxidant molecule that participates in various cellular functions in the human brain. Treatment with vitamin C may prove to be useful against the NDDs associated with cognitive and memory impairments. Consumption of vitamin C is associated with a reduced risk of PD. It can reduce dopamine and levodopa-induced neurotoxicity. Several studies suggest that vitamin C can have a protective effect on dopaminergic neurons against excitotoxicity. Ascorbate is also known to delay the locomotor deficits in the α-synuclein fly model. One of the studies suggests that administration of vitamin C to PD patients resulted in a reduction in the need for levodopa. However, the inadequate availability of vitamin C in the CNS is one of the major constraints in its therapeutic application in PD [173,184–186].

7.3.8 Vitamin D

Vitamin D is a lipid-soluble hormone that can be synthesized. Vitamin D exists in nature in its two major forms, *viz.* vitamin D2 (ergocalciferol), photochemically synthesized in plants and vitamin D3 (cholecalciferol), synthesized in the skin of animals on sunlight exposure. Calcitriol (1,25-dihydroxy-vitamin D3) is the active form of vitamin D. Vitamin D deficiency is considered a major health problem affecting billions of people worldwide. Vitamin D is known to have a direct role in the progression of PD as it increases GSH levels, regulates calcium homeostasis, reduces NO synthase, shows anti-apoptotic and immunomodulatory activities and regulates dopamine levels. Vitamin D reduces the dose of levodopa and improves motor symptoms in PD patients [187,188].

Newmark et al. (2007) hypothesized the role of vitamin D in the progression of PD. Vitamin D receptor knockout mice demonstrated increased motor defects. They found that vitamin D plays a potential role in reducing the 6-OHDA- and MPP+-induced neuronal toxicity by upregulating glial cell-derived neurotrophic factor (GDNF) and restoring the tyrosine hydroxylase/ nuclear receptor-related factor 1 immunoreactivity in the SN region [189]. In another study, Knekt et al. (2010) studied the relationship between serum vitamin D levels and the risk of developing PD. Their results demonstrated that people with elevated vitamin D levels had a lesser risk of developing PD [190]. Suzuki et al. (2013) showed that consumption of vitamin D prevented deterioration of Hoehn and Yahr (HY) rating in PD patients [191]. Thus, we can conclude that vitamin D can act as a neuroprotective agent by various mechanisms.

7.3.9 Vitamin E

Vitamin E (d-α-tocopherol) is a fat-soluble vitamin that acts as an antioxidant by scavenging free radicals and thus preventing lipid peroxidation. Recommended dietary intake for vitamin E is between 3 and 15 mg in different countries, and it varies depending on the age of a person. Various studies have reported the effect of vitamin E intake on the CNS function and progression of NDDs. Regular intake of vitamin E slows the progression of dementia, reduces cognitive deficits, enhances vascular functions and advances CNS functions [185,192].

In AD, vitamin E can counteract the oxidative stress caused by Aβ. It prevents Aβ_{1-42}-induced neurotoxicity by reducing ROS production and scavenging free radicals. Vitamin E supplementation prevents cognitive deficits and apoptosis and lowers the risk of AD. Clinical studies in which subjects were administered higher doses of vitamin E showed a delay in the requirement for pharmacologic treatment due to reduced degeneration of catecholaminergic neurons [193–195]. Vitamin E has also been tested for its efficacy in the progression of PD. Findings of various studies showed that vitamin E-rich diets are associated with a lower incidence of PD. The protective effects of vitamin E are higher when intake is not through supplementation but through diet owing to the enhanced bioavailability of vitamin E and thus, enhanced neuroprotection [196,197]. In a clinical study reported by Stanley Fahn, in individuals who received higher doses of antioxidant vitamin E, there was a delay of 2.5–3 years in receiving levodopa therapy [198].

7.3.10 Ginsenosides

Ginsenosides are a class of phytoestrogens extracted from several species of the plant ginseng. Traditionally, Ginseng has been used to treat various ailments in traditional Chinese medicine, Indian herbal and ayurvedic practices and other Asian cultures. It is well-known for its antiaging, antioxidant, anti-inflammatory and neuroprotective effects. It acts as an antioxidant by restoring the GSH levels and as an anti-inflammatory agent by regulating various inflammatory pathways namely ROS-NFκB, ERK, PI3K/Akt, JNK and estrogen receptor pathway. Ginsenosides have been researched for their potential role in the treatment of various NDDs. Rg1 ginsenoside is particularly isolated from the roots of *Panax ginseng* and found to reduce the 6-OHDA-mediated and MPTP-induced neurotoxicity. It attenuates neurotoxicity mainly by restoring the GSH levels and mitochondrial membrane potential. Another neuroprotective mechanism of Rg1 is the attenuation of c-Jun phosphorylation and thus, regulation of proapoptotic JNK signaling [142,199–201].

7.3.11 Polyunsaturated fatty acids

Polyunsaturated fatty acids (PUFAs) are molecules having long hydrocarbon chains with two or more double bonds in their backbone. PUFAs consist of omega-3 (ω-3) and omega-6 (ω-6) fatty acids. ω-3 fatty acids include α-linolenic acid, eicosapentaenoic acid (EPA) and docosahexaenoic acid (DHA), and ω-6 fatty acids include linoleic acid and arachidonic acid (ARA). ω-3 fatty acids are well-known for their anti-inflammatory and antiaging properties. DHA is

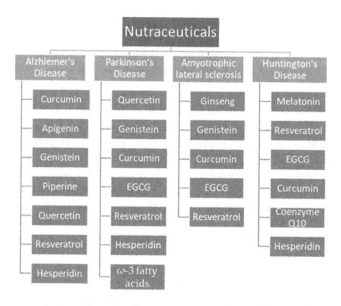

Figure 7.3 *Summary of nutraceuticals explored against various NDDs.*

one of the most important ω-3 fatty acids in the brain, mainly incorporated in phospholipids in mitochondria and ER. It constitutes over 90% of the ω-3 PUFAs. DHA modulates various cellular and physiological processes in the body [202–205].

Treatment with DHA leads to an improvement in mitochondrial function in *in vivo* and *ex vivo* experiments using animal models of AD, PD and HD. DHA was found to attenuate the Aβ, Tau or synaptic neuropathologies in animal models of AD. High DHA intake was associated with lower levels of Aβ in the brain in APP transgenic mice. DHA improved mitochondrial dysfunction in AD models [206,207]. ω-3 fatty acid-rich diet resulted in enhanced neuroprotection in MPTP-induced PD in mice. A study reported that PUFAs protects against motor deficits in animal models of HD [208].

Figure 7.3 depicts a summary of emerging nutraceuticals in the management of various NDDs like AD, PD, ALS and HD. The health benefits of various nutraceuticals with their proposed mechanisms and implications are summarized in Table 7.2. These compounds are showing huge potential to become therapeutic candidates for the treatment of various NDDs in various *in vitro* and preclinical studies.

7.4 Concluding remarks

NDDs such as AD, PD, ALS and HD are one of the greatest challenges worldwide. Various newer approaches are needed to understand the causal and

Table 7.2 Summary of Molecular Neuronal Effects of Nutraceuticals Discussed in this Chapter

S. No.	Nutraceuticals	Activity	Targeted Mechanism	Implication	Ref.
1.	Curcumin	Anti-inflammatory, antioxidant, anticancer and anti-protein aggregation activities	• Scavenges ROS and neutralizes nitric oxide (NO⁻) free radicals • Reduces the cytotoxicity, oxidative stress and apoptotic cell death • Prevents the deposition of Aβ plaques • Restores the mitochondrial membrane potential • Restores the glutathione (GSH) levels • Inhibits the pro-inflammatory signaling pathways through NF-κB or TLRs.	• Ameliorates 6-OHDA-mediated neurotoxicity • Prevents Aβ-induced neuronal death in SH-SY5Y cells • Protects SH-SY5Y cells against dopaminergic neurotoxicity induced by MPTP or MPP⁺.	[145,151,152,213]
2.	Resveratrol	Antioxidant, anti-inflammatory, antiaging, anticancer, antiviral, anti-diabetic, antidepressant, anti-hyperlipidemic, cardioprotective and neuroprotective properties	• Prevents Tau protein aggregation • Prevents the aggregation of the α-synuclein protein • Downregulates the expression of NF-κB • Reduces oxidative damage and conserves dopamine • Increased 5-HT activity	• Reduces cognitive deficits and neuroinflammation • Prevents the formation of Lewy bodies • Inhibits Aβ₁₋₄₂-mediated neuroinflammation • Protects dopaminergic neurons against MPTP⁻, MPP⁺, 6-OHDA⁻ and LPS-induced toxicity in rodent models • Antidepressant activities	[157,158,160,161]
3.	EGCG	Antioxidant, antitumoral, antibacterial and neuroprotective activities	• Scavenges the free radicals and reduces neuroinflammation, oxidative stress and autophagy • Inhibits the formation of amyloid fibrils and binds amyloid precursor protein (APP) and Tau protein and inhibits aggregation • Enhances the mitochondrial restoration • Reduces the α-synuclein accumulation • Restoring dopamine levels • Inhibits pro-inflammatory signaling through NF-κB or TLRs	• Neuroprotective activities in the treatment of AD • Improvement in the motor functions in PD patients and reduces neuronal toxicity	[162–165]

(Continued)

Table 7.2 (*Continued*) Summary of Molecular Neuronal Effects of Nutraceuticals Discussed in this Chapter

S. No.	Nutraceuticals	Activity	Targeted Mechanism	Implication	Ref.
4.	Coenzyme Q10	Antioxidant	• Prevents apoptosis and maintains the mitochondrial membrane potential • Inhibits the formation of Aβ and α-synuclein fibrils and destabilizes the preformed fibrils • Preserves mitochondrial functions	• Effective against rotenone-induced mitochondrial dysfunction • Reduces MPTP-induced neurotoxicity	[166–169]
5.	Quercetin	Antioxidant, anti-inflammatory, anticancer and neuroprotective properties	• Inhibits several aggregation proteins, including Tau protein, Aβ and α-synuclein *in vitro* • Reduces ROS production, • Enhances the glutathione levels • Enhances antioxidant enzyme function • Inhibits the activation of NF-κB	• Reduces cognitive impairments • Alleviates neurodegeneration • Neuroprotective against AD and PD	[173,175–177]
6.	Hesperidin	Antioxidant, anti-inflammatory, antihypertensive, antiviral, anticarcinogenic and neuroprotective activities	• Inhibits the depletion of dopamine • Restores GSH levels • Attenuates ROS production • Restores the mitochondrial enzyme complex activities • Decreases capillary permeability (vitamin P), leakiness, and fragility • Reduces Nrf2-mediated oxidative stress, neuroinflammation and Aβ-mediated neurodegeneration • AChE inhibitor	• Inhibits the APP expression *via* the NF-κB pathway • Improves the memory and cognitive impairments in various mice and rat models of AD • Attenuates LPS-induced neurodegeneration and cognitive impairments in the mouse model of AD	[178–183]
7.	Vitamin C	Antioxidant	• Reduces dopamine and levodopa-induced neurotoxicity • Protective effect on dopaminergic neurons against excitotoxicity	• Protective in patients with AD and PD.	[173,184–186,198]

(*Continued*)

Table 7.2 (Continued) Summary of Molecular Neuronal Effects of Nutraceuticals Discussed in this Chapter

S. No.	Nutraceuticals	Activity	Targeted Mechanism	Implication	Ref.
8.	Vitamin D	Anti-inflammatory, anti-apoptotic and immunomodulatory activities	• Increases GSH levels, • Regulates calcium homeostasis, • Reduces NO synthase, • Regulates dopamine levels • Upregulates GDNF and restores the tyrosine hydroxylase (TH)/ Nuclear receptor-related factor 1 (NURR1) immunoreactivity in the SN region	• Protective in patients with PD and AD • Reduces the dose of levodopa and improves motor symptoms in PD patients. • Reduces the 6-OHDA- and MPP+- induced neuronal toxicity	[187–190]
9.	Vitamin E	Antioxidant	• Scavenges free radicals and prevents lipid peroxidation • Decreases the level of pro-inflammatory cytokines such as IL-1β and TNF-α • Counteracts the oxidative stress caused by Aβ	• Prevents cognitive deficits, apoptosis and lowers the risk of AD • Enhances vascular functions, • Decreases neuroinflammation and neuronal degeneration in the brain of rats	[185,192–197]
10.	Ginsenosides	Antiaging, antioxidant, anti-inflammatory and neuroprotective activities	• Restores the GSH levels • Restores mitochondrial membrane potential • Regulates various inflammatory pathways, namely, ROS-NFκB, ERK, PI3K/Akt, JNK and estrogen receptor pathway • Attenuation of c-Jun phosphorylation, and thus regulation of proapoptotic JNK signaling.	• Reduces 6-OHDA-mediated and MPTP-induced neurotoxicity	[142,199–201]
11.	ω-3 PUFAs	Antioxidant, anti-inflammatory and antiaging activities	• Improvement in mitochondrial functions and physiology • Attenuate the Aβ, Tau or synaptic neuropathologies in animal models of AD	• Protects neurons against chemotherapy, hypoxia, Aβ, diabetic neuropathy and peripheral neuropathy • Enhanced neuroprotection in MPTP-induced PD in mice • Protects against motor deficits in animal models of HD	[202–208]

mechanistic factors of these NDDs. Generation of new meaningful models to understand the disease pathology and test the novel therapeutic agents is the need of the hour. Overall, there is a severe lack of treatment options for patients suffering from NDDs. AD and PD are the most widely occurring and researched NDDs, yet only symptomatic treatments are available which do not halt the underlying pathology. ALS has worse prognosis with only two FDA-approved drugs, *i.e.*, riluzole and edaravone, which are minimally effective. Novel nutraceutical compounds like curcumin, CoQ10, resveratrol, EGCG, hesperidin, vitamin D, vitamin E and ω-3 fatty acids have been used to treat various neurological disorders. They have multiple applications with several advantages over marketed therapeutics and have limited adverse reactions. Many of these compounds act by scavenging the free radicals or by attenuating the oxidative stress owing to their ability to regulate various intracellular signaling pathways. They can also inhibit apoptotic cell death by blocking the intrinsic and extrinsic apoptotic pathways. The major limitations of nutraceuticals are low bioavailability, inability to cross BBB and duration of therapy. Therefore, further research is needed to identify the target, enhance the bioavailability and reduce the adverse effect of nutraceuticals. Thus, the future holds much potential for nutraceuticals to be developed as novel therapeutic agents for better management of NDDs.

References

1. R. Hussain, H. Zubair, S. Pursell and M. Shahab, Neurodegenerative diseases: Regenerative mechanisms and novel therapeutic approaches, *Brain Sciences* 8 (2018), p. 177.
2. A. de Felice, L. Ricceri, A. Venerosi, F. Chiarotti and G. Calamandrei, Multifactorial origin of neurodevelopmental disorders: Approaches to understanding complex etiologies, *Toxics* 3 (2015), pp. 89–129.
3. R.W. Levenson, V.E. Sturm and C.M. Haase, Emotional and behavioral symptoms in neurodegenerative disease: A model for studying the neural bases of psychopathology, *Annual Review of Clinical Psychology* 10 (2014), pp. 581–606.
4. L.G. Apostolova, Alzheimer disease, *Continuum Lifelong Learning in Neurology* 22 (2016), pp. 419–434.
5. F. Magrinelli, A. Picelli, P. Tocco, A. Federico, L. Roncari, N. Smania et al., Pathophysiology of motor dysfunction in Parkinson's disease as the rationale for drug treatment and rehabilitation, *Parkinson's Disease* 2016 (2016), pp. 1–18.
6. B.L. Tan, M.E. Norhaizan, W.P.P. Liew and H.S. Rahman, Antioxidant and oxidative stress: A mutual interplay in age-related diseases, *Frontiers in Pharmacology* 9 (2018), p. 1162.
7. T. Wyss-Coray, Ageing, neurodegeneration and brain rejuvenation, *Nature* 539 (2016), pp. 180–186.
8. V.L. Feigin, E. Nichols, T. Alam, M.S. Bannick, E. Beghi, N. Blake et al., Global, regional, and national burden of neurological disorders, 1990–2016: A systematic analysis for the Global Burden of Disease Study 2016, *The Lancet Neurology* 18 (2019), pp. 459–480.
9. *Dementia*. Available at https://www.who.int/news-room/fact-sheets/detail/dementia.
10. *Dementia statistics | Alzheimer's Disease International (ADI)*. Available at https://www.alzint.org/about/dementia-facts-figures/dementia-statistics/.

11. A. Khan, S. Jahan, Z. Imtiyaz, S. Alshahrani, H.A. Makeen, B.M. Alshehri et al., Neuroprotection: Targeting multiple pathways by naturally occurring phytochemicals, *Biomedicines* 8 (2020), p. 284.
12. G.G. Kovacs, Molecular pathological classification of neurodegenerative diseases: Turning towards precision medicine, *International Journal of Molecular Sciences* 17 (2016), p. 189.
13. H. Chi, H.Y. Chang and T.K. Sang, Neuronal cell death mechanisms in major neurodegenerative diseases, *International Journal of Molecular Sciences* 19 (2018), p. 3082.
14. K.G. Yiannopoulou and S.G. Papageorgiou, Current and future treatments for Alzheimer's disease, *Therapeutic Advances in Neurological Disorders* 6 (2013), pp. 19–33.
15. G. Perry, A.D. Cash and M.A. Smith, Alzheimer disease and oxidative stress, *Journal of Biomedicine and Biotechnology* 2002 (2002), pp. 120–123.
16. Alzheimer Association, Early signs and symptoms of Alzheimer's, *Alzheimer's and Dementia* (2019), pp. 1–88.
17. W.R. Markesbery, The role of oxidative stress in Alzheimer disease, *Archives of Neurology* 56 (1999), pp. 1449–1452.
18. F. Coppedè and L. Migliore, DNA damage and repair in Alzheimer's disease, *Current Alzheimer Research* 6 (2009), pp. 36–47.
19. D.J. Bonda, X. Wang, G. Perry, A. Nunomura, M. Tabaton, X. Zhu et al., Oxidative stress in Alzheimer disease: A possibility for prevention, *Neuropharmacology* 59 (2010), pp. 290–294.
20. X. Du, X. Wang and M. Geng, Alzheimer's disease hypothesis and related therapies, *Translational Neurodegeneration* 7 (2018), pp. 1–7.
21. Y. An, C. Zhang, S. He, C. Yao, L. Zhang and Q. Zhang, Main hypotheses, concepts and theories in the study of Alzheimer's disease, *Life Science Journal* 5 (2008), pp. 1097–8135.
22. A. Ahuja, K. Dev and P. Tyagi, Alzheimer's disease, oxidative stress, and neuroprotective approaches, in: Shamim I. Ahmad (ed), *Reactive Oxygen Species in Biology and Human Health*, CRC Press, Boca Raton, 2016, pp. 123–133.
23. B. Dubois, H. Hampel, H.H. Feldman, P. Scheltens, P. Aisen, S. Andrieu et al., Preclinical Alzheimer's disease: Definition, natural history, and diagnostic criteria, *Alzheimer's and Dementia* 12 (2016), pp. 292–323.
24. E.N. Cline, M.A. Bicca, K.L. Viola and W.L. Klein, The amyloid-β oligomer hypothesis: Beginning of the third decade, *Journal of Alzheimer's Disease* 64 (2018), pp. S567–S610.
25. I.C. Stancu, B. Vasconcelos, D. Terwel and I. Dewachter, Models of β-amyloid induced Tau-pathology: The long and "folded" road to understand the mechanism, *Molecular neurodegeneration* 9 (2014), p. 51.
26. W.J. Huang, X. Zhang and W.W. Chen, Role of oxidative stress in Alzheimer's disease (review), *Biomedical Reports* 4 (2016), pp. 519–522.
27. R. Sultana and D.A. Butterfield, Role of oxidative stress in the progression of Alzheimer's disease, *Journal of Alzheimer's Disease* 19 (2010), pp. 341–353.
28. G. DeMaagd and A. Philip, Parkinson's disease and its management part 1: Disease entity, risk factors, pathophysiology, clinical presentation, and diagnosis, *P and T* 40 (2015), pp. 504–532.
29. A. Kouli, K.M. Torsney and W.-L. Kuan, Parkinson's disease: Etiology, neuropathology, and pathogenesis, in: Thomas B. Stoker and Julia C. Greenland (eds.), *Parkinson's Disease: Pathogenesis and Clinical Aspects*, Codon Publications, Brisbane (Australia) 2018, pp. 3–26.
30. S.Y. Chen and S.T. Tsai, The epidemiology of Parkinson's disease, *Tzu Chi Medical Journal* 22 (2010), pp. 73–81.
31. A. Ascherio and M.A. Schwarzschild, The epidemiology of Parkinson's disease: Risk factors and prevention, *The Lancet Neurology* 15 (2016), pp. 1257–1272.
32. J. Jankovic, Parkinson's disease: Clinical features and diagnosis, *Journal of Neurology, Neurosurgery and Psychiatry* 79 (2008), pp. 368–376.

33. J.A. Obeso, M. Stamelou, C.G. Goetz, W. Poewe, A.E. Lang, D. Weintraub et al., Past, present, and future of Parkinson's disease: A special essay on the 200th anniversary of the Shaking Palsy, *Movement Disorders* 32 (2017), pp. 1264–1310.

34. O. Hwang, Role of oxidative stress in Parkinson's disease, *Experimental Neurobiology* 22 (2013), pp. 11–17.

35. K. Hassanzadeh and A. Rahimmi, Oxidative stress and neuroinflammation in the story of Parkinson's disease: Could targeting these pathways write a good ending? *Journal of Cellular Physiology* 234 (2019), pp. 23–32.

36. R.M. Meade, D.P. Fairlie and J.M. Mason, Alpha-synuclein structure and Parkinson's disease - Lessons and emerging principles, *Molecular Neurodegeneration* 14 (2019), pp. 1–14.

37. G.E. Alexander, Biology of Parkinson's disease: Pathogenesis and pathophysiology of a multisystem neurodegenerative disorder, *Dialogues in Clinical Neuroscience* 6 (2004), pp. 259–280.

38. L. Stefanis, α-Synuclein in Parkinson's disease, *Cold Spring Harbor Perspectives in Medicine* 2 (2012), p. a009399.

39. K.F. Winklhofer and C. Haass, Mitochondrial dysfunction in Parkinson's disease, *Biochimica et Biophysica Acta - Molecular Basis of Disease* 1802 (2010), pp. 29–44.

40. S.R. Subramaniam and M.F. Chesselet, Mitochondrial dysfunction and oxidative stress in Parkinson's disease, *Progress in Neurobiology* 106–107 (2013), pp. 17–32.

41. B. Murray, Amyotrophic lateral sclerosis, *Encyclopedia of the Neurological Sciences* (2014), pp. 165–167.

42. M.A. van Es, O. Hardiman, A. Chio, A. Al-Chalabi, R.J. Pasterkamp, J.H. Veldink et al., Amyotrophic lateral sclerosis, *The Lancet* 390 (2017), pp. 2084–2098.

43. B. Oskarsson, T.F. Gendron and N.P. Staff, Amyotrophic lateral sclerosis: An update for 2018, *Mayo Clinic Proceedings* 93 (2018), pp. 1617–1628.

44. *Motor Neuron Diseases Fact Sheet | National Institute of Neurological Disorders and Stroke.* Available at https://www.ninds.nih.gov/Disorders/Patient-Caregiver-Education/Fact-Sheets/Motor-Neuron-Diseases-Fact-Sheet.

45. E.F. Smith, P.J. Shaw and K.J. de Vos, The role of mitochondria in amyotrophic lateral sclerosis, *Neuroscience Letters* 710 (2019), p. 132933.

46. Y. Sato, E. Nakatani, Y. Watanabe, M. Fukushima, K. Nakashima, M. Kannagi et al., Prediction of prognosis of ALS: Importance of active denervation findings of the cervical-upper limb area and trunk area, *Intractable & Rare Diseases Research* 4 (2015), pp. 181–189.

47. L. le Gall, E. Anakor, O. Connolly, U.G. Vijayakumar, W.J. Duddy and S. Duguez, Molecular and cellular mechanisms affected in als, *Journal of Personalized Medicine* 10 (2020), pp. 1–34.

48. R. Mejzini, L.L. Flynn, I.L. Pitout, S. Fletcher, S.D. Wilton and P.A. Akkari, ALS genetics, mechanisms, and therapeutics: Where are we now? *Frontiers in Neuroscience* 13 (2019), pp. 1310.

49. P.J. Shaw, Molecular and cellular pathways of neurodegeneration in motor neurone disease, *Journal of Neurology, Neurosurgery and Psychiatry* 76 (2005), pp. 1046–1057.

50. O. Komine and K. Yamanaka, Neuroinflammation in motor neuron disease, *Nagoya Journal of Medical Science* 77 (2015), pp. 537–549.

51. F. Gros-Louis, C. Gaspar and G.A. Rouleau, Genetics of familial and sporadic amyotrophic lateral sclerosis, *Biochimica et Biophysica Acta - Molecular Basis of Disease* 1762 (2006), pp. 956–972.

52. S. Ajroud-Driss and T. Siddique, Sporadic and hereditary amyotrophic lateral sclerosis (ALS), *Biochimica et Biophysica Acta - Molecular Basis of Disease* 1852 (2015), pp. 679–684.

53. J.C. Schymick, K. Talbot and B.J. Traynor, Genetics of sporadic amyotrophic lateral sclerosis, *Human Molecular Genetics* 16 (2007), pp. R233–R242.

54. A.E. Volk, J.H. Weishaupt, P.M. Andersen, A.C. Ludolph and C. Kubisch, Current knowledge and recent insights into the genetic basis of amyotrophic lateral sclerosis, *Medizinische Genetik* 30 (2018), pp. 252–258.

55. M. van Blitterswijk, M. Dejesus-Hernandez and R. Rademakers, How do C9ORF72 repeat expansions cause amyotrophic lateral sclerosis and frontotemporal dementia: Can we learn from other noncoding repeat expansion disorders?, *Current Opinion in Neurology* 25 (2012), pp. 689–700.

56. S.H. Appel and D.R. Beers, Immune dysregulation in amyotrophic lateral sclerosis: Mechanisms and emerging therapies, *Lancet Neurol* 18 (2019), pp. 211–231.

57. S.A. Goutman, Diagnosis and clinical management of amyotrophic lateral sclerosis and other motor neuron disorders, *Continuum Lifelong Learning in Neurology* 23 (2017), pp. 1332–1359.

58. A. Hogden, G. Foley, R.D. Henderson, N. James and S.M. Aoun, Amyotrophic lateral sclerosis: Improving care with a multidisciplinary approach, *Journal of Multidisciplinary Healthcare* 10 (2017), pp. 205–215.

59. R. Bhandari, A. Kuhad and A. Kuhad, Edaravone: A new hope for deadly amyotrophic lateral sclerosis, *Drugs of Today* 54 (2018), pp. 349–360.

60. A. Wexler, E.J. Wild and S.J. Tabrizi, George Huntington: A legacy of inquiry, empathy and hope, *Brain* 139 (2016), pp. 2326–2333.

61. K.B. Bhattacharyya, The story of George Huntington and his disease, *Annals of Indian Academy of Neurology* 19 (2016), pp. 25–28.

62. P. McColgan and S.J. Tabrizi, Huntington's disease: A clinical review, *European Journal of Neurology* 25 (2018), pp. 24–34.

63. A. Kumar and V.K. Garg, A review on Huntington's disease, *Journal of Pharmaceutical Research International*, 13 (2016), pp. 1–15.

64. A. Reiner, I. Dragatsis and P. Dietrich, Genetics and neuropathology of Huntington's disease, in: Jonathan Brotchie, Erwan Bezard and Peter Jenner (eds.), *International Review of Neurobiology*, Academic Press Inc., 2011, pp. 325–372.

65. C. Rangel-Barajas and G. v. Rebec, Dysregulation of corticostriatal connectivity in Huntington's disease: A role for dopamine modulation, *Journal of Huntington's Disease* 5 (2016), pp. 303–331.

66. R.H. Myers, Huntington's disease genetics, *NeuroRx* 1 (2004), pp. 255–262.

67. D.C. Rubinsztein and J. Carmichael, Huntington's disease: Molecular basis of neurodegeneration, *Expert Reviews in Molecular Medicine* 5 (2003), pp. 1–21.

68. C. Zuccato, M. Valenza and E. Cattaneo, Molecular mechanisms and potential therapeutical targets in Huntington's disease, *Physiological Reviews* 90 (2010), pp. 905–981.

69. J.M. Gil and A.C. Rego, Mechanisms of neurodegeneration in Huntington's disease, *European Journal of Neuroscience* 27 (2008), pp. 2803–2820.

70. J. Schulte and J.T. Littleton, The biological function of the Huntingtin protein and its relevance to Huntington's Disease pathology., *Current Trends in Neurology* 5 (2011), pp. 65–78.

71. I. Han, Y. You, J.H. Kordower, S.T. Brady and G.A. Morfini, Differential vulnerability of neurons in Huntington's disease: The role of cell type-specific features, *Journal of Neurochemistry* 113 (2010), pp. 1073–1091.

72. A. Fazl and J. Fleisher, Anatomy, physiology, and clinical syndromes of the Basal Ganglia: A brief review, *Seminars in Pediatric Neurology* 25 (2018), pp. 2–9.

73. S. Mason and R. Barker, Novel targets for Huntington's disease: Future prospects, *Degenerative Neurological and Neuromuscular Disease* 6 (2016), p. 25.

74. K.M. Shannon, Recent advances in the treatment of Huntington's disease: Targeting DNA and RNA, *CNS Drugs* 34 (2020), pp. 219–228.

75. C.Y. Guo, L. Sun, X.P. Chen and D.S. Zhang, Oxidative stress, mitochondrial damage and neurodegenerative diseases, *Neural Regeneration Research* 8 (2013), pp. 2003–2014.

76. L.D. Osellame, T.S. Blacker and M.R. Duchen, Cellular and molecular mechanisms of mitochondrial function, *Best Practice and Research: Clinical Endocrinology and Metabolism* 26 (2012), pp. 711–723.

77. M. Kowalska, T. Piekut, M. Prendecki, A. Sodel, W. Kozubski and J. Dorszewska, Mitochondrial and nuclear DNA oxidative damage in physiological and pathological aging, *DNA and Cell Biology* 39 (2020), pp. 1410–1420.

78. R.W. Taylor and D.M. Turnbull, Mitochondrial DNA mutations in human disease, *Nature Reviews Genetics* 6 (2005), pp. 389–402.

79. N.Z. Lax, D.M. Turnbull and A.K. Reeve, Mitochondrial mutations: Newly discovered players in neuronal degeneration, *The Neuroscientist* 17 (2011), pp. 645–658.

80. A. F. C. Lopes, Mitochondrial metabolism and DNA methylation: A review of the interaction between two genomes, *Clinical Epigenetics* 12 (2020), p. 182.

81. P. Sharma, A.B. Jha, R.S. Dubey and M. Pessarakli, Reactive oxygen species, oxidative damage, and antioxidative defense mechanism in plants under stressful conditions, *Journal of Botany* 2012 (2012), pp. 1–26.

82. E. Birben, U.M. Sahiner, C. Sackesen, S. Erzurum and O. Kalayci, Oxidative stress and antioxidant defense, *World Allergy Organization Journal* 5 (2012), pp. 9–19.

83. W. Wang, F. Zhao, X. Ma, G. Perry and X. Zhu, Mitochondria dysfunction in the pathogenesis of Alzheimer's disease: Recent advances, *Molecular Neurodegeneration* 15 (2020), pp. 1–22.

84. Y. Cheng and F. Bai, The association of tau with mitochondrial dysfunction in Alzheimer's disease, *Frontiers in Neuroscience* 12 (2018), p. 163.

85. N. Callizot, M. Combes, A. Henriques and P. Poindron, Necrosis, apoptosis, necroptosis, three modes of action of dopaminergic neuron neurotoxins, *PLoS One* 14 (2019), p. e0215277.

86. D. Trinh, A.R. Israwi, L.R. Arathoon, J.A. Gleave and J.E. Nash, The multi-faceted role of mitochondria in the pathology of Parkinson's disease, *Journal of Neurochemistry* (2020), p. jnc.15154.

87. K. Nuytemans, J. Theuns, M. Cruts and C. van Broeckhoven, Genetic etiology of Parkinson disease associated with mutations in the SNCA, PARK2, PINK1, PARK7, and LRRK2 genes: A mutation update, *Human Mutation* 31 (2010), pp. 763–780.

88. J.S. Park, R.L. Davis and C.M. Sue, Mitochondrial dysfunction in Parkinson's disease: New mechanistic insights and therapeutic perspectives, *Current Neurology and Neuroscience Reports* 18 (2018), pp. 1–11.

89. K.J. Thomas, M.K. McCoy, J. Blackinton, A. Beilina, M. van der Brug, A. Sandebring et al., DJ-1 acts in parallel to the PINK1/parkin pathway to control mitochondrial function and autophagy, *Human Molecular Genetics* 20 (2011), pp. 40–50.

90. P.M.J. Quinn, P.I. Moreira, A.F. Ambrósio and C.H. Alves, PINK1/PARKIN signalling in neurodegeneration and neuroinflammation, *Acta Neuropathologica Communications* 8 (2020), p. 189.

91. J. Huai and Z. Zhang, Structural properties and interaction partners of familial ALS-associated SOD1 mutants, *Frontiers in Neurology* 10 (2019), p. 527.

92. W. Tan, P. Pasinelli and D. Trotti, Role of mitochondria in mutant SOD1 linked amyotrophic lateral sclerosis, *Biochimica et Biophysica Acta - Molecular Basis of Disease* 1842 (2014), pp. 1295–1301.

93. M.C. Zimmerman, L.W. Oberley and S.W. Flanagan, Mutant SOD1-induced neuronal toxicity is mediated by increased mitochondrial superoxide levels, *Journal of Neurochemistry* 102 (2007), pp. 609–618.

94. P. Wang, J. Deng, J. Dong, J. Liu, E.H. Bigio, M. Mesulam et al., TDP-43 induces mitochondrial damage and activates the mitochondrial unfolded protein response, *PLoS Genetics* 15 (2019), p. e1007947.

95. C. Huang, S. Yan and Z. Zhang, Maintaining the balance of TDP-43, mitochondria, and autophagy: A promising therapeutic strategy for neurodegenerative diseases, *Translational Neurodegeneration* 9 (2020), pp. 1–16.

96. H. Muyderman and T. Chen, Mitochondrial dysfunction in amyotrophic lateral sclerosis – A valid pharmacological target? *British Journal of Pharmacology* 171 (2014), pp. 2191–2205.

97. J. Labbadia and R.I. Morimoto, Huntington's disease: Underlying molecular mechanisms and emerging concepts, *Trends in Biochemical Sciences* 38 (2013), pp. 378–385.

98. R. Bagur and G. Hajnóczky, Intracellular Ca2+ Sensing: Its role in calcium homeostasis and signaling, *Molecular Cell* 66 (2017), pp. 780–788.

99. P. Marambaud, U. Dreses-Werringloer and V. Vingtdeux, Calcium signaling in neurodegeneration, *Molecular Neurodegeneration* 4 (2009), pp. 1–15.

100. M.R. Mattson, Calcium and neurodegeneration, *Aging Cell* 6 (2007), pp. 337–350.

101. M. Gleichmann and M.P. Mattson, Neuronal calcium homeostasis and dysregulation, *Antioxidants and Redox Signaling* 14 (2011), pp. 1261–1273.

102. G. Zündorf and G. Reiser, Calcium dysregulation and homeostasis of neural calcium in the molecular mechanisms of neurodegenerative diseases provide multiple targets for neuroprotection, *Antioxidants and Redox Signaling* 14 (2011), pp. 1275–1288.

103. E. Pchitskaya, E. Popugaeva and I. Bezprozvanny, Calcium signaling and molecular mechanisms underlying neurodegenerative diseases, *Cell Calcium* 70 (2018), pp. 87–94.

104. T. Calì, D. Ottolini and M. Brini, Mitochondrial Ca2+ and neurodegeneration, *Cell Calcium* 52 (2012), pp. 73–85.

105. J. Grosskreutz, L. van den Bosch and B.U. Keller, Calcium dysregulation in amyotrophic lateral sclerosis, *Cell Calcium* 47 (2010), pp. 165–174.

106. S.S. Leal and C.M. Gomes, Calcium dysregulation links ALS defective proteins and motor neuron selective vulnerability, *Frontiers in Cellular Neuroscience* 9 (2015), pp. 1–6.

107. V. Meszlényi, R. Patai, B. Nógrádi, J.I. Engelhardt and L. Siklós, Calcium in the pathomechanism of amyotrophic lateral sclerosis-Taking center stage? *Biochemical and Biophysical Research Communications* 2 (2017), pp. 1–4.

108. H.-J. Kim, W. Im, S. Kim, S.H. Kim, J.-J. Sung, M. Kim et al., Calcium-influx increases SOD1 aggregates via nitric oxide in cultured motor neurons, *Experimental and Molecular Medicine* 39 (2007), pp. 574–582.

109. H. Kawamata and G. Manfredi, Mitochondrial dysfunction and intracellular calcium dysregulation in ALS, *Mechanisms of Ageing and Development* 131 (2010), pp. 517–526.

110. Y.A. Kolobkova, V.A. Vigont, A.V. Shalygin and E.V. Kaznacheyeva, Huntington's disease: Calcium dyshomeostasis and pathology models, *Acta Naturae* 9 (2017), pp. 34–46.

111. M. Giacomello, R. Hudec and R. Lopreiato, Huntington's disease, calcium, and mitochondria, *BioFactors* 37 (2011), pp. 206–218.

112. R.A. Quintanilla, C. Tapia and M.J. Pérez, Possible role of mitochondrial permeability transition pore in the pathogenesis of Huntington disease, *Biochemical and Biophysical Research Communications* 483 (2017), pp. 1078–1083.

113. B. Uttara, A. Singh, P. Zamboni and R. Mahajan, Oxidative stress and neurodegenerative diseases: A review of upstream and downstream antioxidant therapeutic options, *Current Neuropharmacology* 7 (2009), pp. 65–74.

114. F. Cioffi, R.H.I. Adam and K. Broersen, Molecular mechanisms and genetics of oxidative stress in Alzheimer's disease, *Journal of Alzheimer's Disease* 72 (2019), pp. 981–1017.

115. P. Mao and P.H. Reddy, Aging and amyloid beta-induced oxidative DNA damage and mitochondrial dysfunction in Alzheimer's disease: Implications for early intervention and therapeutics, *Biochimica et Biophysica Acta - Molecular Basis of Disease* 1812 (2011), pp. 1359–1370.

116. E. Tönnies and E. Trushina, Oxidative stress, synaptic dysfunction, and Alzheimer's disease, *Journal of Alzheimer's Disease* 57 (2017), pp. 1105–1121.

117. V. Dias, E. Junn and M.M. Mouradian, The role of oxidative stress in Parkinson's disease, *Journal of Parkinson's Disease* 3 (2013), pp. 461–491.
118. T. Oeda, S. Shimohama, N. Kitagawa, R. Kohno, T. Imura, H. Shibasaki et al., Oxidative stress causes abnormal accumulation of familial amyotropic lateral sclerosis-related mutant SOD1 in transgenic Caenorhabditis elegans, *Human Molecular Genetics* 10 (2001), pp. 2013–2023.
119. S.C. Barber, R.J. Mead and P.J. Shaw, Oxidative stress in ALS: A mechanism of neurodegeneration and a therapeutic target, *Biochimica et Biophysica Acta - Molecular Basis of Disease* 1762 (2006), pp. 1051–1067.
120. G.J. Harry and A.D. Kraft, Neuroinflammation and microglia: Considerations and approaches for neurotoxicity assessment, *Expert Opinion on Drug Metabolism and Toxicology* 4 (2008), pp. 1265–1277.
121. M.J. Carson, J. Cameron Thrash and B. Walter, The cellular response in neuroinflammation: The role of leukocytes, microglia and astrocytes in neuronal death and survival, *Clinical Neuroscience Research* 6 (2006), pp. 237–245.
122. J. Drouin-Ouellet and F. Cicchetti, Inflammation and neurodegeneration: The story "retolled", *Trends in Pharmacological Sciences* 33 (2012), pp. 542–551.
123. M.M. Esiri, The interplay between inflammation and neurodegeneration in CNS disease, *Journal of Neuroimmunology* 184 (2007), pp. 4–16.
124. M.L. Block and J.S. Hong, Microglia and inflammation-mediated neurodegeneration: Multiple triggers with a common mechanism, *Progress in Neurobiology* 76 (2005), pp. 77–98.
125. W.Y. Wang, M.S. Tan, J.T. Yu and L. Tan, Role of pro-inflammatory cytokines released from microglia in Alzheimer's disease, *Annals of Translational Medicine* 3 (2015), p. 136.
126. Y. Sawikr, N.S. Yarla, I. Peluso, M.A. Kamal, G. Aliev and A. Bishayee, Neuroinflammation in Alzheimer's disease: The preventive and therapeutic potential of polyphenolic nutraceuticals, *Advances in Protein Chemistry and Structural Biology* 108 (2017), pp. 33–57.
127. P.L. McGeer and E.G. McGeer, Inflammation and neurodegeneration in Parkinson's disease, *Parkinsonism and Related Disorders* 10 (2004), p. S3.
128. J.R. Thonhoff, E.P. Simpson and S.H. Appel, Neuroinflammatory mechanisms in amyotrophic lateral sclerosis pathogenesis, *Current Opinion in Neurology* 31 (2018), pp. 635–639.
129. M. A. Thevandavakkam, R. Schwarcz, P. J. Muchowski and F. Giorgini, Targeting Kynurenine 3-Monooxygenase (KMO): Implications for therapy in Huntingtons disease, *CNS & Neurological Disorders - Drug Targets* 9 (2012), pp. 791–800.
130. K. v. Sathyasaikumar, C. Breda, R. Schwarcz and F. Giorgini, Assessing and modulating kynurenine pathway dynamics in Huntington's disease: Focus on kynurenine 3-monooxygenase, in: Sophie V. Precious, Anne E. Rosser and Stephen B. Dunnett, *Methods in Molecular Biology*, Humana Press Inc., New York, NY, 2018, pp. 397–413.
131. F. Coppedè and L. Migliore, DNA damage in neurodegenerative diseases, *Mutation Research - Fundamental and Molecular Mechanisms of Mutagenesis* 776 (2015), pp. 84–97.
132. R.L. Rolig and P.J. McKinnon, Linking DNA damage and neurodegeneration, *Trends in Neurosciences* 23 (2000), pp. 417–424.
133. R. Madabhushi, L. Pan and L.H. Tsai, DNA damage and its links to neurodegeneration, *Neuron* 83 (2014), pp. 266–282.
134. L.J. Martin, DNA damage and repair: Relevance to mechanisms of neurodegeneration, *Journal of Neuropathology and Experimental Neurology* 67 (2008), pp. 377–387.
135. C.P. Gonzalez-Hunt and L.H. Sanders, DNA damage and repair in Parkinson's disease: Recent advances and new opportunities, *Journal of Neuroscience Research* 99 (2021), pp. 180–189.
136. Y. Sun, A.J. Curle, A.M. Haider and G. Balmus, The role of DNA damage response in amyotrophic lateral sclerosis, *Essays in Biochemistry* 64 (2020), pp. 847–861.

137. F. Coppedè, An overview of DNA repair in amyotrophic lateral sclerosis, *The Scientific World Journal* 11 (2011), pp. 1679–1691.
138. S. Ayala-Peña, Role of oxidative DNA damage in mitochondrial dysfunction and Huntington's disease pathogenesis, *Free Radical Biology and Medicine* 62 (2013), pp. 102–110.
139. J.K. Aronson, Defining 'nutraceuticals': Neither nutritious nor pharmaceutical, *British Journal of Clinical Pharmacology* 83 (2017), pp. 8–19.
140. S.K. Gupta, S. Kumar Yadav and S.M.M. Patil, Nutraceutical – A bright scope and oppourtunity of Indian healthcare market, *International Journal of Research and Development in Pharmacy & Life Sciences* 2 (2013), pp. 478–481.
141. A.K. Singh, A.K. Chaturvedani, N.P. Singh and A. Baranawal, Nutraceuticals: Meaning and regulatory scenario, *The Pharma Innovation Journal* 7 (2018), pp. 448–451.
142. R. Makkar, T. Behl, S. Bungau, G. Zengin, V. Mehta, A. Kumar et al., Nutraceuticals in neurological disorders, *International Journal of Molecular Sciences* 21 (2020), pp. 1–19.
143. V. P. Dadhania, P. P. Trivedi, A. Vikram and D. Nand Tripathi, Nutraceuticals against neurodegeneration: A mechanistic insight, *Current Neuropharmacology* 14 (2016), pp. 627–640.
144. H.F. Chiu, K. Venkatakrishnan and C.K. Wang, The role of nutraceuticals as a complementary therapy against various neurodegenerative diseases: A mini-review, *Journal of Traditional and Complementary Medicine* 10 (2020), pp. 434–439.
145. A. Monroy, G.J. Lithgow and S. Alavez, Curcumin and neurodegenerative diseases, *BioFactors* 39 (2013), pp. 122–132.
146. A.B. Kunnumakkara, D. Bordoloi, G. Padmavathi, J. Monisha, N.K. Roy, S. Prasad et al., Curcumin, the golden nutraceutical: Multitargeting for multiple chronic diseases, *British Journal of Pharmacology* 174 (2017), pp. 1325–1348.
147. I. Solanki, P. Parihar, M.L. Mansuri and M.S. Parihar, Flavonoid-based therapies in the early management of neurodegenerative diseases, *Advances in Nutrition* 6 (2015), pp. 64–72.
148. A. Olivera, T.W. Moore, F. Hu, A.P. Brown, A. Sun, D.C. Liotta et al., Inhibition of the NF-κB signaling pathway by the curcumin analog, 3,5-Bis(2-pyridinylmethylidene)-4-piperidone (EF31): Anti-inflammatory and anti-cancer properties, *International Immunopharmacology* 12 (2012), pp. 368–377.
149. Z.J. Liu, Z.H. Li, L. Liu, W.X. Tang, Y. Wang, M.R. Dong et al., Curcumin attenuates beta-amyloid-induced neuroinflammation via activation of peroxisome proliferator-activated receptor-gamma function in a rat model of Alzheimer's disease, *Frontiers in Pharmacology* 7 (2016), p. 261.
150. R. B. Mythri and M. M. Srinivas Bharath, Curcumin: A potential neuroprotective agent in Parkinson's disease, *Current Pharmaceutical Design* 18 (2012), pp. 91–99.
151. H.-F. Ji and L. Shen, The multiple pharmaceutical potential of curcumin in Parkinson's disease, *CNS & Neurological Disorders - Drug Targets* 13 (2014), pp. 369–373.
152. S.K. Kulkarni and A. Dhir, An overview of curcumin in neurological disorders, *Indian Journal of Pharmaceutical Sciences* 72 (2010), pp. 149–154.
153. M.D. Cas and R. Ghidoni, Dietary curcumin: Correlation between bioavailability and health potential, *Nutrients* 11 (2019), p. 2147.
154. N.A. Kelsey, H.M. Wilkins and D.A. Linseman, Nutraceutical antioxidants as novel neuroprotective agents, *Molecules* 15 (2010), pp. 7792–7814.
155. N.Z. Ramli, M.F. Yahaya, I. Tooyama and H.A. Damanhuri, A mechanistic evaluation of antioxidant nutraceuticals on their potential against age-associated neurodegenerative diseases, *Antioxidants* 9 (2020), pp. 1–39.
156. C. Calfio, A. Gonzalez, S.K. Singh, L.E. Rojo and R.B. MacCioni, The emerging role of nutraceuticals and phytochemicals in the prevention and treatment of Alzheimer's disease, *Journal of Alzheimer's Disease* 77 (2020), pp. 33–51.
157. K.C. Yu, P. Kwan, S.K.K. Cheung, A. Ho and L. Baum, Effects of resveratrol and morin on insoluble tau in tau transgenic mice, *Translational Neuroscience* 9 (2018), pp. 54–60.

158. X.-Y. Sun, Q.-X. Dong, J. Zhu, X. Sun, L.-F. Zhang, M. Qiu et al., Resveratrol rescues tau-induced cognitive deficits and neuropathology in a mouse model of tauopathy, *Current Alzheimer Research* 16 (2019), pp. 710–722.

159. H.F. Zhao, N. Li, Q. Wang, X.J. Cheng, X.M. Li and T.T. Liu, Resveratrol decreases the insoluble Aβ1-42 level in hippocampus and protects the integrity of the blood-brain barrier in AD rats, *Neuroscience* 310 (2015), pp. 641–649.

160. F. Jin, Q. Wu, Y.F. Lu, Q.H. Gong and J.S. Shi, Neuroprotective effect of resveratrol on 6-OHDA-induced Parkinson's disease in rats, *European Journal of Pharmacology* 600 (2008), pp. 78–82.

161. P. Kumar, S.S.V. Padi, P.S. Naidu and A. Kumar, Effect of resveratrol on 3-nitropropionic acid-induced biochemical and behavioural changes: Possible neuroprotective mechanisms, *Behavioural Pharmacology* 17 (2006), pp. 485–492.

162. T. Mori, N. Koyama, J. Tan, T. Segawa, M. Maeda and T. Town, Combined treatment with the phenolics ()-epigallocatechin-3-gallate and ferulic acid improves cognition and reduces Alzheimer-like pathology in mice, *Journal of Biological Chemistry* 294 (2019), pp. 2714–2731.

163. Q. Xu, M. Langley, A.G. Kanthasamy and M.B. Reddy, Epigallocatechin Gallate has a neurorescue effect in a mouse model of Parkinson disease, *Journal of Nutrition* 147 (2017), pp. 1926–1931.

164. T. Zhou, M. Zhu and Z. Liang, (-)-Epigallocatechin-3-gallate modulates peripheral immunity in the MPTP-induced mouse model of Parkinson's disease, *Molecular Medicine Reports* 17 (2018), pp. 4883–4888.

165. D.E. Ehrnhoefer, M. Duennwald, P. Markovic, J.L. Wacker, S. Engemann, M. Roark et al., Green tea (-)-epigallocatechin-gallate modulates early events in huntingtin misfolding and reduces toxicity in Huntington's disease models, *Human Molecular Genetics* 15 (2006), pp. 2743–2751.

166. C. Shults, Coenzyme Q10 in neurodegenerative diseases, *Current Medicinal Chemistry* 10 (2005), pp. 1917–1921.

167. X. Yang, Y. Zhang, H. Xu, X. Luo, J. Yu, J. Liu et al., Neuroprotection of coenzyme Q10 in neurodegenerative diseases, *Current Topics in Medicinal Chemistry* 16 (2015), pp. 858–866.

168. M. Spindler, M. Flint Beal and C. Henchcliffe, Coenzyme Q10 effects in neurodegenerative disease, *Neuropsychiatric Disease and Treatment* 5 (2009), pp. 597–610.

169. M.F. Beal, Therapeutic effects of coenzyme Q10 in neurodegenerative diseases, *Methods in Enzymology* 382 (2004), pp. 473–487.

170. H. Takahashi, Coenzyme Q10 in neurodegenerative disorders: Potential benefit of CoQ10 supplementation for multiple system atrophy, *World Journal of Neurology* 4 (2014), p. 1.

171. L. Pogačnik, A. Ota and N. Poklar Ulrih, An overview of crucial dietary substances and their modes of action for prevention of neurodegenerative diseases, *Cells* 9 (2020), p. 576.

172. C. Cleren, L. Yang, B. Lorenzo, N.Y. Calingasan, A. Schomer, A. Sireci et al., Therapeutic effects of coenzyme Q10 (CoQ10) and reduced CoQ10 in the MPTP model of Parkinsonism, *Journal of Neurochemistry* 104 (2008), pp. 1613–1621.

173. H.J. Heo and C.Y. Lee, Protective effects of quercetin and vitamin C against oxidative stress-induced neurodegeneration, *Journal of Agricultural and Food Chemistry* 52 (2004), pp. 7514–7517.

174. S. Hasanbašić, A. Jahić, S. Berbić, M.T. Znidarič and E. Zerovnik, Inhibition of protein aggregation by several antioxidants, *Oxidative Medicine and Cellular Longevity* 2018 (2018), pp. 1–12.

175. H. Khan, H. Ullah, M. Aschner, W.S. Cheang and E.K. Akkol, Neuroprotective effects of quercetin in Alzheimer's disease, *Biomolecules* 10 (2020), p. 59.

176. S.S. Karuppagounder, S.K. Madathil, M. Pandey, R. Haobam, U. Rajamma and K.P. Mohanakumar, Quercetin up-regulates mitochondrial complex-I activity to protect against programmed cell death in rotenone model of Parkinson's disease in rats, *Neuroscience* 236 (2013), pp. 136–148.

177. S. Singh, S. Jamwal and P. Kumar, Neuroprotective potential of Quercetin in combination with piperine against 1-methyl-4-phenyl-1,2,3,6-tetrahydropyridine-induced neurotoxicity, *Neural Regeneration Research* 12 (2017), pp. 1137–1144.

178. S. Cirmi, N. Ferlazzo, G.E. Lombardo, E. Ventura-Spagnolo, S. Gangemi, G. Calapai et al., Neurodegenerative diseases: Might citrus flavonoids play a protective role? *Molecules* 21 (2016), pp. 1–25.

179. A. Khan, M. Ikram, J.R. Hahm and M.O. Kim, Antioxidant and anti-inflammatory effects of citrus flavonoid hesperetin: Special focus on neurological disorders, *Antioxidants* 9 (2020), pp. 1–15.

180. A. Justin Thenmozhi, T.R. William Raja, T. Manivasagam, U. Janakiraman and M.M. Essa, Hesperidin ameliorates cognitive dysfunction, oxidative stress and apoptosis against aluminium chloride induced rat model of Alzheimer's disease, *Nutritional Neuroscience* 20 (2017), pp. 360–368.

181. E. kheradmand, A. Hajizadeh Moghaddam and M. Zare, Neuroprotective effect of hesperetin and nano-hesperetin on recognition memory impairment and the elevated oxygen stress in rat model of Alzheimer's disease, *Biomedicine and Pharmacotherapy* 97 (2018), pp. 1096–1101.

182. M.S. Antunes, A.T.R. Goes, S.P. Boeira, M. Prigol and C.R. Jesse, Protective effect of hesperidin in a model of Parkinson's disease induced by 6-hydroxydopamine in aged mice, *Nutrition* 30 (2014), pp. 1415–1422.

183. E.T. Menze, M.G. Tadros, A.M. Abdel-Tawab and A.E. Khalifa, Potential neuroprotective effects of hesperidin on 3-nitropropionic acid-induced neurotoxicity in rats, *NeuroToxicology* 33 (2012), pp. 1265–1275.

184. S. Dixit, D.C. Consoli, K.C. Paffenroth, J.M. Wilcox and F.E. Harrison, Vitamin C in Neurological Function and Neurodegenerative Disease, in: Qi Chen and Margreet C.M. Vissers (eds.), *Vitamin C*, CRC Press, Boca Raton, 2020, pp. 183–211.

185. A. Martin, K. Youdim, A. Szprengiel, B. Shukitt-Hale and J. Joseph, Roles of vitamins E and C on neurodegenerative diseases and cognitive performance, *Nutrition Reviews* 60 (2002), pp. 308–326.

186. M. Moretti, D.B. Fraga and A.L.S. Rodrigues, Preventive and therapeutic potential of ascorbic acid in neurodegenerative diseases, *CNS Neuroscience & Therapeutics* 23 (2017), pp. 921–929.

187. P. Koduah, F. Paul and J.-M. Dörr, Vitamin D in the prevention, prediction and treatment of neurodegenerative and neuroinflammatory diseases, *The EPMA Journal* 8 (2017), pp. 313.

188. D. Gezen-Ak and E. Dursun, Molecular basis of vitamin D action in neurodegeneration: the story of a team perspective, *Hormones* 18 (2019), pp. 17–21.

189. H.L. Newmark and J. Newmark, Vitamin D and Parkinson's disease – A hypothesis, *Movement Disorders* 22 (2007), pp. 461–468.

190. P. Knekt, A. Kilkkinen, H. Rissanen, J. Marniemi, K. Sääksjärvi and M. Heliövaara, Serum vitamin D and the risk of Parkinson disease, *Archives of Neurology* 67 (2010), pp. 808–811.

191. M. Suzuki, M. Yoshioka, M. Hashimoto, M. Murakami, M. Noya, D. Takahashi et al., Randomized, double-blind, placebo-controlled trial of vitamin D supplementation in Parkinson disease, *American Journal of Clinical Nutrition* 97 (2013), pp. 1004–1013.

192. R. Ricciarelli, F. Argellati, M.A. Pronzato and C. Domenicotti, Vitamin E and neurodegenerative diseases, *Molecular Aspects of Medicine* 28 (2007), pp. 591–606.

193. A. Lloret, D. Esteve, P. Monllor, A. Cervera-Ferri and A. Lloret, The effectiveness of vitamin E treatment in Alzheimer's disease, *International Journal of Molecular Sciences* 20 (2019), pp. 879.

194. D. Browne, B. McGuinness, J. v. Woodside and G.J. McKay, Vitamin E and Alzheimer's disease: What do we know so far? *Clinical Interventions in Aging* 14 (2019), pp. 1303–1317.

195. A. Kontush and S. Schekatolina, Vitamin E in neurodegenerative disorders: Alzheimer's disease, *Annals of the New York Academy of Sciences* 1031 (2004), pp. 249–262.

196. M.W. Fariss and J.G. Zhang, Vitamin E therapy in Parkinson's disease, *Toxicology* 189 (2003), pp. 129–146.

197. T. Schirinzi, G. Martella, P. Imbriani, G. di Lazzaro, D. Franco, V.L. Colona et al., Dietary vitamin E as a protective factor for Parkinson's disease: Clinical and experimental evidence, *Frontiers in Neurology* 10 (2019), p. 148.

198. S. Fahn, A pilot trial of high-dose alpha-tocopherol and ascorbate in early Parkinson's disease, *Annals of Neurology* 32 (1992), pp. S128–S132.

199. L. Hang, A.H. Basil and K.L. Lim, Nutraceuticals in Parkinson's disease, *NeuroMolecular Medicine* 18 (2016), pp. 306–321.

200. N. Mukherjee, D.R. Vayeda, B.C. Spoorthi and A.K. Maiti, Neurotherapeutic efficacy of nutraceuticals in combating Parkinson's disease: A promising alternative, *Journal of Pharmacy Research* 11 (2017), pp. 1127–1134.

201. A. Khan, S. Jahan, Z. Imtiyaz, S. Alshahrani, H.A. Makeen, B.M. Alshehri et al., Neuroprotection: Targeting multiple pathways by naturally occurring phytochemicals, *Biomedicines* 8 (2020), p. 284.

202. D. Sugasini, R. Thomas, P.C.R. Yalagala, L.M. Tai and P.V. Subbaiah, Dietary docosahexaenoic acid (DHA) as lysophosphatidylcholine, but not as free acid, enriches brain DHA and improves memory in adult mice, *Scientific Reports* 7 (2017), pp. 1–11.

203. G.P. Eckert, U. Lipka and W.E. Muller, Omega-3 fatty acids in neurodegenerative diseases: Focus on mitochondria, *Prostaglandins Leukotrienes and Essential Fatty Acids* 88 (2013), pp. 105–114.

204. O. Kerdiles, S. Layé and F. Calon, Omega-3 polyunsaturated fatty acids and brain health: Preclinical evidence for the prevention of neurodegenerative diseases, *Trends in Food Science and Technology* 69 (2017), pp. 203–213.

205. G.Y. Sun, A. Simonyi, K.L. Fritsche, D.Y. Chuang, M. Hannink, Z. Gu et al., Docosahexaenoic acid (DHA): An essential nutrient and a nutraceutical for brain health and diseases, *Prostaglandins Leukotrienes and Essential Fatty Acids* 136 (2018), pp. 3–13.

206. T.A. Ajith, A recent update on the effects of omega-3 fatty acids in Alzheimer's disease, *Current Clinical Pharmacology* 13 (2018), pp. 252–260.

207. T.L. Huang, Omega-3 fatty acids, cognitive decline, and Alzheimer's disease: A critical review and evaluation of the literature, *Journal of Alzheimer's Disease* 21 (2010), pp. 673–690.

208. B.K. Puri, Treatment of Huntington's disease with eicosapentaenoic acid, in: Shlomo Yehuda and David I. Mostofsky (eds.), *Nutrients, Stress, and Medical Disorders*, Humana Press Inc., Totowa, 2006, pp. 279–286.

209. S. Sveinbjornsdottir, The clinical symptoms of Parkinson's disease, *Journal of Neurochemistry* 139 (2016), pp. 318–324.

210. S. Zarei, K. Carr, L. Reiley, K. Diaz, O. Guerra, P.F. Altamirano et al., A comprehensive review of amyotrophic lateral sclerosis, *Surgical Neurology International* 6 (2015), p. 171.

211. S. Mathis, C. Goizet, A. Soulages, J.M. Vallat and G. le Masson, Genetics of amyotrophic lateral sclerosis: A review, *Journal of the Neurological Sciences* 399 (2019), pp. 217–226.

212. F.O. Walker, Huntington's disease, *Lancet* 369 (2007), pp. 218–228.

213. A. Chongtham and N. Agrawal, Curcumin modulates cell death and is protective in Huntington's disease model, *Scientific Reports* 6 (2016), pp. 1–10.

214. M. Rakotoarisoa and A. Angelova, Amphiphilic nanocarrier systems for curcumin delivery in neurodegenerative disorders, *Medicines* 5 (2018), p. 126.

8

Dietary Supplements and Nutraceuticals in the Management of Endocrine Disorders, Endocrinological Challenges in Aging and Nutraceuticals

Remya Jayakumar, Namrata Joshi, and Manoj Dash
Banaras Hindu University

Contents

DOI: 10.1201/9781003110866-8

8.1 Introduction

Annath bavanthi boothani... when the gospels from Vedic literature hails food, the subsistence of all material bodies [1], ancient treatise by Sage *Kashyapa* emphasized the food factor as medicine itself [2]. Hippocrates's quote "Let food be thy medicine and medicine be thy food" preceded the very concept [3]. The framework of food as medicine gets later highlighted by Stephen de Felice by coining the term NUTRACEUTICAL in 1989 [4]. Nutraceuticals started reverberating the baseline history of food as medicine and nowadays can be seen conjoined with any conventional medical prescription and health concept. The loosened legalities regarding the new trend were the added advantage for the upcoming wave leaving behind the questions of safety. This nutraceutical key to health when thoroughly shuffled might be suiting the antiaging process on a preventive schedule.

Ultimate humanhood might be life without aging and disease, which seems to be an elixir, and the health matters than anything. Stretching the lifespan without qualified parameters seems worthless when a subjective consideration is implied. The world is getting older in statistical ratios suggesting an upheaval of 2 billion in 2050 with population of 60 years and above from the 900 million in 2015 [5]. This logically recommends a high pressure to healthy aging, to be practised from every point of view including diet, lifestyle changes, medicines, etc. If life is counted as a short period between birth and death, then healthy aging is the concept of the century. The development of science has bestowed increased lifespan but to remain in full health remains with the concept behind ANTIAGING.

Hormone replacement therapy is regarded as one of the cornerstones in the antiaging theory [6]. Practically, aging is associated with the reduced secretions of hormones and especially of pituitary, adrenals and gonads [7]. Human growth hormone (HGH) administration reduces αβ-amyloid accumulation, increases cognitive performance but is associated with carpel tunnel syndrome, gynecomastia and other discomforts when taken by healthy elderly patients, and not much data exist for the long-term effects of GH supplementation [8]. In women population, the oestrogen and progesterone hormones were getting implicated extensively considering the osteo status in menopausal period, but the regulated supplementation began after the reports from Women's Health Initiative randomized control trials published in 2002 [9]. Testosterone also holds the red label in initiating prostate cancer along with the beneficial point outs in the cognition skills in the elderly [10]. Hormone replacement as such is always associated with side effects and disease manifestations.

Apart from the numerical aging, the aging process gets its start early nowadays creating a population with reduced productivity and life skills. If the success of the antiaging mission is concentrated on this early aging phenomenon, the result might get exaggerated positively on a country's social and economic status too. In total, antiaging theories should get focussed on eradicating the early onset of aging and improving the quality of geriatric life through healthy aging practices.

8.2 Aging mannerisms and endocrine applicability

The human system with increasing age gets subjected to wear and tear which makes alteration in the molecular structure and hence the function too. Glycation theory by Louis-Camille Maillard in 1912 depicted the high level of glucose speeding up the aging process. The theory explains the diabetic encroachment on subjects making them prone to subsequent aging changes. The process explains spontaneous reaction happening between the free reducing sugars and free amino group of proteins, lipids and DNA ending up with advanced glycation end products (AGEs). These AGEs cause loss of elasticity in blood vessels, skin, tendons, etc. and also irreversible protein degradation [11].

The telomere theory suggests the shortening of length of the protein DNA complex to end up in apoptosis. The telomere protects the genome from degradation and prevents inter-chromosomal fusion. Each cell division winds up a small portion of it, and the shortened length causes cell death. Many lifestyle factors, inputs from aging and diseases like cancer, all cause hastening of this lengthwise shortening [12].

Mutations always lead to evolution of new species in which a balance between DNA damage and repair is lost. The fitness of an organism to fit in the ever-changing niche is being challenged. The mitochondrial changes when prominent lead to lifestyle disorders and manifestation of many other diseases too [13].

The proteins get folded or aggregated in a disease process, and the mechanism remains nonspecific to be recognized. A study revealed the presence of this nonspecificity with monoclonal antibodies (mABs). The carboxypeptidase A of the pancreas and beta amyloid antibodies of Alzheimer's were identified with this technique in a study and was found to be matching with the protein folding theory and disease spurt [14].

The discovery of SOD (superoxide dismutase) and phenomenon of synergism suggested the presence of production of reactive iron from superoxide and hydrogen peroxide according to the Fenton's reaction gearing up the process of aging [15]. The uncertainty in the theories of aging can blunt the convergence of solution. The endocrine pathway might be able to find out the route to escape disease launch as shown by the precision of hormone therapy already in practice and benefits attained outwardly.

The hormone replacement therapy conjoined with the post menopause, after hysterectomy, family planning, thyroid manifestations, etc. are some of the already existing models which are a boon to mankind. The underlying side effects to these therapies are also well expected and so the caution to prevention and cure from most diseases now focus with dietary pattern and application of nutraceuticals. The augmentation or synergistic effect of nutraceuticals or dietary supplements together with conventional therapy strategy can attenuate the disease. The knowledge of these commodities as prevention categories might lead to full reverse of the launch of a disease.

8.2.1 Ayurveda concept of antiaging

Ayurvedic perception of human body extends to macro- and micro-aspects. The concept evidences the material body as the miniature personification of the entire universe. Fritjof Capra when published his book in 1975, TAO OF PHYSICS, opened up a new era in the doctrines of contemporary physical science by inclusions from the Indian philosophical principles in science [16]. The ancient text of *Charaka samhitha* declares this depiction by equating the human body with basic elements in universe *Loka Purusha Vadam* [17]. The five elemental theory or *Pancha bootha sidhanta* holds importance in this way. The *Pruthvi* (earth), *Ap* (water), *Tejo* (light), *Vayu* (wind) and *Akash* (space) are the five basic elements. These elements then contribute to the *Tridosha sidhantha (kapha, pitha, vata)* – tri humoral theory, the homeostasis of which maintains the body in equilibrium and the peaks and valleys lead to disease conditions. The *kapha, pitha* and *vatha* collaboration builds up the entire human body, and thus, an approach can be retrieved functionally and anatomically. The *Pruthvi* and *ap* elements constitute *Kapha* portion, the *Teja* element becomes *Pitha* and the *vayu* and *aakasha* comprise *Vatha* portion. These theories give certain ideological equations that suit probable series of disease emergence for which solutions can be made from nature itself. The *pancha bootha sidhanta* holds not only to human beings but to every element in the universe and so to medicinal plants, minerals and to anything that can be converted to medicine.

Sarvam dravyam panchabouthikam asmin arthe...

Cha. Sam.Soo. (26:10)

This equalization helps health and disease approach in many accessible ways.

Ayurveda concludes treatment term to two aspects, one of which considers the aim as health preserving (*Swasthasya oorjaskaram*) and the second one as disease eradication (*Athurasya vikaranuth*) manuals [18]. The health preservation includes two more categories known as *Rasayana* and *Vajeekarana*. *Rasayana* is coined by the word rasa mentioning all the seven elemental tissues, and the *ayana* means the pathway for which the nutritional factor to the body has to be traversed. Shortly, *rasayana* is an entity to keep all the physiological elements intact so that whole body is nourished and well defended properly. *Rasayana* is a physiological clearance to whole body channels, and so, ample health is achieved. *Vajeekarana* is the next option where the concept underlines the fact that when the seventh, the *shukra dhathu* (seminal tissue) is nourished properly, the end product, the *Ojus*, is naturally formed and that *ojus* helps in the immunity deliverance [19]. *Vajeekarana*, therefore, is a cellular concept, and rasayana is the process of clearance of the cellular pathways in achieving the end result the *ojus*, the essence of *dhathus* (primary elemental tissues) [20]. In conclusion, the aim of the *rasayana* and *vajeekarana* modes of treatment is the cellular level clearance of each metabolic pathways and keeping the body acceptable in proper usage of the end products of the reactions.

Rasayana and *vajeekarana* are to be done in a particular age as per acharya. He specifies the words by depicting the below versus....

Poorve vayasi madhye va...

The age must be not much young or not too old, and so the middle age is a beneficial one to take *rasayana* and *vajeekarana* forms of medicine. The process starts with certain preprocedures such as *shodhana* or purificatory therapies. This includes emesis and purgation to be induced with suitable medicines and so in conceptually clearing the body from the accumulated metabolic wastes which does not get eliminated normally. After the conductance of proper purificatory therapies only one must be entering to *rasayana* and *vajeekarana* form of treatment. The person after performing certain rituals is made to enter a particularly designed house with ample but regulated amount of light and wind exposure. The person is made to have certain medications in meal doses, and his actual meal is to be taken when only hunger is initiated. This procedure is to be continued till 3 months, and the person is believed to surpass aging. Technically, the process is called *kuti praveshika*. At the present era, such an arrangement is made in a place called PADINHARKKARA AYURVEDA HOSPITAL AND RESEARCH CENTRE (PAHRC), Palakkad District, Kerala, India.

The above format is the systematic practising of *rasayana* and *vajeekarana* which is unapproachable to a common man in his chores of busy life. Acharya thus mentions the importance of daily regimens (*dinacharya*) and seasonal regimens (*ritucharya*) to be practised for healthy living. These practises solely rest upon the three pillars, which are named *Ahara* (food), *Nidra* (sleep) and *Brahmacharya* (celibacy).

Traya upasthambha ithi ahara swapno brahmacharya mithi.....

(Cha.Sam.Soo.11:35)

The word *ahara* means anything getting ingested, mainly food. The word is an elaborate one and includes all the sensational inputs we are getting from the external environment, becoming a part of our memory and influencing our way of thinking. *Swapna* is literally the sleep but in wide sense includes the circadian rhythm that manipulates our day and night cycle. *Brahma charya* as such means practicing celibacy, but the inner meaning points on the healthy sexual habits and preservation of sex hormones. The three pillars when preserved religiously, the body might be able to propagate through normal aging and remain healthy.

The struggle for antiaging concept comes from the extreme wish to surpass disease conditions. Ayurveda emphasizes any disease condition as an inability of the digestive system to incorporate the ingested materials.

Sarve roge api mande agnau.....

(ashtanga hrudaya. Nidana sthana.12:1)

The concept of *agni* thus gains importance above all concepts. An individual greatly represents the very status of his digestive power. The *agni* if deranged welcomes the chain of disease to crouch upon the body. The weak digestive power accumulates toxins in our body called ama in Ayurveda wordings. This gets cumulative and paves the way to further deterioration of digestive power and ultimately ill health. Any lifestyle diseases are exaggerated versions of this accumulated ama conjoined by the practices such as sedentary lifestyle, junk foods, untimely food habits, etc. All these unhealthy practices end up the body to accept aging at an early phase due to mounting of free radicals creating the bombarding at cellular levels if the free radical theory is accepted as the cause of aging.

The ayurvedic emphases on *agni*, *ahara*, *nidra* and *brahmacharya* all point out the hormonal play in the storyline of health. The hormones bring highly sensitive reactions, and the whole human body physiology rests upon these tiny messenger molecules. Each cell is upon the comment of these compounds and thus interlaces each element of the body. The entire endocrine system when intact leads to normal ongoing, and single derangement suddenly gets manifested in hormonal levels. The stress manipulations and flight and fight hormones are examples.

The modern parameters and scientific data converge on growth hormone, melatonin, testosterone and DHEA as the four hormones having a crucial role in the aging process [21]. As the hormonal replacement therapy is already practised in reverting the aging process but associated with side effects, the alternate solutions hold specificity. The herbal remedies are thus accepted being safe, economical and free from debilitating side effects. The nutraceuticals hold impact in this outline, and the market trends made it widely popular to be acceptable among the world population. The *agni* stands for a conversion mechanism; here, growth hormone represents the anabolic conversion in the young ages and remedial treatments in the medical ailments. Agni also extends to the thyroid hormones, as the basal metabolic rate is greatly pulsated on this hormone. The *Swapna/nidra* word constitutes the melatonin hormone which is highly reactive to day and night patterns and maintains the circadian rhythm. The testosterone and the DHEA denote the sex hormone maintenance, and so, the *brahmacharya* word also strongly points out the same.

The modern science and ancient ayurvedic knowledge thus conclude the same elements as holding the key for the healthy aging and better geriatric environment. The focus of attention for antiaging parameters through the hormonal concept can be evaluated as per the validation of these hormones and finding out better herbal remedies together with the application of *rasayana vajeekarana* knowledge.

8.2.2 Endocrine hormones and antiaging process

Endocrine system with aging factors often exhibits mixed responses. When master members like pituitary shrink down in size, parathyroid hormones scale up ending in osteoporosis. Thyroid hormones and cortisol almost remain stable, while testosterone, oestrogens and progestogens descend in amount.

8.2.2.1 Growth hormone

Growth hormone, a potent anabolic marker in normal course, is in peak spurts till pubertal stage and thereafter declines in levels. Recent scientific data suggest the applicability of hormone with antiaging aspects. Growth hormone affects the IGF1 in the liver, and then, the associated changes bring about morphological characterization. It causes lipolysis and increases somatic growth especially of the epiphyseal bone regions and thus the linear axis of the growth attained. The retrieval of the hormone causes physiological downstream and then the somatic pause to the length axis of development. So after puberty, hormone spurt declines. The elderly subject when administered with the rhGH was found with increased lean body mass, thigh muscle cross sectional area and limb girdle strength. These parameters amplify the aerobic capability, and so, the movement disability might be solved, and added with the lipolysis effect, better carbohydrate and lipid metabolism and improved cognitive function are seen in elders [22].

The irony associated with the hormone starts here. The laboratory mice when made GH-deficient were associated with increased lifespan [23]. Laron syndrome-affected individuals exhibited increased lifespan [24]. Besides the antiaging effect, the hormone is able to remove the disabilities during aging and found to affect even the cardiac incident patients. Our way of hormone applicability in this method will be beneficial to the geriatric and ailment populations. The recombinant ones achieved the result but were not free from the side effects such as oedema, arthralgia, increased blood glucose level, carpal tunnel syndrome, etc. Here, the role of herbal combination might prove better practices.

The literature from the ancient treatises does not hold an actual growth hormone supplementation but hints the stimulation factors especially when the regimens toward the conception and pregnancy schedule are reshuffled. A lot of herbs are described in the initial stages of pregnancy and in the month-wise recommendations. Analytical parameters on to the phytoconstituents of the herbs reveal an antidiabetic protocol. Growth hormone action stimulates IGF-1 (Insulin like growth factor-1) which in turn causes insulin stimulation and glucose uptake from the peripheral tissues [25]. Insulin action even in the presence of auto antibodies to insulin is the action due to IGF-1. This peptide molecule shares the structural similarity to insulin with α and β chain disulphide bondage. So a hypothesis can be formularized with ayurvedic regimens toward the obstetric protocols holding the key to growth hormone substitution. Daf-2 and InR signalling molecules in the pathway of either growth hormone, insulin or IGF-I are also associated with the longevity factors [26]. These herbals can thus be promoted as nutraceutical or functional foods that might suit the elderly difficulties and antiaging medicines.

Ipomoea sepiaria gets mentioned several times in the regimen protocol, and the molecular docking technology identified TCF7L2 (Transcription factor 7 L2) gene regulation factors from the drug. The TCF7L2 gene regulates proglucagon gene, and glucagon peptide I product aids in insulin inhibition. The alteration in the gene presents a risk situation to develop the diseases. Out of the 25 phytoconstituents from the plant, quercetin and 1-monolinoleolglycerol trimethyl silyl ether is seen as a potential inhibitor against TCF7L2 causing type 2 diabetes mellitus (T2DM). The potential α glucosidase inhibitors also recognized from the plant are rutin, myricetin, etc. The quercetin factor in animal model checked the diabetic neuropathy development by lipid peroxidation inhibition and levelling-up of antioxidant enzymes [27]. Ficus benghalensis: the aqueous extract of the aerial roots exhibited hypo-glycaemic effect in a sub and mild diabetic model. LIBS points out the peak to Mg and Ca presence in the drug. The calcium responsive element binding protein (CERB) causes exocytosis of stored insulin by calcium ion uptake [28]. Vernonia cineria: leaf extract exhibits phenolic acids, phenolic aldehyde, flavonoids and caffeoylquinic acid derivative. α-Glucosidase inhibition action is seen with caffeoylquinic acid derivative which controls PPBS (postprandial blood sugar). The β-glucogallin with gallic acid and apocynin which effects atherosclerosis treatment with NADPH oxidase cessation are also reported from the plant [29]. Grewia tenax: Highest antioxidant action from the Grewia species and source of flavonoids and phenolics [30]. Solanum indicum: The alloxan-induced diabetic Wistar rats were supplemented with aqueous extract of the drug and found the β cell regeneration among the animals [31]. Nymphae stellate: The leaf extract was experimented in alloxan-induced diabetes and found with positive results. The drug is also a source of amino acids and saponins [32]. Nymphae pubescens: The tuber of the plant in extract form caused anti-diabetic effect in alloxan-induced rats [33]. Glycyrrhizin glabra: Glycyrrhizin nanoparticles in nicotinamide-streptozotocin-induced diabetic rats had hypo-glycaemic effect [34]. Achyranthes aspera: Alloxan-induced diabetic rats were supplied with the stem and leaf dried powder extract. The phytoconstituents in the plant include quercetin, oleanolic acid, etc., like aglycones. Quercetin, when causes β cell regeneration, the triterpenoid oleanolic acid inhibits α glucosidase and stimulates TGR5- G protein-coupled receptor that increases insulin secretion. Oleanolic acid inhibits Na/glucose co-transport system located in the intestinal brush border that aids in glucose absorption [35]. Convolvulus pluricaulis: The leaf extract of the plant caused free-radical scavenging as the standard drug ascorbic acid and might be the presence of phytoconstituents such as kaempferol, scopoletin, etc. Scopoletin is found in the literature to support antidiabetic effect being a coumarin [36]. Barleria prionitis: Alcoholic leaf and root extract in alloxan-induced diabetes was with antihyperglycemic effect. The flavonoids, sterols, triterpenoids, tannins and phenols present with the drug might be the effective agents as they are all have known antidiabetic action [37]. Strobilanthes ciliates: Aqueous and alcoholic extract of the whole plant exhibited α glucosidase and α amylase inhibition action. The latter one dominated in action [38]. Limonia acidissima: Methanolic extract of fruit pulp exhibited antihyperglycemic effect in alloxan-induced rats [39]. *Tribulus terrestris*: Hepatoprotective action against oxidative stress in streptozotocin-induced rats [40]. Grewia asiatica: The phalsa fruit has to be more promoted as a potential functional food [41]. Uraria picta: The plant extract remained as a content for checking the antidiabetic activity in streptozotocin-induced diabetes and exhibited positive result. The phytochemical array in the plant includes alkaloids, flavonoids, phenols, tannins, saponins, triterpenoids, etc. in all parts of the plant. Tannin and saponin stay for antidiabetic activity, and tannin content was absent in stem and roots. Magnesium was the highest mounting mineral element found more in the leaves and linked with lowering hyperglycaemia [42]. Red rice extracts are found to inhibit α glucosidase and α amylase activity and thats why the recommendation goes to the usage such *shali* (*red rice*) as diet in pregnant ladies [43].

In short, some of the herbal suggestions were with antidiabetic activity and can be used as nutraceuticals based on the phytochemical screening.

8.2.3 Melatonin

The hormone from pineal gland best known as the circadian rhythm manipulator is found to be an oldest known molecule present universally in animals, plants and human beings. The organ inevitability of production of the hormone was shattered when the presence was seen in a single cell organism.

Gonyaulax polyhedral (Lingulodinium polyhedrum) reacts to day-and-night patterns. The mitochondria are also found to be the producer of this hormone, and its receptor is seen on the organelle membrane [44]. The melatonin entry to cells is usually avoided with receptor and takes place with gradient nature. The free radical theory of aging supports the action of this hormone in bringing out more beneficial effect as it stimulates the antioxidant enzymes glutathione peroxidase, superoxide dismutase, etc. The hormone is found in lower concentrations, but because of its presence in mitochondria, it becomes the free-radical scavenger in the vicinity and so the first counterpart at the production site of the ROS. Melatonin hormone exclusively relates to sleep disorders, and hormone supplementation improves sleep degrees [45].

Sleep deprivation causes oxidative damage to the brain from the hypothalamic-pituitary-adrenal axis getting stimulated and corticosterone production which aids in free radical overproduction and further neurodegeneration. The inhibition of certain nitric oxide synthase-like enzymes that produce nitric oxide might help in protecting from the nerve damage. Centella asiatica water extract inhibited the nitric oxide synthase formation [46]. Convolvulus pluricaulis is found to reduce brain plasticity [47]. The synaptic plasticity is lined to sleep, and consolidation of a good amount of sleep helps in achieving memory build-up and stress regulation [48].

Blood flow increases during sleep, and thus, the mild hypercapnia due to reduced ventilation might be drained out. This prevents the irregularities in respiration and thus presents ample amount of undisturbed sleep [49]. Glycyrrhiza glabra is found to increase the blood flow to brain during sleep [50]. REM sleep is associated with acetylcholine production and acetylcholine esterase inhibitors like donepezil, galantamine, etc. increase the production.

Prolonged use in Alzheimer's-like disease will disturb REM sleep when the memory consolidation mostly happens. Tinospora cordifolia is found to increase the cognition with enhancement on acetylcholine and might be a better substitute than ACEIs because of other qualities that are vested upon its antioxidant potential [51].

Charaka describes the aforesaid four drugs as *medhya rasayana* (brain tonic), and as sleep needs a multifactorial approach for smooth conduction, these herbals might help in many involved pathways which need to be analysed with phytoconstituents [52].

8.2.4 Testosterone

The handling of the hormone seems to be as old as history. Records depict the usage with ancient Egyptians and Romans belief that products from testis can be an aid in aphrodisiac enhancement, and so, aging can be reversed [53]. The practice continued even when "internal secretions" of modern-day endocrinology was being established. Later in 1889, French physiologist Charles Edward and Brown Sequard found their physical might enhancement and aging feature reversal on using injections of an extract from the testicles of dogs and guinea pigs. The Nobel prize for chemistry owned by Leopold Ruzicka and Adolf Butenants in 1939 for isolation of testosterone along with other reproductive hormones changed the practice of using gonadal preparation [54].

The peak in puberty attributes the male secondary sexual characteristics, sexual behaviour and function along with sperm production. The plasma levels mount for 300–1,000 ng/dL by age 17, and thereafter, decline about 1.2% starts with each forwarding age [55]. Testosterone also maintains muscle mass and strength, fat distribution, bone mass, red blood cells products, libido, etc. The testosterone activity in females even though is maintained by oestrogen and progesterone, the hormone level in females has to be managed for perfect homeostasis. Pregnancy is associated with a 70% increase in testosterone, and levels are more in primigravidae. PCOS and preeclampsia exhibit even higher hormone levels and very less in assisted reproductive techniques. The aromatase enzyme converts the maternal testosterone to oestrogen in foetus [56].

The abuse on testosterone products is high in market despite their limited bioavailability through oral route. The gel, patch and injection routes of applicability are also available to combat the oral route [57]. The internal and external ways of hormone is not free from side effects, so alternate ways of hormone sustenance need to be evaluated. The Ayurveda approach to testosterone comprises variety of herbal combinations. The combinations exhibit limited evidence to specify the target sites but get mentioned by many technical Sanskrit terms that need to be evaluated under the light of modern-day scientific technology. *Acharya Shargadhara* mentions this in his 13th-century literature as

Vajeekaran, Sukrakaram, Sukrapravarthakam, Sukrasthambanam, Shukra rechakam and *Shukra shoshanam.*

Vajeekran includes *Nagabala* and *kapikachu beejam* [58]. Little evidence exists regarding the *Nagabala*/Sida verocaefolia action on the reproductive system, but the other member, the velvet beans, gets sound support under various in vivo and clinical experiments. The Parkinsonism individuals were found with low testosterone levels, and the decline becomes more profound with the progressive pathogenesis with the disease. A study on male Parkinson patients with control, promiprazole and L-dopa administered grouping found to have adequate plasma levels of testosterone in the medicine groups and control with declining levels [59]. The male albino rats when given methanolic extract of Mucuna pruriens was with increased testosterone, LH and FSH levels. The LH and FSH surge implies the gonadotropin hormone from anterior pituitary [60].

Shuklakara oushadha includes increasing the semen quality of the individual. The drugs involved in this group are ashwagandha (Withania somnifera), musali (Curculigo orchioides), sarkara (Saccharum officinarum) and shathavari (Asparagus racemosus). NO-arginine pathway is involved in stress-induced infertility. NO, the free-radical gas, is produced from L-arginine by the NO synthases (NOS). NOS in the male reproductive system aids in normal spermatogenesis. The formed NO in low concentration enhances the sperm motility, and high concentration affects the motile sperm [61].

Withania somnifera methanolic extract caused the nitric acid production in J774 macrophages [62]. The normozoospermic infertile men were given the root powder in milk and were found with positive result [63]. Curculigo orchioides increased the spermatogenesis as evident in the experiment done with the ethanolic extract of the rhizome in albino rats. The increase of spermatids, spermatocytes and vigorous sexual activity than the untreated group was seen [64]. Asparagus racemosus is a known endometrial proliferator and ovarian hormone regulator. The lyophilized extract together with curculigo orchioides increased the sexual behaviour based on seven parameters experimented. The NO-interacted manipulation exhibited the stress reducing-effect with drug [65]. Saccharum officinarum juice caused a significant increase in testosterone and sperm motility, whereas the processed sugar inversely affected the semen quality [66].

Shukla pravarthaka group includes milk, masha (*Vigna mungo*), *Bhallatha phala majja* (Semicarpus anacardium), and *Amalaki.* Embilica officinalis in male albino rats against the oxidative stress induced by organophosphorus pesticide, Chlorpyrifos (CPF). The embilica only treated group did not show much significance than the control, but the CPF and amla group did not show an increase in sperm count, but motility and sperm density increased. The moderate decline in the testosterone level was also noted in the same group and indicated the protective role of the drug against the pesticide effect and preservation of healthy sperm [67]. Ethanolic extract of the Semicarpus anacardium administered in the male albino rats caused spermatogenic arrest but brought out anti-inflammatory and antioxidant activity. The TNF-α, NO and myeloperoxidase were decreased in a cohort study of arthritic patients [68]. The rest of the components in the group include milk and Vigna mungo. Vigna mungo is with more calcium, less sodium, source of glutamic acid and aspartic acid. The essential amino acids, tryptophan and sulphur were not present. The less digestibility property increases the releasing time of glucose and so suits hyperglycaemic situation too. The source of tocopherols, β-sitosterol, flavonoids, condensed tannins and free-radical scavenging action is also noted. The tyrosinase-inhibiting action prevents the aging manifestations of human skin. These properties suggest that the functional food aspect of Vigna mungo needs to be employed regarding the infertility conditions [69].

Shukra rechaka property is seen in *bruhathi phala* (Solanum nigra), and the aqueous leaf extract increased the sperm count and motility and decreased abnormal sperms in adult male Sprague-Dawley rats. The slight increase in haemoglobin percent also was noted. The flavonoid percent of a drug prevents oxidative damage lesions in living organisms, and flavonoids in the solanum plant thus contributed to the antioxidant activity being exhibited [70].

Shukra sthambaka is represented by *Jaatiphala/Myristica fragrans* which on experimentation improved aphrodisiac activity in male mice in terms of mounting and mating frequency with ethanolic extract [71]. The standard drug sildenafil citrate and nutmeg extract was checked by the same authors in terms of mounting frequency (MF), intromission frequency (IF), ejaculatory latency (EL) and post ejaculatory latency (PEL). Nutmeg extract significantly increased the aphrodisiac activity by neuronal stimulation [72].

The *Shukra shoshana* effect was mentioned by *Harithaki/*Terminalia chebula. The aqueous-ethanolic extract of fruit of the plant was given for 28 days in male Wistar strain rats. The sperm count and motility were significantly reduced than control group. These alarming results point out the cautious use of the medicine and establish the findings of ancient treatises [73].

8.2.5 Dihydroepiandrosterone

This steroid from Zona reticularis synthesized by P450c17 is an individually varying entity. The high levels after birth sourced from the foetal adrenal activity faces a decline and then a spurt in between the 6th and 10th year of life called adrenarche. The high levels thus in the puberty continue till the third decade of life, and then the decline starts, and after 70 years, the adreno-pause happens. Thus, the hypothesis was formulated based on the proportion in lifetime that the administration in the descent time might be useful [74]. The challenge lies in the fact that the rodent adrenals are devoid of the steroid and so limited access to experiment models. The models but exist where large doses of DHEA administration to rodents were beneficial in clearing carcinoma, diabetes, obesity, etc. [75]. But the lack of evidence did not make the mob stay back from the usage, and the USA is reported to consume it under the antiaging principle [74].

So apart from the aging proportion in the antiaging framework, the steroid is significant in the conversion to androstenedione. The androstenedione is acted by 17βHSD and P450 aromatase to form testosterone and oestradiol, respectively. The proportion-wise and sex hormone precursor stages make the DHEA significantly placed in the antiaging concept [76]. The natural sources of the DHEA precursor aid in the artificial synthesis of the steroid which exists in the wild yam. The maintenance and sex hormone production make the DHEA component inevitable. The lipid metabolism with cholesterol manipulation signifies the regular intake of fat constituents. Here, the application of *Nithya rasayana* from Ayurveda holds key position as treatise specify the ghee and milk intake regularly and counted it as an antiaging practice [77].

The ghee effect was experimented in male Wistar albino rats for both lipid profiles and testosterone levels. The TG, HDL and LDL did not show any difference in both control and test drug groups. The test drug was also with testosterone decline [78]. The study did not include the dose-dependent pattern because the 10% dietary ghee fed on Fischer rats for 4 week did not increase the total cholesterol [79]. So more experiments are the need of the hour to establish the correlation if existing is positively or negatively associated. Ghee is also a rich source of DHA (docosahexaenoic acid) which in absence causes the neuronal derangement and leads to many degenerative diseases like Parkinson's, Alzheimer's, dementia, etc. [80]. Ghee-fed rats did not pass the elevated plus-maze test and cognition pattern were not achieved but cannot be concluded because of the short duration of the test [81].

8.2.6 Endocrine disorders and nutraceuticals

When the internal milieu fails to get regulated by the mighty endocrine chemicals, the pathway then paves to procession of diseases. The 2019–2020 data from WHO suggest the endocrine entity diabetes mellitus and the senile disability Alzheimer's disease as the inclusions among the top ten leading causes of death and alarm the necessity of focus to be directed against such conditions. Though most dealt ailments include dyslipidaemia, obesity, diabetes, osteoporosis, thyroid problems, etc., there are many rare and perplexing endocrine diseases [82].

8.2.7 Dyslipidaemia and obesity

Dysregulation of lipids causes CVD, obesity, hypertension, cancer, metabolic syndrome and many more lifestyle disorders. The statin group of medications remarkably lowers the lipid profile but not exempted from side effects [83]. A long run of complications are associated with statin build-up including statin intolerance, DM, cancer, memory loss, kidney and liver disorders, gall stone formation, rhabdomyolysis, GI disturbances, etc. [84]. The combination of statin with nutraceutical duo augmented the desired effects in many clinical and in vitro experiments. Obesity and metabolic syndrome are linked to this irregular lipid management because of the insulin resistance happening from adipokines, free fatty acids (FFA) and cytokine intervention.

Ayurveda deals with the conditions of dyslipidaemia, obesity and metabolic syndrome under the *Medas dhathu* (tissue) management. The relevant manipulations under '*medas*' or lipid component is found to cure such disorders. One of the chapters of *Charaka Samhitha* is dedicated to this *meda* management [85]. The nutraceuticals benefitting dyslipidaemia might be acting through synergistic or scavenging activity in cases of herbal supplements. The effect of ayurvedic formulations with herbal combinations has to be exploited thoroughly to satisfy the existing methodology of patient intervention in the lipid disorder scenario.

8.2.7.1 Tinospora cordifolia

Tinospora is one such element experimented for hypolipidemic action. The effect was compared with ROSOVASTATIN, and significant forceful action on lowering LDL-C, VLDL-C and increment on HDL-C level was seen. The percentage of atherosclerotic action was almost similar in comparison. Flavonoids in the plant extract increased the LCAT (lecithin cholesterol acyl transferase), which incorporates free cholesterol into HDL-C component. Saponins of the drug increased the faecal cholesterol excretion. The saponin action on increasing lipoprotein lipase activity decreased the free fatty acids from the circulation and thus lowered the TC. Tannin component increased the lipoprotein lipase activity near the endothelium lining and so hydrolysed the triglycerides portion. Plant sterols decreased the cholesterol absorption and increased its excretion. Antioxidant component causes lipid peroxidation and ROS scavenging simultaneously [86].

8.2.7.2 Cyperus rotundus

The effect of the plant on lipid abnormalities was found to be nonstatistically significant with SIMVASTATIN. The aqueous extract of the rhizome was experimented in this type of studies [87]. SREBP-1c (sterol regulatory element binding protein 1c) is a master gene in the lipogenesis pathway [88]. The hexane fraction of the tuber was found with regulating this gene. Obese Zucker rats were fed with tuber powder, and weight gain was seen prevented [89].

8.2.7.3 Takrarishta

Takrarishta is a fermented product with some herbs and probiotic culture. In hypercholesterolemia patients, the bacterial diversity of intestinal microbiota was less. The experiments in clinical studies revealed the physical exercise and fermented probiotic effect increasing the HDL-C constituent. The probiotic culture always domains in the gut microbiota either by competing with pathogenic strains for nutrition and existence. The isoflavones in fermented soy products decreased the electronegative LDL which is produced from the oxidation of atherosclerotic products. The body mass index, waist circumference, conicity index and waist height ratio also were decreased. The fermentation happened on bile salt hydrolases causing deconjugation of bile salts. This causes lower cholesterol absorption and lessens the enterohepatic circulation. The action on cholesterol was the excretion effect. Cholesterol was solubilized and excretion increased. Encroachment on lipids is less than statins as found in comparison data [90].

8.2.7.4 Honey

Honey as an adjuvant or mainstream medicine can affect upon triglycerides. When honey was administered for 56 days in diabetic subjects, the lipid profile met the desired ratio. The polyphenols in honey were found to prevent nerve degeneration from the oxidative stress. The endothelial proneness to atherosclerosis was also seen inhibited [91].

8.2.7.5 Vidanga

Aqueous extract of the fruit in Wistar albino rats exhibited normal fibrillary nerve appearance in the treated group when the experimentation was looked upon for methionine-induced hyperhomocysteinemia. Antioxidant action removed the lipid peroxidation level and decreased the formation of thiobarbituric acid reactive substances [92].

8.2.7.6 Hordeum vulgare

The name in classics is *yava*, a fibre-rich commodity that increases the gastric emptying time. The satiety feeling thus originates and also does not absorb cholesterol fraction [93].

8.2.7.7 Emblica officilnalis

Fresh juice of the fruit was administered in cholesterol-fed rabbits for 60 days. The resultant action was seen as 82% reduction in serum cholesterol, 60% triglycerides, 77% phospholipids and 90% reduction in LDL than the control group. Aortic plaque rejection together with excretion of more cholesterol and phospholipids were noted. This shows the absorption defects related to cholesterol metabolism. The ascorbic acid constitutes more in amount in amla. Ascorbic acid reaction results in lowering the LDL cholesterol, therefore lowering the atherosclerosis. Subjects with a high amount of Vit C concentration in plasma had low risk of atherosclerosis. Amla contains a high amount of Vit C in natural form and also cytokine-like substances – Zeatin, Z-nucleotide, flavonoid pectin and 30% tannins. Amla action was assumed to be either due to tannins retarding the oxidation or either by Vit C and pectin decreasing the serum cholesterol levels. Flavonoids are the potent hypolipidemic agents. The constituents interfere with the cholesterol absorption and inhibits HMG Co A reductase activity [94]. The clinical study conducted in 60 patients of the SSG Hospital in Vadodara was seen with a comparable result between SIMVASTATIN and dried amla fruit juice powder in capsule form. Both the entities showed equivalent results, but the VLDL lowering was more seen on the SIMVASTATIN-treated group [95].

8.2.7.8 Terminalia chebula

The fruit has well-known rasayana action, and the components constituting toward the hyperlipidaemia-alleviating action are to be evaluated. The methanolic bark extract of the tree was compared with the atorvastatin-treated group. The HDL increment was seen with the methanolic bark extract-treated group. The fruit is rich in ellagic acid, gallic acid, chebulinic acid, chebulagic acid and corilagin. The alkaloids, phytosterols, saponins and tannins are present in high amounts in the fruit. The action is directly on the adipose tissue which is a dynamic organ constituting of adipocytes. Adipocytes are the major endocrine organs with secretion to lipid and protein factors. They have an impact on metabolism of other tissues, regulation of appetite, immunological responses and vascular diseases. Adipose tissue inflammation is a hyperlipidaemia marker. The study comprising whole fruit dried powder and gallic acid was assessed in vitro with results showing the whole fruit dried powder more effective than the gallic acid alone-treated group. Herbal treatment decreased hypertrophy of adipocytes, and the fibre richness obstructed the fat absorption [96].

8.3 Osteoporosis

The disease is a well-known hit in the postmenopausal period as the most debilitating presentation. The surprise lies in the fact that the disease not only affects the old-age population but at any time in life. The predominance rate is seen with women category, and the postmenopausal period augments the symptoms with deficiency of oestrogen. Shortly, OA can be regarded as an oestrogen-deficient secondary manifestation. OA appears together with damaged cartilage, inflamed synovium and eroded chondrocytes. Inflammatory cytokines which cause erosion of cartilage and subchondral bone are found in synovial fluid. Pain and synovial inflammation trigger the physical distress and weakens a person. Arthritic pain is seen after the inflammations of joint cartilage after serious damage. The condition worsens when the bones collide after the synovial protection is lost. The trabecular bone microarchitecture gets affected leading to considerable loss of bone mineral density affecting the mechanical strength and later leading to the lumbar, forearm and hip fractures. The socioeconomic impacts due to fractures are a matter of concern, and the mortality also needs to be evaluated in the situation [97]. The OA treatment in the conventional method starts with steroidal and nonsteroidal methods which has good control over inflammation and bone health protection but are associated with mounting side effects ranging from gastrointestinal to cardiac and renal manifestations. The combating options for the disease range from hormone therapy, calcitonin, bisphosphonates, strontium ranelate to selective oestrogen receptor modulator. The herbal counterpart might be a better suggestion as seen with the various in vitro and in vivo experiments carried over in the decades behind [98].

8.3.1 Cedrus deodara

The drug is mentioned for the pacification of vata, and old age is a vata predominant stage. The osteoporosis-associated inflammation might be alleviated by the usage of this drug. The aqueous extract of air-dried stem bark of the plant was administered in the carrageenan-induced inflammation, and the effect was compared with the standard treatment drugs like betamethasone and phenylbutazone. The effect of Cedrus deodara was seen less than that of the standard drugs. The same study involved the granuloma pouch and cotton pellet method and found that the Cedrus deodara effect reduced the exudate but less than betamethasone. Antiarthritic activity was also checked upon and found that the ulceration was minimum with Cedrus deodara. The volatile oil from the plant was more effective with local application. The drug might be able to alleviate the inflammatory part associated with the disease [99].

8.3.2 Gmelina arborea

The rats with ovariectomy done where given the standard drug and the Gmelina arborea extract. The femur ash weight and cancellous bone appearance were appreciable when compared to the standard drug treated group [100].

8.3.3 Vitis vinifera

Grapes are enriched with polyphenols like quercetin, resveratrol, catechins, anthocyanins, proanthocyanins, etc. Lumbar bone mineral density was modified positively on consumption of red wine, a resveratrol supplement [101]. Several studies point to the bone mineral density of hip, spine and femur getting improved on intake by flavanols, catechin, anthocyanins, total flavonoids, etc. [102]. Bone calcium retention was achieved with supplementation of grape-enriched diet [103].

8.3.4 Asparagus racemosus

Asparagus racemosus root powder methanolic extract was given for 40 days in ovariectomized Wistar rats. The biomechanical strength was equivalent to the oestrogen-supplemented group. Osteoblastic dominance was indicated by the ALP activity decrease. Urinary calcium excretion was also seen minimized. The authors admit a need of longer duration of this study to get a more precise knowledge on the drug benefit. The phytoestrogens are thought to be the beneficiary elements here with diphenol ring similar to endogenous oestrogen. The flavonoids and sterols of asparagus are competent enough to supplement the oestrogen receptor in the absence of natural oestrogen supply [104].

8.3.5 Boerhavia diffusa

The Wistar strain was supplied for 5 weeks with Boeravinone B, a content of Boerhavia diffusa with prior ovariectomy. The Tartrate-resistant acid phosphatase (TRAP), alkaline phosphatase (ALP), Collagen Type 1 fragment (CTX) and serum osteocalcin (OC)-like parameters were reduced than the control group. The TNF-α, IL-β increased after ovariectomy reduced after Boeravinone B administration. The osteoblast activity was increased with the NF-κB P65 reduction with the test drug, and IκB-α and SIRT-1 inhibition reduced the osteoclast formation. Thus, the drug shows promising benefits to suit osteoporotic condition [105].

8.3.6 Cynodon dactylon

The lyophilized plant product was powdered and was compared with metformin in the letrozole-induced PCOS condition. The alterations from normal oestrus phases and vaginal cell cytology in PCOS were returned to normal both in the treated and conventional medicine group. The increase in body weight decreased only in the drug-treated groups. The uterine mass was reduced than the metformin group due to the antihyperlipidemic and insulin resistance action of the Cynodon dactylon group [106].

8.3.7 Curcumin longa

A study was conducted among spinal cord-injured patients in Iran with curcumin for 6 months. The bone resorption markers like procollagen type 1N-terminal pro peptide, serum carboxy-terminal telopeptide of type 1 collagen, osteocalcin and ALP were analysed in the study. Curcumin-intervened group exhibited better BMD than the other groups [107]. In the ovariectomized Sprague-Dawley rats, curcumin was given and compared against Premarin, the conjugated oestrogen. Trabecular bone volume was preserved, and the free-radical scavenging activity reduced the oxidative stress that could arise from the osteoclast proliferation after ovary removal surgery [108].

8.3.8 Terminalia chebula

An in vitro analysis was checked for the ethanolic extract of the dry fruit for the periodontal disease-affected dental plaque bacteria. The osteoclast precursors were inhibited, and osteoblast proliferation was stimulated to prevent the bone resorption [109]. Aqueous extract of the fruit was given as a dietary supplementation for joint discomfort patients. The hydrolyzable tannins (chebulagic acid, chebulinic acid, gallic acid) prevented the oxidative stress for better repairing activities as evident from the significant reduction in the cartilage oligomeric matrix protein (COMP). This biomarker is indicative of the matrix degradation which was more in the placebo that the treated group [110]. An ovariectomized study could be evident for the estrogenic action if existing with the drug.

8.3.9 Glycyrrhiza glabra

The glycyrrhizic acid was checked against the glucocorticoid-induced osteoporosis in 3-month-old rats after the adrenalectomy. The plasma osteocalcin and pyridinoline levels were reduced and 11β—HSD dehydrogenase activity increased in the treated group [111]. But data suggest the nil effect of glabridin and glycyrrhizic acid in Wistar rats ovariectomized osteoporosis model [112]. Breast cancer cell line exhibited the estrogenic effect of the glabridin [113]. The glabridin and glabrene supplemented in the post-menopausal women proved that the estrogenic effect of glabridin and glabrene was similar to action in raloxifene. The conjoined conventional therapies with glabrene can be a more promising future in the vascular injury, and the atherogenesis modulation in the cardiovascular disease management [114]. In vitro analysis of glycyrrhizin exhibited action upon inhibiting the osteoclast formation [115]. The root extract of the drug experimented in the ovariectomized Wistar rats inhibited the osteoclast formation [116].

Thus, many of the medicines quoted here come from the *prajastapana maha Kashaya*/procreation agents depicted by *Acharya Charaka*. The conception and pregnancy greatly depend upon hormonal interplay, and thus, the medicines might be supporting the oestrogen, progesterone and many more hormonal substitute effect [117].

8.4 Hypothyroidism and hyperthyroidism

The thyroid abnormalities manifest as the second common endocrine diseases with hyper- and hypo-demonstration in 2% and 1%, respectively [118].The hormonal judgement arena includes digestion, reproduction and cognitive function of an individual and prevalence exists more in women population. The T3 and T4 overexpression causes reduced secretion of the TSH from the anterior pituitary, and underproduction from thyroids causes over-production of TSH in blood serum. A twist in the regulation mechanisms seen with mild thyroid failure where the peripheral smear carries normal levels and TSH remains slightly elevated presents as the subclinical cases undercover and are seen especially in elderly persons [119].

The myoinositol is found to be the TSH stimulator and regulator of H_2O_2-mediated iodination. The former belief was that this nutrition element belonged to Vitamin B group but later was found producing by the body itself. The external sources are found to be citrus foods. Studies exist about myoinositol and selenium curing the Hashimoto's thyroiditis [120]. Red rice is also the source of this content promoting the functional food aspect [121].

Resveratrol, the name stands next to the grapes and the wine extracted from them. The compound is a natural polyphenol belonging to the flavonoid family. The particularity aiding thyroid gland is the arrest it brings about to proliferation of thyroid cancer cells. The abundance causing phosphorylation to p53 is found out to be the mechanism. The iodine trapping support earned it the name anti-thyroid compound and regulates TSH secretion on administration. *Drakshasava* is an ayurvedic formulation made under the *asava* dosage forms with dominant ingredient as grapes and the self-generated alcohol sort of preparation arising from them. The HPLC peaks simulate resveratrol and pterostilbene. *Draksharisht* also comes under the same mode of resveratrol source, and studies need to confirm the presence and support to thyroid manipulations [122].

The chemical form 3-Hydroxy-4 *trimethylazaniumyl*, the carnitine, is present as a natural isomer, the L-carnitine, 25% of which is produced by the body and rest to be supplied from the outer source [123]. Carnitine aids in the β oxidation of the fatty acids by exchanging long chain of fatty acids across the mitochondrial membrane and liberates energy. The cardiac microenvironment was supported by lessening inflammation, necrosis, oxidation, etc. by the L-carnitine administration. This supports osteoblast formation and osteocalcin secretion [124]. The hyperthyroid patients are prone to beneficiaries than hypoincidents. The thyroid storm incidents were reduced with the L-carnitine. The Grave's disease in an elderly patient met with reduction in high BMR on giving L carnitine supplement on withdrawal caused the rebound of high BMR [125].

VEGF (Vascular Endothelial Growth Factor) is a glycoprotein that exhibits angiogenic property and promotes endothelial permeability. The thyroid epithelial cells are with this entity, and in vitro thyroid cancer cell lines suggest high hormone concentrations paving favourable to the increased serum levels [126]. The Hashimoto's thyroiditis promotes VEGF expression with high hormone levels. The drugs directing the downregulation might be suitable synergisms in the treatment for such hyperthyroid-like situations. The *Kantya dashaemani*, the drugs with action on neck region, are grouped by *Acharya Charaka*, including Piper nigrum, Glycyrrhiza glabra, dried grapes, etc. and seven more [127]. The Piper nigrum extract intraperitoneal administration to

C57BL/6 mice with VEGF-induced B16F-10 melanoma cells reduced the capillary formation [128]. The grape seed extract inhibited the kinase activity of purified VEGF receptors due to polyphenol fraction in the breast cancer cell lines [129]. Glycyrrhiza glabra aqueous extract was tested in the Ehrlich ascites tumour cells, and VEGF inhibition was found [130].

8.5 Diabetes mellitus

A noncommunicable disease getting epidemic status was seen with diabetes mellitus, and the numbers mount up to 422 million as per the latest revisions from WHO. Though the disorder from Islets of Langerhans dominates in the presence of the disease, many adjoined symptoms make the body threatened to morbidities. The insulin and metformin pharmacology though were able to control key points of disease progress, many factors affecting the quality of life were unanswered such as microvascular alterations of retina, lens, kidneys, atherothrombosis, etc. The veil of lifestyle disease made the patient counselling effective with diet and regular exercise, but the majority of patient population itself kept the advice out of practices contributing to the vulnerability of the situation. The invasion to nutraceutical defensive methods might be a solution to such ailments when the pathogenesis is taken into consideration. Inflammation and oxidative stress are the known precursors of the disease proceedings. Pancreatic beta cell failure has a preceding inflammation history rendering the cells unable to functionally advance further. Oxidative stress from the ROS adds fuel to the inflammation process and aids in insulin resistance too. If the foremost target of nutraceuticals is able to surpass this inflammation and oxidative stress, the disease development process might be delayed [131].

8.5.1 Emblica officinalis

Amla or Indian gooseberry is a rich source of vitamin c and thus is recommended by any health practitioner regarding the ongoing or preventive aspect of diabetes. Vitamin C or ascorbic acid scavenges the ROS directly and thus the cessation of further chain of actions and reduces the incident of protein glycation. The further development of comorbidities such as hypertension resulting from the stiffening of the collagen with the glycation of proteins is thus made to pause. Tannin provides antioxidant properties, and gallic acid stands for the immune modulating actions being the polyphenols which usually defence the ultraviolet radiation and guards against pathogens. The pectin dietary fibre delivers well regulation to bowel movements [132].

8.5.2 Symplocus racemosus

The methanolic extract from bark created reduction in blood glucose levels in streptozotocin-induced diabetic rats. The proceeding pathway is either by supporting the glucose using up from peripheral tissues or by inhibiting hepatic gluconeogenesis. The in vitro analysis hinted it as α-glucosidase inhibition. Antioxidant action was seen on DPPH, hydroxyl scavenging performance, and the total reducing power assay was comparable with standard drug, ascorbic acid. The hepatic protective action was by reducing the levels of liver enzymes, total bilirubin and total proteins, GSH, catalase and SOD in dose-dependent fashion. These results were obtained with DMBA-induced hepatocellular carcinoma, carbon tetrachloride liver damage and toxicity. Symposide, symplososide, ellagic acid, betulinic acid and oleanolic acid are some of the chemical constituents present with the plant [133].

8.5.3 Terminalia chebula

Terminalia chebula seed extract was experimented for the streptozotocin-induced diabetes. The normal serum creatinine levels give a promising effect on the diabetic nephropathy as excess albumin and abnormal renal function were reversed. Biologically active ingredients include gallic acid, chebulic acid, 1,6-di-O-galloyl-β-D-glucose, punicalagin, 3,4,6-tri-O-galloyl-β-D-glucose, casuarinin, chebulanin, corilagin, neochebulinic acid, terchebulin, ellagic acid, chebulagic acid, chebulinic acid and 1,2,3,4,6-penta-O-galloyl-β-D-glucose. The action includes decreasing the blood glucose and glycosylated haemoglobin, stimulation of surviving or remnant beta cells of Islets of Langerhans, increasing the plasma insulin and C-peptide. (i) The blood glucose levels were decreased by regulation to carbohydrate-metabolizing enzymes. (ii) The beta cell stimulation causes more insulin secretion. (iii) The C- peptide levels were increased which are the modulators of insulin action. C-peptide action is found out to be by increasing glycogen and by using up amino acid. (iv) The proteolysis is seen affecting the skeletal tissues in a diabetic atmosphere, and the extract supply increased the total protein content. (v) The renal impairment from increased serum albumin and creatinine levels was noted. The blood urea and creatinine level returned to normal on extract introduction. (vi) The sialic acid acts as a marker for the glycolysis and reduced levels promises the fruit extract action on the molecule [134].

8.5.4 Curcuma longa

One of the initial drugs mentioned to treat diabetes in ancient treatises with Indian gooseberry is Curcuma longa. Curcuma longa attenuates tumour necrosis factor (TNF-α) and plasma FFA (free fatty acids). The protein carbonyl and NF-κB get inhibited by curcumin. Cessation of lipid peroxidation and lysosomal enzyme activities are also supported. The curcumin activation of enzymes in liver causes glycolysis, gluconeogenesis and lipid metabolism. The majority action seen is with initial disease development adjoined with antioxidant defence setting up [135].

8.5.5 Cedrus deodara

The ethanolic extract of the drug was tested against streptozotocin-induced DM. The prior administration before the induction drug increased glucose tolerance level. The continuous administration thereafter decreased the serum glucose levels. Pancreatic type of action is more pronounced in the drug as the regeneration of damaged islets and retrieving of size of enlarged (hyperplasia) islet cells are observed with EECD [136]. The alkaloids, flavonoids, phenol, glycoside, saponin, tannin and proteins might be allocating multiple actions to counter the disease. Flavonoids might be the damaged β-cell regenerator, and effects on post prandial glucose levels are also noticed. In alloxan-induced diabetes, the petroleum ether extract of the drug confronting might be promising to Type 1 DM and found discarding α-glucosidase action [137].

8.5.6 Tinospora cordifolia

The phytoconstituents in Tinospora were examined under the molecular docking technology. Nine constituents including alkaloids, terpenes and steroids were found to affect the diabetic pathway [138]. The isoquinoline alkaloid-rich fraction from the stem of the plant and palmatine, jatorrhizine and magnoflorine were analysed in vitro in rat pancreatic β-cell line, the RINm5F. The gluconeogenesis arrest was similar to the standard drug tolbutamide [139]. The hexane, ethyl acetate and methanol extract of the drug was supplied for the 100 days to check the effect in chronic diabetes. The methanol extract reduced the fasting blood glucose than the other extracts. The reversal of reduced glucokinase, increased glucose 6 phosphate action, and reduced glycosylated Hb levels were achieved [140].

In vitro analysis of the dried leaf methanolic extract revealed the antioxidant saponarin exhibiting the α-glucosidase action [141].

8.5.7 Terminalia bellirica

The aqueous extract was examined in pancreatic β cell line, BRIN-BD11. The study revealed the insulin-like activity of the drug. The protein glycation was inhibited, and starch digestion was reduced by the drug part. The striking effect was the absence of extracellular Ca and inhibitors of cellular calcium uptake reducing the action of the drug. The calcium and vitamin D supplements enhancing the cellular uptake of insulin have been seen in the molecular environment [142].

8.5.8 Plumbago zeylanica

The plumbagin from the root of the plant was found to reduce the blood glucose in streptozotocin-induced diabetes in rats. Increase of hexokinase activity and decrease of glucose-6-phosphatase and fructose-1,6-bisphosphatase are also found with the drug portion. The GLUT4mRNA translocation is linked with the glucose homeostasis located in skeletal muscle fibres. Plumbagin augmented the protein expression for effective glucose regulation [143].

8.5.9 Holarrhena antidysenterica

The streptozotocin-induced diabetes was examined with the ethanolic extract of the seed. The starch metabolism hindrance and inhibition of α glucosidase activity are thought to be the reason behind the hypoglycaemic effect [144]. The aqueous seed extract also exhibited the antidiabetic action in a correlation study with antihyperlipidemic action [145].

8.5.10 Berberis aristata

The ethanolic extract of the root was checked in streptozotocin-induced diabetic Wistar strains with standard drug metformin. The phytoconstituents responsible for the antidiabetic action might be the insulin-like effect. The peripheral glucose uptake, enhancement of hepatic gluconeogenesis and reduction of endogenous glucose production also might be contributing to the overall antidiabetic action [146].

8.5.10.1 Honey

A diabetic patient is benefitted with honey in many ways, if the adulterated form is taken off from the market and so promoting the local beekeepers. Honey has the carbohydrate fraction occupied by fructose, glucose-like monosaccharide. These increase the gastric emptying time and produces satiety feeling. Synergistically, the food intake is made less by and lengthens the intestinal absorption. The oligosaccharide in honey, the palatinose, also has the abovementioned effect [147].

The drugs mentioned here come from the depictions in *Prameha chikitsa/* diabetic syndrome of the classic *Astanga hrudaya* by *Vaghbata Acharya*. The chapter revises handful of formulations still in practice and effect in many adjunct manifestations of the diabetic syndrome. These drugs come in the initial versus where the applicability of nutraceutical might be strongly experienced [148].

8.6 Challenges in the promotion of nutraceuticals as antiaging

The health-promoting natural benefits from nutraceuticals have become a welcome step to any health-care specialty, but the reality behind the delivery of target sites is a matter of concern. The nutraceuticals in long-time run for chronic ailments or antiaging purpose need to be scrutinized to avoid mishappening. When the nutraceutical concept underlies the care taken for ingestion of medicines as food supplements, there is also emphasis on physical activity, lifestyle modification, etc., to the wholesome health concept. The applicability of nutraceuticals needs to be combined with this parallel aspect for better outcomes.

The highlight criteria to be fulfilled by any health-care commodity should be that the side effect must be negligible from the usage protocol. The antiaging and aging experimental data always present the adult and elderly with bundles of medicine. The lifestyle diseases are another major field for exposure to different medicines. Together, the situation presents with lots of drugs with little knowledge of their interaction background. The pseudobelief that herbal supplements and medicines are on safe sides favours their over-the-counter sale without any regulations. The herbals as dietary supplements, functional foods and nutraceuticals have unavailable data of interaction with conventional medicines. Drug-Drug Interaction (DDI) and Herb-Drug Interaction (HDI) have to be constantly shuffled under the light of novel strategies. The antiaging *Triphala* is found to interact with Warfarin, the blood coagulant agent, in elderly people [149]. Similarly, garlic, with its phytoconstituents, also intervenes with Warfarin complexity resulting in bleeding-like manifestations [150]. Once, the calcium supplements were encouraged with diabetic medications by physicians pointing out the calcium efflux for insulin uptake by the cells. Recent studies evidence the cardiovascular manifestations happening from such type of combinations and discarded greatly [151].

The antiaging concept presents with chronic use of certain medications like *Chyavanprash*. This semisolid medicine is greatly sold under the nutraceutical lead [152]. The trials need to be focussed on the long-term use of this medication and verify on the basis of age-wise differences to the formulation. The formulation is enriched with lipids, and sugar or jaggery becomes the base for preservation and presence of honey too. The adulterated honey can bring about many diseases rather than curing the ailments together with lowering the digestive capacity. The daily use of such formulations is not encouraged by Ayurvedic principles in the antiaging category. The testosterone-enhancing products are the next group which need to be scrutinized due to chronic usage. The Terminalia chebula ingredient in *triphala* is not enhancing the sperm count and motility rather than reducing the same. This fact might be taken into consideration when the nutraceutical concept is applied.

Indian gooseberry/*amla* is a rich source of vitamin C, in juice form or administered as raw. The heat stability of vitamin C needed to be taken into consideration if the product prepared out of amla is made available to the patient. The vitamin C content in sun-dried, shade-dried and refrigerated material was taken into consideration in an observation, and the shade-dried sample kept the vitamin proportion more and refrigerated sample also kept the ample ratio suggesting a processing and storage technique to the raw material on nutraceutical applicability. A single fruit is found to have 600–700 mg of ascorbic content more than a tablet can supply [153].

Ayurveda always considers herb as a whole and not the fragmented portion that is capable to interact in a specific pathway. The drug as a whole acts in multiple pathways and attenuates many diseases. The time, age, digestive enzyme, etc. influence the drug absorption criteria. The nutraceuticals include many fragmented drug portions and so the disease attenuating might be not always satisfied. The bioavailability is the other issue with nutraceutical contents. The data suggesting the target approach or serum levels are many times not reachable. The curcumin is such an entity where low serum levels, half-life, short circulation, etc. are seen [154]. Ginger powder is found to cause thyroiditis in a single case study incident, showing the unethical use of a nutraceutical commodity without prior knowledge [155]. Many innovations such as specially designed food matrices, engineered nanoparticles, probiotic encapsulation technology, etc. have been fabricated in the field to achieve the desired effect. These all point out the need of extensive research in the nutraceutical field and tailoring new regulations for the safety and efficacy regarding the nutraceuticals.

References

1. A.C Bhakthivedanta Swami Srila Prabhupad, Bagavat gita as it is, Chapter 3, Text 14.
2. Jivaka V, Samhita K. In: *Khila Sthana*. 8th edition. 6. Sharma Pandit Hemaraja., editor. Vol. 4. Chaukhamba Sanskrit Sansthana; 2002. revised by Vatsya.
3. Smith R, editor, "Let food be thy medicine...." *BMJ* 2004 Jan 24; 328(7433). https://www.ncbi.nlm.nih.gov/pmc/articles/PMC318470/.
4. Kalra EK. Nutraceutical-definition and introduction. *Aaps Pharmsci*. 2003 Sep;5(3):27–8.
5. https://www.who.int/news-room/fact-sheets/detail/ageing-and-health.
6. Rinaldi A, Hormone therapy for aging, *EMBO Rep*. 2004 Oct, 5(10): 938–941 https://www.ncbi.nlm.nih.gov/pmc/articles/PMC1299164.
7. Jones CM, Boelaert K. The endocrinology of ageing: A mini-review. *Gerontology*. 2015;61(4):291–300.
8. Lee Vance M. Growth hormone for the elderly? *N Engl J Med*. 1990; 323:52–54 DOI: 10.1056/NEJM199007053230109.
9. Lawton B, Rose S, McLeod D, Dowell A. Changes in use of hormone replacement therapy after the report from the Women's Health Initiative: cross sectional survey of users. *BMJ* 2003 Oct 9;327(7419):845–6.
10. Institute of Medicine (US) Committee on Assessing the Need for Clinical Trials of Testosterone Replacement Therapy. *Testosterone and Aging: Clinical Research Directions*. Liverman CT, Blazer DG, editors. Washington (DC): National Academies Press (US); 2004. PMID: 25009850.
11. Monnier VM. Toward a Maillard reaction theory of aging. *Prog Clin Biol Res*. 1989 Jan 1;304:1–22.
12. Jin K. Modern biological theories of aging. *Aging Dis*. 2010 Oct;1(2):72.
13. Miquel J. An update on the oxygen stress–mitochondrial mutation theory of aging: genetic and evolutionary implications. *Exp Gerontol*. 1998 Jan 1;33(1–2):113–26.
14. Ladiges W. The quality control theory of aging. *Pathobiol Aging Age Relat Dis*. 2014 May 23;4. doi: 10.3402/pba.v4.24835. PMID: 24891937; PMCID: PMC4033319.
15. Liochev SI. Reactive oxygen species and the free radical theory of aging. Free Radical Biology and Medicine. 2013 Jul 1;60:1–4.
16. Capra F. Tao of Physics: An Exploration of the Parallels Between Modern Physics and Eastern Mysticism ISBN1570625190 (ISBN13: 9781570625190).

17. Agnivesha, Charaka, Drdabala, Pandit Kashinadha Pandey and Dr, Gorakhnadh Pandey, Vidyodhithini Hindi Vyakhya, Charaka Samhitha, Chaukhamba Visvabharati, Varanasi, Shareera stanam 5:3 Pg:886.
18. Agnivesha, Charaka, Drdabala, Pandit Kashinadha Pandey and Dr, Gorakhnadh Pandey, Vidyodhithini Hindi Vyakhya, Charaka Samhitha, Chaukhamba Visvabharati, Varanasi, Chikitsa sthanam1:4, Pg:3.
19. Priyavat S. *Sushruta Samhita Dalhana Vyakhya Chaukhambha Orientelia*, 4th edition reprint, soothrasthana15:19.
20. Sharma PV. Dalhana commentary, Sushrutha samhitha, soothra sthana, 15/19.
21. Shomali ME. The use of anti-aging hormones. Melatonin, growth hormone, testosterone, and dehydroepiandrosterone: consumer enthusiasm for unproven therapies. *Md Med J*. 1997 Apr;46(4):181–6. PMID: 9114695.
22. Thomas SG, Esposito JG, Ezzat S. Exercise training benefits growth hormone (GH)-deficient adults in the absence or presence of GH treatment. *J Clin Endocrinol Metab*. 2003 Dec;88(12):5734–8. doi:10.1210/jc.2003-030632. PMID: 14671161.
23. Bartke A. Growth hormone and aging: updated review. *World J Men's Health*. 2019 Jan;37(1):19.
24. Laron Z. Do deficiencies in growth hormone and insulin-like growth factor-1 (IGF-1) shorten or prolong longevity? *Mech Age Dev*. 2005 Feb 1;126(2):305–7.
25. Friedrich N, Thuesen B, Jørgensen T, Juul A, Spielhagen C, Wallaschofksi H, Linneberg A. The association between IGF-I and insulin resistance: a general population study in Danish adults. *Diabetes care*. 2012 Apr 1;35(4):768–73.
26. Kimura KD, Tissenbaum HA, Liu Y, Ruvkun G. daf-2, an insulin receptor-like gene that regulates longevity and diapause in Caenorhabditis elegans. *Science*. 1997 Aug 15;277(5328):942–6.
27. Menakha M, Sangeetha M, Mani P, Al-Aboody MS, Vijayakumar R. In silico prediction of drug molecule from Ipomoea sepiaria against Type 2 diabetes. *Prog Med Sci*. 2018;3:9e14.
28. Singh RK, Mehta S, Jaiswal D, Rai PK, Watal G. Antidiabetic effect of Ficus bengalensis aerial roots in experimental animals. *J Ethnopharmacol*. 2009 May 4;123(1):110–4.
29. Alara OR, Abdurahman NH, Ukaegbu CI, Azhari NH. Vernonia cinerea leaves as the source of phenolic compounds, antioxidants, and anti-diabetic activity using microwave-assisted extraction technique. *Indus Crops Prod*. 2018 Oct 15;122:533–44.
30. Sharma C, Malgaonkar M, Sangvikar SG, Murthy SN, Pawar SD. In vitro evaluation of antimicrobial and antioxidant profile of Grewia L. root extracts. *J Appl Life Sci Int*. 2016 Aug 5:1–9.
31. Umamageswari MS, Karthikeyan TM, Maniyar YA. Antidiabetic activity of aqueous extract of Solanum nigrum linn berries in alloxan induced diabetic wistar albino rats. *JCDR* 2017 Jul;11(7):FC16.
32. Dhanabal SP, Raja MM, Ramanathan M, Suresh B. Hypoglycemic activity of Nymphaea stellata leaves ethanolic extract in alloxan induced diabetic rats. *Fitoterapia*. 2007 Jun 1;78(4):288–91.
33. Rushender CR, Eerike M, Madhusudhanan N, Konda VG. Antidiabetic activity of Nymphaea pubescens ethanolic extract-in vitro study. *J Pharm Res*. 2012;5(7):3807–9.
34. Rani R, Dahiya S, Dhingra D, Dilbaghi N, Kim KH, Kumar S. Evaluation of anti-diabetic activity of glycyrrhizin-loaded nanoparticles in nicotinamide-streptozotocin-induced diabetic rats. *Eur J Pharm Sci*. 2017 Aug 30;106:220–30.
35. Talukder FZ, Khan KA, Uddin R, Jahan N, Alam MA. In vitro free radical scavenging and anti-hyperglycemic activities of Achyranthes aspera extract in alloxan-induced diabetic mice. *Drug Discov Ther*. 2012 Dec 31;6(6):298–305.
36. Agarwal P, Sharma B, Jain SK, Fatima A, Alok S. Effect of Convolvulus pluricaulis chois. On blood glucose and lipid profile in streptozocin induced diabetic rats. *Int J Pharm Sci Res*. 2014 Jan 1;5(1):213.

37. Dheer R, Bhatnagar P. A study of the antidiabetic activity of Barleria prionitisLinn. *Ind J Pharmacol.* 2010 Apr;42(2):70.
38. Nair AK, Chandrasekar MJ, Shijikumar PS. Phytochemical and pharmacological aspects of Strobilanthes ciliatus Nees (Bremek.): A review. *Int J Res Ayurveda Pharm.* 2016;7:72–7.
39. Vasant RA, Narasimhacharya AV. Limonia fruit as a food supplement to regulate fluoride-induced hyperglycaemia and hyperlipidaemia. *J Sci Food Agr.* 2013 Jan 30;93(2):422–6.
40. Li M, Qu W, Wang Y, Wan H, Tian C. Hypoglycemic effect of saponin from Tribulus terrestris. *Zhong yao cai= Zhongyaocai= Journal of Chinese Medicinal Materials.* 2002 Jun 1;25(6):420–2.
41. Khatune NA, Rahman BM, Barman RK, Wahed MI. Antidiabetic, antihyperlipidemic and antioxidant properties of ethanol extract of Grewia asiatica Linn. bark in alloxan-induced diabetic rats. *BMC Compl Alter Med.* 2016 Dec;16(1):1–9.
42. Rastogi C, Paswan SK, Verma P, Vishwakarma V, Srivastava S, Rao CV. Chapter-6 Uraria picta: A comprehensive review and its pharmacological action. *Rec Adv Pharm Sci.* 2011; 76: 93.
43. Boue SM, Daigle KW, Chen MH, Cao H, Heiman ML. Antidiabetic potential of purple and red rice (Oryza sativa L.) bran extracts. *J Agr Food Chem.* 2016 Jul 6;64(26):5345–53.
44. Karasek M. Melatonin, human aging, and age-related diseases. *Exp. Gerontol.* 2004 Nov 1;39(11–12):1723–9.
45. Review Mitochondria: Central Organelles for Melatonin0s Antioxidant and Anti-Aging Actions Russel J. Reiter 1,*, Dun Xian Tan 1, Sergio Rosales-Corral 2, Annia Galano 3, Xin Jia Zhou 1 and Bing Xu.
46. Chanana P, Kumar A. Possible involvement of nitric oxide modulatory mechanisms in the neuroprotective effect of Centella asiatica against sleep deprivation induced anxiety like behaviour, oxidative damage and neuroinflammation. *Phytother Res.* 2016 Apr;30(4):671–80.
47. Das R, Sengupta T, Roy S, Chattarji S, Ray J. Convolvulus pluricaulis extract can modulate synaptic plasticity in rat brain hippocampus. *NeuroReport* 2020 May 22;31(8): 597–604.
48. Wang G, Grone B, Colas D, Appelbaum L, Mourrain P. Synaptic plasticity in sleep: learning, homeostasis and disease. *Trends Neurosci.* 2011 Sep 1;34(9):452–63.
49. Santiago TV, Guerra E, Neubauer JA, Edelman NH. Correlation between ventilation and brain blood flow during sleep. *J Clin Investig.* 1984 Feb 1;73(2):497–506.
50. Rathee P, Chaudhary H, Rathee S, Rathee D. Natural memory boosters. *Phcog Rev.* 2008;2:249–56.
51. Asuthosh A, Malini S, Bairy KL, Muddanna SR. Effect of Tinospora cordifolia on learning and memory in normal and memory deficits rats. *Indian J Pharmacol.* 2000;34:339–49.
52. Agnivesha, Charaka, Drdabala, Pandit Kashinadha Pandey and Dr, Gorakhnadh Pandey, Vidyodhithini Hindi Vyakhya, Charaka Samhitha, Chaukhamba Visvabharati, Varanasi, Chikitsa sthanam 1/3/30–31
53. Hoberman JM, Yesalis CE. The history of synthetic testosterone. *Sci Am.* 1995 Feb 1;272(2):76–81.
54. Institute of Medicine (US) Committee on Assessing the Need for Clinical Trials of Testosterone Replacement Therapy. *Testosterone and Aging: Clinical Research Directions.* Liverman CT, Blazer DG, editors. Washington (DC): National Academies Press (US); 2004. PMID: 25009850.
55. Stanworth RD, Jones TH. Testosterone for the aging male; current evidence and recommended practice. *Clin Inter Aging.* 2008 Mar;3(1):25.
56. Kallak TK, Hellgren C, Skalkidou A, Sandelin-Francke L, Ubhayasekhera K, Bergquist J, Axelsson O, Comasco E, Campbell RE, Poromaa IS. Maternal and female fetal testosterone levels are associated with maternal age and gestational weight gain. *Eur J Endocrinol.* 2017 Oct 1;177(4):379–88.

57. Singh J, Handelsman DJ. The effects of recombinant FSH on testosterone-induced spermatogenesis in gonadotrophin-deficient (hpg) mice. *J Androl.* 1996 Jul 8;17(4):382–93.

58. Sharangadhara A, Samhita S. Commented by Adhamalla and Kashiram. Chaukhambha Orientalia, Varanasi. 2005. Poorva Khanda, 4th Adhyaya.

59. Okun MS, Wu SS, Jennings D, Marek K, Rodriguez RL, Fernandez HH. Testosterone level and the effect of levodopa and agonists in early Parkinson disease: results from the INSPECT cohort. *J Clin Mov Dis.* 2014 Dec;1(1):1–5.

60. Ashidi JS, Owagboriaye FO, Yaya FB, Payne DE, Lawal OI, Owa SO. Assessment of reproductive function in male albino rat fed dietary meal supplemented with Mucuna pruriens seed powder. *Heliyon.* 2019 Oct 1;5(10):e02716.

61. Eskiocak S, Gozen AS, Taskiran A, Kilic AS, Eskiocak M, Gulen S. Effect of psychological stress on the L-arginine-nitric oxide pathway and semen quality. *Braz J Med Biol Res* [Internet]. 2006 May [cited 2021 Mar 10]; 39(5):581–588. Available from: scielo.br/scielo.php? script=sci_arttext&pid=S0100-879X2006000500003&lng=en. doi:10.1590/S0100-879X2006000500003.

62. Iuvone T, Esposito G, Capasso F, Izzo AA. Induction of nitric oxide synthase expression by Withania somnifera in macrophages. *Life Sci.* 2003 Feb 21;72(14):1617–25.

63. Ahmad MK, Mahdi AA, Shukla KK, Islam N, Rajender S, Madhukar D, Shankhwar SN, Ahmad S. Withania somnifera improves semen quality by regulating reproductive hormone levels and oxidative stress in seminal plasma of infertile males. *Fert Steril.* 2010 Aug 1;94(3):989–96.

64. Chauhan NS, Dixit VK. Spermatogenic activity of rhizomes of Curculigo orchioides Gaertn in male rats. *Int J Appl Res Nat Prod.* 2008 Jun;1(2):26–31.

65. Pandey AK, Gupta A, Tiwari M, Prasad S, Pandey AN, Yadav PK, Sharma A, Sahu K, Asrafuzzaman S, Vengayil DT, Shrivastav TG. Impact of stress on female reproductive health disorders: Possible beneficial effects of shatavari (Asparagus racemosus). *Biomed Pharmacother.* 2018 Jul 1;103:46–9.

66. Ogunwole E, Kunle-Alabi OT, Akindele OO, Raji Y. Saccharum officinarum juice alters reproductive functions in male Wistar rats. *J Basic Clin Physiol Pharmacol.* 2020 Apr 28;31(4):/j/jbcpp.2020.31.issue-4/jbcpp-2019-0235/jbcpp-2019–0235.xml. doi: 10.1515/jbcpp-2019-0235. PMID: 32755099.

67. Sharma A, Verma PK, Dixit VP. Effect of Semecarpus anacardium fruits on reproductive function of male albino rats. *Asian J Androl.* 2003 Jun;5(2):121–4. PMID: 12778323.

68. Bhat, Harshith P. et al. Indian medicinal plants as immunomodulators: scientific validation of the ethnomedicinal beliefs. in: Ronald Ross Watson and Victor R. Preedy (eds). *Bioactive Food as Dietary Interventions for Arthritis and Related Inflammatory Diseases.* Academic Press. 2013. pp. 215–24.

69. Zia-Ul-Haq M, Ahmad S, Bukhari SA, Amarowicz R, Ercisli S, Jaafar HZ. Compositional studies and biological activities of some mash bean (Vigna mungo (L.) Hepper) cultivars commonly consumed in Pakistan. *Biol Res.* 2014;47:1–4.

70. Adelakun SA, Ogunlade B, Olawuyi TS, Aniah JA, Omotoso OD. Histomorphology, sperm quality and hormonal profile in adult male sprague-dawley rats following administration of aqueous crude extract of solanum nigrum by gastric gavage. *JBRA Assist Reprod.* 2018 oct;22(4):338.

71. Tajuddin, Ahmad S, Latif A, Qasmi IA. Aphrodisiac activity of 50% ethanolic extracts of *Myristica fragnas* Houtt. (nutmeg) and *Syzygium aromaticum* (L.) Merr. & Perry. (clove) in male mice: a comparative study. *BMC Complement Altern Med.* 2003;3:6. doi:10.1186/1472-6882-3-6.

72. Ahmad S, Latif A, Qasmi IA, Amin KM. An experimental study of sexual function improving effect of *Myristica fragrans* Houtt. (nutmeg). *BMC Complement Altern Med.* 2005;5:1–7. doi:10.1186/1472-6882-5-16.

73. Ghosh A, Jana K, Pakhira BP, Tripathy A, Ghosh D. Anti-fertility effect of aqueous-ethanolic (1: 1) extract of the fruit of Terminalia chebula: Rising approach towards herbal contraception. *Asian Pac J Reprod.* 2015 Sep 1;4(3):201–7.

74. Arlt W. Dehydroepiandrosterone and ageing. *Best Pract Res Clin Endocrinol Metabol.* 2004 Sep 1;18(3):363–80.
75. Svec F, Porter JR. The actions of exogenous dehydroepiandrosterone in experimental animals and humans. *Proc Soc Exp Biol Med.* 1998 Jul;218(3):174–91.
76. Miller WL. Androgen biosynthesis from cholesterol to DHEA. *Mol Cell Endocrinol.* 2002 Dec 30;198(1–2):7–14. doi: 10.1016/s0303–7207(02)00363-5. PMID: 12573809.
77. Agnivesha, Charaka, Drdabala, Pandit Kashinadha Pandey and Dr, Gorakhnadh Pandey, Vidyodhithini Hindi Vyakhya, Charaka Samhitha, Chaukhamba Visvabharati, Varanasi, Chikitsa sthanam1: 4.
78. The impact of Ghee on Serum Lipids, Sex Hormones and Spermogram of Wistar rats Heydari O1, Mortazavi SA2, Zhaleh M3*, Abdollahzad H4
79. Sharma H, Zhang X, Dwivedi C. The effect of ghee (clarified butter) on serum lipid levels and microsomal lipid peroxidation. *Ayu.* 2010 Apr;31(2):134.
80. Horrocks LA, Yeo YK. Health benefits of docosahexaenoic acid (DHA). *Pharmacol Res.* 1999 Sep;40(3):211–25. doi: 10.1006/phrs.1999.0495. PMID: 10479465.
81. Karandikar YS, Bansude AS, Angadi EA. Comparison between the effect of cow ghee and butter on memory and lipid profile of wistar rats. *JCDR* 2016 Sep;10(9):FF11.
82. https://www.who.int/news-room/fact-sheets/detail/the-top-10-causes-of-death.
83. Zodda D, Giammona R, Schifilliti S. Treatment strategy for dyslipidemia in cardiovascular disease prevention: Focus on old and new drugs. *Pharmacy.* 2018 Mar;6(1):10.
84. Golomb BA, Evans MA. Statin adverse effects. *Am J Cardiovasc Drug.* 2008 Nov;8(6):373–418.
85. Agnivesha, Charaka, Drdabala, Pandit Kashinadha Pandey and Dr, Gorakhnadh Pandey, Vidyodhithini Hindi Vyakhya, Charaka Samhitha, Chaukhamba Visvabharati, Varanasi, Sutra sthanam. 21
86. Manjunath SE, Nayak RP, Venkatappa KG, Rai MS. Evaluation of hypolipidemic effect of Tinospora cordifolia in cholesterol diet induced hyperlipidemia in rats. *Int J Basic Clin Pharmacol.* 2016 Jun 29;5(4):1286–92.
87. Chandratre RS, Chandarana S, Mengi SA. Effect of aqueous extract of Cyperus rotundus on hyperlipidaemia in rat model. *Int J Pharm Biol Arch.* 2012;3(3):598–600.
88. Oh GS, Yoon J, Lee GG, Kwak JH, Kim SW. The Hexane fraction of Cyperus rotundus prevents non-alcoholic fatty liver disease through the inhibition of liver X receptor α-mediated activation of sterol regulatory element binding protein-1c. *Am J Chin Med.* 2015 May 5;43(03):477–94.
89. Lemaure B, Touché A, Zbinden I, Moulin J, Courtois D, Macé K, Darimont C. Administration of Cyperus rotundus tubers extract prevents weight gain in obese Zucker rats. *Phytother Res.* 2007 Aug;21(8):724–30.
90. Marimuthu Anandharaj, Balayogan Sivasankari, Rizwana Parveen Rani, "Effects of probiotics, prebiotics, and synbiotics on hypercholesterolemia: a review", *Chinese Journal of Biology*, vol. 2014, Article ID 572754, 7 pages, 2014. https://doi.org/10.1155/2014/572754.
91. Terzo S, Mulè F, Amato A. Honey and obesity-related dysfunctions: a summary on health benefits. *J Nutr Biochem.* 2020 Aug; 82:108401. doi: 10.1016/j.jnutbio.2020.108401. Epub 2020 Apr 17. PMID: 32454412.
92. Bhandari U, Ansari MN, Islam F, Tripathi CD. The effect of aqueous extract of Embelia ribes Burm on serum homocysteine, lipids and oxidative enzymes in methionine induced hyperhomocysteinemia. *Ind J Pharmacol.* 2008 Aug;40(4):152.
93. Idehen E, Tang Y, Sang S. Bioactive phytochemicals in barley. *J Food Drug Anal.* 2017 Jan 1;25(1):148–61.
94. Mathur R, Sharma A, Dixit VP, Varma M. Hypolipidaemic effect of fruit juice of Emblica officinalis in cholesterol-fed rabbits. *J Ethnopharmacol.* 1996 Feb 1;50(2):61–8.
95. Gopa B, Bhatt J, Hemavathi KG. A comparative clinical study of hypolipidemic efficacy of Amla (Emblica officinalis) with 3-hydroxy-3-methylglutaryl-coenzyme-A reductase inhibitor simvastatin. *Ind J Pharmacol.* 2012 Mar;44(2):238.

96. Maruthappan V, Shree KS. Hypolipidemic activity of Haritaki (Terminalia chebula) in atherogenic diet induced hyperlipidemic rats. *J Adv Pharm Technol Res*. 2010 Apr;1(2):229.

97. Pacifici R. Estrogen, cytokines, and pathogenesis of postmenopausal osteoporosis. *J Bone Min Res*. 1996 Aug;11(8):1043–51.

98. Khosla S, Hofbauer LC. Osteoporosis treatment: recent developments and ongoing challenges. *Lancet Diab Endocrinol*. 2017 Nov 1;5(11):898–907.

99. Gupta S, Walia A, Malan R. Phytochemistry and pharmacology of cedrus deodera: an overview. *Int J Pharm Sci Res*. 2011 Aug 1;2(8):2010.

100. Wayal, Sandesh. (2013). The osteoprotective effect of gmelina arborea extract in ovariectomized rats. 974–9446.

101. Cantos E, Espin JC, Tomás-Barberán FA. Varietal differences among the polyphenol profiles of seven table grape cultivars studied by LC– DAD– MS– MS. *J Agr Food Chem*. 2002 Sep 25;50(20):5691–6.

102. Welch A, MacGregor A, Jennings A, Fairweather-Tait S, Spector T, Cassidy A. Habitual flavonoid intakes are positively associated with bone mineral density in women. *J Bone Min Res*. 2012 Sep;27(9):1872–8.

103. Hohman EE, Weaver CM. A grape-enriched diet increases bone calcium retention and cortical bone properties in ovariectomized rats. *J Nutr*. 2015 Feb;145(2):253–9. doi:10.3945/jn.114.198598. Epub 2014 Dec 3. PMID: 25644345.

104. Chitme HR, Muchandi IS, Burli SC. Effect of Asparagus racemosus Willd root extract on ovariectomized rats. *Open Nat Prod J*. 2009 Feb 26;2(1):16–23.

105. Zhang J, Zong L, Bai D. Boeravinone B promotes fracture healing in ovariectomy-induced osteoporotic rats via the regulation of NF-kappa B p65/I kappa B-alpha/ SIRT-1 signaling pathway. *Trop J Pharm Res*. 2019 May 1;18(5):955–60.

106. Nallathambi A, Bhargavan R. Regulation of estrous cycle by Cynodon dactylon in letrozole induced polycystic ovarian syndrome in Wistars albino rats. *Anat Cell Biol*. 2019 Dec;52(4):511.

107. Hatefi M, Ahmadi MR, Rahmani A, Dastjerdi MM, Asadollahi K. Effects of curcumin on bone loss and biochemical markers of bone turnover in patients with spinal cord injury. *World Neurosurg*. 2018 Jun 1;114:e785–91.

108. Farida Hussan, Nawwar Ghassan Ibraheem, Taty Anna Kamarudin, Ahmad Nazrun Shuid, Ima Nirwana Soelaiman, Faizah Othman. Curcumin Protects against ovariectomy-induced bone changes in rat model. *Evidence-Based Complementary and Alternative Medicine*, vol. 2012, Article ID 174916, 7 pages, 2012. https://doi.org/10.1155/2012/174916.

109. Lee J, Nho YH, Yun SK, Hwang YS. Use of ethanol extracts of Terminalia chebula to prevent periodontal disease induced by dental plaque bacteria. *BMC Compl Alter Med*. 2017 Dec;17(1):1–0.

110. Lopez HL, Habowski SM, Sandrock JE, Raub B, Kedia A, Bruno EJ, Ziegenfuss TN. Effects of dietary supplementation with a standardized aqueous extract of Terminalia chebula fruit (AyuFlex®) on joint mobility, comfort, and functional capacity in healthy overweight subjects: A randomized placebo-controlled clinical trial. *BMC Compl Alter Med*. 2017 Dec;17(1):1–8.

111. Ramli ES, Suhaimi F, Asri SF, Ahmad F, Soelaiman IN. Glycyrrhizic acid (GCA) as 11β-hydroxysteroid dehydrogenase inhibitor exerts protective effect against glucocorticoid-induced osteoporosis. *J Bone Min Metabol*. 2013 May 1;31(3):262–73.

112. Kaczmarczyk-Sedlak I, Klasik-Ciszewska S, Wojnar W. Glabridin and glycyrrhizic acid show no beneficial effect on the chemical composition and mechanical properties of bones in ovariectomized rats, when administered in moderate dose. *Pharmacol Rep*. 2016 Sep;68(5):1036–41.

113. Tamir S, Eizenberg M, Somjen D, Stern N, Shelach R, Kaye A, Vaya J. Estrogenic and antiproliferative properties of glabridin from licorice in human breast cancer cells. *Cancer Res*. 2000 Oct 15;60(20):5704–9.

114. Somjen D, Knoll E, Vaya J, Stern N, Tamir S. Estrogen-like activity of licorice root constituents: glabridin and glabrene, in vascular tissues in vitro and in vivo. *J Ster Biochem Mol Biol*. 2004 Jul 1;91(3):147–55.

115. Li Z, Chen C, Zhu X, Li Y, Yu R, Xu W. Glycyrrhizin suppresses RANKL-Induced osteoclastogenesis and oxidative stress through inhibiting NF-κB and MAPK and activating AMPK/Nrf2. *Calc Tissue Int*. 2018 Sep;103(3):324–37.

116. Galanis D, Soultanis K, Lelovas P, Zervas A, Papadopoulos P, Galanos A, Argyropoulou K, Makropoulou M, Patsaki A, Passali C, Tsingotjidou A, Kourkoulis S, Mitakou S, Dontas I. Protective effect of Glycyrrhiza glabra roots extract on bone mineral density of ovariectomized rats. *Biomedicine* (Taipei). 2019 Jun;9(2):8. doi: 10.1051/bmdcn/2019090208. Epub 2019 May 24. PMID: 31124454; PMCID: PMC6533940.

117. Agnivesha, Charaka, Drdabala, Pandit Kashinadha Pandey and Dr, Gorakhnadh Pandey, Vidyodhithini Hindi Vyakhya, Charaka Samhitha, Chaukhamba Visvabharati, Varanasi, sutra sthanam 4:49, p. 97.

118. Taylor PN, Albrecht D, Scholz A, Gutierrez-Buey G, Lazarus JH, Dayan CM, Okosieme OE. Global epidemiology of hyperthyroidism and hypothyroidism. *Nat Rev Endocrinol*. 2018 May;14(5):301–6. doi:10.1038/nrendo.2018.18. Epub 2018 Mar 23. PMID: 29569622.

119. Shahid MA, Ashraf MA, Sharma S. Physiology, thyroid hormone. StatPearls [Internet]. 2020 May 18.

120. Nordio M, Pajalich R. Combined treatment with Myo-inositol and selenium ensures euthyroidism in subclinical hypothyroidism patients with autoimmune thyroiditis. *J Thyroid Res*. 2013;2013:424163. doi: 10.1155/2013/424163. Epub 2013 Oct 2. PMID: 24224112; PMCID: PMC3809375.

121. Inositol hexaphosphate, a natural substance found in whole kernel corn and brown rice, activates natural killer cell function – Inhibits cancer. *Posit Health News*. 1998 Fall;(No 17):23–5. PMID: 11366552.

122. Paul B, Masih I, Deopujari J, Charpentier C. Occurrence of resveratrol and pterostilbene in age-old darakchasava, an ayurvedic medicine from India. *J Ethnopharmacol*. 1999 Dec 15;68(1–3):71–6. doi:10.1016/s0378-8741(99)00044-6. PMID: 10624864.

123. Benvenga S, Feldt-Rasmussen U, Bonofiglio D, Asamoah E. Nutraceutical Supplements in the Thyroid Setting: Health Benefits beyond Basic Nutrition. *Nutrients* 2019 Sep;11(9):2214.

124. Defelice SL, Gilgore SG. The antagonistic effect of carnitine in hyperthyroidism. Preliminary report. *J New Drug*. 1966 Nov 12;6(6):351–3.

125. Benvenga S, Ruggeri RM, Russo A, Lapa D, Campenni A, Trimarchi F. Usefulness of L-carnitine, a naturally occurring peripheral antagonist of thyroid hormone action, in iatrogenic hyperthyroidism: a randomized, double-blind, placebo-controlled clinical trial. *J Clin Endocrinol Metabol*. 2001 Aug 1;86(8):3579–94.

126. Klein M, Catargi B. VEGF in physiological process and thyroid disease. *Ann Endocrinol (Paris)*. 2007 Dec;68(6):438–48. doi:10.1016/j.ando.2007.09.004. Epub 2007 Nov 7. PMID: 17991452.

127. Agnivesha, Charaka, Drdabala, Pandit Kashinadha Pandey and Dr, Gorakhnadh Pandey, Vidyodhithini Hindi Vyakhya, Charaka Samhitha, Chaukhamba Visvabharati, Varanasi, Sutra sthana 4:9

128. Sunila ES, Kuttan G. Piper longum inhibits VEGF and proinflammatory cytokines and tumor-induced angiogenesis in C57BL/6 mice. *Int Immunopharmacol*. 2006 May 1;6(5):733–41.

129. Wen W, Lu J, Zhang K, Chen S. Grape seed extract inhibits angiogenesis via suppression of the vascular endothelial growth factor receptor signaling pathway. *Cancer Preven Res*. 2008 Dec 1;1(7):554–61.

130. Sheela ML, Ramakrishna MK, Salimath BP. Angiogenic and proliferative effects of the cytokine VEGF in Ehrlich ascites tumor cells is inhibited by Glycyrrhiza glabra. *Int Immunopharmacol*. 2006 Mar 1;6(3):494–8.

131. Davì G, Santilli F, Patrono C. Nutraceuticals in diabetes and metabolic syndrome. *Cardiovasc Ther.* 2010 Aug;28(4):216–26.

132. D'souza JJ, D'souza PP, Fazal F, Kumar A, Bhat HP, Baliga MS. Anti-diabetic effects of the Indian indigenous fruit Emblica officinalis Gaertn: Active constituents and modes of action. *Food Funct.* 2014 Apr;5(4):635–44. doi:10.1039/c3fo60366k. PMID: 24577384.

133. Acharya N, Acharya S, Shah U, Shah R, Hingorani L. A comprehensive analysis on Symplocos racemosa Roxb.: Traditional uses, botany, phytochemistry and pharmacological activities. *J Ethnopharmacol.* 2016 Apr 2;181:236–51.

134. Kumar GP, Arulselvan P, Kumar DS, Subramanian SP. Anti-diabetic activity of fruits of Terminalia chebula on streptozotocin induced diabetic rats. *J Health Sci.* 2006;52(3):283–91.

135. Zhang DW, Fu M, Gao SH, Liu JL. Curcumin and diabetes: a systematic review. *Evid Based Complement Alternat Med.* 2013;2013:636053. doi: 10.1155/2013/636053. Epub 2013 Nov 24. PMID: 24348712; PMCID: PMC3857752.

136. Singh P, Khosa RL, Mishra G. Evaluation of antidiabetic activity of ethanolic extract of Cedrus deodara (Pinaceae) stem bark in streptozotocin induced diabetes in mice. *Nig J Exp Clin Biosci.* 2013 Jan 1;1(1):33.

137. Devmurari V, Shivanand P, Vaghani S, Jagganath K, Goyani M, Jivani NP. Antihyperglycemic activity of ethanolic extract of Cedrus deodara wood in alloxan induced hyperglycemic rat. *Int J Chem Sci.* 2010;8(1):483–8.

138. Khanal P, Patil BM, Mandar BK, Dey YN, Duyu T. Network pharmacology-based assessment to elucidate the molecular mechanism of anti-diabetic action of Tinospora cordifolia. *Clin Phytosci.* 2019 Dec;5(1):1–9.

139. Patel MB, Mishra S. Hypoglycemic activity of alkaloidal fraction of Tinospora cordifolia. *Phytomedicine* 2011 Sep 15;18(12):1045–52.

140. Rajalakshmi M, Eliza J, Priya CE, Nirmala A, Daisy P. Anti-diabetic properties of Tinospora cordifolia stem extracts on streptozotocin-induced diabetic rats. *Afr J Pharm Pharmacol.* 2009 May 31;3(5):171–80.

141. Sengupta S, Mukherjee A, Goswami R, Basu S. Hypoglycemic activity of the antioxidant saponarin, characterized as α-glucosidase inhibitor present in Tinospora cordifolia. *J Enzy Inhib Med Chem.* 2009 Jun 1;24(3):684–90.

142. Kasabri V, Flatt PR, Abdel-Wahab YH. Terminalia bellirica stimulates the secretion and action of insulin and inhibits starch digestion and protein glycation in vitro. *Br J Nutr.* 2010 Jan;103(2):212–7. doi:10.1017/S0007114509991577. Epub 2009 Sep 1. PMID: 19723351.

143. Sunil C, Duraipandiyan V, Agastian P, Ignacimuthu S. Antidiabetic effect of plumbagin isolated from Plumbago zeylanica L. root and its effect on GLUT4 translocation in streptozotocin-induced diabetic rats. *Food Chem Toxicol.* 2012 Dec 1;50(12): 4356–63.

144. Keshri UP. Antidiabetic efficacy of ethanolic extract of holarrhena antidysenterica seeds in streptozotocin - induced diabetic rats and its influence on certain biochemical parameters. *J Drug Deliv Ther.* 2012 Jul 15;2(4), pp 159–162.

145. Ali KM, Chatterjee K, De DBT, Ghosh D. Efficacy of aqueous extract of seed of Holarrhena antidysenterica for the management of diabetes in experimental model rat: A correlative study with antihyperlipidemic activity. *Int J Appl Res Nat Prod.* 2(3): 13-21, Sep-Oct 2009.

146. Pareek A, Suthar M. Antidiabetic activity of extract of Berberis aristata root in streptozotocin induced diabetic rats. *Pharmacologyonline* 2010;2:179–85.

147. Erejuwa OO, Sulaiman SA, Ab Wahab MS. Honey - a novel antidiabetic agent. *Int J Biol Sci.* 2012;8(6):913.

148. Acharya Vagbhat. Prame chikitsa Adhaya. In Paradakara HSS, editor. Ashtanga Hrudaya with Sarvangasundara commentary of Arunadatta and Ayurvedarasayana commentary of Hemadri. Chaukambha Orientalia: Varanasi; Reprint 2005.p.502

149. Awortwe C, Makiwane M, Reuter H, Muller C, Louw J, Rosenkranz B. Critical evaluation of causality assessment of herb–drug interactions in patients. *Br J Clin Pharmacol.* 2018 Apr;84(4):679–93.

150. Borrelli F, Capasso R, Izzo AA. Garlic (Allium sativum L.): Adverse effects and drug interactions in humans. *Mol Nut Food Res.* 2007 Nov;51(11): 1386–97.
151. Song Y, Xu Q, Park Y, Hollenbeck A, Schatzkin A, Chen H. Multivitamins, individual vitamin and mineral supplements, and risk of diabetes among older US adults. *Diab Care.* 2011 Jan 1;34(1):108–14.
152. Sharma R, Martins N, Kuca K, Chaudhary A, Kabra A, Rao MM, Prajapati PK. Chyawanprash: A traditional Indian bioactive health supplement. *Biomolecules* 2019 May;9(5):161.
153. Thankitsunthorn S, Thawornphiphatdit C, Laohaprasit N, Srzednicki G. Effects of drying temperature on quality of dried Indian gooseberry powder. *Int Food Res J.* 2009;16(3):355–61.
154. Anand P, Kunnumakkara AB, Newman RA, Aggarwal BB. Bioavailability of curcumin: Problems and promises. *Mol Pharm.* 2007 Dec 3;4(6):807–18.
155. Sanavi S, Afshar R. Subacute thyroiditis following ginger (Zingiber officinale) consumption. *Int J Ayu Res.* 2010 Jan;1(1):47.

Molecular Mechanisms to Understand Aging and Immune Function and Nutraceutical Interventions

Salwa and Lalit Kumar
Manipal College of Pharmaceutical Sciences

Contents

DOI: 10.1201/9781003110866-9

9.1 Introduction

Significant advancements in mitigating, slowing, or treating human pathologies are responsible for an exceptionally longer lifespan in the advanced parts of our world, and it is indeed highly frequent today to hit eight to nine decades of life. Aging, a universal phenomenon, that begins in the initial stages of adulthood, is a stable, continuing phase of natural adaptation and not a disease by itself during which many bodily functions begin to gradually decrease due to progressive dysregulation of certain molecular processes [1]. It is characterized by deterioration in physiological functions, as well as higher rate of morbidity and mortality. Almost every nation in the world is experiencing rise in both, the size and the proportion of older population. At present, the world population of people aged 65 years and older is estimated at 728 million, which is anticipated to increase than double its current value, reaching almost 1.5 billion by 2050 [2]. Aging is a dynamic process taking place in all the organisms due to genetic, epigenetic and environmental conditions and is associated with alterations at the molecular, cellular and tissue levels [3]. Random molecular damage drives the aging process at cellular level that gradually gets accumulated upon aging. While cells possess processes to restore or eliminate injury, they really aren't 100% efficient, and their capacity begins to decline with age [4]. The involvement of certain molecular mechanisms and exogenous factors contributes to the aging process. In existing aging research, the key challenge lies in identifying the origin of aging processes that enable multiple pathologies and dysfunction, mainly among the elderly population. Stem cell fatigue, impaired intracellular connectivity, genetic changes and telomere erosion, epigenetic changes, lack of protein homeostasis, detection of altered nutrients and growth factor, nonfunctioning of mitochondria and cellular senescence are features of aging [5]. The commonality among these aforementioned hallmarks is linked to the immune system.

Amidst all the plausible consequences of aging, impairment of the immune system is believed to play a vital role. A well-functioning immune system is deemed essential for the prolonged sustainability of host against the regular attack of new species and microorganisms. But it has been recognized in humans as in many other animals that perhaps the efficacy of the immune system decreases profoundly with age, leading to gradual decline in the capabilities to cope with infections and to establish resistance after vaccination, and vulnerability to age-related inflammatory diseases, that are linked to higher death rates in the aged. A variety of protection networks have been built in innate and adaptive immune systems to defend people from detrimental pathogens such as viral, bacterial, fungal and microparasite and to remove broken, harmful and dysfunctional host cells, like senescent cells and poisonous or allergenic materials that pose a major threat to survival [6,7]. Due to the clinical impact, changes that take place in humans after 50 years of age have received particular attention, and these changes have been globally termed as "immunosenescence". The term "immunosenescence" was coined by Roy Walford in 1969 [8,9], and it is referred to as an age-related progressive decrease in immune functioning and homeostasis at the molecular, cellular and organelle level, characterized by decreased immunocompetence (impaired capacity to respond to new antigen), unsustained responses from memory, increased rate of infection, autoimmune disease, inflammation and neoplasia [10]. It influences both innate (natural) and humoral (acquired) immunity, though T lymphocytes are adversely impacted. Immunosenescence promotes development of inflammatory phenotype known as "inflammaging". The term "inflammaging" was coined by Franceshi et al., to define a poor-grade, asymptomatic, persistent and systemic inflammation associated with low degree of chronic immune cell invasion and increased concentrations of pro-inflammatory circulatory cytokines and chemokines inside the tissue microenvironment and systemic environment [11,12]. Aging-related fall in immune functioning includes change in the amount of monocytic and dendritic cells in the circulation, thymic involution, polyfunctionality of T cell, or generation of pro-inflammatory cytokines [13] (Figure 9.1). They reduce the potential to cause successful antibody and cellular responses against various infections and vaccinations [8]. Three components that can be portrayed upon consideration of impact of aging on critical elements of the immune system include various immune cells, lymphoid organs and circulating factors [14].

In order to identify the most effective techniques for immune restoration and successful induction of vaccination-mediated immunity in elderly adults, to create a healthy state in later years and to develop promising therapeutic approaches, a better interpretation of immunosenescence and the pathways accountable for established deleterious changes is essential. Multiple studies

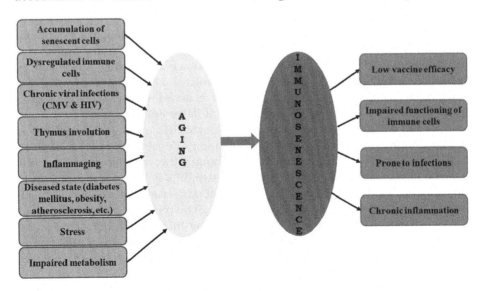

Figure 9.1 *Various mechanisms involved in aging and immunosenescence and the possible effects on the aged individual.*

of the underlying processes of age-related immune dysfunction have established the groundwork for identifying targeted interventions in recent years. The basic discernment of the molecular mechanisms involved in immunosenescence and its impact on aging will be completely clarified in this chapter so as to help progression of research and develop new therapeutic interventions for the compensation of age-associated immunological dysfunction.

9.2 Innate (nonspecific) immunity

The innate immune system has always been more recognized since the early 1990s for both its vital role in overall immunity and its substantial complexity. The innate immune system offers a standard system of protection against toxic pathogens and materials entering the body, perhaps through the skin or digestive system [15]. They rely on a set of proteins and phagocytic cells which identify the retained characteristics of pathogens and quickly get activated to chase away invaders [16]. It includes neutrophils, monocytes/macrophages, dendritic cells, natural killer (NK) cells and microglia. The phenotype and tasks of these cells are profoundly diminished with aging, yet, in comparison, an age-related hyperactivity of innate immunity might also be demonstrated.

9.2.1 Neutrophils

Neutrophils, also known as polymorphonuclear leukocytes, are produced in bone marrow ($\sim10^{11}$ cells/day) and are widely present in human blood. Under normal circumstances, neutrophils enter the blood stream, travel to tissues where they execute their tasks and are ultimately destroyed by the macrophages. They are the first ones to be recruited during any damage or inflammation. The organism is continuously patrolled by neutrophils for any indications of infectious agents, and these cells rapidly attack and destroy the invading pathogens when identified. Three major antimicrobial activities of neutrophils are phagocytosis, degranulation and nuclear material release [15]. For antibacterial action, they also generate several degradative enzymes, reactive oxygen species and antimicrobial peptides. Granulocytes are a group of white blood cells constituting of neutrophils in combination of eosinophils and basophils. Several studies have demonstrated that though the number of neutrophils is normal, the activation or function of neutrophils is severely compromised upon aging, mainly those related to chemotaxis, phagocytosis and intracellular killing through free-radical production. This may be partly blamed for increased vulnerability of elderly people to the infections ultimately leading to high rates of mortality and morbidity. Susceptibility to spontaneous and induced apoptosis of neutrophils increases causing imbalance in the homeostasis. Imbalance in the functionality is accompanied by changes in signaling of molecule traffic and in signaling of toll-like receptors (TLRs) [17]. The concentration of free calcium ions (Ca^{2+}) in the cytosol exhibits an important part in the management of functions of the neutrophil. During phagocytosis, the elevated levels of calcium in the cytosol spread through neutrophils and with the control of actin mediate the fusion of phagosome and lysosome. Drop-off in the ability of calcium mobilization leads to decreased chemotaxis, superoxide anion production and lytic enzyme action due to reduced chemotactic peptide-induced transmembrane signaling. Along with calcium ion concentration, carbohydrate metabolism of neutrophils has also been demonstrated to affect their function. Findings by Wenisch et al. suggest that increase in intracellular concentrations of calcium ion in resting neutrophils and/or decreased uptake of hexose will lead to reduced phagocytic potential and reduced neutrophil bactericidal activity in the aged [17]. Certain microbiota-derived signals also trigger neutrophil aging via pathways mediated by TLR2, TLR4 and MyD88 [18].

9.2.2 Macrophages

Macrophages are specialized immune effector cells originating from monocytes and are associated in the identification, phagocytosis and wrecking of harmful pathogens. Additionally, they can also present antigens to T cells and release cytokines that activate other cells in order to initiate inflammation. They also produce reactive oxygen species, such as nitric oxide, which can destroy phagocytosed bacteria. The main function of macrophages is to clear the interstitial environment of extracellular material [19]. They travel to and communicate with almost all the tissues, guarding for pathogens or getting rid of dead cells. The two different phenotypes of macrophages include: the classical (M1) and the alternative (M2). They persist in steady state in normal healthy population, but during the existence of chronic inflammation, there is a disparity which contributes to comorbidities and age-associated disease development. The aging process is accelerated due to the accumulation of senescent macrophages. Macrophages show intact phagocytic activity and decreased percentage of CD68 positive cells in bone marrow of adults. Certain studies have also shown enhancement in lipopolysaccharide (LPS)-induced cytokine secretion, whereas others have shown unaltered or reduced secretion. Upon stimulation with agonists of TLR1/2 heterodimer, an age-related reduction in TNF-α and IL-6 production and an increased production of IL-10 in macrophages were also reported. There is some evidence of decrease in TLR1/2-mediated cytokine production, reduction in CD16- and increase in CD16+ cells with age. The number of macrophages in elderly people is not affected, but few important tasks such as phagocytosis, chemotaxis, superoxide production, signal transduction, apoptosis, TLR expression and function, major histocompatibility complex (MHC) II expression and cytokine production seem to be reduced (Table 9.1). On the contrary, PGE production was found to increase by macrophages upon aging [20,21]. The effect of aging on macrophages is decreased expression of TLR1, 2 and 4, with decreased generation of proinflammatory cytokines [22].

Table 9.1 Aging Factors That Contribute to Macrophage/Microglia Dynamics

Factors	Young	Old
Microenvironment	Supportive factors and signaling of normal cellular activities, effective clearance of debris	Misfolded proteins, free radicals, impaired clearance of debris
Intrinsic	Normal physiological activities	Cellular senescence, epigenetic changes, genomic instability
Macrophage/microglia	Efficient response upon activation, phagocytosis	Reduced response upon activation, impaired phagocytosis and chemotaxis
Cytokine/chemokine and other factors	CCL2, CX3CR1, CX3CL1, CD200, CD200R	Dysregulation of TNF-α, TGF-β, CCL5, CCL11, IL-6, IL-1β, MHC-II, CD68, INFs and several TLRs
Effects	Proper cellular functions, dynamics and interactions	Neurodegeneration and impaired repair

9.2.3 Microglia

Microglia are the immune cells residing in the central nervous system (CNS) possessing the capacity to discern materials of injured CNS cells or attack penetration of foreign substances by recognizing the receptors inherent on their surface. After detection, pro-inflammatory signaling cascade will be induced which stimulates microglia to get activated. During aging, microglia show enhanced release of proinflammatory cytokines and proliferative capacity, along with reduced phagocytosis of amyloid β (Aβ) fibrils and chemotaxis. Possible mechanisms underlying loss of immune function of microglia upon aging are as follows:

a. Inhibitory ligand receptor interactions with microglia will be lost as neurons get damaged with age.
b. Accumulation of misfolded proteins such as Aβ during aging elevates proinflammatory cytokines in microglia [23].
c. Increase in the expression of transforming growth factor β with age and long-term exposure of microglia to the cytokine impairs the ability of microglia to secrete anti-inflammatory cytokines [24].

The transforming growth factor β-mediated impairment leads to decreased levels of interferon regulatory factor-7 (IRF-7), a transcription factor that is necessary in switching microglia from a proinflammatory to an anti-inflammatory phenotype. With age, the amount of anti-inflammatory cytokine IL-4 increases at the choroid plexus inducing epithelial cells to produce an increased amount of CCL11 that might drag microglia toward more proinflammatory state [25]. Aged microglia represent structural alterations such as cytoplasmic hypertrophy, fragmentation and disappearance of certain functions (Table 9.1). There is enhancement in the expression of TLR1, 2, 4, 5, 7 and CD14 in microglial cells with increasing age [26], while the signaling of CX3CL1 (chemokine (C-X3-C motif) ligand 1)-CX3CR1 (receptor 1), CD (cluster of differentiation) 200-CD200R and CD200, CX3CR1 decreases in aged microglia, ultimately leading to stimulation of proinflammatory cytokines [27].

9.2.4 Dendritic cells

Dendritic cells (DCs) are the most powerful antigen presenting cells of the immune system representing a link between innate and adaptive immune response. DCs are found in all tissues of the body, where they detect imbalance in the homeostasis and process the antigens for presentation to T cells [28]. Aging is correlated with many alterations in the cytokine microenvironment which will either have stimulatory or inhibitory effect on the activation and/or maturation of DCs [29]. The antigen uptake capacity of DC is altered due to premature activation as a result of enhanced TNF-α and prostaglandins [30]. Similarly, activation of DCs is suppressed because of increased levels of IL-10 and glucocorticoid on aging [31]. No change has been reported in number and phenotype of DCs in aged humans [32,33]. But progressive decline in the number of circulating myeloid DCs (mDC) was reported by Della-Bella et al., while no change in the number of plasmacytoid DCs (pDC) was observed [34]. In older population, pDCs exhibit lesser production of IFN I/III and low capacity for the presentation of antigens, whereas mDCs exhibit reduced TLR-mediated signaling, presentation of antigens, chemotaxis and endocytosis. CD141 mDC subset is essential to defend the viral infections and tumors [35]. Recent study suggested reduction in the percentage of CD141 mDC subset in the aged, and this may be the plausible mechanism leading to increased prevalence of diseases with the advancement of age [36]. The cell functions of DCs undergo modification with age ultimately leading to increased secretion of proinflammatory cytokines. Susceptibility to infections increases due to reduced phagocytic activity and migration in the elderly. Finally, impaired function of DCs may contribute to immunosenescence of T and B cells and chronic inflammation connected upon aging [37].

9.2.5 Natural killer cells

NK cells are described as large granular innate lymphocytes accountable for recognition and defense in opposition to virally infected, transformed or senescent, and cancerous cells. Depending on the surface expression of CD56, NK cells are classified into two groups: CD56[bright] cells (immature) and CD56[dim] cells (mature). During the process of aging, the components of NK subsets might show certain changes in concentration and functional activity [38]. These changes play a vital part in weakened retaliation to influenza infection and vaccination in elderly population. Alteration in NK cell function will lead to impairment of cytotoxicity and secretion of immune regulatory cytokines and chemokines resulting in a condition known as NK cell immunosenescence [39]. Several research studies have highlighted phenotypic changes in NK cells upon aging, mainly increase in CD56[dim] cells (seen in CD16+ subset), fall in CD56[bright] cells (seen in CD 16– subset) and higher expression of immunosenescence marker, CD57. This modification reflects improper interaction of innate and adaptive immunity, along with reduced production of chemokine and cytokine-influenced expansion. Reduction in the amount of NK cells expressing NKp30 or NKp46 receptors has been reported in the aging process [40]. Significantly higher expression of sirtuin 1 (SIRT1) and heat shock protein 70 (HSP70) was found in both stimulated and nonstimulated human NK cells, and they were resistant to further stimulation with IL-2, LPS or PMA with ionomycin. However, manganese superoxide dismutase (SOD2) expression was less in nonstimulated cells, and their sensitivity to stimulation became high with aging [41]. Also, existence of senescent cells has been linked to reduction in clearance activity of NK cells by the recent findings [42]. Features of the aging process that are attributed to decline in NK cells upon aging include the following:

a. Increase in the rate of re-activation of latent Mycobacterium tuberculosis
b. Low resolution of inflammatory responses
c. Enhanced incidence of bacterial and fungal infections

Age-related impairment in NK cell cytotoxicity (NKCC) is quite controversial. It all depends on the protocol and the study design. When PBMCs were used as effector cells, the NKCC was equivalent between young and old donors [43], whereas in the case of purified NK cells, decrease in lytic activity was observed [44]. Certain studies suggest that age-associated impairment in NKCC is due to post-binding defect. Migration of NK cell is impaired with age. Cytokine and chemokine stimulation markedly increase NKCC by upregulating their production of IFN-γ, MIP-1α and IL-8. Antibody-dependent cell cytotoxicity (ADCC) remains unaffected by the aging process [40].

9.3 Adaptive (specific) immunity

The adaptive immune system produces antibodies and utilizes them to wrestle against particular pathogens that the body has encountered previously. The body is also able to fight against pathogens that change over the period of time by using adaptive immunity, as this system is continuously learning and adapting. The two major concerns of aged population are increased sensitivity to infection and reduced reaction to vaccination contributing to reduction in control of infectious diseases in late life and are consequence of senescent adaptive immune system. The major impact of aging on the adaptive immune system is reduction in the spontaneous generation of B and T lymphocytes exhibiting major effect on the capability to retaliate to the immune challenges (Table 9.2). The adaptive immune system is associated with two main weapon systems: extremely diversified antigen-recognizing (naïve) lymphocytes and very long-lived antigen-trained (memory) lymphocytes. The former guarantees a particular reaction to any promising challenges from the world of foreign antigens, and the latter ensures a quicker and more robust approach

Table 9.2 Age-Related Alterations in Innate Immune Functions

Type of Cell	Effect	Activity
Innate Immune Cells		
Neutrophils and macrophages	↑	Number
	↑	TLR expression
	↓	Phagocytic activity
	↓	Chemotaxis
	↓	MFC II expression
	↓	ROS production
	↓	Production of cytokines
NK cells	↑	Number
	↓	Cytotoxicity
	constant	Ab dependent cytotoxicity
	↓	IL-2 dependent IFN-γ and IL-12 induced chemokine secretion
	↓	CD56^{dim}
	↓	Production of cytokines and chemokines
	↑	CD56^{bright}
Monocytes	↑, ↓ or constant	Production of cytokine induced by LPS
	↓	TLR1/2 induced production of IL-6 and TNF-α
	↓	Phagocytosis
	↓	Surface expression of TLR1 and TLR4
	↓	CD68+ macrophages in bone marrow
Dendritic cells	↓	Langerhans cell density in skin
	↓ or constant	Number of pDCs
	↑ or constant	Number of mDCs
	constant	Trans-endothelial transfer, conserved capability of antigen pulsed DCs to trigger T-cell multiplication
	↓	Pinocytosis or endocytosis, migration induced by chemokines
	↓	Production of IFN-α in PBMCs
	↑	IL-6 and TNF-α generation induced by TLR4 and TLR8 in MDDCs
	↓	IL-2 generation
	↓	Presentation of antigens
	↓	TLR-mediated signaling
Adaptive Immune Cells		
B cells	↑	Memory B cells
	↓	Number of naïve cells
	↓	Production of Abs
	↓	Ab specificity

(Continued)

Table 9.2 Age-Related Alterations in Innate Immune Functions

Type of Cell	Effect	Activity
T cells	↑	TCR expression
	↑	Production of cytokines
	↑	CD28-
	↓	Amount of naïve cells
	↓	CD8+ cytotoxicity
	↓	Function of CD4+
	↓	Replicative capacity

IL, interleukin; MIP, macrophage inflammatory protein; TLR, toll-like receptor; TNF, tumor necrosis factor; mDC, myeloid dendritic cell; IFN, interferon; pDC, plasmacytoid dendritic cell; NK, natural killer; PBMC, peripheral blood mononuclear cell; LPS, lipopolysaccharide; MDDC, monocyte-derived dendritic cell; Ab, antibody.

to succeeding experiences of an earlier encountered antigen. The adaptive immune system adapts to these age-related transitions and defends the body effectively against several foreign materials for almost the entire adult life, despite a significant drop in the production of naïve lymphocytes and an inadequate up-keeping of memory lymphocytes post puberty. The gradual reduction in immune function causes vulnerability only in the late stage of life, with a consequent rise in morbidity and mortality owing to infection in older people [45].

9.3.1 B cells

Humoral immune response mediated by B cells is crucial for adaptive immune function as they give rise to a diverse set of antibodies that aid in proficiently clearing antigens including pathogens. Additionally, they play a special part in the immune system via antigen presentation to CD4+ T cells and secretion of cytokines [46]. The development of B cells begins with hematopoietic stem cells (HSCs). Aging has been accompanied with substantial reduction in B cell generation in bone marrow, contributing toward immunosenescence. The most significant impairments that affect B cells during the process of aging are the decreased number of naïve B cells, weakened ability to respond against newer antigens, decrease in clonal expansion ability of memory cells and weak antibody functioning such as less affinity and opsonizing ability [13]. The amount of B cell precursors in bone marrow decreases during aging along with reduction in the percentage and absolute number of total CD19+ B cells. The number of HSCs increases with age but possesses functional defects including self-renewal and homing defects, and they are less effective at generating B cells in comparison to younger population [47]. The human memory B cell comprises two distinct populations: IgM memory (IgG-IgA-CD27+) and switch memory (IgG+IgA+) B cells. IgM memory B cell carries somatically hypermutated iGV region genes which controls *Streptococcus pneumoniae* infections, being the major source of pneumonia in elderly people. On aging, increase in serum IgG and IgA levels is observed, although the number of peripheral B cells and their ability to produce antibodies are decreased. This contradiction is partnered by IgM reduction and unchanged IgD serum levels. Specificity, affinity and isotype switch of antibodies are overblown during aging, which determines enhanced sensitivity of the older people to serious infections and reduces the safeguarding function of vaccines. B cell switch in IgM to IgG, IgE or IgA is reduced during the aging process due to the existence of faults in E2A-encoded transcription factor E47 which is answerable for explaining the diversity of antibody and downregulation of activation-induced cytidine deaminase and class switch recombination (CSR) in B cells [48]. In mature B cell compartments, enhanced expression of activation markers CD27 and CD38 is demonstrated which is established by lower amounts of IgM and IgD in aged people, causing a fundamental transfer from naïve (CD27−) B cell subset to memory (CD27+) component [49].

9.3.2 T cells

Increasing investigation has been laid on the functioning of T cells during the course of aging because of their major effect on overall immune responses. T cell precursors emanate from HSCs in the bone marrow and travel to the thymus for differentiation into naïve T cells. Thymus is answerable for the development and production of mature naïve T cells. Some of the effects of aging on T cells include constant reduction in the production of naïve T cells, minimal repository of T cell receptor (TCR) and weaker activation of T cells. Naïve T cells are necessary for fighting against new exposures in older population. When certain older populations were studied for adaptation theme, the ones with higher *in vitro* CD8+ T cell-mediated proinflammatory reactions to CMV antigens relished survival advantage [50]. The thymus gland deteriorates on aging starting from the puberty known as "thymus involution". This natural process results in the reduction of the amount of naïve T cells with increase in age. Reduction in the amount and frequency of naïve T cell and increase in differentiated T lymphocytes and reduced T cell receptor take place due to thymus involution and impaired functioning. Decline in the proliferation of CD4+ naïve T cell is observed in elderly people and mice along with alterations in cytokine secretion and reduction in responsiveness to stimulation of TCR [45]. Deprivation of CD28 in CD4+ and CD8+ T cells is one of the hallmarks of aging, because this loss alters the production of second messengers and activation of signal pathway, thereby reducing immune reaction to vaccine in geriatric people. Apart from the notable effect of thymic involution on naïve T cells, certain other functional defects observed include reduction in T cell repository, production of IL-2 and enhanced memory T cell population due to low-grade viral infection having a conspicuous impact on the immune functions of the elderly [51]. The recurrence of naïve T cells is diminished within CD8+ T cell compartment, but CD4+ compartment has been found to be more stable during aging, and it is responsible for maintaining the homeostasis. Healthy adults possess several millions of TCR β sequence in the circulating

T cells, but this number is seen to reduce in old age. This reduction in the number of TCR repository forms another aspect characterizing aging T cells [52]. The term "anergy" is used to define the unresponsive T cells during the absenteeism of co-stimulatory signals.

9.4 Intervention of nutraceuticals in aging

Stephen De Felice, founder and chairman of the Foundation for Innovation in Medicine, coined the term "nutraceutical" in 1989 [53]. The term refers to products extracted from herbal products, dietary supplements (nutrients) and refined foods, such as cereals, soups and drinks, which, along with nutrition, are often used as medicine. A substance that provides physiological benefit or protection against chronic diseases is known as a nutraceutical product. They can be used to promote health, slow the progression of aging, avoid chronic diseases, extend the lifespan or enhance the body's structure and functioning [54]. Optimal nutrition is important for healthy aging and maintenance of immune function. The risk of malnutrition increases with age contributing to impaired immune function in elderly people. Nutraceuticals contain several compounds that have the ability to repair immune dysfunction in aging. Several studies have demonstrated that the bioactive ingredients such as phytochemicals, probiotic bacteria and omega-3-fatty acids work against cellular senescence and immunosenescence which go beyond enhancing immune functionality and clear up old and damaged cells (Figure 9.2). Probiotics, prebiotics and dietary fatty acids when provided to elderly population show

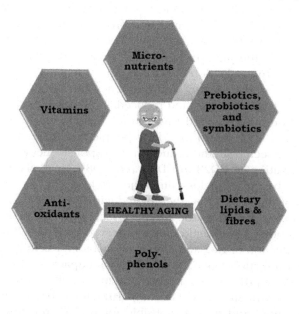

Figure 9.2 *Intervention of nutraceuticals leading to healthy aging.*

anti-inflammatory activities along with improvement in innate and adaptive immune functions and reconstitution of intestinal microbiome. Liberation of nitric oxide, a potent vasodilator and exertion of anti-inflammatory actions, either by activating T regulatory cells or by reducing leukocyte respiratory burst is promoted by the polyphenols.

9.4.1 Micronutrients

Micronutrients such as vitamins and minerals are required for a well-organized performance of the immune system. They are required in trace amounts due to smaller homodynamic range, but the maintenance of required quantity is imbalanced in elderly people. Everyday intake of micronutrients is not sufficient for the aged, due to several reasons like poor socio-economic circumstances, alterations in taste receptors, lack of teeth, alteration in intestinal absorption of food, loss of appetite, gut disorders, changes in metabolism and low energy requirement [55]. This results in deficiency of micronutrients leading to impairment of immune function, although supplementation of micronutrients helps in recovery of cellular activities. Major micronutrients with immunomodulatory effects include zinc, copper, iron and selenium.

9.4.1.1 Zinc

Zinc is an essential trace element which plays an important role in many biochemical reactions and molecular processes having significant effects on synthesis of DNA, apoptosis, signal transduction, differentiation and proliferation of cellular components of the immune system. Several studies have confirmed the decline of zinc levels with increasing age due to insufficient consumption, improper metabolism, infection and inflammation. Zinc plays an important role in many aspects of immune function and is required for several tasks such as suppression of generation of proinflammatory cytokines by monocytes/macrophages and reduce ROS production. Zinc deficiency also affects antibody production. Marginal deficiency of zinc leads to compromise in the immune function and gets balanced in turn on supplementation of zinc along with efficient downregulation of chronic inflammatory responses in aged people. Normal serum zinc concentration decreases the incidence and duration of pneumonia leading to lesser use and duration of antimicrobial therapy, thereby reducing associated morbidity. It has also shown to reduce the incidence of infection in elderly population and reversal of immunosenescence by improving NK cell cytotoxicity, changes in Th1/Th2 balance [56], restoring serum thymulin activity and improved response to vaccines. The incidence of infection was comparatively lower after supplementation of zinc for a period of 12 months in the participants supplemented with elemental zinc gluconate with a dose of 45 mg/day than in test category. Zinc concentration in plasma was found to be high, and production of TNF-α and oxidative stress markers was low in zinc-supplemented participants.

9.4.1.2 Copper

Copper takes active participation in various reactions that promote growth and development. Meat is the prime source of copper in food. Copper is stored in liver as metallothioneins which is in a membrane-bound form. Less consumption of food and beverages especially milk that promotes absorption of copper from the intestine will result in lower concentration of copper in aged people. Deficiency of copper in diet results in immune dysfunction such as neutropenia, impairment in NK cell functioning and decrease in IL-2 production. Complete restoration of immune activity was achieved after copper supplementation in deficient population [57]. Severe copper deficiency lads to impaired immune response, antioxidant activity and altered metabolism in aged people.

9.4.1.3 Iron

Iron is one more important element for the differentiation and proliferation of cells. It forms a part of the process of catalyzation of hydroxy radical formation which is used in the actions of transcription factors like hypoxia-inducible factor-1 or NF-κB. Deficiency of iron results in impaired immune functions and anemia in aged population due to thymic atrophy and reduction of T cells and NK cells. Iron supplementation will maintain immune activities in the elderly and prevent the birth of degenerative disorders.

9.4.1.4 Selenium

Selenium is known to exhibit antioxidant activity, which in turn manages ROS and redox homeostasis, thereby inflammation and immune functions [58]. Decline in the selenium concentration leads to the enhancement of IL-6-mediated inflammation, impairment in calcium flux and protein misfolding. Oxidative damage increases in aging and supplementation of selenium will help in overcoming this damage along with increase in CD4+ T cells and NK cells.

9.4.2 Prebiotics, probiotics and symbiotics

Gut microbiota are compromised in elderly people because of the use of several medications, inadequate supply of nutrients and immunosenescence. Prebiotics (nondigestible oligosaccharides), probiotics (specific strains of *Lactobacilli* and *Bifidobacterium*) and symbiotics (combination or pro and prebiotics) act as immunomodulators, which has proven to be helpful in preventing several disease conditions and promoting healthy aspects in geriatric population. They are useful in cases of malnutrition, lactose intolerance, absorption of calcium and constipation. Both prebiotics and probiotics have been shown to boost immunity, intestinal barrier functions and increased resistance to diseases in elderly people. They are responsible for decreased production of TNF-α, IL-1β and IL-6 and increased generation of anti-inflammatory cytokine IL-10, thereby controlling inflammation in aged people. Antibiotic treatment will cause imbalance in gut microbiota leading to diarrhea and other diseases. Use of prebiotics and probiotics will help in restoration of the good bacteria. Combinational use of prebiotics and probiotics has shown synergistic effect in improving immune functions and facilitating intestinal barrier function. They are also known to enhance innate immune functions by phagocytosis and cytotoxicity against particular bacteria such as *Staphylococcus aureus*, enhance peripheral blood NK cells and reduce expression of CD25 by resting T lymphocytes [59]. A study reported improvement in functional ability of peritoneal immune cells and redox state in aged mice fed with probiotic fermented milk [60].

9.4.3 Dietary lipids

The presence of polyunsaturated fatty acids (PUFAs) in the diet, especially omega-3-fatty acids such as α-linolenic acid (ALA), docosahexaenoic acid (DHA) and eicosapentaenoic aid (EPA), exerts several benefits on inflammatory processes and aging [61]. Omega-3 fatty acids are associated with the maturation and management of immune functions by getting incorporated into the cell membranes of immune cells which straightaway influence receptor-ligand signaling and reduce proliferation of those cells [62]. Upon omega-3-fatty acid supplementation to humans for a period of 4 months, markers of inflammation such as TNF-α and IL-6 in the systemic circulation had decreased. It was found to also restore the Th1/Th2 disparity in aged mice by reducing the production of Th2 cytokines and increasing IL-2 secretion [63].

9.4.4 Polyphenols

Polyphenols are a complex and heterogenous group of secondary metabolites which confer many favorable effects on human health which includes anticancer, anti-diabetes, anti-inflammatory, antioxidant and immunomodulatory properties. Polyphenols are naturally occurring compounds. Flavonoids and nonflavonoids are the two major categories of polyphenols (Table 9.3). The ability of polyphenols to modulate immune functions has been proven in rodent models and humans. The sources of polyphenols are fruits, vegetables, legumes, cereals, cocoa and beverages. The metabolism of anthocyanin produces protocatechuic acid, which in combination with isothiocyanate sulforaphane influences dendritic cells by impairing the generation of proinflammatory cytokines such as IL-6, 8, 12 and 23 in response to LPS stimulation. This suggests the major effect on the NF-κB signaling pathway because DC maturation and stimulation of T cell was unaffected by sulforaphane. Grape polyphenols ameliorated chemokinetic function of neutrophils by modifying CD16 and CD66b expression *in vitro*. Neutrophil bactericidal activity in elderly people was reduced by the consumption of carotenoids. Green tea

Table 9.3 Classification of Polyphenols [55]

Classification of Polyphenols	Source of Origin	Active Ingredient
Flavonoids		
Flavanol	Cocoa, green tea, barley	Catechin, gallocatechin
Flavanol	Grape, green tea,	Epicatechin-3-gallate
Flavanone	Lemon	Eriodyctiol
Flavone	Celery, carrots, parsley	Apigenin, luteolin
Isoflavone	Peanuts, soy	Daidzein, genistein
Flavonol	Apple, cranberry, tomato, wine	Quercetin, kaempferol
Anthocyanin	Blueberry, red apple	Cyanidin, delphinidin
Nonflavonoids		
3,4',5-trihydroxy-trans-stilbene	Wine, nuts, grape seed and skin	Resveratrol

polyphenols, mainly epigallocatechin, exerts antioxidant, anti-inflammatory and anti-cancer benefits. In aging mice model, it was found to improve the number of CD8+ T cells and increase the expression of CD28, a co-receptor molecule on PBMCs. Inflammatory activity was reduced after administration of cocoa powder (40 g/day) for 4 weeks to human subjects by modulating the activation of monocytes which was noticeable by reduced expression of VLA-4, CD36 and CD40 in these cells and reduction of inflammaging, regulated antibodies consequently providing strong anti-immunosenescence activities. Supplementation of stilbenes, resveratrol and arachidin-1 to old mice resulted in an increment in the amount of positive protein-4-associated cytotoxic T-lymphocyte cells and gene expression levels of CTLA-4, interleukin-10, transforming growth factor-β, and Forkhead box P3, hence promoting victorious immune functioning during aging. Consumption of green tea and soybean polyphenols in the daily diet enhanced immune function and redox homeostasis.

9.5 Conclusion

Aging is a biological and physiological phenomenon that is quite complicated. The rapidly increasing global aging population, new infectious agents, and growing care costs have increased the need for alternative health management approaches to be developed. With aging leading to decrease in effectiveness with increasing years, the immune system is significantly remodeled, resulting in an increased risk of chronic disorders, cancers, autoimmunity and vaccine failure. Immunomodulation is also a promising clinical approach to improving older adult wellbeing. As illustrated in this chapter, the fundamental nutritional transistors, such as phytomolecules, essential fatty acids and probiotic bacteria are evolving to alleviate various aspects of age-related detrimental effects on immune system and cell death. It also features a newer outlook on our perception of not only aging development, yet additionally how nutritional influences could be beneficial in helping to boost some of aging's deleterious aspects. Many studies have shown promising results for these compounds in various complications. In conclusion, a balanced mixture of nutraceuticals in the human diet may have a beneficial impact on healthy aging.

References

1. Overview of aging - Older people's health issues. MSD Manual Consumer Version. [cited 2020 Nov 25]. Available from: https://www.msdmanuals.com/home/older-people%E2%80%99s-health-issues/the-aging-body/overview-of-aging.
2. Government policies to address population ageing. 2019;(2020):4.
3. Khan SS, Singer BD, Vaughan DE. Molecular and physiological manifestations and measurement of aging in humans. *Aging Cell.* 2017;16(4):624–33.
4. Mc Auley MT, Guimera AM, Hodgson D, Mcdonald N, Mooney KM, Morgan AE, et al. Modelling the molecular mechanisms of aging. *Biosci Rep.* 2017;37(1):BSR20160177.
5. López-Otín C, Blasco MA, Partridge L, Serrano M, Kroemer G. The hallmarks of aging. *Cell.* 2013;153(6):1194–217.
6. Shanley DP, Aw D, Manley NR, Palmer DB. An evolutionary perspective on the mechanisms of immunosenescence. *Trends Immunol.* 2009;30(7):374–81.
7. Chaplin DD. Overview of the immune response. *J Allergy Clin Immunol.* 2010;125(2):S3–23.
8. Aiello A, Farzaneh F, Candore G, Caruso C, Davinelli S, Gambino CM, et al. Immunosenescence and its hallmarks: How to oppose aging strategically? A review of potential options for therapeutic intervention. *Front Immunol.* 2019;10:2247.
9. Effros RB. Roy Walford and the immunologic theory of aging. *Immun Ageing.* 2005;2(1):7.
10. DeWitt JC, Luebke RW. Immunological aging. In: *Reference Module in Biomedical Sciences.* Elsevier; 2015 [cited 2020 Dec 2]. Available from: http://www.sciencedirect.com/science/article/pii/B9780128012383020067.
11. Franceschi C, Bonafè M, Valensin S, Olivieri F, De Luca M, Ottaviani E, et al. Inflammaging: An evolutionary perspective on immunosenescence. *Ann N Y Acad Sci.* 2006;908(1):244–54.
12. Qin L, Jing X, Qiu Z, Cao W, Jiao Y, Routy J-P, et al. Aging of immune system: Immune signature from peripheral blood lymphocyte subsets in 1068 healthy adults. *Aging.* 2016;8(5):848–59.
13. Costantini E, D'Angelo C, Reale M. The role of immunosenescence in neurodegenerative diseases. *Mediators Inflamm.* 2018;2018:1–12.
14. Nikolich-Žugich J. The twilight of immunity: Emerging concepts in aging of the immune system. *Nat Immunol.* 2018;19(1):10–9.
15. Information NC for B, Pike USNL of M 8600 R, MD B, Usa 20894. How does the immune system work? InformedHealth.org. Institute for Quality and Efficiency in Health Care (IQWiG); 2020 [cited 2020 Dec 4]. Available from: https://www.ncbi.nlm.nih.gov/books/NBK279364/.
16. Alberts B, Johnson A, Lewis J, Raff M, Roberts K, Walter P. Innate immunity. *Mol Biol Cell* 4th Ed. 2002 [cited 2020 Dec 4]; Available from: https://www.ncbi.nlm.nih.gov/books/NBK26846/.
17. Panda A, Arjona A, Sapey E, Bai F, Fikrig E, Montgomery RR, et al. Human innate immunosenescence: causes and consequences for immunity in old age. *Trends Immunol.* 2009;30(7):325–33.
18. Visan I. Aging neutrophils. *Nat Immunol.* 2015;16(11):1113–1113.

19. Mosser DM, Edwards JP. Exploring the full spectrum of macrophage activation. *Nat Rev Immunol.* 2008;8(12):958–69.
20. Linton P-J, Thoman ML. Immunosenescence in monocytes, macrophages, and dendritic cells: Lessons learned from the lung and heart. *Immunol Lett.* 2014;162(1):290–7.
21. Rawji KS, Mishra MK, Michaels NJ, Rivest S, Stys PK, Yong VW. Immunosenescence of microglia and macrophages: impact on the ageing central nervous system. *Brain.* 2016;139(3):653–61.
22. Shaw AC, Joshi S, Greenwood H, Panda A, Lord JM. Aging of the innate immune system. *Curr Opin Immunol.* 2010;22(4):507–13.
23. Perry VH, Holmes C. Microglial priming in neurodegenerative disease. *Nat Rev Neurol.* 2014;10(4):217–24.
24. Cohen M, Matcovitch O, David E, Barnett-Itzhaki Z, Keren-Shaul H, Blecher-Gonen R, et al. Chronic exposure to TGF β1 regulates myeloid cell inflammatory response in an IRF 7-dependent manner. *EMBO J.* 2014;33(24):2906–21.
25. Baruch K, Schwartz M. CNS-specific T cells shape brain function via the choroid plexus. *Brain Behav Immun.* 2013;34:11–6.
26. Letiembre M, Hao W, Liu Y, Walter S, Mihaljevic I, Rivest S, et al. Innate immune receptor expression in normal brain aging. *Neuroscience.* 2007;146(1):248–54.
27. Bachstetter AD, Morganti JM, Jernberg J, Schlunk A, Mitchell SH, Brewster KW, et al. Fractalkine and CX3CR1 regulate hippocampal neurogenesis in adult and aged rats. *Neurobiol Aging.* 2011;32(11):2030–44.
28. Patente TA, Pinho MP, Oliveira AA, Evangelista GCM, Bergami-Santos PC, Barbuto JAM. Human dendritic cells: Their heterogeneity and clinical application potential in cancer immunotherapy. *Front Immunol.* 2019;9:3176.
29. Bruunsgaard H, Pedersen M, Pedersen BK. Aging and proinflammatory cytokines. *Curr Opin Hematol.* 2001;8(3):131–6.
30. Jonuleit H, Kühn U, Müller G, Steinbrink K, Paragnik L, Schmitt E, et al. Pro-inflammatory cytokines and prostaglandins induce maturation of potent immuno-stimulatory dendritic cells under fetal calf serum-free conditions. *Eur J Immunol.* 1997;27(12):3135–42.
31. Caux C, Massacrier C, Vanbervliet B, Barthelemy C, Liu Y-J, Banchereau J. Interleukin 10 inhibits T cell alloreaction induced by human dendritic cells. *Int Immunol.* 1994;6(8):1177–85.
32. Agrawal A, Agrawal S, Cao J-N, Su H, Osann K, Gupta S. Altered innate immune functioning of dendritic cells in elderly humans: A role of phosphoinositide 3-Kinase-signaling pathway. *J Immunol.* 2007;178(11):6912–22.
33. Uyemura K, Castle SC, Makinodan T. The frail elderly: Role of dendritic cells in the susceptibility of infection. *Mech Ageing Dev.* 2002;123(8):955–62.
34. Della Bella S, Bierti L, Presicce P, Arienti R, Valenti M, Saresella M, et al. Peripheral blood dendritic cells and monocytes are differently regulated in the elderly. *Clin Immunol.* 2007;122(2):220–8.
35. Flinsenberg TWH, Compeer EB, Koning D, Klein M, Amelung FJ, van Baarle D, et al. Fcγ receptor antigen targeting potentiates cross-presentation by human blood and lymphoid tissue BDCA-3+ dendritic cells. *Blood.* 2012;120(26):5163–72.
36. Agrawal S, Ganguly S, Tran A, Sundaram P, Agrawal A. Retinoic acid treated human dendritic cells induce T regulatory cells via the expression of CD141 and GARP which is impaired with age. *Aging.* 2016;8(6):1223–35.
37. Agrawal A, Agrawal S, Gupta S. Role of Dendritic Cells in Aging. In: Fulop T, Franceschi C, Hirokawa K, Pawelec G, editors. *Handbook of Immunosenescence: Basic Understanding and Clinical Implications.* Cham: Springer International Publishing; 2017 [cited 2020 Dec 6]. p. 1–15. Available from: doi:10.1007/978-3-319-64597-1_25-1.

38. Witkowski JM, Larbi A, Le Page A, Fülöp T. Natural killer cells, aging, and vaccination. In: Weinberger B, editor. *Interdisciplinary Topics in Gerontology and Geriatrics.* S. Karger AG; 2020 [cited 2020 Dec 6]. p. 18–35. Available from: https://www.karger.com/Article/FullText/504493.

39. Przemska-Kosicka A, Childs CE, Maidens C, Dong H, Todd S, Gosney MA, et al. Age-related changes in the natural killer cell response to seasonal influenza vaccination are not influenced by a synbiotic: A randomised controlled trial. *Front Immunol.* 2018;9:591.

40. Hazeldine J, Lord JM. The impact of ageing on natural killer cell function and potential consequences for health in older adults. *Ageing Res Rev.* 2013;12(4):1069–78.

41. Kaszubowska L, Foerster J, Kaczor JJ, Schetz D, Ślebioda TJ, Kmieć Z. NK cells of the oldest seniors represent constant and resistant to stimulation high expression of cellular protective proteins SIRT1 and HSP70. *Immun Ageing.* 2018;15(1):12.

42. Sagiv A, Burton DGA, Moshayev Z, Vadai E, Wensveen F, Ben-Dor S, et al. NKG2D ligands mediate immunosurveillance of senescent cells. *Aging.* 2016;8(2):328–44.

43. Almeida-Oliveira A, Smith-Carvalho M, Porto LC, Cardoso-Oliveira J, Ribeiro ADS, Falcão RR, et al. Age-related changes in natural killer cell receptors from childhood through old age. *Hum Immunol.* 2011;72(4):319–29.

44. Miyaji C, Watanabe H, Minagawa M, Toma H, Kawamura T, Nohara Y, et al. Numerical and functional characteristics of lymphocyte subsets in centenarians. *J Clin Immunol.* 1997;17(5):420–9.

45. Weng N. Aging of the Immune System: How much can the adaptive immune system adapt? *Immunity.* 2006;24(5):495–9.

46. Ma S, Wang C, Mao X, Hao Y. B cell dysfunction associated with aging and autoimmune diseases. *Front Immunol.* 2019;10:318.

47. Holodick NE, Rothstein TL. B cells in the aging immune system: time to consider B-1 cells: Aging of B cells. *Ann N Y Acad Sci.* 2015;1362(1):176–87.

48. Frasca D, Landin AM, Lechner SC, Ryan JG, Schwartz R, Riley RL, et al. Aging down-regulates the transcription factor E2A, activation-induced cytidine deaminase, and Ig class switch in human B cells. *J Immunol.* 2008;180(8):5283–90.

49. Colonna-Romano G, Bulati M, Aquino A, Pellicanò M, Vitello S, Lio D, et al. A double-negative (IgD−CD27−) B cell population is increased in the peripheral blood of elderly people. *Mech Ageing Dev.* 2009;130(10):681–90.

50. Pawelec G. T-cell immunity in the aging human. *Haematologica.* 2014;99(5):795–7.

51. Salam N, Rane S, Das R, Faulkner M, Gund R, Kandpal U, et al. T cell ageing: Effects of age on development, survival & function. *Indian J Med Res.* 2013;138(5):595–608.

52. Yoshida K, Cologne JB, Cordova K, Misumi M, Yamaoka M, Kyoizumi S, et al. Aging-related changes in human T-cell repertoire over 20 years delineated by deep sequencing of peripheral T-cell receptors. *Exp Gerontol.* 2017;96:29–37.

53. JUL 2000 TPJ. 1. What is a nutraceutical? *Pharm J.* [cited 2020 Dec 8]. Available from: https://www.pharmaceutical-journal.com/cpd-and-learning/learning-article/1-what-is-a-nutraceutical/20002095.article.

54. Nasri H, Baradaran A, Shirzad H, Rafieian-Kopaei M. New concepts in nutraceuticals as alternative for pharmaceuticals. *Int J Prev Med.* 2014;5(12):1487–99.

55. Magrone T, Jirillo E. Nutraceuticals in immunosenescence. In: Neves D, editor. *Anti-Ageing Nutrients.* Chichester, UK: John Wiley & Sons, Ltd; 2015 [cited 2020 Dec 8]. p. 183–202. Available from: http://doi.wiley.com/10.1002/9781118823408.ch5.

56. Uciechowski P, Kahmann L, Plümäkers B, Malavolta M, Mocchegiani E, Dedoussis G, et al. TH1 and TH2 cell polarization increases with aging and is modulated by zinc supplementation. *Exp Gerontol.* 2008;43(5):493–8.

57. Bonham M, O'Connor JM, Hannigan BM, Strain JJ. The immune system as a physiological indicator of marginal copper status? *Br J Nutr.* 2002;87(5):393–403.

58. Huang Z, Rose AH, Hoffmann PR. The role of selenium in inflammation and immunity: From molecular mechanisms to therapeutic opportunities. *Antioxid Redox Signal.* 2012;16(7):705–43.
59. Landete JM, Gaya P, Rodríguez E, Langa S, Peirotén Á, Medina M, et al. Probiotic bacteria for healthier aging: Immunomodulation and metabolism of phytoestrogens. *BioMed Res Int.* 2017;2017:1–10.
60. Hunsche C, Cruces J, De la Fuente M. Improvement of redox state and functions of immune cells as well as of behavioral response in aged mice after two-week supplementation of fermented milk with probiotics. *Curr Microbiol.* 2019;76(11):1278–89.
61. Shahidi F, Ambigaipalan P. Omega-3 polyunsaturated fatty acids and their hhealth benefits. *Annu Rev Food Sci Technol.* 2018;9(1):345–81.
62. Fan Y-Y, Fuentes NR, Hou TY, Barhoumi R, Li XC, Deutz NEP, et al. Remodelling of primary human CD4+T cell plasma membrane order by n -3 PUFA. *Br J Nutr.* 2018;119(2):163–75.
63. Lim BO, Jolly CA, Zaman K, Fernandes G. Dietary (n-6) and (n-3) fatty acids and energy restriction modulate mesenteric lymph node lymphocyte function in autoimmune-prone (NZB×NZW)F1 mice. *J Nutr.* 2000;130(7):1657–64.

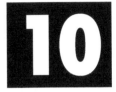

A Transdisciplinary Approach for Ocular Aging Based on Nutritional Principles in Ayurveda

Pankaj Wanjarkhedkar
Deenanath Mangeshkar Hospital & Research Center

Pravin Bhat
Sumatibhai Shah Ayurveda Mahavidyalaya

Anagha Ranade
Regional Ayurveda Research Institute for Fundamental Research

Contents

DOI: 10.1201/9781003110866-10

10.1 Introduction

Ayurveda is a traditional clinical science known as the Indian system of medicine and also is a healing art for life which is in practice since centuries to prevent and treat diseases. It describes cause and effect relationship to all biological activities. Ayurveda outlines the basic need to maintain health and prevents the disease (*swasthasya swasthya rakshanam*) [1].

Ancient Ayurvedic classics describe vision as drishti which is anatomical and the functional unit of eye. The surgical and medical management of ophthalmic diseases demands the understanding of anatomy and physiology of the eye. The knowledge of aetiology, characteristic and pathogenesis of ophthalmic diseases are important for the diagnosis, prevention as well as treatment of the ophthalmic diseases.

10.2 *Netra* (EYE) – Ayurvedic perspective

Eyes are the highly specialized sense organs among the five sense organs in human beings. It has a prime position in all sense organs. Other sense organs perceive the sensation only after senses reach to that organ, but eyes need to focus on the sense object to perceive the image/sense. Loss of function of this sense organ may lead to serious disability in humans rendering them blind. Therefore, it is very important to protect eyes from various diseases [2].

Eyes are organs with a very finer and intricate structure on which the efficient working of all other structures depends to a greater extent. The development of the human eye is a complex series of sequential steps that begins on the 22nd day following fertilization of the ovum and continuous until the postnatal period. The embryonic development of the eye is derived from ectoderm and mesoderm. The neurosensory retina is developed from the neuroectoderm, corneal stroma and endothelium, and choroid is derived from the neural crest, while surface ectoderm gives rise to conjunctival epithelium and lens [3]. The three elements which are important in embryonic development of the eye are growth factors, neural crest cells and homeobox genes. Visual acuity is the most important factor of eyes which depends on the spatial arrangement of the cells of the eye.

10.2.1 Etymological derivations and synonyms of the eye in Ayurveda texts

The Ayurvedic classics described the etymological derivation of the synonyms of eye which have a scientific meaning.

Akshi – Source of reaching to seeing. [Shabdakalpadrum]
Chakshu – Which is responsible for sight. [Vachaspatyam]

Drishti – Source or tool with which one can see. [Shabdakalpadrum]
Netra – Which takes or drives toward knowledge. [Shabdakalpadrum]
Lochana – With which one can see.
Nayan – Which drives toward the subject.

10.2.2 Predominance of *Mahabhoota* in the eye [4]

Like all other organs of body, eyes also exhibit properties of five basic elements, i.e., *Panchamahabhoota* wherein *Teja/Agni* (i.e., fire) is the main predominant *Mahabhoota* which is responsible for sight (Table 10.1).

10.2.3 Association of *Tridosha* and ocular health

Vata, *Pitta* and *Kapha* are the three *Doshas* (basic humours) of the body and are responsible for normal functioning of the body. When these *Doshas* are vitiated, it leads to diseases [5]. The functions of these *Tridoshas* vary from organ to organ, and the altered equilibrium state of these *Doshas* triggers the genesis of the disease pathology.

10.2.3.1 Vata Dosha

Vata is of five types, and their relation with the eye is as follows:

a. **Prana Vayu**: *Prana Vayu* plays an important role in perceiving the sense of an object and carries information to brain through the optic nerve.
b. **Udana Vayu**: *Udana Vayu* gives lustre and strength to the eye.
c. **Vyana Vayu**: *Vyana Vayu* does the function of opening and closure of eyelids and blood circulation in eyes and circulates and propagates body elements *Rasa* and *Rakta* (i.e., plasma and blood) in the body.
d. **Samana Vayu**: *Samana Vayu* nourishes the Jatharagni (i.e., digestive fire). If it is in the equilibrium state, it nourishes the eyes and is responsible for normal functioning of vision.
e. **Apana Vayu**: *Apana Vayu* is responsible for the excretion of waste products from the body. The same way, it does the function of elimination of excessive tears and waste products in eyes.

Table 10.1 Parts of Eye and Predominant *Mahabhoota*

Parts of Eye	Predominant *Mahabhoota*
Muscular part	*Prithvi* (i.e., earth)
Blood	*Teja/Agni* (i.e., fire)
Black part of eye	*Vata* (i.e., air)
White part of eye	*Jala* (i.e., water)
Tear channels	*Akasha* (i.e., space)

10.2.3.2 Pitta dosha

Pitta has been classified into five types as follows:

a. *Pachaka Pitta* – *Pachaka Pitta* functions along with *Samana Vayu*, and it digests the food and divides it into *Saara* (i.e., essence part of food) and *Kitta* (i.e., excreta). This essence portion is responsible for generation of basic body humour, i.e., *Tridosha* in body for normal functioning of body tissue like eyes.

b. *Ranjaka Pitta* – *Ranjaka Pitta* facilitates in appropriate formation of blood components and is the main component of body which is responsible for life.

c. *Sadhaka Pitta* – *Sadhaka Pitta* resides in heart and is responsible for the normal mental status of human beings. This gives strength to the other body tissues like eyes.

d. *Alochaka Pitta* [6] – *Alochaka Pitta* plays an important role for vision. It nourishes the *Chakshu*. When vitiated, eyes are unable to perceive the images which leads to diminution or loss of vision. *Alochaka Pitta* is of two types: *Chakshu Vaisheshik*; this type carries the images from cornea to macula. It is responsible for normal refractive status of eyes. *Buddhi Vaisheshik*: this type of *Alochaka Pitta* carries the image sense from retina to visual cortex and is responsible for the knowledge of an object through afferent and efferent pathways.

e. *Bhrajaka Pitta* – *Bhrajaka Pitta* is located in skin and responsible for lustre, color of the skin and around the eye. *Bhrajaka Pitta* also plays an important role in normal functioning of retina as it is one of the complex forms of skin situated inside the eye.

10.2.3.3 Kapha dosha

Kapha has also been classified into five types but function in eyes maintained by Kledak Kapha and Tarpaka Kapha as follows:

a. *Kledaka Kapha* – *Kledaka Kapha* does the function of unctuousness, healing, moistening in eyes.

b. *Tarpaka Kapha* – *Tarpaka Kapha* is located in Shira (head region). This type of *Kapha* nourishes the structures and centres of the brain and hence is responsible for vision.

10.3 Physiology of vision [7]

Eye is one of the main sensory organs and plays an important role in formation of vision. Its functions are taken as functions of *Dnyanendriya* (sense organ). The function of the eye is to perceive comprehensive knowledge of the external object in the form of an image. The stages of physiology of vision are as follows:

10.3.1 Contact of an object with the sense organ (Indriyarthasannikarsha)

In this stage, the externally situated object is transformed into the form of image in the biological element in the eye.

The mechanism involved in this stage are the following:

a. Conduction of light rays reflected by object to the eye
b. Refraction of light rays into the eye
c. Convergence of light rays inside the eye on macula.

The conduction of light rays is possible in clear media like cornea, lens, aqueous, vitreous. Any opacity in media leads to functional loss of eye. This convergence results in formation of image on macula which represents an object by all means. From Ayurvedic perspective, *Vata* aids in conduction of rays from object to photosensitive retina, whereas *Kapha* is responsible for maintaining the aqueous humour and vitreous humour and thus helps to uphold the normal refractive status of the eye.

10.3.2 Analysis of object (Roopalochanam)

This stage consists of photochemical, electrical changes and nervous stimulation. The photochemical changes are concerned with the rods and cones of retina. The rhodopsin present in the rod cells is a chromoprotein and consists of a reactive part, i.e., chromophore which is responsible for the preferential absorption of light. This chromophore belongs to a family of carotenoids. Sunlight exposure causes the breakdown of the chromophore through several processes and form retinol which is a colourless vitamin A. The visual process is initiated due to the photochemical changes. These photochemical changes give rise to stimulation of nerve endings called as electrical potential. A nerve impulse is formed because of the photochemical and electrical changes which represents the stimulation of retina in turns represents the light rays converged on it. Impulse can be considered as *Indriyasamvedana* (knowledge of an object to sensory organ). *Alochaka Pitta* with the help of mind analyses the object and forms a miniature image of an object.

10.3.3 Stage of knowledge (Dnyanotpatti)

In this stage the visual impulse formed are converted into actual visual sense. This visual sense is transported in brain with the help of *Buddhivaisheshik Alochaka Pitta* and can be reproduced whenever necessary.

The stage of knowledge consists of

a. Conduction of impulse from *Drishtipatala* (retina) to the *buddhi* (i.e., visual cortex)
b. Transformation of visual impulse (*Indriyasamvedana*) to visual sense (*Indriyadnyana*).

Conduction of impulse is confined to visual pathways which are the structural path through which the visual impulses are carried to visual cortex in the form of afferent and efferent pathway. Bipolar cells, optic chiasma, optic tract, lateral geniculate body, optic radiations and visual cortex are the component of visual pathway. The conduction of impulses is done by *Vayu*; especially, it's a function of *Prana Vayu*. The seat of *Prana Vayu* is the brain, so it functions for conduction of impulses.

The conversion of impulse into sense is done by *Buddhivaisheshika Alochaka Pitta*. It receives the impulses sent by optic pathway and gives determination and confirmation of an object. This process is called stage of knowledge.

10.3.4 Visual perceptions

Visual perceptions are of four types as follows:

a. **Light sense**: light sense is the sense through which one can process light in all gradations of intensity. The light minimum (the minimum intensity of light perceived by retina) and the dark adaptation (ability of eye to adapt itself to decreasing illumination).
b. **Form sense**: the ability of an eye by which we can perceive the shape of object is called as form sense. The object seen in bright light are clearer than in dim light. *Pitta Dosha* is more concerned for this phenomenon than *Kapha Dosha*.
c. **Color sense**: the ability of an eye to distinguish between the different colours as exited by light of different wavelengths is called as color sense. The color sense depends upon the functional capacity of *Alochaka Pitta*. So dysfunction of *Alochaka Pitta* may lead to loss of color sense.
d. **Sense of contrast**: the sense by which the objects are distinguished in contrast is called as sense of contrast. It is the ability to perceive small changes in brightness between regions not separated by a defined boundary.

10.4 Theory of aging in conventional science [8]

Gerontologist defines that aging is a complex phenomenon and a process of age-related increase in death rate or failure rate. Biologists define aging as the complete changes that occur in a living organism with passage of time that impact the ability to survive stress, functional impairment and death.

There are two components of aging as follows.

10.4.1 Chronological aging

This is the actual age of a person which is calculated in terms of years, months and days. This is an unstoppable and irreversible process of aging which cannot be changed by medicine.

10.4.2 Biological aging

This is also called as physiological aging which refers to an individual's development and changes based on cellular and molecular parameter. The biological aging is the set of processes that triggers the deterioration of health and leading to death as a function of chronological age. The modern biological theories of aging in humans are divided into programmed and damage or error theories.

10.4.3 Programmed theory

The programmed theory states that aging follows a biological timetable while damage or error theory describes the environmental assaults to the human being that induce the cumulative damage at various levels as a course of aging. The programmed theory is divided into three categories as follows:

10.4.3.1 Programmed longevity

It includes the process of sequential switching on and off of certain genes, while senescence is the time when age-related changes are manifested.

10.4.3.2 Endocrine theory

The pace of aging is controlled by the hormones, and insulin/IGF1 signalling pathway plays an important role.

10.4.3.3 Immunological theory

The immune system in the human being decreases over the period of time in life, and humans become susceptible to infections and aging causes death. Clinical evidence suggests that the immune system in humans is at peak during the middle age of life that is at puberty and adolescent age while as age progresses it declines during geriatric age. This causes the decrease in effectiveness of antibodies hence geriatric population succumbs to newer diseases which leading to cellular stress resulting into death. However the direct association has not been established yet.

10.4.4 Damage/error theory

The damage or error theory has sub categories as follows.

10.4.4.1 Wear and tear theory

Dr. August Weismann, a German biologist, in 1882 proposed the theory of wear and tear which is induced by wear and tear of vital organs resulted due to repeated usage and aging.

10.4.4.2 Rate of living theory

This theory proposes that an organism's rate of oxygen and basal metabolism is indirectly proportional to lifespan of that organism.

10.4.4.3 Cross-linking theory

Cross-linking theory postulates that an accumulation of cross-linked protein damages cells and tissue which slows down the bodily processes resulting into in aging.

10.4.4.4 Free radical theory

According to this theory, the free radicals and superoxide cause damage to the macromolecular parts of the cell, giving rise to accumulated damage cessation of cellular and organic functions. Free radicals attack on macromolecules like nucleic acid, lipids, sugar and proteins.

10.4.5 Somatic DNA damage theory

This theory proposes that aging results from damage to the genetic integrity of body cells.

10.5 Aging in Ayurveda

As described before, Ayurveda is a clinical science that emphasizes on maintenance of health. It comprises eight major clinical disciplines, wherein *Jara* exclusively deals with preventive and curative measures for aging. *Rasayana* therapy, i.e., rejuvenation is the base of prevention of aging described in Ayurveda. *Jara* is also called as *Vriddhavastha* and is the last part of life span caused due to degenerative changes in body. Ayurveda divided the total lifespan of human beings into three parts as *Balyavastha* (i.e., childhood – 0–16 years), *Madhyavastha* (i.e., adolescent age – 16–60 years) and *Vardhakyavastha* (i.e., geriatric or old age – 60 years and above). *Acharya Sharangdhara* typically described the degenerative changes occurring in an individual in various stages. The sequential senescence in aging is an interesting phenomenon (Table 10.2).

Table 10.2 Milestone of Aging/Sequential Loss

Decade	Years of Life	Milestone of Aging
First	1–10	*Bala* (strength)
Second	11–20	*Vriddhi* (growth)
Third	21–30	*Chavi* (aura)
Fourth	31–40	*Medha* (intellect)
Fifth	41–50	*Twak* (skin)
Sixth	51–60	*Drishti* (vision)
Seventh	61–70	*Shukra*
Eight	71–80	*Vikram*
Ninth	81–90	*Buddhi*
Tenth	91–100 & above	*Karmendriya*

10.5.1 *Ayu*

Ayu word is derived from *'Etigaccatiiti Ayu'* indicating the nature of continuation. The measures adapted are for healthy continuity of life [9]. The motor activity and the psyche are maintained by the sensory apparatus called *Indriya*. The functioning of sense is the manifestation from *Dnyanendriya* (sense organs of perception) receives knowledge while *Karmendriya* (organ of action) are responsible for motor functions.

10.5.2 Physiology of aging in Ayurveda [10]

In old age, many diseases may occur due to altered equilibrium state of all the body humour, i.e., *Vata*, *Pitta* and *Kapha*. This altered equilibrium state is a result of factors such as lifestyle, habits, age, etc. The normal functioning of five types of *Vata* is deteriorated with old age (Tables 10.3–10.5).

Table 10.3 Functions Affected by *Vata* in Old Age

Types of *Vata*	Function Affected in Old Age	Ocular Manifestation
Prana	Difficulty in deglutition, delayed digestion, *diminished sensory functions*, breathlessness on slight exertion, etc.	Diminution of vision, loss of function of neurosensory retinal layer
Udana	Slurred speech, memory loss, weakness, loss of normal skin tone	Loss of lustre of eyes
Vyana	Unsteady gate, palpitation, impaired circulation of blood and plasma to various tissue	Ptosis, lagophthalmos, flickering of eyelids
Samana	Decreased or loss of appetite, delayed digestion, reduced metabolic activities related to digestion	Refractive errors (~ Timira)
Apana	Urinary track disorders such as incontinence, disorders related to lower abdomen and pelvic region.	Loss of vision if natural urges are suppressed, diminution of vision

Table 10.4 Functions Affected by *Pitta* in Old Age

Types of Pitta	Function Affected in Old Age	Ocular Manifestation
Pachaka	Loss of appetite, indigestion, formation of *Aama* (i.e., toxins formation within the body) due to indigestion	Refractive errors ~ Timira
Ranjaka	Anaemia, diseases of haemopoietic system, skin diseases	Bitot's spot
Alochaka	Visual disorders, cataract, glaucoma, age-related macular degeneration	Age-related macular degeneration, macropsia, metamorphopsia, cataract, refractive errors, glaucoma
Bhrajaka	Loss of skin lustre, atrophy, wrinkles of skin, loss of elasticity of tissue	Conjunctival xerosis, retinal xerosis, retinitis pigmentosa
Sadhaka	Loss of memory, psychosomatic diseases, state of depression, confusion, delirium	Loss of sense perception of eyes, diminution of vision

Table 10.5 Functions Affected by *Kapha* in Old Age

Types of Kapha	Function Affected in Old Age	Ocular Manifestation
Avalambaka	Cardiovascular diseases	Connective tissue disorders, scleritis
Tarpaka	Improper functioning of sense organs	Sunken eyes, loss of lustre of eyes, cataract, diabetic retinopathy
Bodhaka	Loss of taste sensation, various oral diseases	-
Shleshaka	Locomotor disorders, osteoarthritis, rheumatic arthritis	Blepharitis, arcus senilis
Kledaka	Gastro-intestinal disorders	Refractive errors ~ Timira

10.5.3 Aging and *Dhatu*

Dhatu (i.e., body tissue) is an important component of *Sharir* along with *Dosha*. *Dhatu* is important to maintain the state of equilibrium of body with *Dosha*. These *Dhatu* performs two important functions as *Dharana* (to hold the body) and *Poshana* (nourishment of body). Due to the process of aging, *Dhatu* undergoes functional alterations resulting in sequential weakness of all *Dhatu* (body tissue) (Table 10.6).

10.5.4 *Oja vis-à-vis* aging

The control of homeostasis is done by the important structure in brain and is known as the hypothalamus. The autonomic nervous system, neuroendocrine system and limbic system are controlled and maintained by hypothalamus. The neuroendocrine system also controls the immune system. The release of cytokines and immune mediators activates the immune cells which is responsible for physiological and pathological conditions in the body. The glucocorticoids are the immunomodulatory hormone that can stimulate as well as suppress the immune function. It depends on the type of immune response and the cell involved.

Table 10.6 Functions Affected by Weak Dhatu in Old Age

Dhatu	Function Affected in Old Age	Ocular Manifestation
Rasa	Anaemia, digestion problems, loss of taste, greying and falling of hairs	Sunken eyes, loss of lustre of eyes, asthenopia,
Rakta	Skin diseases, anaemia, hypertension, vertigo, decrease of lustre	Choroidal diseases, retinal vascular disorders, corneal vascularization
Mamsa	Muscular disorder	Squint, sunken eyes
Meda	Prediabetic conditions, splenomegaly	Sunken eyes
Asthi	Diseases of bone	Cataract
Majja	Diseases of joints, functional disorders of brain and eye	Hemianopia, refractive errors, diminution of vision, optic nerve disorders
Shukra	Anaemia, loss of libido	Loss of lustre of eyes, diminution of vision,

Oja maintains the homeostasis with the help of *Vayu* and *Agni*. Nrf-2, i.e., nuclear factor erythroid -2 protein is a transcription factor in human and regulates the expression of antioxidant proteins that protects against the oxidative damage due to injury or inflammation. During the oxidative stress, the Nrf-2 is not degraded and binds to DNA promoter and initiates transcription of oxidative genes and their proteins. Hence the Nrf-2 pathway repair the damage and production of antioxidant enzymes and surviving the genes. When Nrf-2 activator releases the Nrf-2 protein it migrates into cell nucleus and bonds to the DNA at the location of Antioxidant Response Element (ARE) known as Human ARE (hARE). This hARE system is a master regulator of antioxidant system in the human cell. This system deranges once the body undergoes degeneration or aging changes, disease manifestation resulting in cellular damage. This phenomenon is known as oxidative stress and causes production of free radicals. The oxidative stress and associated free radicals cause diseases and symptoms of aging. The self-defence mechanism system of body helps in this condition to fight with released free radicals. The activated Nrf-2 produced antioxidant enzymes like catalase, glutathione and superoxide dismutase (SOD) neutralizes the free radicals in 1:10,00,000 ratio causes the defence against disease and combating the aging. This cellular defence mechanism is known as the *Vyadhi-Utpaad Pratibandakatva* [11].

Ojo-Visramsa is similar to the inactive state of immune system which does not responds when diseases manifested. In this condition *Kapha Dosha* lost its primary function of stability and vitiation of *Vata Dosha* which creates the symptoms like general debility and degeneration in the body tissue succumbs to disease manifestation and symptoms of aging. Loss of normal functions of the body cell and altered immune response are some of the factors seen due to *Ojovisramsa* in old age. *Agnidushti*, i.e., dysfunctioning of the digestive fire also plays a major role in vitiation of *Tridosha* leading to *Ojodushti* causing altered immune response in old age [12].

10.5.5 *Oja vis-à-vis* immunity

Body undergoes degeneration continuously throughout the lifespan. Every cell in the body as well as the body as a whole would be considered as *Sharira* based on the derivation of word *Sharira*. All the cells in the body are having *Dosha Prakriti*, *Dhatu Prakriti*, *Manas* and *Atma*. Each cell has its own channel, i.e., *Srotas* for nourishment. This nourishment is taken or done as per the requirements of metabolic needs determined by the core part of tissue, i.e., nucleus (DNA) and its *Manas* and the metabolic waste expulsion prompted by *Manas*. A normal living cell is having healthy Manas (i.e., knowledge) includes desire and disgust according to the state and metabolic need of a cell. The equilibrium state of *Dosha* decides the normal functioning of a healthy cell. The activation of the *Agni* of cell which is in accordance with the *Prakriti* of cell results in nourishment of cellular structure which performs anabolic (*Kapha*), metabolic (*Pitta*) and catabolic (*Vata*) activities. So there is a difference between every cell regarding the nourishment and metabolism.

Oja is a pure and clear component of *Hridaya*, i.e., heart. It is a quintessence of all the body tissue and is important part of the body to stabilize the structures and tissue in body. The ultimate distillation of each tissue combines together and determines the main immune system of the body which resists the diseases. *Bala*, i.e., *Vyadikshamatva* is the combinative action of *Udana Vayu*, and *Agni* and is a functional component of *Oja*. The state of *Oja* (i.e., somatic health) is determined by the state of *Manas* and *Hridaya*. The core of *Dhatu*, i.e., *Oja* and the last *Dhatu*, i.e., *Shukra* (responsible for reproduction) forms the *Pravara Bala* in body. The *Sanhanana*, i.e., *Vyadhibalavirodhitva*, is achieved with the help of immune activity which is performed by the *Oja*. The innate or acquired immunity develops the resistance to the diseases of the body, known as *Vyadhi Utpadaka Pratibandhakatva*, while humoral or cell mediated immunity determines the *Vyadhi Bala Virodhitva*. In the inflammatory response in immune-mediated mechanism is one of the forms of *Vyadhibala Virodhitva*. The complete immune mechanism is done by *Oja* and controlled by heart (neuroendocrine mechanism). The strength of immune cells, i.e., differentiation power, retention (suppressor T-cell) and memory are due to *Udana Vayu* [13].

Vyadhikashamatva is correlated with concept of immunity in conventional science. *Vyadhikashamatva* is known as the prevention of diseases and ability to resist the diseases [14].

The nutritional status of an individual decides the condition of *Vyadhikashamatva*. *Bala* is an important component of *Vyadhikashamatva* and depends on the *Dhatu, Prakriti, Dosha, Kala* and *Oja*. This *Bala* is further divided into *Sahaj Bala* (i.e., since birth), *Kalaj Bala* (acquire), and *Yuktikruta* (i.e., acquire active and passive immunity). The inheriting characteristic property of human being which is present since birth is called as *Sahaj Bala*. The effect is found to be at chromosomal level. The defects can be pacified with the help of Ayurvedic treatment modalities is the only option in this type.

The *Bala* which is depends upon season, age, time, place of birth is known as *Kalaj Bala*. Place with an abundance of water, ponds, having pleasant climatic conditions is called *Anup Desha* and in *Kapha* dominant area contributes to stronger immunity.

The *Bala* depends upon the acquired health by consumption of wholesome diet, following *Dinacharya* and *Ritucharya, Rasayana* (rejuvenation) and *Vajikarana* (aphrodisiac) therapy [15] is called as *Yuktikruta Bala*. The *Yuktikruta Bala* targeted for enhancing or acquiring the immunity. *Satmya* is adapting the wholesome diet and giving up the unwholesome diet promotes the immune status of an individual.

The consumption of wholesome diet enhances the tissue metabolism thereby promoting optimum formation of *Oja*.

10.5.6 *Dosha* and Immunity

The three *doshas* in the state of equilibrium act like a pillar of the body. The antibodies functions in the body to defeat pathogens and resists the disease, similarly the normalcy of the *Dosha* in the body make the person healthy. *Dosha* function as antibodies as they play the same role in the body for defeating the disease pathology in normalcy state [16].

10.6 Ocular immunity

In 1940, Sir Peter Medawar contributed the term Ocular Immune privilege which suggest a special relationship between the eye and immune system [17].

The immune system protects the body from the invasion of various microbes and toxins within body and thus provides the health. The immune system contains the well-organized defence mechanism in the body in which polymorphonuclear leucocytes, specific killer T-cells, natural killer cells and microphages attacks the invaded pathogen. It induces the inflammatory response to protect the tissue from pathogens, but the inflammation itself causes the functional damage to the tissue leading to necrosis and fibrosis of the tissue. The eyes are the very sensitive organ, and a very little damage to any tissue like cornea, retina and macula may lead to mild to severe impairment of vision [18].

The ocular immune response is the specially developed system by the eye which help to protect the damage to the tissue from inflammatory responses. The ocular immune response is an expression of compromise between the protective immunity to pathogens and the potential injury to the ocular tissue which undergoes irreversible damage. J. Wayne Streilein, who characterized the immune response in the eye as "a dangerous compromise between the immune system and the eye" [19].

The immune system is composed of two functionally distinct components: the innate or nonspecific immune system which is a first line of defence and the adaptive or specific immune system which is a second line of defence and provides protection against the re-exposure of pathogen [20].

Each of the component of Immune system has a subcomponent of cellular and humoral immunity. Innate immune system also has characteristic feature functioning as a barrier to infection [21].

There are two phases of immune response as pathogen recognition and pathogen removal. The adaptive immune system requires some time to react to an infecting agent, while innate immune system reacts to acute infections. The adaptive immune system is antigen-specific and has immunological memory, while innate immunity is not an antigen specific and neither have an immunological memory.

10.6.1 Mucosal immunity

Mucosal surface occupies over $400\,ft^2$ of surface area in the human body [22], which is more than that of surface area of skin. The ocular mucosal surface is having a specialized local immune system. Mucosal immunity of ocular surface acts to provide protection from pathogens and minimizing the risk of inflammation.

10.6.2 Anterior chamber

Anterior chamber is having a specific phenomenon responsible for dynamic immunoregulatory process is Anterior Chamber Associated Immune Deviation (ACAID) which is characterized by an active, antigen specific suppression of immune-mediated inflammation [23].

10.6.3 Cornea

In last 100 years, the Keratoplasty had 90% of success rate. The acceptance of allograft is greater in corneal transplants. If the immune privilege is not perfect, then the chances of graft rejection are greater in keratoplasty. There are numerous mechanisms contributing to the immune privilege of cornea. Immune-mediated ocular disorders and inflammatory diseases.

10.6.4 Ocular allergy

The incidence of allergic eye diseases is known to be increased, and ocular allergy affects 20% of the population annually [24]. Atopy is the term used for allergies to the mucosal surface and skin. The forms of allergic eye diseases are seasonal allergic conjunctivitis (SAC), perennial allergic conjunctivitis (PAC), vernal keratoconjunctivitis (VKC), atopic keratoconjunctivitis (AKC), and giant papillary conjunctivitis (GPC). The SAC and PAC are the commonest forms of ocular allergies, while VKC, AKC and GPC are the other rare forms noted in population of allergic eye diseases. AKC is the chronic form and may leads to vision loss in patients than the other forms. Environmental exposure is an important contributing factor in severity of ocular allergies.

The basic phenomenon in all ocular allergies is the mast cell activation and degranulation which creates the symptoms like itching. The use of mast cell stabilizers, antihistamines, nonsteroidal anti-inflammatory drugs (NSAID), corticosteroids, and cyclosporine is the treatment option in ocular allergies.

10.6.5 Dry eye syndromes

National Eye Institute/Industry Workshop on Dry Eye defined Dry Eye Syndrome (DES) as a group of conditions affecting the ocular surface and tear film characterized by reduced tear secretion and/or excessive tear evaporation associated with symptoms of ocular discomfort [25]. The tear film contains various immunoglobulin and tears are secreted by the lacrimal gland which has CD4+ and CD8+ lymphocytes, dendritic cells, macrophages, and mast cells; in humans, plasma cells in lacrimal tissue [26]. The damage to the autoimmune mechanism may leads to lacrimal gland dysfunction seen in Sjogren's syndrome. Along with patient's education, use of artificial tears like carboxymethyl cellulose eye drops, gels, and emulsions can be used. Warm compress application is also useful. The molecules like cyclosporine are used to prevent the T-cell activation and inflammatory cytokine production in dry eye.

10.6.6 Infections to the eye

The eye is most commonly exposed to various organisms in the external environment and having a defence mechanism against it. Bacterial, viral and fungal keratitis and conjunctivitis are the commonest infectious forms in the eye. The various enzymes in tears which are bacteriostatic in nature plays important role in defence mechanism. Antibiotics and anti-inflammatory eye drops play an important role in such conditions.

Uveitis is an inflammation of the uveal tract of the eye. Uveal track includes iris tissue, ciliary body and choroid. According to affected anatomical structures uveitis is divided into three types as: anterior uveitis (iritis) (Figures 10.1 and 10.2), intermediate uveitis (cyclitis) and posterior uveitis (choroiditis). Whenever all ocular components are involved with inflammatory process, it is called as pan uveitis/iridocyclitis. Apart from the location involvement, uveitis is also classified as infectious and noninfectious.

The infectious uveitis is caused by various microorganisms like bacteria, viruses, fungus, helminths, protozoa, etc., and a group of toxoplasma and mycobacterium tuberculosis are the major specific organism involved in the pathogenesis. The noninfectious uveitis involves a mechanism of autoimmune

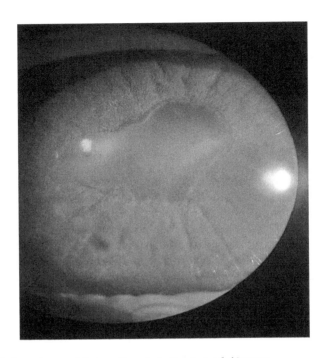

Figure 10.1 Anterior uveitis in a female patient aged 40 years.

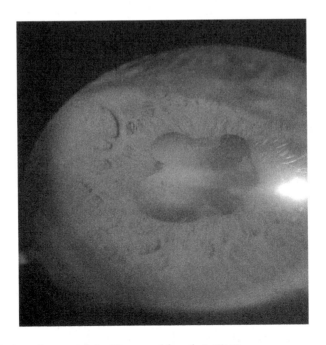

Figure 10.2 Anterior uveitis in 63-year-old male patient.

response to the tissue specific antigen in uveal tract and retinal tissue. The retina-specific CD4⁺ T-cells breaks the blood retina barrier by targeting the antigen in the eye [27].

Toxoplasmosis is having around 20%–60% of total posterior uveitis and manifest symptomatic ocular infection caused due to specific immunity [28].

10.7 Ocular aging [29]

As the body undergoes degenerative changes in a lifespan of human being, eyes are also not exception to this. In fact, the age-related changes are most of the time manifested first in eyes. All the anatomical structures and components of eye undergoes aging changes causing visual problems in human being. There is need of an hour to differentiate the changes due to aging and other eye diseases in human being. The understanding of various theories in modern science is explained earlier in this chapter. The different changes occur in the eye due to aging are as follows:

10.7.1 Eyelids and lacrimal system

Skin folds and wrinkles appear on eyelids due to tissue atrophy in which mesodermal content of body begins to shrink. As the skin of eyelid is thinnest in the body, shrinkage and wrinkles lead to loss of structural support to tarsal plate, canthal tendon and orbicularis oculi muscle as well causes orbital fat prolapse, eyelid malposition, blepharoptosis and tearing. A pinch test can be performed to see the strength in lower lid laxity. The amount of eyelid pinched away from the eyeball and the relative delay and the absence of snap in the lower lead to regain in its normal anatomical position is noted. Reduction in orbital fat because of aging causes the sunken appearance of eyeball.

Punctal eversion, entropion, and ectropion (Figure 10.3) are some of the abnormalities caused due to progressive laxity of eyelids as an aging process. Age-related eyebrow ptosis or involutional eyelid ptosis are caused due to disinsertion of levator palpebrae superioris muscle. Dermatochalasis or pseudoptosis manifested due to anterior migration of preaponeurotic fat. Eyelid malposition's can cause continuous watering and recurrent infections of the lacrimal apparatus, resulting in decrease cystitis.

10.7.2 Corneal changes

The corneal curvature changes lead to astigmatism. This causes the difficulty in focusing the target without glasses. Due to aging, cornea undergoes changes like loss of corneal lustre, corneal sensitivity, and increase in corneal fragility occurs. Age-related structural dystrophic changes occurs in corneal

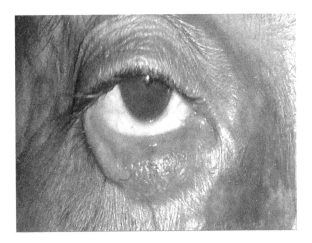

Figure 10.3 *Senile ectropion in a female patient aged 72 years.*

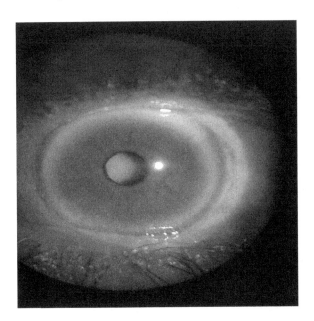

Figure 10.4 *Arcus senilis with immature cataract in a male patient aged 67 years.*

epithelium, stroma and endothelium. The most common aging change noted is Arcus senilis (Figure 10.4), which is seen in the form of white prominent line around the limbus on cornea. Hudson-Stahli line, Hassle Henley bodies, Krukenberg Spindle, and corneal guttata are some other asymptomatic degenerative changes noted in cornea.

Corneal endothelial layer is the innermost layer of cornea which, once get degenerated cannot get regenerated again. The maintenance of corneal deturgescence is done by endothelial cells. The average endothelial cell count is around 3,000 cells/mm^2 at birth, which may decrease up to 1,000 cells/mm^2 at old age, resulting in Fuch's endothelial dystrophy, corneal opacity and decrease in quality of vision.

10.7.3 Trabecular meshwork and uveal changes

Uveal tissue like ciliary muscles plays an important role in accommodation. Zonules/suspensory ligaments are attached to the ciliary muscles and encapsulated lens, which changes the shape of lens during near and distant vision. Due to aging process, decrease in amplitude of ciliary muscles results in presbyopia, which is a physiological refractive error. Iris tissue also loosen its pigments results in atrophic changes of iris. Increased pigmentation in trabecular meshwork may precipitate glaucoma due to blocked outflow.

10.7.4 Lens

Lens is an integral part of eye which is responsible for refraction along with cornea. It is made up of outer cortex, and central nucleus part. Due to aging and increased oxidative stress in lens fibres, transparent and crystalline lens undergoes degenerative changes and it loosen its transparency causing the sclerotic changes in nucleus resulted in cataract. Cataract is in the first position to cause reversible blindness in world and seen in geriatric age group due to aging and metabolic changes.

10.7.5 Vitreous

Vitreous is a gel like structure in the posterior segment of eye which maintains the integrity and shape by its volume. Vitreous is a collagen fibril which may undergo liquefaction process and cause posterior vitreous detachment due to aging process. The collagen fibrils and hyaluronic acid also undergoes irreversible changes, causing a formation of band of vitreous manifested as floaters in eye in elder people. It can also be manifested in young adults due to degenerative process in vitreous.

10.7.6 Retina

Neurosensory retina is the most sensitive structure of visual apparatus which provides sense of vision. The neuro sensory elements like rods and cone cells, retinal nerve fibre layer, and retinal ganglionic cells constitute the visual apparatus. The process of aging leads to degeneration of these neuro sensory elements resulting in decreased visual acuity and contrast sensitivity, the visual field, retinal ganglion cell loss, increased dark adaptation threshold, retinal thinning, tessellation, etc. The process of apoptosis is also one of the factors resulted because of the process of aging and leads to loss of vision in glaucoma. Apoptosis is a genetically controlled programmed cell death. The important part of retina is macula, where cone cells are found in abandoned quantity and are responsible for the visual acuity. The process of aging causes destruction of cytoplasmic material by retinal pigment epithelium and collection of debris in macular region results in formation of drusen and causing age-related macular degeneration (ARMD). ARMD is of two types as dry and wet ARMD. Dry ARMD accounts for 90% and associated with maculopathy and geographical atrophy of retina.

10.8 Clinical conditions due to aging and immunity

1. Aging process involves the controlled and chronic inflammatory process and dysregulation in immune system mechanism. Hence this dysregulation leads to functional loss of lacrimal gland resulted in decreased innervation and secretory activity [30].
2. Age-related macular degeneration is a complex multifactorial degenerative disease that causes irreversible loss of vision in old-age peoples. The structural and functional changes in retinal pigmentary epithelium play an important role in pathogenesis of ARMD. The immune system dysfunction establishes the onset of changes of ARMD in retina due to old age (Figure 10.5). The macro- and microglia which are the part of retinal glial cells play a major role in the pathogenesis of ARMD [31].

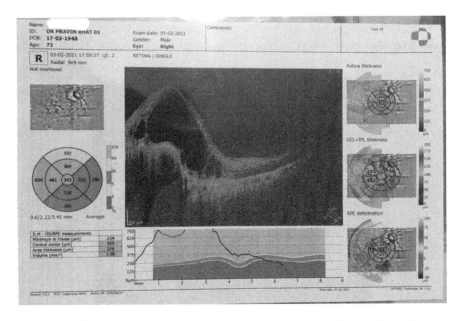

Figure 10.5 *Ocular coherence tomography image of choroidal neovascular membrane in age-related macular degeneration in male patient aged 72 years.*

3. Uveitis in the geriatric population is 14.7% of the total uveitis population reported worldwide. The developing countries are the sufferer representing 18.6% of the uveitis population. Some of the studies quoted that the female predominance is more in geriatric uveitic population [32].

4. Senile age-related cataract (ARC) is the leading cause of reversible blindness and seen in geriatric population widely across the globe. Many research has been done on this disease, but there is no nonsurgical treatment available till date. There are many factors including age, sex, oxidation, physical trauma, diet, and medications contribute the disease pathology [33] (Figures 10.6 and 10.7).

5. Presbyopia is the physiological refractive error having loss of accommodation to see near objects. Presbyopia develops over the period

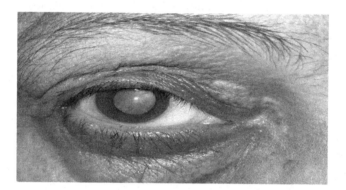

Figure 10.6 Hypermature cataract in a 65-year-old female patient.

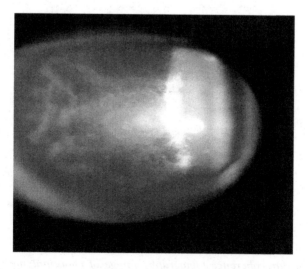

Figure 10.7 Mature cataract in a 70-year-old male patient.

of time and progresses with aging. The symptoms are usually noted after the age of 40. Headache or fatigue after reading or doing close work is the presenting symptom. Patients with presbyopia hold reading materials at arm's length. Correction of presbyopia can be done with reading glasses.

6. Floaters in vitreous indicate aging of the vitreous which is a complex biochemical and structural process. The opacities in the vitreous body are called floaters and are form the shadow on retina. Floaters are seen in the form of small objects in the visual field and are perceived as lines, circles, dots, cobwebs, clouds, flies or of any other shape. Floaters have random movement in the eye and are termed as kinetic opacities. Floaters are distinctly noted on white and bright background while looking at the sky. The perception of floaters is known as myodesopsia (muscae volitantes in Latin) [34].

7. Dry eye is a multifactorial disease and is prevalent eye disorder affecting many people worldwide. Meibomian Gland Dysfunction is one of the contributing factors in dry eye. The meibomian gland dysfunction leads to evaporative type of dry eye as the secretion of lipid layer decreases leading to evaporation of aqueous layer of tear film. Aging is the major risk factor for Meibomian gland dysfunction. Dryness may lead to foreign body sensation, itching, burning and, in some patients, loss of vision due to keratitis [35] (Figure 10.8).

8. Retinitis pigmentosa is a genetic disease in which retinal pigmentary epithelium undergoes degeneration leading to loss of peripheral vision. The macular thickness decreased in RP patients between 45 and 55 years old, whereas it increased in RP patients older than 55 years [36].

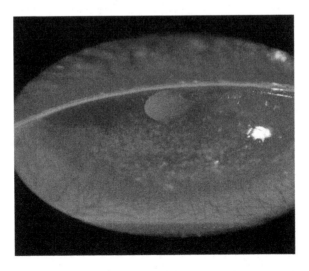

Figure 10.8 *Fluorescein-stained image of dry eye in a female patient aged 40 years associated with rheumatic arthritis.*

9. Retinal pigmentary epithelium undergoes degenerative changes during aging process. The age-related changes in retina leads to visual impairment. The first protein database enumerated in some studies which gives future directions to treat the age-related retinal changes [37].

10. Refractive error occurs due to change in the axial length of eyeball. But the anterior equatorial dimensions also play an important role which seems to be due to the aging process and are seen in adult eyes [38].

11. Aging results in impaired ocular surface response to infections leading to immunodeficiency, increased reactivity to self-antigen. This results into chronic inflammation and autoimmunity [39]. Some studies have shown the association between aging and decreased tear production as well as alteration in surface immunity [40] (Figure 10.9).

12. The eye is called as the window to the soul of the immune system and gives clues to understand the mechanisms of immune responses in transplantation and autoimmunity. The understanding of the pathways of ocular immune regulation is helpful to develop the therapies as the eye is having a special immune privilege [41].

10.8.1 Cataract: The most common condition in ocular aging

Lens is a clear, avascular optical structure situated behind iris in posterior chamber encapsulated in anterior and posterior elastic capsule. The elastic anterior capsule contains epithelial layer which gives rise to the newer

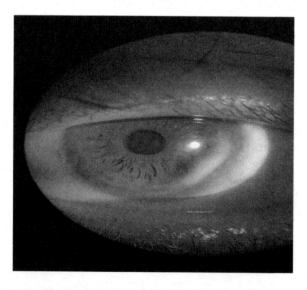

Figure 10.9 *Corneal changes in a 38-year-old male patient after vernal keratoconjunctivitis.*

lens fibres. The nucleus possesses the older lens fibres and are compactly arranged. The lens fibres lost its transparency as the aging process starts and the derangement in the pathway and physiology of lens leads to formation of Cataract. Cataract is the leading cause of reversible blindness worldwide. The senile age group prevalence rate is very high [42].

Along with the aging, smoking, alcohol consumption, exposure to UV light, nutritional deficiencies and lower socioeconomic status are the contributing factors in cataractogenesis. The Framingham Eye Study reported the higher number older population of more than 75 years of age (45.9%) suffering from loss of vision of 20/30 (6/9) or worse [43].

The Beaver Dam Eye Study reported 38.8% of men and 45.9% of women older than 74 years [44]. In India, 82% of the geriatric population in the age group between 75 and 85 years suffered from cataract [45].

The number of cases of reversible blindness are increasing worldwide due to less number of ophthalmologist and more the disease burden in society. The only possible treatment is surgery which is advanced to Femtosecond laser cataract surgery from couching technique invented by Sushruta in 600 BC.

In Ayurveda, *Linganash* is the term used for loss of vision. *Linganash* is broadly divided into endogenous and exogenous types. The endogenous type of *Linganash* describes the anatomical and etiological description. According to *Dosha*, i.e., body humour involved, *Kaphaj Linganash* is the only surgically curable type described in Ayurvedic classics [46].

The plant based drugs having high potency and less side effects are gaining interest in researches for cataract. The nutraceutical extracts of roots, fruits, leaves of some plants like *Vaasa (Adhatoda vasica), Allium cepa, Angelica dahurica, Biophytum sensitivum, Cassia fistula, Citrus aurantium, Cochlospermum religiosum, Haridra (Curcuma longa), Amalaki (Embelica officinalis), Karela (Momordica charantia), Shigru (Moringa oleifera), Tulasi (Ocimum sanctum), Origanum vulgare, methika (Trigonella foenum) and Nirgundi (Vitex negundo)* are studied for their anticataract activity. The polyphenols, vitamins and carotenoids are the major antioxidant component of the Ayurvedic plants useful in prevention or delaying the cataractogenesis. Hence the natural antioxidant biomolecules are effective in cataract [47].

Turmeric is the widely used spice and herbal medicine in India is having antioxidants, xenobiotic and tumour inhibition activity and proven in delaying cataractogenesis in rats [48].

The rejuvenating therapy like *Rasayana* medicines described in Ayurvedic classics are rich source of antioxidants, polyphenols, flavonoids, adaptogenic, immunomodulatory, immunostimulant, cytoprotective and rejuvenating properties. *Rasayana* medicines are having a high therapeutic potential in delaying the aging process and thus cataractogenesis. *Chyavanprash, Medhya Rasayan, Brahmi Rasayan, Guduchi (Tinospora cordifolia), Ashwangdha*

(*Withania somnifera*), *Yashtimadhu* (*Glycyrrhiza glabra*), *Vacha* (*Acorus calamus*), and *Triphala* are some of the reported drugs having DNA repair properties and telomerase activator and protective effect [49].

10.8.2 Ocular malignancies

The incidence for retinoblastoma, uveal melanoma, conjunctival melanoma, and lacrimal gland carcinomas was studied. Age-conditional probability of developing cancer is a conceptually friendly means of understanding and communicating risk. It is particularly useful in comparing the risks of uncommon or rare ocular cancers. The assessment of risk in terms of age-conditional probability is a versatile and an unutilized pedagogical tool. The risk of each malignancy displayed age-dependent variation. For adult malignancies, males are having higher risk in all age intervals. Uveal melanoma had the greatest cumulative lifetime risk. The probability of developing retinoblastoma declines precipitously after the age of 3 years [50].

Compared with mid adults and older adults, young patients manifested a higher proportion of iris melanoma. Compared with older adults, young and mid adults showed smaller melanoma basal dimension and lower tumour-related metastasis and death [51].

10.9 Aetiology as per Ayurveda in current lifestyle

In case of ocular diseases in Ayurveda, there is a description of subtle etiological factors in the verse *Ushn-abhitaptasya-jalapraveshaat* [52]. Many of these are closely related to the present faulty lifestyle habits. The aging phenomenon is closely associated with lifestyle regimens. The same holds true in case of ocular diseases, viz. *Ushnabhitaptasyajalapraveshaat* is nothing but the sudden exposure to cold conditions after being previously in hot climatic conditions, or drinking cold water before or after drinking hot tea or coffee. The consumption of very cold water after being in sun or exposure toward cold showers after strenuous exercise/activities. This refers to the *svedawaha-srotasa-dushti* due to faulty practice of *sheeta/ushna*. *Sveda* is closely associated with *alochaka pitta* in case of eyes. *Doorekshanaat*, i.e. regular or repeatedly concentrating the distant object for a longer time which is commonly seen in drivers, army and air-force personnel, etc. *Swapana-viparyaya, Kopa, shoka, Klesha* (~undue stress), *Sukshma-nirikshanaat* refers to looking at minute things for a longer time repeatedly as in cases of biology scientist who are using microscopes, manuscriptologist dealing with manuscripts having a very small font, gemologist, IT professionals using laptops or PCs for longer hours without break, and even children using mobile phones for a longer time. *Atisvedana* refers to exposure to excessive sudation, which is familiar in case of trendy sauna baths, excessive gym, people working near furnaces, mine workers, local hotel chefs, and costal tourism. Dietary factors include *Shuktarnala, amla nishevanan,* i.e., excessive/ abnormal consumption of fermented foodstuffs, viz. alcoholic drinks, bakery products, etc., and thus, we see that all these faulty lifestyle habits are the prime cause of ocular aging too. These disrupt the equilibrium of the three *dosha*, and thus, the diseases start manifesting.

10.10 Pathogenesis vis-à-vis dietary misconduct in ophthalmic disorders

Ayurveda focuses more on dietary conduct as a major factor in prevention as well as management of disease. In case of ocular disorders, consumption of sour foods, fermented foodstuffs, eating *vidahiahara* and wrong meal timings have been indicated as prime etiological factors. It is believed to hamper function of *Alochaka pitta* which further leads to perception related vision deficits. The nutritional insult occurs in two ways as described in compendia. Santarpanam, i.e., overnutrition, or *Apatarpanam*, i.e., malnutrition/under nutrition.

The connection of diet, gut function and eyes is a unique feature of Ayurvedic ophthalmology. Ayurveda always emphasizes the importance of dietary conduct which when not followed hampers the *tridosha function* and metabolism up to tissue levels which then sets in different pathologies.

Scientists are now trying to unveil the influential role of dietary factors in ocular health. The retina itself is the most active metabolic part of the eye which is functional counterpart of *Alochak pitta*. The gut microbiota research has helped establish the holistic facts of Ayurveda to a certain extent. The *agnimandya* or *dhatuvaishamya* is entitled to be the aetiology for pathologies as per Ayurveda. This holds true as dysbiosis in gut microbiome has an impact on ocular health. For instance, the connection between dysbiosis in gut which manifest the development of bacterial keratitis in an Indian cohort. Dysbiosis increases the susceptibility of ocular pathogens in projecting the disease more pronouncedly [53]. In another study gut microbial diversity and abundance in patients of uveitis was different than that of healthy individuals. This clearly indicates the possible links of *mahasrotasa, ahara* and *netra roga* as per Ayurveda [54,55].

Faulty dietary habits comprising of high-fat diet [56], high glycaemic index diet [57] are leading causes for macular degeneration.[58]. These have close resemblance to *vishamaashana, Samashana, Guru ahara, Shuktaahar*. The *doshaprakopa* that is vitiation, in case of ocular diseases occurs probably due to the cascade of events occurring in gut which develop sub clinical inflammatory state [59]. The healthy butyrate producing gut microbiota, viz. those affiliated to Lachnospiraceae and Ruminococcaceae and to the genera Megasphaera, Roseburia, Lachnospira, Acidaminococcus, and Mitsuokellamultacida are found decreased in fungal keratitis patients and pathogenic were increased in the consortium [59–63].

Further involvement of links in gut-to-ocular axis has been established wherein it has been observed that gut dysbiosis (~*Doshavaishamya* due to *Agnimandya*) modulates the ocular surface inflammatory response.

In metabolic diseases lie diabetes and obesity, ocular manifestations are linked to gut dysbiosis wherein a lower proportion of bacteroides has been correlated with a higher blood glucose concentration and thus posing risk of retinopathy [64].

In humans, relative abundances of gut microbiota, namely, Ruminococcaceae and Prevotella, are higher in AMD patients as compared to controls without disease [65]. In another study, higher relative abundances of Anaerotruncus, Oscillibacter, Ruminococcus torques, and Eubacterium ventriosum were documented in individuals with AMD, whereas Bacteroides eggerthii was enriched in controls [66]. Interestingly, Ruminococcus has mucin degradation abilities, Oscillibacter reduces tight junction strength, and Eubacterium induces production of IL-6 and IL-8 cytokines, which would result in increased gut permeability and inflammation whose effects may reach target organs such as the eye.

10.11 Ayurveda guidelines for ocular diseases with nutraceutical perspectives

Ayurveda has a unique management of diseases which again target the strengthening of gut function. *Langhana*, i.e., intermittent fasting is readily prescribed in Ayurveda in case of *santarpanjanyavyadhi*.

In an animal study on diabetic retinopathy, intermittent fasting was adopted which lead to restoration of Bacteroides to firmicutes ratio thus correcting the pathology and preventing the manifestation of retinopathy [67].

10.12 Do's and don'ts in eye diseases as per Ayurveda

The basis of all functions of the body is Ahara (diet) and hence the most important etiological factor of eye diseases. The functional elements of the body, i.e., Dosha and Dhatu (tissue), are created, maintained and destroyed by the dietary factors. The dietary factor which adversely affect the eyes are known as *Achakshyushya Ahara* (diet affecting the functional component of eye, i.e., vision). The following is the list of beneficial and nonbeneficial dietary and other factors list (Table 10.7).

Table 10.7 Beneficial Dietary Regime as Recommended in Texts of Ayurveda

Sanskrit Name	English/Latin Name	Food Category
Surana	Elephant foot yam Amorphophallus companulatus	Vegetable/Medicinal
Patola	Snake gourd Trichosanthesdioeca	Vegetable/Medicinal

(Continued)

Sanskrit Name	English/Latin Name	Food Category
Vartaka	Brinjal	Vegetable/Dietary
Karvellaka	Momordica charantia L.	Vegetable/Dietary
Kadali	Unripped Banana	Fruit
Mulaka	Raphanaus sativus L.	Vegetable/Dietary
Meghanada (Tandulaja)	Amaranthus blitum	Vegetable/Dietary
Dhanyaka	Coriandrum sativum L.	Vegetable/Dietary
Dadima	Pomegranate Punica granatum	Fruit
Draksha	Grapes – Vitis vinifera L.	Fruit
Shigru	Drumstick Moringa oleifera Lam.	Vegetable/Dietary + Medicinal
Ghritam	Ghee	Dairy product
Godugdha	Cow's Milk	Dairy product
Ajadugdha	Goat Milk	Dairy product
Saindhava	Rock salt	Salt
Mudga	Vigna radiate L.	Cereals
Godhuma	Wheat	Dietary
Kulattha	Macrotyloma uniflorum Lam.	Cereals
RaktaShali	Brown Rice	Dietary
Yava	Barley	Dietary
Triphala	Combination of Terminalia chebula, Terminalia bellerica, Emblica officinalis	Medicinal
Katak	Strychnos potatorum L.	Medicinal
Amalaki	Indian gooseberry Emblica officinalis	Medicinal & Dietary
Kumari	Aloe vera L.	Medicinal
Punarnava	Boerhavia diffusa L.	Medicinal
Kakamachi	Solanum americanum Mill.	Medicinal
Shatavari	Asparagus racemosus willd.	Medicinal
Jeevanti	Holostemmaada kodien Schult.	Medicinal
Vastuka	Dysphania ambrosioides L.	Medicinal

10.13 Dietary recommendations for maintaining healthy ocular functions

Cereals, rice and wheat must be preferred followed by barley.

Pulses: green gram and dolichos are suggested.

Herbs: *Kumari* (Aloe vera), *jeevanti* (Leptadenia reticulata), *punarnava* (Boerhavia procumbens), *patola* (Trichosanthesdioca), *karvella* (bitter gourd),

Table 10.8 Nonbeneficial for Eyes as Documented in Texts of Ayurveda

Food	Life Style
Too sour & Spicy food	Day-time sleeping and night awakening
Baked food items	Overeating
Over cooked food items	Daily hot water head bath
Fried food items	Smoking tobacco
Milk with fish	Suppression of natural urges
Milk with fruit	Reading/sleeping in wrong position
Hypercaloric food items	Looking too small or too distant objects continuously
Refined Carbohydrates	Excessive indulgence in sex
Sea food	
Masha (Vigna mungo L.)	
Sour gruel	
Alcohol	
Pineapple	
Sour Mango	

grapes, *triphala*, seeds of coriander, Brown rice, *yava* (barley), *mugda* (green gram), *vanyakultha* (Dolichosbiflorus) (Table 10.8)

The word Chakshyushya means nourishment of the sense organ, i.e., eye. The sedentary lifestyle and ignorance to proper diet putting ocular health at risk. The prevention and promotion of ocular health is described in various Ayurvedic classics. The regular intake of Chakshyushya diet along with changes in lifestyle can prevent the ocular diseases and reduces the chances of ocular aging. The Chakshyushya class of diet and lifestyle in Ayurvedic classics is as follows [68,69]:

- *Triphala* (tri of T. chebula, T. bellarica, and E. officinalis): *Triphala* is a combination of three fruits, i.e., *Haritaki* (T. chebula), *Bibhitak* (T. bellarica), and *Amalaki* (E. officinalis) in equal proportion. This combination is having rejuvenation properties especially in eyes. It balances the body humour, i.e., *Vata, Pitta*, and *Kapha. Triphala* is having antioxidant, anti-inflammatory and immune modulatory properties [70].
- *Ghrita* (ghee/clarified butter): Ghee is one of the types of unctuous substance mentioned in Ayurvedic classics. It is a rich source of omega 3 fatty acids, omega 6 fatty acids and vitamin A, vitamin D, vitamin E and vitamin K which are very essential for maintenance of vision. The plain ghee and medicated ghee are having high utility in prevention of ocular disease. The ghee is having a lipophilic action and by virtue of its action it reaches the cell membrane which also contains lipid. The lipophilic action helps to penetrate the corneal layers and hence

nourishes the eye. Ghee reduces the oxidative stress in the tissue and prevents the further damage of tissue [71].

- *Madhu* (honey): Honey is having antioxidant and anti-inflammatory properties. Local instillation of honey stimulates the epithelialization of the tissue and important in wound healing. It contains flavonoids and phenolic acid.
- *Yava* (barley): It is a Hordeum vulgare from family Poaceae. *Yava* are rich in calcium, phosphorous and iron and having antioxidant property. It is a rich source of biologically active nutrients like tocopherol, vitamins, phenolic acid, minerals, etc., which plays a vital role in age-related macular degeneration [72].
- *Padabhyanga* (foot massage): Regular practice of foot massage with the help of bronze metal pot is proven to be beneficial for the eyes. It rejuvenates the ocular tissue as the lens and skin is having the same surface ectodermal origin. So application of ghee for foot massage or sesame oil for body massage and head massage increases the vision and delays the aging process.
- *Shatavari* (Asperagus racemosus): *Shatavari* is having the anti-inflammatory, antioxidant and immunostimulant property. Shatavari is having a neuroprotective effect in neurodegenerative diseases. It rejuvenates the body tissue by virtue of its action and said to be beneficial for eyes in Ayurvedic classics. The steroidal saponins present in the A. racemosus is proven to have an immune stimulant action [73].
- *Mudga* (Green gram): Green grams are from Fabaceae family and are rich source of vitamin A, vitamin B6, niacin, and vitamin K. It also contains carbohydrates, proteins, calcium and iron. Green gram is a complete package of nutrients and can be consumed in the form of noodles, papad, fried green gram, daal, and soup [74].

The metabolic activity of the gut microbiota is depends on the dietary content, i.e., macronutrients, micronutrients and various phytochemicals. Eating a variety of plant food like drumsticks, curcumin, buttermilk, different lentils especially green gram, cow's milk and ghee which are sources of vitamin A is useful in preventive ophthalmology. The use of *Thali* diet is supposed to provide diverse different ingredients through the contents, and one may include Chakshyushya diet for prevention of ocular aging and protection of immunity [75].

In nutshell, Chakshyushya Dravyas are having an immune modulatory property which is useful for prevention of ocular aging and protection from various ocular diseases. The oxidative damage of lens tissue is prevented by the physiological action of presence of glutathione and ascorbate in Chakshyushya Dravya. The presence of various vitamins, polyphenols, tannins and zinc in Chakshyushya Dravya are useful for protection of eyes from free radical damage and degenerative diseases of eye like ARMD.

10.14 Ocular surface microbiome (OSM) – A link for therapeutic activity of *Kriya-kalpa* in *netraroga*

Proteobacteria, Firmicutes and Actinobacteria are the three dominant phyla in the ocular surface microbiome. Any alterations in the bacterial community on the scleral and corneal surface has been documented in development of red eye in contact lens wearers, endopthalmitis, dry eye, keratitis, etc. [76].

This can establish a connection to the possible link of therapeutics of *bidalak, anjana, Akshi tarpan, Aschyotana, Parisheka*. Toll-like receptors play a pivotal role specially in innate and adaptive immune responses on the ocular surface. These responses are closely associated with *Sahaj Bala* and *Yuktikruta Bala*, respectively, in Ayurvedic parlance. Intracellularly expressed (toll-like receptors) TLR2s and TLR4s contribute to an immune-silent environment at the ocular mucosal epithelium [77].

The medicated oils and ghee preparations in Ayurveda prescribed in *Kriya kalpas* probably mediate in the TLR mechanism of balancing the interplay between innate and adaptive immune responses on ocular surface. Also, ocular secretory IgA levels depend on the commensal microbiome [78]. These practices must be a part of daily as well as seasonal regimen (*Dinacharya* and *Rutucharya*).

10.15 Summary

Most of the ocular diseases, whether benign or malignant, have an etiological impact of aging and immunity. The management of ocular aging needs to be considered with the multidimensional approach as recommended in Ayurveda, including the concepts of ocular immunity, *Tridosha* equilibrium, *Chakshushya* medicines, diet with nutritional principles and lifestyle modifications to prevent the diseases primarily. A prospective cohort study shall contribute to generate robust evidence supporting these observations and experiences in the classic texts.

References

1. Acharya JT (Ed). *Charak Samhita by Agnivehsa*. Sutrasthana Arthedashamahamuliya Chapter. 30, Verse 26. 3rd ed. Bombay: Nirnay Sagar Press; 1941. p. 187.
2. Kunte A, Navre K, Paradkar H. (Ed). *Ashtang Hridaya by Vagbhata*. Uttartantra Timirpratishedha, Chapter-13, Verse-98. 6th ed. Bombay: Nirnay Sagar Press; 1939. p. 825.
3. Yanoff M, Duker J. *Ophthalmology*. Chapter-3. 2nd ed. London: Mosby; 2004. pp. 23–24.
4. Acharya JT (Ed). *Sushrut Samhita by Sushruta*. Uttaratantra Aupadravikamadhyaya, Chapter-1, Verse-11. 2nd ed. Bombay: Nirnay Sagar Press; 1931. p. 538.
5. Kunte A, Navre K, Paradkar H. (Ed). *Ashtang Hridaya by Vagbhata*. Sutrasthana, Ayushkamiya, Chapter-1, Verse-20. 6th ed. Bombay: Nirnay Sagar Press; 1939. p. 14.

6. Kunte A, Navre K, Paradkar H. (Ed). AshtangHridaya by Vagbhata. Sutrasthana Doshabhediya, Chapter-12, Verse-14. 6th ed. Bombay: Nirnay Sagar Press; 1939. p. 194.
7. Shanthakumari P. *Textbook of Ophthalmology in Ayurveda.* Chapter 2. 1st ed. Trivandrum; 2002. p. 27–33.
8. Jin K. Modern biological theories of aging. *Aging and Disease.* 2010;1(2):72–74.
9. Kunte A, Navre K, Paradkar H. (Ed). *Ashtang Hridaya by Vagbhata.* Sutrasthana. Ayushkamiya, Chapter-1, Verse-1. 6th ed. Bombay: Nirnay Sagar Press; 1939. p. 4.
10. Bhat S, Rajashekhar K. Physiology of aging according to Ayurveda – A review. *International Ayurvedic Medical Journal.* 2018;6(5):1099–1104.
11. Pawar N, Kulkarni A. Concept of vyadhikshamatva in Ayurveda. *International Journal of Research -Granthaalayah.* 2020;8(8):239–243.
12. KC Rajkumar. *Unveiling the Truths in Ayurveda.* 1st ed. Bangalore: SBEBA Wisdom Series; 2017. p. 137–141.
13. KC Rajkumar. *Unveiling the Truths in Ayurveda.* 1st ed. Bangalore: SBEBA Wisdom Series; 2017. p. 133.
14. Acharya JT. (Ed). *Charak Samhita by Agnivesha.* SutrasthanaKriyantshirasiya, Chapter-17,Verse-73–74. 3rd ed. Bombay: Nirnay Sagar Press; 1941. p. 103.
15. Byadgi PS. Concept of immunity in Ayurveda. *Journal of Applied Pharmaceutical Science.* 2011;1(05):21–24.
16. Byadgi PS. Critical appraisal of immunity in Ayurveda. *Journal of Homeopathy & Ayurvedic Medicine.* 2014;3:153. doi:10.4172/2167-1206.1000153.
17. Medawar PB. Immunity to homologous grafted skin; the fate of skin homografts transplanted to the brain, to subcutaneous tissue, and to the anterior chamber of the eye. *British Journal of Experimental Pathology.* 1948;29:58–69.
18. Smith R, Godfrey W, Kimura S. Complications of chronic cyclitis. *American Journal of Ophthalmology.* 1976;82(2):277–282.
19. Streilein J. Immune regulation and the eye: A dangerous compromise. *The FASEB Journal.* 1987;1(3):199–208.
20. Paulsen F, Zierhut M. Einführung in die immunologie. In: Erb C (Ed). *Search on Glaucoma.* Amsterdam: Excerpta Medica/Elsevier; 2008. p. 4–11.
21. Male D, Brostoff J, Roth D, et al. *Immunology.* 7th edition. Amsterdam: Elsevier; 2006. Chapter. 1, p. 19–28; Chapter. 6, p. 203–6 and p. 212–213.
22. Staats HF, Jackson RJ, Marinaro M, Takahashi I, Kiyono H, McGhee JR. Mucosal immunity to infection with implications for vaccine development. *Current Opinion in Immunology.* 1994 Aug;6(4):572–583. doi:10.1016/0952-7915(94)90144-9. PMID: 7946045.
23. Streilein JW, Niederkorn JY. Induction of anterior chamber-associated immune deviation requires an intact, functional spleen. *Journal of Experimental Medicine.* 1981 May 1;153(5):1058–1067. doi:10.1084/jem.153.5.1058. PMID: 6788883; PMCID: PMC2186172.
24. Abelson MB, Schaefer K. Conjunctivitis of allergic origin: immunologic mechanisms and current approaches to therapy. *SurvOphthalmol.* 1993 Jul-Aug;38 Suppl:115–132. doi: 10.1016/0039-6257(93)90036-7. PMID: 7901917.
25. De Haas EB. The pathogenesis of keratoconjunctivitis sicca. *Ophthalmologica.* 1964;147:1–18. doi:10.1159/000304560. PMID: 14113264.
26. Wieczorek R, Jakobiec FA, Sacks EH, Knowles DM. The immunoarchitecture of the normal human lacrimal gland. Relevancy for understanding pathologic conditions. *Ophthalmology.* 1988 Jan;95(1):100–109. doi:10.1016/s0161-6420(88)33228-8. PMID: 3278257.
27. Prendergast RA, Iliff CE, Coskuncan NM, Caspi RR, Sartani G, Tarrant TK, Lutty GA, McLeod DS. T cell traffic and the inflammatory response in experimental autoimmune uveoretinitis. *Investigative Ophthalmology & Visual Science.* 1998 Apr;39(5):754–762. PMID: 9538882.
28. Bowling B, Kanski J. *Kanski's Clinical Ophthalmology.* Chapter 11. 8th ed. Erscheinungsortnichtermittelbar: Elsevier; 2016. p. 428.

29. Salvi S. Ageing changes in the eye. *Postgraduate Medical Journal*. 2006;82(971):581–587.
30. de Souza RG, de Paiva CS, Alves MR. Age-related autoimmune changes in lacrimal glands. *Immune Network*. 2019 Feb 27;19(1):e3. doi:10.4110/in.2019.19.e3. PMID: 30838158; PMCID: PMC6399097.
31. Telegina DV, Kozhevnikova OS, Kolosova NG. Changes in retinal glial cells with age and during development of age-related macular degeneration. *Biochemistry (Mosc)*. 2018 Sep;83(9):1009–1017. doi:10.1134/S000629791809002X. PMID: 30472939.
32. Abdulaal MR, Abiad BH, Hamam RN. Uveitis in the aging eye: Incidence, patterns, and differential diagnosis. *Journal of Ophthalmology*. 2015, Article ID 509456, 8 pages. doi:10.1155/2015/509456.
33. Shinohara T, Singh DP, Chylack LT, JR. Review: Age-related cataract: Immunity and lens epithelium-derived growth factor (LEDGF). *Journal of Ocular Pharmacology and Therapeutics*. 2000;16(2):181–191.
34. Lumi X, Hawlina M, Glavač D, Facskó A, Moe MC, Kaarniranta K, Petrovski G. Ageing of the vitreous: From acute onset floaters and flashes to retinal detachment. *Ageing Research Reviews*. 2015 May;21:71–77. doi:10.1016/j.arr.2015.03.006. Epub 2015 Apr 2. PMID: 25841656.
35. Ding J, Sullivan DA. Aging and dry eye disease. *Experimental Gerontology*. 2012 Jul;47(7):483–490. doi:10.1016/j.exger.2012.03.020. Epub 2012 Apr 28. PMID: 22569356; PMCID: PMC3368077.
36. Chen YF, Wang IJ, Su CC, Chen MS. Macular thickness and aging in retinitis pigmentosa. *Optometry and Vision Science*. 2012 Apr;89(4):471–82. doi: 10.1097/OPX.0b013e31824c0b0b. PMID: 22388669.
37. Gu X, Neric NJ, Crabb JS, Crabb JW, Bhattacharya SK, Rayborn ME, Hollyfield JG, Bonilha VL. Age-related changes in the retinal pigment epithelium (RPE). *PLoS One*. 2012;7(6):e38673. doi:10.1371/journal.pone.0038673. Epub 2012 Jun 11. PMID: 22701690; PMCID: PMC3372495.
38. Richdale K, Bullimore MA, Sinnott LT, Zadnik K. The effect of age, accommodation, and refractive error on the adult human eye. *Optometry and Vision Science*. 2016 Jan;93(1):3–11. doi:10.1097/OPX.0000000000000757. PMID: 26703933; PMCID: PMC4692191.
39. Mashaghi A, Hong J, Chauhan SK, Dana R. Ageing and ocular surface immunity. *British Journal of Ophthalmology*. 2017 Jan;101(1):1–5. doi:10.1136/bjophthalmol-2015-307848. Epub 2016 Jul 4. PMID: 27378485; PMCID: PMC5583682.
40. Furukawa RE, Polse KA. Changes in tear flow accompanying aging. *American Journal of Optometry and Physiological Optics*. 1978;55:69–74.
41. Perez VL, Saeed AM, Tan Y, Urbieta M, Cruz-Guilloty F. The eye: A window to the soul of the immune system. *Journal of Autoimmunity*. 2013 Sep;45:7–14. doi:10.1016/j.jaut.2013.06.011. Epub 2013 Jul 17. PMID: 23871641.
42. Lee CM, Afshari NA. The global state of cataract blindness. *Current Opinion in Ophthalmology*. 2017 Jan;28(1):98–103. doi:10.1097/ICU.0000000000000340. PMID: 27820750.
43. Kahn HA, Leibowitz HM, Ganley JP, Kini MM, Colton T, Nickerson RS, Dawber TR. The framingham eye study. I. Outline and major prevalence findings. *American Journal of Epidemiology*. 1977 Jul;106(1):17–32. doi:10.1093/oxfordjournals.aje.a112428. PMID: 879158.
44. Klein BE, Klein R, Linton KL. Prevalence of age-related lens opacities in a population. The Beaver Dam Eye Study. *Ophthalmology*. 1992 Apr;99(4):546–52. doi:10.1016/s0161-6420(92)31934-7. PMID: 1584573.
45. Hankinson SE. Epidemiology of age-related cataract. In: Albert DM, Jakobiec FA, eds. *Principles and Practice of Ophthalmology*, 2nd edn. Philadelphia, PA: WB Saunders, 2000: 511–519.

46. Dhiman KS, Dhiman K, Puri S, Ahuja D. A comprehensive review of Cataract (Kaphaja Linganasha) and its surgical treatment in Ayurvedic literature. *Ayurveda*. 2010 Jan;31(1):93–100. doi:10.4103/0974-8520.68197. PMID: 22131692; PMCID: PMC3215330.

47. Sunkireddy P, Jha SN, Kanwar JR, Yadav SC. Natural antioxidant biomolecules promises future nanomedicine based therapy for cataract. *Colloids Surfaces B: Biointerfaces*. 2013 Dec 1;112:554–62. doi:10.1016/j.colsurfb.2013.07.068. Epub 2013 Aug 14. PMID: 24001900.

48. Krishnaswamy K. Traditional Indian spices and their health significance. *Asia Pacific Clinical Nutrition*. 2008;17 Suppl 1:265–268 PMID: 18296352.

49. Sharma R, Martins N. Telomeres, DNA damage and ageing: Potential leads from Ayurvedic Rasayana (anti-ageing) drugs. *Journal of Clinical Medicine*. 2020 Aug 6;9(8):2544. doi:10.3390/jcm9082544. PMID: 32781627; PMCID: PMC7465058.

50. Nittmann M, Margo C, E: Age conditional probability of ocular and ocular adnexal malignancies. *Ocular Oncology and Pathology*. 2020. doi:10.1159/000511364.

51. Shields CL, Kaliki S, Furuta M, Mashayekhi A, Shields JA. Clinical spectrum and prognosis of uveal melanoma based on age at presentation in 8,033 cases. *Retina*. 2012 Jul;32(7):1363–1372. doi:10.1097/IAE.0b013e31824d09a8. PMID: 22466491.

52. Acharya JT. (Ed). *Sushrut Samhita by Sushruta*. Uttaratantra. Aupadravik. Chapter-1, Vesre-26–27. 2nd ed. Bombay: Nirnay Sagar Press; 1931. p. 539.

53. Jayasudha R, Chakravarthy SK, Prashanthi GS, Sharma S, Garg P, Murthy SI, Shivaji S. Alterations in gut bacterial and fungal microbiomes are associated with bacterial Keratitis, an inflammatory disease of the human eye. *Journal of Biosciences*. 2018 Dec;43(5):835–856. PMID: 30541945.

54. Horai R, Zárate-Bladés CR, Dillenburg-Pilla P, Chen J, Kielczewski JL, Silver PB, Jittayasothorn Y, Chan CC, Yamane H, Honda K, Caspi RR. Microbiota-dependent activation of an autoreactive T cell receptor provokes autoimmunity in an immunologically privileged site. *Immunity*. 2015 Aug 18;43(2):343–53. doi:10.1016/j.immuni.2015.07.014. PMID: 26287682; PMCID: PMC4544742.

55. Huang X, Ye Z, Cao Q, Su G, Wang Q, Deng J, Zhou C, Kijlstra A, Yang P. Gut microbiota composition and fecal metabolic phenotype in patients with acute anterior uveitis. *Investigative Ophthalmology & Visual Science*. 2018 Mar 1;59(3):1523–1531. doi:10.1167/iovs.17-22677. PMID: 29625474.

56. Andriessen EM, Wilson AM, Mawambo G, Dejda A, Miloudi K, Sennlaub F, Sapieha P. Gut microbiota influences pathological angiogenesis in obesity-driven choroidal neovascularization. *EMBO Molecular Medicine*. 2016 Dec 1;8(12):1366–1379. doi:10.15252/emmm.201606531. PMID: 27861126; PMCID: PMC5167134.

57. Rowan S, Jiang S, Korem T, Szymanski J, Chang ML, Szelog J, Cassalman C, Dasuri K, McGuire C, Nagai R, Du XL, Brownlee M, Rabbani N, Thornalley PJ, Baleja JD, Deik AA, Pierce KA, Scott JM, Clish CB, Smith DE, Weinberger A, Avnit-Sagi T, Lotan-Pompan M, Segal E, Taylor A. Involvement of a gut-retina axis in protection against dietary glycemia-induced age-related macular degeneration. *Proceedings of the National Academy of Sciences of the United States of America*. 2017 May 30;114(22):E4472–E4481. doi:10.1073/pnas.1702302114. Epub 2017 May 15. PMID: 28507131; PMCID: PMC5465926.

58. Zinkernagel MS, Zysset-Burri DC, Keller I, Berger LE, Leichtle AB, Largiadèr CR, Fiedler GM, Wolf S. Association of the intestinal microbiome with the development of neovascular age-related macular degeneration. *Scientific Reports*. 2017 Jan 17;7:40826. doi:10.1038/srep40826. PMID: 28094305; PMCID: PMC5240106.

59. Yang H, Huang X, Fang S, Xin W, Huang L, Chen C. Uncovering the composition of microbial community structure and metagenomics among three gut locations in pigs with distinct fatness. *Scientific Reports*. 2016 Jun 3;6:27427. doi:10.1038/srep27427. PMID: 27255518; PMCID: PMC4891666.

60. Załęski A, Banaszkiewicz A, Walkowiak J. Butyric acid in irritable bowel syndrome. *Przeglad Gastroenterologiczny*. 2013;8(6):350–353. doi:10.5114/pg.2013.39917. Epub 2013 Dec 30. PMID: 24868283; PMCID: PMC4027835.

61. Jumas-Bilak E, Carlier JP, Jean-Pierre H, Mory F, Teyssier C, Gay B, Campos J, Marchandin H. Acidaminococcusintestini sp. nov., isolated from human clinical samples. *International Journal of Systematic and Evolutionary Microbiology*. 2007 Oct;57(Pt 10):2314–2319. doi:10.1099/ijs.0.64883-0. PMID: 17911303.

62. Morgan XC, Tickle TL, Sokol H, Gevers D, Devaney KL, Ward DV, Reyes JA, Shah SA, LeLeiko N, Snapper SB, Bousvaros A, Korzenik J, Sands BE, Xavier RJ, Huttenhower C. Dysfunction of the intestinal microbiome in inflammatory bowel disease and treatment. *Genome Biology*. 2012 Apr 16;13(9):R79. doi:10.1186/gb-2012-13-9-r79. PMID: 23013615; PMCID: PMC3506950.

63. Shivaji S. Connect between gut microbiome and diseases of the human eye. *Journal of Biosciences*. 2019 Oct;44(5):110. PMID: 31719219.

64. Delzenne NM, Cani PD, Everard A, Neyrinck AM, Bindels LB. Gut microorganisms as promising targets for the management of type 2 diabetes. *Diabetologia*. 2015 Oct;58(10):2206–2217. doi: 10.1007/s00125-015-3712-7. Epub 2015 Jul 31. PMID: 26224102.

65. Lin P. The role of the intestinal microbiome in ocular inflammatory disease. *Current Opinion in Ophthalmology*. 2018 May;29(3):261–266. doi:10.1097/ICU.0000000000000465. PMID: 29538183.

66. Zinkernagel MS, Zysset-Burri DC, Keller I, Berger LE, Leichtle AB, Largiadèr CR, Fiedler GM, Wolf S. Association of the intestinal microbiome with the development of neovascular age-related macular degeneration. *Scientific Reports*. 2017 Jan 17;7:40826. doi:10.1038/srep40826. PMID: 28094305; PMCID: PMC5240106.

67. Beli E, Yan Y, Moldovan L, Vieira CP, Gao R, Duan Y, Prasad R, Bhatwadekar A, White FA, Townsend SD, Chan L, Ryan CN, Morton D, Moldovan EG, Chu FI, Oudit GY, Derendorf H, Adorini L, Wang XX, Evans-Molina C, Mirmira RG, Boulton ME, Yoder MC, Li Q, Levi M, Busik JV, Grant MB. Restructuring of the gut microbiome by intermittent fasting prevents retinopathy and prolongs survival in *db/db* mice. *Diabetes*. 2018 Sep;67(9):1867–1879. doi:10.2337/db18-0158. Epub 2018 Apr 30. PMID: 29712667; PMCID: PMC6110320.

68. Tripathi J. (Ed). *Chakrapanidatta*. Netraroga Chikitsa, Verse-92. 6th ed. Varanasi: Choukhambha Sanskrit Series; 2008. p. 479.

69. Anuja Singh V, Sumithra T. Gowda. Critical analysis on Chakshushya Varga. *Journal of Ayurveda and Integrated Medical Sciences*. 2017;4:138–141. doi:10.21760/jaims.v2i4.9339.

70. Kumar NS, Nair AS, Nair AM, Murali M. Pharmacological and therapeutic effects of triphala – A literature review. *Journal of Pharmacognosy and Phytochemistry*. 2016;5(3):23–27.

71. Sarashetti KS. R. vision and ghee. *Journal of Biological & Scientific Opinion*. 2015;3(3):143–146.

72. Kumari R, Singh M, Kotecha M. Yava (Hordeum Vulgare Linn.): A review. *International Research Journal of Pharmacy*. 2016;7(3):5–9.

73. Singh R. Asparagus racemosus: A review on its phytochemical and therapeutic potential. *Natural Product Research*. 2016 Sep;30(17):1896–908. doi:10.1080/14786419.2015.1092148. Epub 2015 Oct 13. PMID: 26463825.

74. Adsule RN, Kadam SS, Salunkhe DK. Chemistry and technology of green gram (Vigna radiata [L.] Wilczek). *Critical Reviews in Food Science and Nutrition*. 1986;25(1):73–105. doi:10.1080/10408398609527446. PMID: 3539530.

75. Shondelmyer K, Knight R, Sanivarapu A, Ogino S, Vanamala JKP. Ancient *Thali* diet: Gut microbiota, immunity, and health. *Yale Journal of Biology and Medicine*. 2018 Jun 28;91(2):177–184. PMID: 29955222; PMCID: PMC6020729.

76. Cavuoto KM, Banerjee S, Galor A. Relationship between the microbiome and ocular health. *Ocular Surface.* 2019 Jul;17(3):384–392. doi:10.1016/j.jtos.2019.05.006. Epub 2019 May 21. PMID: 31125783.
77. Gilger BC. Immunology of the ocular surface. *Veterinary Clinics of North America: Small Animal Practice.* 2008 Mar;38(2):223–31, v. doi:10.1016/j.cvsm.2007.11.004. PMID: 18299004.
78. Kugadas A, Gadjeva M. Impact of microbiome on ocular health. *Ocular Surface.* 2016 Jul;14(3):342–349. doi:10.1016/j.jtos.2016.04.004. Epub 2016 May 14. PMID: 27189865; PMCID: PMC5082109.

Nutritional Psychiatry as Basis of Nutraceutical Development for Mental Illness in Aging Population

Rupali Joshi Panse

Ayurveda

Contents

11.1 Introduction

Ayu (Life) is the combination of body, senses, mind and soul.

(Charaksamhita)

The subtleness and oneness both are the identities of mind and mind is responsible for both presence and absence of knowledge due to its existence in the communication within senses organ, objects and self.

(Charakasamhita)

DOI: 10.1201/9781003110866-11

These quotes from Charaksamhita rightly describe the complex relation of physical body and nonphysical entity like mind and knowledge and their wholeness as life.

This chapter involves three major unrecognized, comparatively less funded and researched areas in health sector: nutrition, geriatrics and psychiatry. Some decades show unexpected prevalence of nutritional disorders and impact of nutrition on health. In last 3–4 decades, the surge in noncommunicable diseases and limitations of conventional clinical medical treatment in geriatric population raised demand for alternative medicine and therapies. High and steep rising curve in psychiatry cases and especially increased involvement of geriatric population have raised a demand for more research in geriatric psychiatry too. This chapter is a blend of these critical components of health sector, e.g., geriatric psychiatry and role of nutrition. To climb a step ahead, this chapter discusses the promising future of innovative branch in psychiatry, nutritional psychiatry and its contribution in geriatric psychiatry. Impact of food-based nootropic herbs and getting advantage of nutraceuticals in Ayurveda dietetics is the unique and centralized feature of the topic discussed here. While it is established that the human brain endures diverse insults in the process of aging, food-based nootropics are likely to go a long way in justifying the impacts of these insults.

- **Geriatric Psychiatry**: The present scenario challenges in conventional treatment, limitations, new hopes)

    Population affected: The population of elderly persons is growing with exceptional speed. According to statistics from World Population Prospects, the 2019 Revision, by 2050, one in six people in the world will be over the age of 65 (16%), up from 1 in 11 in 2019 (9%). By 2050, one in four persons staying in Europe and Northern America could be aged 65 or over. In 2018, for the first time in record, persons aged 65 or above outnumbered children under 5 years of age globally. The number of persons aged 80 years or over is projected to triple, from 143 million in 2019 to 426 million in 2050 [1]. Though not all but mass group of older people suffer from multiple illnesses and significant disability. They tend to undergo great medical difficulty and vulnerability. Old ones have illnesses with atypical and unclear presentations. Aging population suffer major cognitive, emotional and functional problems. They are especially at risk to iatrogenic health problems too. Those who are socially isolated, and the poor are at high risk for premature or inappropriate institutionalization. Almost 45% of elderly suffer from some chronic illness and many have 2–3 physical illnesses together with a mental disorder. The prevalence of mental disorders in the elderly ranges from 20% to 30% of which the commonest are depression (10%) and dementia (3%) [2]. The global burden of mental illness (including geriatric population), both in terms of financial cost and debility, rivals that of all cancers combined.

It is estimated that 50 million people worldwide are living with dementia with nearly 60% living in low- and middle-income nations. The overall sum of people with dementia is estimated to rise to 82 million in 2030 and 152 million in 2050 [3].

This fact would necessitate that we foresee and plan for geriatric care both in the health system and in the families and community.

- **Common geriatric psychological disorders and their reasons**:

  Mood disorders, suicidal behavior, anxiety, depression bipolar disorder, Alzheimer's and another dementia, and schizophrenia are the common geriatric psychological diseases. Common reasons for the mental illnesses in old-age population are:
  - Chronic physical illness (e.g., cancer or heart disease, skin disorder arthritis, etc.)
  - Addiction of substances as alcohol or other substance abuse
  - Dementia-causing physical illness (e.g., Alzheimer's disease)
  - Serious Illness or demise of a near person
  - Painful physical condition
  - Complications of some medication
  - Dependency on others in terms of finance and mobility
  - Neglected diet and nutrition
  - Socio economical adversities

- **Challenges in conventional medicinal treatment**:

  The elderly is highly prone to develop psychiatric disorders, probably because of age-related changes in the brain, concomitant physical disorders, as well as increased stress in later life. Psychiatric disorders in this population may have a different presentation than in other groups and some of psychopathologies might be mistaken for normal age-related changes at home or even in primary care level. Identification of these hidden psychological changes and disorders is basic challenge among geriatric psychology. Physical dependency on others affects the quality of day-to-day life at a great extent. The result of this reflects in lack of proper physical exercises, mobility, association and nutrition. Most of the healthcare is concentrated on drug or medicine in geriatric population. Nutrition, emotional health and cognitional supportive therapies can reach a little number of geriatric populations. This led to incomplete management of various physical and mental diseases. The sum of this reflects in the increase numbers of old-age population suffering from mild to moderate psychological conditions. Some of them are recognized many of them remain unnoticed.

  The provision of safe drug therapy is considered one of the greatest challenges in the geriatric health care as patients. This subgroup be inclined to suffer more frequently from multiple physical and psychiatric illnesses. This may interfere and complicate each other's management. On an average, the elderly tends to be taking more medications than other age populations, which outcomes in complicated interactions between the various drugs. Also, pharmacodynamic and pharmacokinetic alterations with aging change the way drugs and the body interact with each other. Associated chronic systemic disorders and therapeutic drugs affects the digestion. Malabsorption of essential nutrients is immediate result of it. Nutritional compromise has direct impact on the mood and emotional health. Chronic nutritional deficiencies are related to central nervous system disorders. Compromised elementary canal is further obstacle in drug management in old population.

Pharmacokinetic limitation in absorption due to reduced gastric activity, delayed emptying of stomach, etc. limits the selection. Poor metabolism, i.e., loss in hepatic mass, reduced blood supply, etc. and excretion (loss of renal mass, thickening of the base of glomeruli, etc.) and distribution of the drug are big challenges in managing the geriatric psychological conditions with medicine.

Apart from these pharmacokinetic limitations and altered physiological changes, almost all the drugs used to treat the psychological conditions have minor to major adverse results which keep the physical health at stake.

List of side effects of drugs as an example [4]

- Hypersalivation
- Sedation (unnecessary/unwanted)
- Gastrointestinal effects such as nausea, constipation and diarrhea
- Effects on the liver
  - Cholestatic jaundice
  - Raised transaminase enzyme activities
- Endocrine effects
  - Weight gain
  - Diabetes mellitus
- Epilepsy in some cases
- Side-consequences like poor attention, impaired memory and behavioral problems may lead to confusion regarding diagnosis and produce further deterioration in patients with pre-existing cognitive decline. Other anticholinergic side-effects such as urinary retention and constipation need to consider. These complications restrict the remedial use in psychotherapy with chemical molecules.
- **New hopes on the horizon of geriatric psychiatry**:

  Role of nutrition in healthy mind is one of the most undervalued concepts in psychiatry till some years ago. Brain and nerve cells need various amounts of complex carbohydrates, essential fatty acids, amino acids, vitamins, minerals and water to remain healthy. To reduce the prevalence of mental disorders, an integrated approach which synchronously echoes the relationship of biological, psychological, spiritual and social aspects of Psychiatry is needed.

In contemporary science, the insights of the gut-brain axis have set off a new component to the way we understand and treat mental illness. This has directed to understanding of potential branches such as "nutritional psychiatry".

Nutritional Psychiatry is an innovative new approach to working with some of the most common issues we see in our world today when it comes eating, body image and weight. Nutritional psychology or psychiatry is a science which studies how nutrients affect mood and behavior. It also studies and implement food or nutrients as therapeutic measures.

This field examines the relationship between food and our internal understanding, revealing the biophysiological mechanisms, influenced by our nutrient intakes that underlie mood and behavior. Dietary choices and meal habits affect our physic and psyche over the days and years. Recently discovered relationships between human intestinal microbiome and the brain seem likely to have influence in psychiatric disorders. Food and mood disorders have revealed close and valid relation of mood alteration with typical food consumption. Research shows that certain types of bacteria or their metabolic products may be associated with depression and lowered excellence of life [5]. The intestinal microbiome participates in the proper functioning of the intestine, functions as part of the immune system, and it also can generate neuroactive molecules. If the intestinal microbiome is interrupted, CNS function disorders may also occur. It is well known that the intestine, to function properly, receives regulatory signals from the central nervous system (CNS). Over the past two decades, research studies have proved that the intestine is also capable of communicating signals to the CNS and collected by the brain. This term is named "gut-brain axis". This two-way communication channel includes both the neuronal pathway as well as the endocrine, nutritional and immune pathways. Under physiological and homeostasis circumstances, the axis is steady in all ways. However, if, for example, there is a microbial overgrowth and pathological situation in the intestine, this fragile balance is disrupted, and this can manifest both at the gastrointestinal or immune level, and at the central level. Thus, an imbalance in the human intestinal microbiota may give rise to the development of apparently isolated central nervous system disease, such as depression. Preserving the ecosystem naturally by good diet is achievable. From a standpoint of mental wellbeing 90% of serotonin receptors are in the gut. This clearly explains the reason why someone on prescribed antidepressant such as sertraline or fluoxetine suffers the most common adverse effects related to gut. Gut flora and nutrition therefore have crucial role in pathology and cure of most of psychological illness.

11.2 Role of various micronutrients on mental nourishment and metabolism in psychology

Nearly 9–10 decades of research reveal the significance of diet and nutrients for psychological health. Many among recent studies on nutrients important to mental illness noticed irritability and mood problems in people having deficiency of vitamin B [6]. Ample supplement shows positive improvements in the symptoms. Some instances with mental illness nutrients such as manganese [7] and nicotinic acid [8] achieved encouraging outcomes irrespective of deficiencies of the same. Interest in Nutritional studies have dropped since the introduction of psychiatric medications around the 1950s. But recent work on folic acid (vitamin B9) suggests that low levels may be blamed for depressive symptomatology and poor response to conventional antidepressant medication. Folate can be used to enhance antidepressant response. In order to combat hyperhomocysteinemia (high homocysteine levels) and reduce depressive symptoms without the use of additional antidepressant medication, folate alone or in combination of Vitamin B 12 can be used.

The brain is an organ with high metabolic and nutrient requirements. On average, the brain uses 20% of an individual's daily caloric intake, approximately 400 calories/day. It is composed of 60% fat and contains high concentrations of cholesterol and polyunsaturated fatty acids (PUFAs) such as omega-3s.

Monoamine neurotransmitters like Serotonin, nor epinephrine and dopamine are produced in the pathophysiology of mental illness to counter it. This depends on enough building blocks of amino acids and mineral-related co-factors. Folate and other B vitamins are vital for the methylation cycle. Methylation cycle produces a co-factor crucial for monoamine neurotransmitter synthesis, BH-4 [9]. Proper function of the methylation cycle also reduces homocysteine elevated levels which are linked to cardiovascular disease and depression.

Omega-3 fatty acids establish an integral part of neuronal cell membranes and influence several critical activities in the central nervous system. More specifically, they synchronize neurotransmission, influence gene expression and directly impact neurogenesis and neuronal survival. They also act as anti-oxidants and have anti-inflammatory properties. Along with omega-3 intake, the balance of omega-6 and omega-3 fatty acids also appears to be appropriate. Western diets tend to be abundant in omega-6 fatty acids, and quite low in omega-3s, this significant change happened due to industrialization and progressive increase in the processed food industry [10]. Omega-6 fatty acids are the primary fatty acid in many vegetable oils. Often the cooking fats of choice in packaged and restaurant food is corn oil, Soy oil or other vegetable oils. Long-chained omega-3 fatty acids are found in fish, seafood and grass-fed beef. Western diet does not contain these typical foods in daily basis and in adequate quantity. Grass-fed beef omega-3 content varies greatly, but generally contains 100 mg of long-chained omega-3 fatty acids per 100 g serving. This is significantly less than a comparable serving of fatty fish [11]. The fact emphasizes the importance of educating patients about meat quality and healthy alternatives. Cow ghee is a rich source of omega-3 fatty acids and a safe option as cooking fat.

Omega-3 fatty acids are supposed to be efficient as either stand-alone or adjunctive treatment for ADHD, depression, bipolar disorders and PTSD (post-traumatic stress disorder). Also, elevation of the amount of omega-6 more than omega-3 fatty acid in the blood has been linked with major depressive disorder and ADHD. Certain indication stresses on the theory that cutting the omega-6 and adding up omega-3 supplements lead to improvement in symptoms of ADHD. The impacts of trace elements on brain, behavior, mood elevations are being validated with the more research work. Zinc, copper and magnesium also perform an essential modulatory position in controlling a subtype of glutamate receptor (NMDA receptor) [12]. Glutamate is a primary transmitter for most excitatory neurons in the cerebral cortex. This NMDA receptor has been linked in various ways of cortical operation; therefore, it seems that reduced levels of these crucial nutrients may yield anomalous NMDA activity and following abnormal behavior.

Vitamin C (ascorbate) is popularly known for its antioxidant properties. It is a co-factor for a group of biosynthetic and monitoring enzymes contribution in essential biological functions. It is required for the normal production of some of the vital chemicals such as monoamine neurotransmitters dopamine, noradrenaline and serotonin [13]. Their deficiencies and improper regulation can be blamed as reason to depression (Figure 11.1).

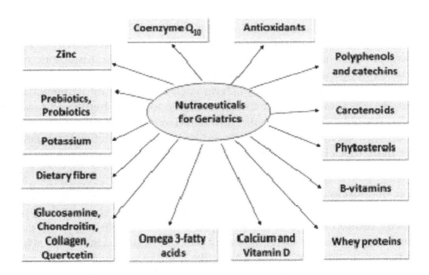

Figure 11.1 *Essential nutrients for geriatric health.*

Vitamin C coordinates the epigenome as it is a supporting component for enzymes involved in both DNA and histone demethylation. Epigenetic alterations provide a system by which environmental indicators, such as stress, can change gene expression and neural function and thereby influence behavior, cognition and mental health [14]. Vitamin C levels are determinedly organized all through the body, and its allocation is generally thought to reflect a functional requirement. Vitamin C concentrations are maximum in the brain and other neuroendocrine tissues such as the pituitary and adrenal glands. It is a vital trace element needed by brain to survive and function appropriately.

Vitamin C is supposed to be actively involved in neuronal maturation and physiological functioning [15].

Recent hypothesis suggests that in existence with internal damage, low-grade inflammation and immune imbalance, due to psychosocial stress, can be able to initiate the pathology and symptoms of depression [16]. Vitamin C has several anti-inflammatory activities and is an excellent antioxidant.

Prebiotics and probiotics: Two-way influence of Gut flora and CNS draws attention of healthy gut bacteria. Gut flora may help reduce inflammatory reactions in gut and in turn stress stimulatory chain of mechanism in CNS. This seems important preventive measure in psychological field. The market of pre and pro biotic synthetic and natural products are in boom. It is important to understand the role of naturally present bacteria in gut and to preserve their harmony. Natural food and diet habits can effectively preserve it. The diet and lifestyle which insults the gut flora should be discouraged, mere external supplements of pre- and probiotic will not sustain the cause in long term health and the results are unsatisfactory in these cases. Understanding the importance of natural prebiotic and probiotic in their original form such as fruits, vegetables, buttermilk, fresh curd, ghee and naturally less fermented food items will certainly contribute more. Alternative medicine such as Ayurveda have mentioned the role of these natural prebiotic food in their most organic form. The science uses this theory in treating many disorders related to dysbiosis of gut bacteria such as lactose intolerance, Crohn's disease, diarrhea and IBS. The use of prebiotic forms of herbs and food such as herbal treated curd, buttermilk, fermented syrups like Takrarishta (buttermilk herbs) in such psychological disorders is highly beneficial. Geriatric gut flora is more susceptible for dysbiosis and may trigger or aggravate various psychological manifestations.

The role of conscious nutrition in psychological health and diseases was identified merely some decades ago. Surprisingly some 1,000 years back Ayurveda identified nutrition as one of the strongest pillars to nourish not only physical but psychological health too. The whole concept of nutrition is kept always in the center while addressing the topics like code of conduct of daily regimen (lifestyle), seasonal impact on human physiology (epigenetics), in order to prevent the disease relapse. The aspect of preventive medicine lies in Ayurveda dietetics and lifestyle. Food consumed is seen as the basic cause of growth and nourishment of the functional components called Doshas in Ayurveda. Three basic physiological entities, i.e., Vata, Pitta and Kapha, governs all the metabolic reactions. Apart from the physical governance, these three Doshas are also responsible for keeping the emotional health. Intellect, thought process, feelings, beliefs and responses are constantly under the influence of Tridosha. Food is supposed to nourish these Doshas. Food is also a threat to these Doshas if the right code of conduct of diet is disrespected. Thus, the integration of diet and psychology has its roots in the theory of inseparability of food with body mind and soul.

Geriatrics: A separate branch in Ayurveda! Ayurveda is a comprehensive stream of science consisting of eight branches of specialization in health and medicine. Among them is "Jara" (geriatrics) which deals with the aging and aging-related health issues. According to the Ayurvedic texts aging is affected by Tridosha and their prevalence in personal lifestyle. Considering the longer living age in that era, the typical old age was assumed after 70 years. At this age, the prominent features of aging like loss of physical strength, debility, loss of sexual competence and other sensory disabilities were described. Surprisingly, mental aging was addressed even much more lately, i.e., after the age of 80 years. Cognitive inability and mental aging were followed by the physical aging. Contradictory to what we see today is mental health is getting affected much earlier than physical health. It is time to take the fact into the consideration about early prevalence of mental health.

What could be the favoring factors for delayed aging in ancient time? Was there any practice or medicine which naturally protected the individual against physical as well as mental aging? The answer is treasured in the simple, scientific and time-trusted way of living. Every day is either contributing or deteriorating the health by each daily routine and diet. Daily practices include physical and mental lifestyle. Diet or nutrition is the largest component of the health influencing factors in lifestyle. Was there any specific type of diet to protect the mental aging and the mental disorders related to aging? To get the answer to the above questions, it is wise to understand the concept of mind, psychology, and how Ayurveda look to the psychological health and diseases in brief.

Ayurveda and psychology: Ayurveda while defining the health includes mental health as an inseparable component along with physical health. It defines health as a sound condition of body, mind and all senses. During discussion of diseases, medicine in various sections of Samhitas like Charaka and Sushruta explain the role of psyche and, factors affecting the emotional health and their management. The sole objective of Ayurvedic science is to prevent the diseases and maintain the quality of health. This preventive approach encourages the parameters like nutrition, code of conducts in lifestyle and practices to prevent physical and mental diseases. There are psychological diseases described in Ayurveda such as Unmada (psychosis), Mada (depression) and Murcha. Sutrasthana in Charaka Samhita is dedicated to the right code of conduct regarding diet, lifestyle and behavior [17]. Ayurveda theories play a vital role in understanding the Ayurveda concept of psychiatry and management of mental health.

Sanskrit shloka: उन्मादपुनर्मनोबुद्धिसञ्ज्ञाज्ञानस्मृतिभक्तिशीलचेष्टाचारवभिर्मंवदि् यात्||५|| (च.चि.९/५)

Meaning: (psychosis/insanity is imbalance in mind, intellect, sensory functions, memory, thoughts, beliefs and behavior.)

1. **Three-pillar theory of life**: Ayurveda describes nutrition (Aahara), sleep (Nidra) and physiological sexual indulgence in limits (Brahmacharya) as three strong pillars which supports the health as a strong foundation if are obeyed properly. But if any of the pillar is weak or violated, it will make this foundation shaky and create many physiological and psychological diseases (Table 11.1).

Trayo upstambha iti, Ahara, swapno, brahmcharyam iti. [18]

Table 11.1 Psychology in Ayurveda: A Holistic Approach

Ayurveda and Nutritional PSYCHIATRY	Lifestyle (Vihara) and Mental Health	Ayurvedic Management of Psychological Disorders
• Aahara: Nutrition for body and mind • Psychological personality and food choices (Satva, Raja, Tama food and Mind nutrition) • Incompatible Diet theory (Virudhahara) • Daily and seasonal diet regime code of conduct (Dincharya/Rutucharya) • Six taste theories and psychological impact • Eight-fold guideline for Nutrition. General diet guidelines. (Ashtvidhi Vidhana) for physical and mental health • Rasayana for geriatrics (restorative nutraceuticals for old age) • Whole and unwholesome food list and significance of mental health • Medhya Rasayana (Nootropic herbs, food/polyherbal combinations)	• Sleep and its impact on psychology • Sleep disorders and their management • Functional food for sleep disorders and their treatment • Voluntary and involuntary physical and emotional urges and their role in psychological diseases (Dharaniya Adharniya Vega theory) • Senses, sense organs and their role in psychological health. Abuse of one or more sense organ and mental illnesses. (Asatmya Indriya Arth Samyoga) • Crime by intellect (Paradnayparadha) and psychological disorders • Code of conduct for behavior, preventive measures in Psychology (Sadvrutta)	• Yuktivyapashraya (counseling) • Sadachara (behavioral therapy, REBT) • Herbo-mineral medicine • Panchakarma • Shirodhara, Shiro abhyanga • Nasya • Dhupan therapy (aroma therapy/herbals smoke therapy) • Rasayana Chikitsa (restorative medicine) • Pathya diet (wholesome nutrition) • Apunarbhav Chikitsa (preventing medicine and therapy to avert relapse, rehabilitation

Diet and nutrition (Aahara): The whole concept of health, diseases and even their cure has underlying solution in nutrition. Aahara is a term in Sanskrit language used for food in Ayurveda. Aahara is the prime source of life as it nourishes every cell in the body. Apart from the physical nourishment, Aahara is also responsible for the nourishment of emotions and psyche.

Tushti, Pushti, Balam, Medha sarvam Anne pratishthitam

While describing the results of good Aahara In Charaksamhita uses term "Prinan" (replenishment), trupti (satisfaction) and tushti (joy/contentment). These have manifestation in mind or feelings. The term Medha means intellect and cognition. The impact in terms of emotions and feelings may not be expressed in physical metabolism but can be felt for sure. Unpleasant sight, smell taste of food in same way develops emotions such as nausea, reluctance toward food, sadness in some cases. Apart from the physical growth, consumed Aahara is also responsible for the nourishment of the feelings and emotions. Though the psychological impacts of food are not visible immediately or confirmed by any definite biomarker yet, it can be experienced and validated by the observations by the person and later in physiological changes as a remote impact. Everything around us is composed of *Pancha Mahabhuta*, i.e., Earth (*Prithvi*), Water (*Ap*), Fire (*Teja*), Air (*Vayu*) and Ether (Akasha). In living and nonliving things, the *Panchamahabhuta* components have different proportions and give them appropriate structures and appearances. Consumed meal nourishes the respective Mahabhuta-dominant tissue elements in the living body.

Vedic science and Ayurveda have categorized the food in three groups based on their traits. These traits are completely linked to psychological aspect. Satwik, Rajasik and Tamasik are three groups according to the properties of the food and how they build psyche. Even the spiritual literature Bhagavat Geeta has grouped the type of Aahara and their impact on the good or bad temperament. Satva, Raja and Tama are three prime sets of behavioral patterns or personalities dominated by the respective guna (trait). These three gunas (properties) rule the psyche of person. The dominance of one guna or the combination of these is responsible for the psychological profile of a human being. Diet has been a significant criterion found in the ancient text for influencing these Trigunas. Ayurvedic literature emphasizes the inseparable dependency of food and mood (nutrition and psyche) and its impact beyond the physical health [19]. Can we consider these Trigunas as etiological and predictive parameter for psychological disorders? What are the physiological and psychological traits of these three major types of personalities? Satva guna is the premium existences of good qualities in a person.

- Satva guna-dominant person is found affection toward food that is fresh, less spicy, less hot, not too sweet and eat only to nourish the bodily elements. Satva guna controls the greed, selfishness, fear and anger and makes the person kind, generous and satisfied. This person usually wears the clean, light-colored clothes and has pleasant aura. He does not overact, take revenge or trouble anyone. He is brave, content and steady in his speech and deeds. Due to the Satva guna, he stays away from anything that can influence his health and psyche in bad way. Usually, normal form of Kapha Dosha forms Satva guna.
- Raja guna person chooses food that is spicy, dry, light and salty. Raja guna person is ambitious and pursues the goal passionately to achieve it by hook or crook. Raja guna likes to wear bright colorful clothes, perfumes, jewelry and other forms of self-pleasing. The person indulges in entertainment and things that please his own body and soul. Raja person can be influenced quickly by their surroundings. There responses are sharp, loud and quick. They are brave and unnecessarily indulge in ambitious ventures. Anger, revenge, ruling and dominating nature are the bold traits of Raja guna-dominant person. Raja guna is dominated by Pitta Dosha. Due to sharp Pitta Dosha, the person tends toward intellectual achievements, innovation and larger-than-life foresight and action. Their psychological profile is vulnerable. These types are like Type A personality.
- Tama guna person likes food, which is too sweet, too spicy, too hot, sticky and does not care whether it is stale or fresh. This kind of person indulges himself in eating and sleeping a lot. Physically not so active, this person tends toward lethargic lifestyle. Tama guna person lives in unhygienic surrounding. He/she is reluctant toward clean body and clothes. The overall aura of this person is unpleasant and depressing. The person thinks and reacts destructively for self or others. The person is lazy and, most of the times, can turn to criminal activities and harmful nature. Selfishness, lack of foresight, zest and enthusiasm are the bold features of the person.

All these traits are determined by minute observation in an enormous number of people. Charaka says that the person who shows consistent trait of any one of these Trigunas can be referred to as a personality of that guna. This Triguna theory is very important to decide the psychological profile of the person in terms of prediction and prevention. The core personality in terms of any above-mentioned guna influences the food choices, behavioral patterns and actions that can either preserve the physical and mental health or obliterate it. It is a unique thing to assess in the patient having psychological disorder. These traits are carried in old age too. Knowing a person's inclination toward Satwik, Rajasik or Tamasik nature can determine the course of the geriatric health profile.

Since Aahara has major influence on these gunas, it's necessary to mention how and which Aahara influences these Trigunas. Because this nutritional influence on the brain can nourish or generate disparities in psychological health.

Satwik Aahara: This type of Aahara is advocated as ideal Aahara for all. Satwik food is freshly cooked, simple and grown in good soil and is in accordance with season. Satwik meal has all six tastes (sweet, sour, salty, pungent, bitter and astringent) in balance. It does not have any taste in excess or less. It is properly cooked (not overcooked/half cooked). It is cooked and served in clean hygienic conditions. It is served in portion as per the person's digestive fire and need. It is consumed with good company and in happy state of mind. Satwik food has sufficient portion of cow ghee and oils. It is not devoid of good fat, too dry, too cold, preserved or adulterated. This type of meal can be termed as Satwik meal. Satwik food nourishes the body as well as intellectuals of person. This type of food keeps the Tridosha in balance and keep the three types of intellectuals normal. It has calming effects on sense organs and brain. It does not produce the undigested toxin or Ama, the Ayurvedic term for toxin. Satwik diet is responsible to keep the emotional state clam and clear. The person is not easily disturbed by the circumstances around them. He can think and act rationally due to balanced Tridosha on physical and mental levels.

Rajasik Aahara: Raja guna meal is exotic, spicy, hot, tangy, tongue pleasing and Pitta nourishing. It excites the taste buds and generates extra heat in the body. It is lavish and consists of multiple cuisines to satisfy the satiety of ambitious Raja guna person. This type of meal is oily and majorly taken with alcohol and other tropical beverages. This type of meal usually consists of many spices and are cooked by various methods of food process. Rajasik meal favors the Pitta Dosha in the body and mind. It nourishes feelings like pride, ambition, bravery and passion. If it is practiced in excess and ignore the rules of dietetics then it increases possessiveness, anger, revenge, violent responses, etc. Rajasik meal tends to have harsh effects on psychology in long-term practice. These people can face anxiety and stress more easily due to already-triggered Pitta Dosha.

Tamasik Aahara: Tamasik meal is known as the unhealthiest type of diet to culminate the physical and mental health. Tamas meal is heavy to digest, cooked in unhygienic way and served in unclean surrounding. The ingredients of such meal are usually not at their good state. Using rotten, stale, sticky and aged things to prepare meal leads to Tama guna. This diet is not fresh and mind pleasing. It is either very sticky or very dry and lifeless. Tamasik diet is devoid of nutrition and leads to indigestion, obesity, laziness and indigested toxins in the body. This type of meal does not please the senses or nourish their capabilities, but it leads to the diminished sensory functions. Persons become physically inactive and mentally non-receptable. The sensory and motor coordination is sluggish due to the absence of quality nutrients in the poor diet habits. The person is sleepy, inactive and pessimistic and also has negative thoughts. The food consumed typically increases the Ama and faulty Kapha Dosha that obscures the sense reception. They can easily slip into the disturbed emotional state. It affects the rational behavioral of intellect in terms of awareness, analysis and memory of incidences and feelings. These people are more susceptible to suffer psychological diseases.

These three gunas can influence the psyche through diet, sense organs and lifestyle. Therefore, Ayurveda science takes Satwik Aahara into consideration while managing the diseases, be either physical or mental. It can also trace the etiology in psychiatric diseases to the Aahara type along with other influencing factors. Importance of conscious nutrition, therefore, plays a very crucial role in psychology. This nutrition can be beyond the caloric measurement and balanced nutrients. There are multiple factors that influence and alter the properties of the food one consumes.

After Triguna Aahara, another theory in Ayurveda is related to the psychology and throws light on the importance of nutrition on psychology. The concept of Virudhhanna, i.e., incompatible food combination, is an innovative approach in Ayurveda science to explain the pathologies of a number of NCDs, immunocompromised diseases and unexplained pathologies in human bodies which reflect physically and psychologically. Virudhhanna is recognized as a prime etiology in various mental disorders [20].

Virudhhanna: A newly emerging science branch called topography exclusively studies the effects of various food combinations on health. Topography reveals about the combination of basic categories of the food and their effects in the body. The similar unique theory is put in Ayurveda called as Virudhhanna. Incompatibility is a unique concept in Ayurveda. "Virudhahara" ie. certain types of combinations s listed in Table 11.2 hinders the metabolism of tissue, and inhibits the process of formation of tissue. The food, which is wrong in combination, has undergone wrong processing, consumed in incorrect quantity, with food of opposite qualities, consumed in incorrect time of the day and in wrong season can become Virudhahara. Apart from numerous mild to serious systemic illnesses, insanity is mentioned as an obvious result of consuming ViruddhaAahara. Application of this theory for prediction and prevention is important. This theory provides a strong foundation to study the recent diet, culinary trends and their incompatibility. For geriatric population being highly prone for the results, this theory becomes most applicable (Table 11.2).

The preventive and curative aspects of Ayurveda revolve around the central theme of *Pathya* Aahara and Vihara. Ayurveda emphasizes basic dietary guidelines in terms of appropriate food, combinations of food, methods of cooking, storage, eating atmosphere, hygiene and etiquette (Ashtvidhi Aahara Vidhi Vishesha Ayatana).

Table 11.2 Few Examples of Incompatible Food Items

- **Fruits + milk** (as in milkshake deserts, ice creams, fruit followed by drinking milk or vice versa)
- **Fish +milk** either by combining or eaten separately followed by each other.
- **Curd heated** and used as an ingredient.
- **Milk +salt** combined in recipes.
- **Milk/milk products +meat** at once
- **Radish +milk** together combined.
- **Milk and melons** together
- **Buttermilk heated** and consumed or used in dishes.
- **Ghee and honey** in equal weight combined.
- **Too Hot and too cold food** together are the examples of Virudhhanna described in Ayurveda.
- Stale, too fermented, too sour, dry food.

Examples of today's trendy incompatible food that may not be mentioned in Ayurveda.

- Almost all the cocktails which are the wildest imagination of mixing the different property bearing juices and alcohol.
- Citrus fruit flavored milkshakes and ice creams
- Use of milk, curd, cream, buttermilk in marinating or preparing curry and gravy.
- Extreme hot and cold things together on dish are hit nowadays like, fried hot ice-cream, hot brownie with cold ice-cream.
- Fruit salad served with custard made from milk. Fruit-flavored rabdi (condensed milk desert) esp. **custard apple thick milk dessert (rabdi)** is highly allergic due to its mucous increasing property.
- Many unusual flavored alcoholic beverages as coffee cream liquor, white chocolate, and cocktails, mocktails, smoothies containing veggies+milk+cream+ yogurt together, etc.
- Sweets, desserts and recipes that have honey as an ingredient and need to be cooked or heated.
- Eating curd, rice and pickle together daily at night.
- Khichadi (cereal rice) and milk together.
- Preserved salty (MSG) synthetic oxidants, preservatives, artificial taste enhancers.

11.3 General Ayurvedic dietary guidelines

1. **Intake of food in time (Kale Bhojana)**: The term "kaal" means time. Time of intake of food is given fair importance in nutrition. The base of Ayurveda dietetics and nutrition is based upon the physiological normal parameters like when, how and what to eat by whom. The time of consumption of food looks after the digestive fire, initiation of digestion absorption and the next refill for food. When Pitta Dosha seated in stomach with help of Vata secrets digestive juice in stomach, the Jatharagni (digestive fire) gets ignited as hunger. This Pitta should never be insulted. Lack of meal or delay in meal frequently can be a considerably metabolic crime in long-term practice. Circadian rhythm is a remarkable symphony played by the Tridosha. Rhythm of metabolism is maintained by the timely consumption of food. Any error like eating meal when one is not hungry, eating meal when the previous meal is not digested completely and infrequent meal timings for a long period are some of the very commonly committed diet mistakes. The time of consumption is important in mental health or psychological pathologies. Gut-brain relation is deeply rooted in emotions and feelings too. Hunger is probably the very first physiological step that gets affected in almost every psychological ailment. The increased or abnormal decrease in hunger is observed in almost every patient of mental illness. All the eating disorders are somewhere related to mental health too. Anorexia, compulsive eating disorder, Bulimias are commonly associated with the psychological pathologies. So, while diagnosing as well as managing these disease the time or frequency of consumption of food should also be given importance. There is a Sanskrit verse which praises the right timing of meal as "Kale Bhojana Tridosha samyakaranaam sreshtham", which literally means that the correct code of conduct and appropriate mealtimes are equal to health. Nutritional psychiatry can assess the abnormalities associated with the meal timing as history and pathologies associated both physically and psychologically. Ayurveda dietetics associates the calorie need of body with Tridosha state in the rhythm of body clock and defines the appropriate mealtime too. In mental illness cases in geriatric patient where there is already-diminished digestion and metabolism, it is very important to decide good timing of their meal according to their body type and pathological condition. This will help reduce load on major metabolic reactions mainly digestion and excretion. Also, timely meal helps build gut bacterial symbiosis with the central autonomous system. Though simple, the time factor has high influence on the physical and mental health in term of nutrition.

2. **Food intake as per suitability (Satmya Bhojana)**: Satmya is suitable in simple language. Everybody according to their unique body type or prakriti get accustomed to certain type of environment lifestyle

and food. The reach of this suitable factors is up to the genetic material or genotype. Ayurveda puts a theory where simple thumb rule is established. "Samanen Samansya Vrudhhi viparite rhasa" means the similar property things and practices to the Dosha in body increase the dominance of related Dosha. The same way the opposite property practices, lifestyle or food will decrease the dominance of that (Vata/Kapha/Pitta) Dosha. Food practices and lifestyle in accordance with the body type promote the health and wellness. On the other hand, if these things are not followed or disobeyed frequently, it causes metabolic errors on physical and mental health. While treating, Pathya food (therapeutic diet) is decided to suit the overall body type and the recovery from diseases.

3. **Food intake as per the Prakriti of individual (Hita Bhojana)**: Keeping Tridosha balanced nourishes the tissue as per the composition requirement. The food compatible with Prakriti helps to combat the diseases causing Dosha by preserving the immunity and healing and avoiding the extra burden of food incompatible with prakriti or body type. Hita Bhojana also refers to the nutrients necessary to be fulfilled. Balanced diet is Hita Bhojana, and Pathya diet is Hita Bhojana. Ayurveda texts like, e.g., Charaksamhita, have categorized the food groups such as Nitya Sevaniya Aahara (the food that one should consume regularly as major portion of diet.) is favorable to all in any form at all times. Such food is considered as gut friendly and can be used as guidelines for general and specific diet requirements.

4. **Proper hygiene (Shuchi Bhojana)**: Excludes one of the criteria of Tama guna meal. Hygiene rules out infectious diseases. Hygienic surrounding and food is appealing to the emotions of person. Cleanliness is not only limited to the dirt or microbes but also refers to the quality of the food, grain, vegetables fruits, etc. Food containing trace amount of pesticides, synthetic fertilizers, hormone, etc. are not considered as pure, and they are therefore not able to give the optimum nutrition as per their nutritive index. Food is clean and pure when it is dirt and microbe free, simple, noncomplex, nonmodified and organic. For example, ready-to-cook, preserved and processed meat may be microbe free and clean, but the nutritive values of them will not be the same as the fresh meat. So according to Ayurvedic theories of dietetics such food is stale and not pure. Proper hygiene, therefore, signifies the overall quality of the food and not just cleanliness.

5. **Intake of food which is unctuous (Snigdha Bhojana)**: It underlines the importance of good fat (essential fatty acids/DHA/omega fatty acids). Proper balance of carbohydrates, proteins and lipids in geriatric ages is very important for metabolic and mental health. The absence of essential fatty acids can damage the myelin sheet of

neurons and can result in errors of sensory and motor conductions. This has a huge impact on cognitional health. Cow ghee, sesame oil, fish oil, coconut oil and olive oil are supposed to have good impacts on brain cells. Ayurveda states ghee, oil and lard (animal fat) as the best Vata Dosha pacifier in an increasing order. In many western recipes, lard is used just as ghee or oil in Asian countries. Ghee is most easily assimilable, and lard is the heavier among the three. In old-age population, appetite and metabolic rate are reduced. Also, the heavier the fat, the more lipid metabolic errors are expected. Therefore, ghee is considered the best choice among all fats. Cow ghee especially is stated as Tridosha pacifier. Food that has not enough lipid content therefore may cause Vata Dosha imbalance according to Ayurveda. The dry-nature food abnormally raises the oxidative stress at tissue level, and tissue nourishment is hampered. The excessive consumption of dry-nature food also is responsible for tissue damage. Increased Vata Dosha is the prime culprit in all the neurological disorders as per the Ayurveda diagnostic theories. So not only lipid but also the good fat should be consumed regularly within normal limits.

6. **Intake of food which is warm (Ushna Bhojan)**: This signifies the nature of food which is fresh and not stored or preserved or refrigerated. Because stale, cold dry meal is supposed to be one of the reasons of Ama (toxin like substance formed due to indigestion or molecular metabolic waste). This Ama is the prime perpetrator for every single physical and mental disorder according to Ayurveda. Also, the warm food is in accordance with the internal temperature of digestive system. Frequent cold-food intake can restrain the digestion and tongue receptors due to the constriction of micro capillaries. Food should be warm and fresh.

7. **Intake of food which is easy to digest (Laghu Bhojan)**: Particularly in geriatric population, this is important to reduce the digestive burden and avoid indigestion. Easy-to-digest diet should also be nutritious. This diet theory is helpful in deciding the wholesome diet for various pathologies especially in old-age population.

8. **Eat while there is interest on food, and while eating, concentrate on food and the process of eating (Tanmana Bhojan)**: Involvement of psyche or mind plays an important role in food intake and its digestive benefits. The food should be mind-pleasing as well as nutritious. Proper attention and recognition to the food also signify that one should be aware of all senses while eating. It makes the person aware of what he or she is eating.

9. **Eat food with six taste components (Shad-Rasa Aahara)**: Six taste components play roles in metabolic activities and body nourishments. Skipping of any of the taste and type of food will generate nutritional deficiency.

The Sanskrit Shloka "Sarv rasa Satmya aarogyakaranam sreshtham, Ikaha rasa Satmya aarogyakaranam" means eating all tastes in balance is the best practice that keeps health. On the other hand, eating food predominantly with a particular taste is the main reason for sickness and diseases.

10. **Food should be primarily sweet in nature (Madhura Praya)**: Sweet taste does not mean dessert or sugary food. According to criteria from Ayurvedic dietetic theory, the sweet taste-dominant food is nourishing and heavy to digest, and promotes growth and healing. Sweet taste promotes anabolism, while other tastes mostly tend to catabolic mechanism at cellular level. Sweet taste has calming and nourishing effect on tissues. Sweet taste belongs to the food group protein. Most of the protein-rich food has sweet taste. Pulses like green mung and lentil and meat like goat meat and seafood have sweetness as its dominant taste. It takes care of the Kapha Dosha which plays a major role in cognitional health. Kapha Dosha dominates the Vata Dosha which is responsible for various catalytic reactions in the body. If there is less sweet rasa or protein in meal, it will cause malnourishment of various tissues. Also, memory, analysis and knowledge holding are the Kapha-initiated activities, and hence it should be preserved. A proper balance of Kapha and Vata Doshas is expected here.

11. **Food should be ingested calmly, neither too slow nor too fast (*Na Ati Druta Vilambita*)**: Involvement of five senses in food ingestion supports the proper satisfaction from food mentally. Also, it removes the possibility of delayed digestion due to slow eating. Eating fast without proper attention can lead to gag reflex or possibility of bolus entering the airway. This rule is equally helpful in diagnosis of psychological disorders. The persons with suppressed feelings, various complexes and depression are seen eating their food in different manners. Many people in depression are slow eaters. They are not in their senses while eating the food. The harmony of smell, taste, sight and hand coordination is hampered. Such people often do not realize how much time they are taking to eat even a small amount of food. On the other hand, some patients with anxiety, fear and personality disorders consume food in an abnormal hurry. The manner how one eats can also help diagnose the Dosha type that involves in psychological disorders. Slow eaters are usually Kapha dominated, and fast eaters are Vata victims. Thus, a simple rule in Ayurveda dietetics can direct in reverse diagnosis as well as an etiquette in dietetics in nutritional psychiatry. Proper counseling of nutrition involves not only the food list but also these food etiquettes which seems so simple but contributes to the deeper level in prevention as well as management of the various mental diseases.

12. **After bathing *(Snatah)***: Food should be consumed after bathing. One should not bathe immediately after eating the meal. Food

digestion requires proper blood supply to the digestive system, and bathing immediately after meal retracts the blood supply toward the limbs and skin. Frequent errors like this can lead to the chronic indigestion and metabolic errors in long term. This practice is also against the Dincharya guideline, and according to Ayurvedic theories, wrong Dincharya (lifestyle) is the root cause for almost all the noninfectious physical and mental illnesses. This humble rule is valuable code in correct lifestyle.

13. **Food intake only when there is sufficient hunger (*Kshudvan*)**: Food according to the digestive fire/capacity is always advocated. Eating without hunger is a big mistake for circadian rhythm too. It places increased burden on the digestive system and encourages Ama production and diseases along the period. Loss of appetite is a common symptom in many psychological disorders. If in such circumstances the meal is consumed forcibly then it may affect the physical condition as well. False hunger or stress hunger is mistaken as increased appetite or hunger in many psychological conditions.

14. **Proper washing of hand, feet and face should be done before food intake (Dhatu Pada-Kara-Anana)**: The simple practice of washing the hands feet is very important to avoid contagious diseases.

15. **Offering prayers and paying obeisance to gods and forefathers (*Pithru -Deva Tarpana*)**: There should be feeling of gratefulness, appreciation and respect toward the food. It generates the calmness in mind and replaces the unwanted emotion if it is there at the time of eating. By doing so, we are bringing our emotions to neutral or positive, and it avoids the impact of disturbed psyche on digestion as mood impacts food and nourishment through Satva Raja Tama properties. This approach also teaches one to look at the meal consciously with all senses at alert state. So one can easily pay attention to the wholeness of food and other described criteria related to the dos and don'ts.

16. **After offering food to guests, teachers and children (*Athithi-Balakaguru Tarpana*)**: This diet rule is more related to the spiritual heath of an individual. This simple self-discipline in ancient times was to make people realize their belonging and duties toward the society and living being around them. Empathy toward people around you is an essential component of emotional health and spiritual personality. Person who is aware of the wellbeing of others and concerns about vital needs of living being can manage own emotions as well. It also teaches one to be patiently sharing. This emotional connection also takes care of mental health. Association with the wise people mentioned above opens the opportunity for person to share problems and get the necessary comfort and counseling. Many times, food is an

excuse for social gathering. This type of design improves the association of the society.

17. **Without disgracing food (*Anindan Bhunjaana*)**: Disgracing denotes here food waste, criticizing food frequently, leaving food in plate, avoiding unfavorite food, keeping it in unhygienic place, etc. These manners show one's illiteracy toward nutrition. Also disgracing frequently can be related to the imbalanced mental health due to various emotions and thoughts. Treating food and food related vectors rightly disciplines the person toward diet habits.

18. **Silently (*Moun*)**: This dietetic rule too suggests the undeviated involvement of person while consuming food. Too much talking and laughing can distract the attention from the essential fact of eating.

These are simple diet rules that contribute to physical and mental health and appropriate nutrition when obeyed as daily practices.

11.4 Role of Rasa (tastes) in psychological health

Apart from the basic nutritive values of food, i.e., proteins, lipids, carbohydrates and other chemical components such as vitamins and minerals, Ayurveda recognizes the substance/food by its various properties and taste (rasa). Rasa is one of the major properties among other 20 properties. Every substance possesses one or more dominant taste, and that taste has a role to imprint the results on every cell throughout the digestion as well as after assimilation.

Rasa (taste) of the substance is the foremost tool in Ayurveda to assess and determine the pharmacological properties and actions of the substance. Similarity in *rasa* is said to signify similar structure and consequently similar pharmacological behavior.

Types of rasas and their functions on systems or organs:

Six types of rasas are described in Ayurveda with their unique properties and their effect on various systems in body [21].

Some of Rasa properties & functions are listed in Table 11.3.

Ayurveda dietetics looks this theory as a reference guideline for choosing various taste-bearing food items or herbs for the treatment and nutritional management.

Sleep (Nidra): Sleep is the second most important pillar for both physical and emotional health. According to Ayurveda, sleep is a blessing for health, and abnormalities in sleep can be a burden leading to physical and mental illnesses. Sleep plays a crucial role in preserving the emotional health and psychological soundness. Strong evidence suggests insomnia is a trigger factor

Table 11.3 Physical and Physiological Impact of Elemental Combinations

Taste and Elemental Combination		Physical Impact	Psychological Impact	Example of Food with Dominant Rasa
Sweet	Earth + water	Nurtures, builds and fortifies body tissues	Soothing, calming, pleasing	Carbohydrates, Protein, Fat Pulpy fruits, Grains, pasta, rice, bread, starchy vegetables, cow milk, meat, chicken, fish, sugar, honey, ghee
		Excessive consumption causes: Adipose tissue diseases, obesity, diabetes	lethargy, anxiety	
Water + fire	Salty	lubricates tissues, softens, maintains mineral balance and holds water	enhances appetite and other tastes, enthusiasm, calms nerves and stops anxiety	Mineral salts rock salt, sea salt, soy sauce, salted meats, fish, seaweed, pickles
		Excess consumption: wrinkles, thirst, loss of strength, hair loss	cravings, anger, impatience, lethargy	
Earth + fire	Sour	stimulates appetite and digestion, strengthens heart, relieves thirst and satiates	enhances intellectual activities, keeps intellectuals alert	Organic acids: ascorbic acid, citric acid, acetic acid Indian gooseberry, Citrus fruits, berries, tomatoes, pickled foods, salad dressing, yoghurt, alcohol
		Excess consumption: loss of strength, feverish feeling, excessive unfulfilling thirst	resentment and jealousy, anger, impatience, hot temper	
Fire + air	Pungent	Maintain body temperature body and promotes sweating, improves metabolism and relieves neurological origin pain	opens mind and senses	Spices and essential oils Peppers, chilies, onions, garlic, cayenne, black pepper, cloves, ginger, mustard, salsa, radish, wasabi
		Excess consumption: thirst, depletion of reproductive fluid and strength, fainting, waist/back pain	irritability, anger, impatience	
Earth + air	Astringent	cleanses blood and helps maintaining healthy blood sugar level, dries moisture and fat	Cooling effect on high temper, clears senses and reactions, reduces laziness	Tannins Betel nut, Java plums gooseberry, Lentils, dried beans, broccoli, green apples, pears, grape skins, cauliflower, cabbage, pomegranates, tea
		Excess consumption: Dried mucosa, flatulence constipation, heaviness or pain in chest, thirst	anxiety, fear, panic, insomnia	
Ether+ air	Bitter	Cleanses and detoxifies, reduces fat and water excess, relieves thirst and fever, antimicrobial	helpful in managing food cravings, clears senses and emotions	Alkaloids or glycosides Green leafy vegetables, green and yellow vegetables, kale, celery, broccoli, sprouts, beets
		Excess consumption: Flatulence or upset stomach, tissue depletion	anxiety, worry, insomnia	

in the occurrence of psychotic experiences and other mental health problems. Ayurveda strongly advocates good sleep to balance the Tridosha. Loss of sleep causes the Vata Dosha imbalance and abnormal dominance of Pitta Dosha. Both cause tissue destruction, abnormal metabolism, and deterioration in sensory and motor functions and dysbiosis in the gut. Chronic insomnia leads to insufficient healing of collateral damages in metabolism in brain cells and immune system. This increases the predisposition of many systemic disorders. Old-age population already is prone due to decreased span and compromised quality of sleep because of aging.

Is there any role of nutrition in sleep disorders? Can sleep be improved with the precise use of nutraceutical? These questions hold tremendous possibilities of new solutions in the field of psychology and geriatric psychiatry.

Among many other physiological, pathological factors and external impacts, diet and nutrition have always played a significant role in normal physiological sleep. Keeping circadian rhythm is a key step in health and wellness. Digestion and sleep are essential tools to fix the cycle.

11.5 Liaison of nutrition and sleep

Melatonin is secreted predominantly by the pineal gland and mainly at nighttime, and it induces sleep and other mechanisms of sleep cycle. The primary physiological function of melatonin is to convey information of the daily cycle of light and darkness to the body. In addition, it may have other health-related functions. Melatonin is an essential dietary amino acid synthesized from tryptophan. It has been demonstrated that some nutritional factors such as intake of vegetables, caffeine, and some vitamins and minerals, could modify melatonin production [22]. Strong influence of food on melatonin synthesis is detected in studies of subjects undergoing periods of fasting. Energy constraint reduces the nocturnal secretion of melatonin, although the number of human studies proving this is limited. Short-term voluntary fasting by total refusal of food or with very limited intake of energy (<300 kcal/day) from 2 to 7 days reduces melatonin concentration in the blood by about 20%. Some food items, especially edible plants, contain melatonin. The presence of melatonin in plants is universal, although with widely varied concentrations from picograms to micrograms per gram of plant tissue, melatonin has been detected in notable amounts for example in tomatoes, olives, barley, rice walnuts and grapes. Wine, beer and coffee have a high amount of melatonin. In geriatric patients, use of alcohol and caffein is not practical. Also, caffein has both stimulatory and inhibitory effects on melatonin secretion. When the short listing continues, the choices for tryptophan- or melatonin-containing food becomes less. Recent trends of supplements for nutritional deficiencies, especially in western countries, include melatonin and tryptophan supplements too. There is limitation due to the adverse effects to these supplements too. L-**tryptophan** is POSSIBLY **SAFE** when taken orally in short term. L-**tryptophan** can cause some side effects such as heartburn, stomach pain, belching and gas, nausea, vomiting, diarrhea and loss of appetite. Melatonin is generally safe for short-term use. With repeated or long-term use of Melatonin one is likely to become substance dependent and can have a diminished response (habituation) and or a hangover effect.

The most familiar melatonin side effects are headache, dizziness, nausea and drowsiness. Other less common melatonin side effects might include short-lasting feelings of depression, slight tremor, minor anxiety, abdominal painful cramps, irritability, abridged alertness, confusion/disorientation and hypotension. In addition, melatonin supplements can interact with various medications, including anticoagulants and anti-platelet drugs, anticonvulsants, contraceptive drugs, diabetes medications and medications that suppress the immune system (immunosuppressants).

Considering the above limitations, increasing the natural nutritional level of melatonin and tryptophan seems the wisest and only left good alternative. Functional foods are the emerging options for it. Appropriate choice of food and form of the meal can be a solution for geriatric patients where sleep is already reduced as a physiological aging effect.

11.6 Ayurvedic view on sleep nutrition and geriatric psychiatry

Nervous system and mind are indulged in reception, analysis and response of innumerable senses and endless metabolic activities throughout the day. Nidra (Sleep) is the result of the fatigue of it, which carries away the brain from cognitive and sensory functions and induces a phase of partial cease for the body and mind. Tridosha plays an important role in sleep. Circadian rhythm has its own ups and down in term of three physiological Doshas. Among them, Kapha Dosha induces sleep. The dominance in a 24-hour cycle of biological clock Kapha Dosha increases with the time of night cycle. As a result, all the activities like circulation, motor functions, secretions in the body are reduced. Metabolic rate gets dropped due to less active Pitta. Kapha Dosha's impact is dominant throughout the sleep cycle. Most of the healing, regenerating and immune built up are also results of the properties of Kapha Dosha. It is important to maintain the Kapha Dosha dominance within limits for physiological sleep. If Kapha Dosha increases pathologically it induces excess sleep which does not benefit but harms. If Kapha Dosha reduces or eventually Vata Dosha and Pitta Dosha increase abnormally, it also affects sleep. Ayurveda emphasizes balanced "sleep awake cycle" as sleep maintains stability in dhatu (tissues), enhances metabolic activities from digestion to excretion, retains energy and keeps enthusiasm up. It promotes growth, builds immunity and increases the life span by reducing catabolism [23]. Sleep is a crucial step in harmony in endocrine activities too. Sleep deprivation, disturbed sleep patterns and insomnia are stated as potent etiology for cognitive health deterioration and sense organ blips. Chronic state of sleep deprivation leads to impaired sense reception and analysis affecting the psyche and thought process of the person. Ayurveda states this condition as a threat to Dhi (intellect of cognition), Dhruti (intellect for analysis) and Smriti (Memory). These are all collectively responsible for psychological pathologies in human beings. Charaka Samhita mentions sleep deprivation as a potent reason for memory deterioration, confusions and sensory impairments [24].

Old age increase Vata Dosha naturally and it can be vitiated very easily by diet lifestyle and other pathological situations. It is highly important to keep it at a balanced state. Kapha Dosha is less active, so overall the quality and quantity of sleep is reduced in old age. In this situation, diet and lifestyle are useful implements to deal with the Dosha imbalance and sleep abnormalities. Most of the treatment protocols emphasize the sleep-promoting drugs and supplements in psychiatric patients. In most cases, use of tranquilizers for long on regular basis is impractical and come along with a handful of serious health hazards. Promoting the quality and quantity of sleep in psychiatric patients further demands more effective, safe and natural solution. Nutraceuticals in their easiest, safest and most natural forms can resolve this problem to a great extent. In a way, it is an effective measure in preventing, treating and maintaining the geriatric psychiatric health.

11.7 Ayurvedic nutraceutical concept for sleep disorders in geriatric psychiatry

A specialized category of medicinal herbs is dedicated to the purpose of sleep in Charaka Samhita and other texts in the Vedic literature. Herbs like Shankhapushpi, Brahmi, Vacha, Sarpgandha, Ashwgandha and Jatamamsi have tranquilizing effects in a safe way. These herbs are nootropics and have a calming effect on Pitta and Vata Doshas. They have pacifying active ingredients which reduce the brain activity. They are potent nerve tonic and relieve the stress in the nervous system. Using these herbs appropriately in other functional foods instead of the artificial nutrients and chemicals will be a positive addition in the functional food for geriatric sleep disorders and natural tranquillizing nutraceutical industry. Other kitchen spices like nutmeg, poppy seeds, cardamom and rose petals hold analgesic, nootropic, anxiolytic, sedative, hypotensive and circulatory stimulant properties. These herbs and spices play major roles as nutraceuticals in geriatric patients suffering from depression, insomnia, REM sleep behavior disorder, anxiety and other psychiatric aliments. These are taken as food rather than drug or medicine. So naturally the unwanted load of tranquilizers and their adverse side effects are surpassed. In the field of geriatric psychiatry, it will be huge value addition if this practice comes in the mainstream management of the field. Efficacy of these nutraceuticals will be constant as the mode of administration is as easy as diet. The benefits can be achieved in long term in required dosages without the concern of hazards. Drug interaction is a major concern in conventional drug management for sleep disorders which is overruled as herbs used as nutraceuticals are from food category and dosages are minimal.

Below is a list of functional food /nutraceuticals:

- **Moon milk**: milk with turmeric/nutmeg/saffron/rose petals/almonds/ poppy seeds induces sleep in geriatric patients. This milk can be prescribed at bedtime. A user-friendly combination of one or more of the above can be put in the form of sachets, milk powder, or dissolving tablet form in desired dosages and frequencies.
- **Ksheerpaka (milk decoction)**: This functional food is a specialized recipe from medicinal food in Ayurveda. Unlike moon milk where just herbs are added in milk, the Ksheerpaka includes milk boiled with certain portion of herb juice, herb decoction, or the herbs itself for a specific time. It is then filtered and used as a potent functional food. Ashwagandha (*Withania somnifera*), Sarpgandha (*Rauwolfia serpentina*), Shatavari (*Asparagus racemosus*), Vacha (*Acorus calamus*), dates and dry figs are example herbs for the Ksheerpaka preparation. The above herbs are easily absorbed in the gut due to quick absorption of milk. They show quick dozing effect without any aftereffects like heavy head, confusion, etc. in elderly persons.
- Rice cooked with certain nerve tonics like Vacha, Ashwagandha, dry ginger and ghee is the simplest form of functional food one can think of.
- Ghee is a potent nerve tonic and good source of DHL. Medicated ghee is an excellent example of nutraceutical. Cow ghee has high tryptophan level (4 mg/100 gm) [25]. Cow ghee is praised for internal healing and as Medhya (nootropic) food item. Cow ghee pacifies Vata Dosha and overcomes the harsh neuron insults in chronic sleep disorders. It is promising and allows frequent, long-term use without any adverse effects. Vacha ghee, Brahmi ghee, Ashwagandha ghee, Shatavari Ghee, Yastimadhu (Glycyrrhiza glabra) ghee [26] and other medicated ghee can be a valuable functional food. The nutritive aspect of ghee can benefit the patients in multiple ways. All the above ghee types come under classification of herbs which are antiaging, memory enhancing and have effects on cognition.
- A slow diffusion method called Fanta in Ayurveda offers a variety of functional drinks like Jatamamsi Fanta and Sariva (**Hemidesmus indicus)** Fanta. These forms of functional food can be consumed just like any sherbet (soft drink).
- Extracted essential oils like sandalwood, jasmine, rose, lavender, prime rose, cinnamon, cardamom and nutmeg extract can be wisely used in small quantity as a flavor enhancer in various recipes to induce calming effect on nerve cells to promote sleep.

In nutshell, sleep disorders are part of geriatric psychiatric ailments and need attention from the beginning itself. This second important pillar can be preserved with the help of Ayurveda dietetic theories and achieve the promising results in psychiatry. Ayurveda functional food can help in reducing a remarkable portion of therapeutic load in management of geriatric psychiatry.

1. **Brahmacharya**: Sexual activity and sexual projection most of the times are ignored in old-age population. But it plays an important role in keeping emotional health sound or otherwise affect it. Sexual act within limit and in harmony with the physical and psychological conditions is favorable for human health. Ayurveda guides the code of conduct regarding sexual health and provides a detailed guideline of dos and don'ts. Old age, physical debility and active mental involvement in sex is a complex triangle. Improper knowledge and wrong ways to handle this situation may lead to some of psychological disorders in old people, especially in males. This is a topic one should not omit from geriatric psychological assessment. This chapter is dedicated to the nutraceutical aspects of geriatric psychiatry. Nutritional intervention with respect to the tissue malnourishment and improved vitality contributes to this area. Psychological aspects in sexual dysfunction cannot be overruled as sex is an important part in old age too. Proper counseling is more needed than medicine in many cases. Increase in Vata Dosha and decrease in Shukra Dhatu (spermatogenesis) are bold features in male old people. Proper application of diet controlling Vata Dosha and Rasayana (rejuvenating herbal preparations) helps to achieve the result satisfactorily in many cases. Sexual activities are observed considering age, physical health, season and frequency. Vajikarana is a specialized area in Ayurveda which is dedicated to the increase in the libido and sexual vitality. Vajikarana diet and herbal preparation work both on endocrine balance and tissue development. Milk and milk derivatives like cream, ghee, condensed milk, meat and high-protein pulses (black urad, mung beans, kidney beans, etc.) are usually prescribed after examining all the physical and psychological aspects and appetite. Rasayana herbs like Ashwagandha, Amalaki, Talimkhana (Asteracantha longifolia), Gokshura (**Tribulus terrestris**) and sesame seeds are used in various combinations to increase vitality and reproductive health.

2. **Daily regime and seasonal regime for health (Dincharya and Rutucharya)**: Lifestyle is a perception of a particular society toward life and the way its people live, think and behave. It includes dietary practices, physical-mental activities, cognitive exposure, and cultural and environmental revelations. Considering the specificity of the topic of this book, this section focuses on the effect of diet, season and psychological health only. Other factors are explained in brief. Effects of

environment on tissue to DNA is being studied in a separate branch called epigenetics. It is well accepted that the surrounding environment and geographical changes do have positive/negative impacts on the physical and psychological health. These effects are not momentary, but these can be stored as a genetic memory which is rooted and carried from generation to generation. This genetic memory of various experiences related to the surrounding environment and its effects at cellular level is crucial especially in chronic lifestyle-related disorders and NCDs (noncommunicable disorders). The attributes of both are expressed when the slightest change in bodily environment, immunity and psyche happens. Ayurveda has a spiritual base to the scientific thoughts to make them more faithfully practicable by common people. This whole knowledge and a set of practices are irrespective of any specific religion. The wholeness of this medical science can be achievable and related globally. Dincharya literally means everyday activities related to personal care, health and hygiene. This personal care consists of both physical and mental health. It includes following the right code of conduct in daily practices. Dincharya offers a standard example of dos and don'ts in everyday activities. Dincharya includes important daily chores like to begin with like simple teeth cleaning, tongue cleaning, hygiene and health of five sense organs, food, sleep sexual life too. Personal and social behaviors are also discussed as a standard guideline which mainly focuses on general ethical practices one should follow in day-to-day life.

In relation to this topic, we can use this theory from Ayurveda for the management of geriatric psychology using the nutraceutical concept.

Importance of Dincharya in geriatric psychology disorders [27]: To understand the relevance of Dincharya (Daily Regime) in the cases of psychiatric ailments in old-age population overview of it is important. The following are the major practices considered important enough to have impacts on physical and mental health. As we know, Vata Dosha is dominant in old age and can easily disturb the circadian rhythm if the daily routine of diet practices, excretion patterns and sleep habits are not kept normal and watched for.

Ayurveda Dincharya starts from the habit of early rise in the morning before sunrise as it is the most active and alert state of Vata Dosha, and it can help the important functions like excretion right after the person awake. This habit initiates hunger on time and is good for alertness of all sense organs. Habit of waking up early keeps the sleep cycle sound as well.

The further step is teeth and tongue cleaning (Dantdhavana and Jinhva nirlekhana) with the astringent taste-dominant herb sticks/twigs. Instead of starting of the day with harmful chemicals in toothpastes, it is a very sensible way to clean. The herbs not only clean but are very beneficial for the oral cavity, reduce extra stickiness in saliva and enhance the function of the taste buds. It keeps oral mucosa healthy. The herbs get easily absorb through saliva and thus improve the oral cavity health. These include neem (*Melia azadirachta*), shigru/drumstick (Moringa pterygosperma), Guguulu (Balsamodendron mukul) and Babul (Vachellia nilotica). The bitter, tonic, antiseptic, astringent and antibacterial qualities make these nutraceuticals efficient. In several indigenous tooth powders, toothpastes and toilet soaps, the extracts from various parts of these herbs are used nowadays. The use of neem twigs as toothbrushes has been endorsed by the dentists to prevent caries. Azadirachta indica mouth wash is reported to inhibit the growth of *S. mutans* and carious lesions. According to Ayurveda, these astringent and bitter taste-dominant teeth cleaners exclude the toxins and sticky Kapha Dosha to promote oral health.

After this, oil pulling (Kavala/Gandusha) practice is done in which coconut oil/sesame oil/ghee or milk is held in the mouth and moved with cheek muscles and tongue thoroughly for 5 minutes. This rinsing action is proved to pull retract many bacteria in oral mucosa due to the fat-soluble nature of bacterial cell membrane. This practice is proved beneficial in many oral cavity disorders in old age. It protects the mucosa, maintains the flexibility and softness, removes the stickiness, heals the bruises due to artificial dentures in old age, etc. The practice can also be used in the nutraceutical aspect. Oils like Yastimadhu oil, Bala oil or any other medicinal oil can be used as per the need and indication of the person's disease. The cold compressed oils are reach in vitamin E, vitamins B6 and B12, and antioxidants and so good sources of essential fatty acids.

After oil pulling, eye and ear drops are instilled. Usually, the purest form of honey or Triphala grit for eyes and for ears sesame oil is used. This practice keeps the sense organs healthy and functional. The practice is followed by the proper advice of Ayurveda Vaidya. The same way Ayurveda has given a significant importance to regular nasal instillation of oil which is called as Nasya. The Sanskrit verse "Nasahi Shiraso Dwaram" literally means the nose (nostrils) is the gateway to the skull base due to anatomical access through nostrils. Nasya is a key procedure in all the psychological diseases too. It controls Vata Dosha and is beneficial to the brain disorders. Simple oils/ghee are used for regular or therapeutic Nasya and can prove much beneficial in psychological diseases. In daily routine, Nasya is administered as a routine practice to enhance the cognitional health through nourishing the five senses. The benefit of Nasya is addressed as follows. The one who regularly does Nasya gets healthy black hair, and all their senses are replenished and nourished. Charaka Samhita/Sutrasthana/Chapter5/shloka 56-61 describes the Nasya in detail.

e.g. Anu tail Nasya gives benefits in conditions like Hemicrania, Facial paralysis, tremors, torticollis, chronic coryza, etc. and such practice is very well described in Charaka Samhita/ Sutrasthana/Chapter 5/shloka 63-70.

External application of herbs treated oil used to be an integral part of daily routine from childhood. The act of massage is termed as Abhyanga. Sesame oil is beneficial when applied externally due to the abundant nutrients it contains. This Abhyanga generates favorable heat, smoothen the skin, removes dead skin, activates the sweat glands. Oil massage reduces joint pain, swelling, muscular ache and weakness. It alerts the senses and also induces sleep when used at different purposes. Oil application on the head and in the ear, nose and umbilicus is advocated for the health of respective sites. Application of oils having specific actions such as aroma oils on the central nervous system is used to relax the body and mind. Oils from Khus (Cetiver sativum), Chandan (sandalwood), rose, Jatamansi and jasmine are mind-relaxing ones. Oils from Bala, Dashmula and Laksha have muscle-relaxant and anti-inflammatory properties. Application of oils can play crucial roles in geriatric psychology to improve sensory and motor health. Regular massage practice is helpful to preserve the cognitive health to some extent along with diet and medicine. Feet massage with cow ghee or oil is encouraged to relive stress, improve circulation and comfort eye pain. It is effectively used by Ayurvedic physicians in the management of sleep disorders too.

3. **Sadvrutta**: Sadvrutta is an integral part of Dincharya. The literal meaning of Sadvrutta is good behavior. Apart from emotional urges and day-to-day stress, there are a number of things that are related to emotional health. Self-control and knowledge of self-body and mind can make a person understand the physiology or possible reasons leading to illnesses. Sadvrutta also relates to the code of conduct in diet habits. These are already discussed in this chapter.

4. **Theory of nonsuppressible and suppressible urges (Dharaniya Adharniya Vega) [28]**:

Various natural/involuntary urges are important parts of the metabolism and physiology. Ayurveda emphasizes the significance and identifies the role of these urges and their influence on health. These natural urges are grouped into suppressible and nonsuppressible urges. Some urges are meant to suppress as they can impact health negatively. On the other hand, some natural urges are meant to be fulfilled to keep the metabolism normal. Resisting, suppressing, or forcibly creating the nonsuppressible urges can be a potent reason of various systemic imbalances and diseases. Neglecting these urges often can create imbalance in Dosha which further can induce various diseases in respective organs or systems. One should know which urges should be held and which should not be. Common urges due to physical stress are sneezing, hungry, thirst, tears, vomiting, urination, defecation, ejaculation burps, sleep, flatulence, yawning and rapid breathing.

Along with these involuntary urges, suppressible urges are mentioned to have a considerable impact on psychological health.

Suppressible urges: Natural emotional urges unlike physiological involuntary urges need to be inspected by conscious mind and intellect and should be held if they are unfavorable. Holding, resisting and redirecting these unwanted harmful emotional urges can break the pathological advancement toward psychological and physical health. The following are the suppressible urges one should channelize.

Greed, grief, fear, anger, ego, shamelessness, envy, jealous, passion or Kama (sexual desire), pride, arrogance, anxiety, anguish and inferiority complex are feelings or responses in mind to various happenings around oneself. If not let go or handled properly, these emotional expressions induce wrong behaviors in persons and thus directly affect the mental health. Extreme expression of these feelings can cause various psychological disorders ranging from simple depression to severe psychosis. People who are not able to handle the extreme feelings can be a potent threat to themselves, family and society too. It will be wise to identify these emotions or urges and direct them in right way. Having knowledge of the facts about theses urges and their relationship with physical and mental health can bring a positive change in the preventive medicine practice. The right Code of conduct and daily regime guides person to keep mental health sound. It also teaches various techniques to deal with these feelings. Counseling by wise experts, Satwik Aahara, good company and exercise (physical and mental) are some of the behavioral therapies in Ayurveda. This approach is very personalized and hence in the current era of spike in psychological illness very needful too. Various eating disorders can be validated by the above theory easily. Thus, the theory of Adharniya (nonsuppressible urges) and Dharaniya Vega (suppressible urges) have relevance in geriatric psychology, nutrition and management too. Interestingly, it can be used as preventive measures if properly introduced as early as possible in childhood.

5. **Pradyaparadha [29]:** The Pradnyaparadha theory can be put at the center of all the etiologies and pathogenesis. Pradnyaparadha means "crime by intellect". Every action taken by the conscious mind with intellect at place is called as Pradnyaaparadha. All the mistakes in diet, lifestyle, emotions and behavior fall under this vast category.

6. **Asatyma Indriya Samyoga:** Like the physiological diseases, the imbalance of Tridosha is the culprit for psychological pathologies.

Sense organs are called Indriya in Sanskrit, and these are the vehicles for knowledge of all senses. Senses are an integral part of physical and mental health. Ayurveda gave immense importance to the balanced relation between sense and sense organs. Any imbalance between sense organs and knowledge and excessive or wrong use of sense organs are termed as Ayoga, Atiyoga and Mithya yoga in Ayurveda. This applies to five sense organs which are termed as Dnyanendriyas (eyes, ear, nose, tongue and skin) and also Karmendriyas (hands, legs, mouth, anus and genital). Any imbalance in this multilevel web of senses, sense organs and motor reactions can impact the physical and mental wellbeing. Most of the addictions like screen (visual) and substance abuse (nasal/oral) are easily seen and potential harmful examples of misuse of one or more sense organs. For this chapter introduction of this theory is adequate.

7. **Ayurvedic nutraceuticals to manage geriatric psychology**: Ayurveda advocates the use of Rasayana (restorative therapy to old age) for physical and mental health. This part of chapter will extend the knowledge of the prime Rasayana herbs, herbal preparation and herbal medicines for psychological disorders (Manasa Vikara). Rasayana or restorative nutraceuticals are exclusively used for the vitality in old-age population. Rasayana are intended to prevent or treat the physical and psychological diseases in old age. It is an interesting fact that Ayurveda has a separate branch dedicated to the preventive measure entirely for geriatric population for thousands of years. All the therapeutic measures are designed according to the needs of declining cognitive ability and physical debility. Restoring the tissue quality through nutrition, systemic health and preserving the neuroendocrine functions is wisely taken into consideration in the Rasayana therapy.

Rasayana cannot be termed as medicine as it comes under the regular practice or portion of lifestyle. It is the finest example of holistic nutraceuticals which are not synthetic molecules but are in their purest organic form. Rasayana is formulated and processed in proven manner and are highly bioavailable. The restorative combinations in the Rasayana therapy have multiple benefits along with their prime indication. All the herbs and media used to prepare are hepatoprotective, gut friendly and does not cause any adverse effects on any other organ or system. This assures the sustainability of the course of therapy. Rasayana can be used in long term as there is no drug interaction or complications due to it. Mode of administration is as simple as eating meal, which again makes it more convenient considering the senile age of the targeted population.

These preparations are classic combination of one or more herbs together with food items such as milk, oil, ghee, etc. These are consumed not as medicines but as a portion of meal. The category of

Rasayana which is dedicated to the mental health is called as Medhya Rasayana (nootropic restorative combinations) which again underlines the authority of Ayurvedic theories in the field of psychology. Some Rasayana combinations are targeted toward increasing memory and muscular tone. Some are targeted toward cosmetic purposes like skincare, haircare, etc. Others are immunomodulators and are effective in chronic disorders.

11.8 Bright features of the nutraceuticals in Ayurvedic preparations

1. **Medium or base for product**: Medium or base is a vehicle to deliver the nutraceutical. It should be easily accessible, available, affordable and more organic. Sesame oil, cow ghee and cow milk are few of the common mediums used. The effectivity of the preparation of any nutraceutical is dependent upon the basic medium or prime ingredient. Major Rasayanas are administered in the form of ghee, cow milk or as oil base. This innovative form of nutraceutical offers the doctor opportunity to apply them in various methods. Oils can be applied externally and consumed orally too. They can be used as nasal instillation and for basti (therapeutic enema). Cow milk treated with herbal nutraceuticals is easy to produce and consume. Innovative methods of packaging and preservation without compromising the nutritive standards can open the endless opportunities for food industries and wellness stores.

The medium used for the administration itself has its own medicinal and nutritional contributions in the process. This factor is eliminated in the above type of nutraceuticals. Among these fortified or treated herbal ghee is the choice of Rasayana in geriatrics. At higher temperature, ghee is more stable than butter because it does not have any proteins or sugars that will burn. Most fatty acids in ghee are saturated, making it a great choice for frying needed dishes and searing at higher heat. Cow milk is expected to be chemical free and unprocessed to keep its original properties intact. Organic A2-type cow milk is advocated for such nutraceutical purposes. Also, Ayurveda advocates heating the milk till it boils and use of it when fresh.

Oils used for Rasayana purposes are cold compressed, non-refined and in their purest form. Sesame, coconut, flaxseed and mustard seed oils are used in general according to indication. Properties of oils are discussed in the same division of this chapter further.

Samskara (preparation/processing method): Samskara or processing of Rasayana nutraceuticals is important. Typically, food processing is responsible for the nutritive loss or inevitable addition of synthetic ingredients which is the of concern in elderly patients. But Ayurvedic nutraceutical and Rasayana formulation are in their most natural forms due to unique preparation methods and devoid of harmful synthetic preservatives or other molecules. Slow heat method and the appropriate utensils used in preparation of ghee and oil increase their shelf life to longer periods than regular oil or ghee. The extract obtained from juices, powder, or decoction of herbs in lipid base increases the potency, active period and bioavailability to a greater extent. Shelf life of ghee and oil is satisfactory.

Chyavanprasha is considered as one of the most potent antioxidants antiaging Rasayana preparation in Ayurveda. Whenever the ingredients are of aromatic spices they lose their essential active medicinal oils if heated at high temperature so they have to be added at the last stage of product manufacturing. Whenever the ingredients are aromatic spices they lose their essential active medicinal oils during heating and therefore are taken care by mixing them at the last stage of product preparation and put as topping spices. These spices are not only aroma enhancers but also potent digestive stimulants that help to digest and assimilate Chvyvanprasha easily. On the contrary, the Ayurvedic herbs and root medicines are converted into decoction and absorbed in the nonrefined organic sugar syrup. Amla (Emblica officinalis) pulp is used instead of the fruit juice to derive the maximum nutritive ingredients. Honey, ghee and oil are added as the best bioavailable form of DHL, nonsaturated fatty acids and other many medicinal effects on multiple systems. The unique stages of preparation with specific herbal ingredients fetch medicinal properties from the product to combat the three Doshas and achieve tissue nutrition. On the contrary, some are just simple combinations like Sandhana. Asava Arishta is a pharmacological process in which the required herbs are treated together and preserved through the process of fermentation. The form of this medicine is liquid. Very mild natural alcohol present in the process acts as preservative and increases the shelf life of active ingredients within. Asava Arishta is medicated wine in its simple form and has less alcohol content than actual wines. They are easy to consume and have appetizing effects with mild calming and sedation. Ayurvedic herbs and spices used can target multiple objectives with its pharmacological act. Saraswataarisht and Ashwagandharisht are two major examples of herbal preparation used in geriatric psychological disorders. Nootropic herbs present in Saraswataarisht take care of the memory, cognition, antipsychotic effects and insomnia or other sleep disorders. Ashwagandharisht has shown improved muscular tone and hypotensive results with improved digestion. This unique process of natural slow fermentation and preserving herbs in alcohol base has good shelf life as long as 7 years when stored at room temperature, in shadow, and in clean glass or wooden barrels.

2. **Administration**: Mode of administration is always thing of concern especially in old age and children. Ayurvedic herbal nutraceuticals

and medicines are prepared in a way that they can be administered in more than single mode. Most of the treated oils and ghee can be applied externally, consumed orally, and administered anally or nasally.

External application: Vitamins and minerals have traditionally been given orally in the form of pills or powders. However, there is no doubt that some people are intolerant to oral synthetic multivitamins and other supplements. There are numerous possible justifications for this, but the two most likely will be allergy and the agitative gut instead of digesting one. Microbes are as hungry for trace elements and vitamins as we are and will gratefully accept such a free lunch, multiply their numbers and ferment even harder! When foods are fermented instead of being digested, this can produce all sorts of noxious products such as alcohol, D-lactate, hydrogen sulfide and probably others, all of which overload the liver detox system and have the potential to inhibit mitochondria and cause foggy brain symptoms. In Ayurveda, these toxins are termed as Ama (unexpected products in the course of digestion).

Delivering these micronutrients through the largest organ skin is an alternate potential option. Of course, this makes perfect sense as the skin is permeable. Massage therapies have been proved to have benefits over thousands of years. Drug patches are effective to deliver medicine through skin. Skin can be considered for nutrients absorption too. Almost in all the mental illness, external medication such as applying various herbal powders, oils and wet powders is recommended in Ayurveda. Medicated oil massage, oil bath, Shirodhara (forehead oil bath) and Shirobasti (holding oil in special cap on head) are the unique therapies appeared in all the Samhitas and treatment modalities. Medicated oils for external application are aromatic, essential oils treated with methods where the active ingredients are extracted from decoction to oils by medium heat. Oil used most of the time is sesame seed oil. Sesame seed contains 50%–60% of high-quality oil which is rich in polyunsaturated fatty acids (PUFA) and natural antioxidants, sesamin, sesamolin and tocopherol homologues [30]. These bioactive components enhance the stability and keeping quality of sesame oil along with numerous health benefits. Sesame seed is high in protein, vitamin B1 and dietary fiber, and is an excellent source of phosphorous, iron, magnesium, calcium, manganese, copper and zinc. According to Ayurvedic wisdom, Tila Tailam (sesame oil) is the best oil to pacify the Vata Dosha which is an inseparable culprit in mental disorders. Apart from this, massage relieves the stiffness, strengthens the muscles, improves the blood circulation in limbs, reduces stress to some extent and promotes peaceful sleep. Various herbs and nutrients can be utilized to get result to desired. Apart from this, massage relieves the stiffness, strengthens the muscles, improves the blood circulation in limbs, reduces stress to some extent and promotes peaceful sleep. Various herbs and nutrients can be utilized to get result to desired extent.

Oral administration: The most conventional and conveniently method used for administration of drugs or nutrients is through the mouth. In geriatric population, Ayurveda nutraceuticals assure easy digestion, palatability and low dose. Ayurvedic psychological restoring preparations are in form of ghee, liquid or semisolid, supplement tablets, in likable forms. E.g., Chyavanprasha nowadays comes in attractive packing and good shelf life. Ghee capsules, oil capsules, ready-to-use herbal spice combinations, herbal tea packs and herbal nutrient supplement decoction pouches are the updated version without compromising the quality and basic ethics of preparation.

There is a promising scope in the food industry to incorporate the Ayurvedic nutraceutical preparation in a more user-friendly form. Grains, pulses, milk, ghee, oil, fresh cookies/biscuits, refreshing drinks, packaged food, snack items and ready-to-eat meal packs can be used as powerful media to fortify with Ayurvedic herbs. To give some examples, 60-day red rice is potent antioxidant. Organic production of it should be promoted. Green mung soup is advised as wholesome diet in almost all the geriatric and other diseases. Making it available in small pouches with required mixture of spices will make it an ideal Ayurvedic fortified food. Market is flooded with flavored milk like chocolate, strawberries and whatnots. Gummies like Ayurvedic Amla (Emblica officinalis) candies are popular in Asia, especially in India. Without using synthetic jelly or other binding agents, simple organic cane sugar or jaggery does wonder in Amla Candy (Indian gooseberry candy). Nutrient-loaded jam with wood apple, Indian gooseberry and mango should be on shelves in western markets too. Ayurveda diet recipes like fresh turmeric pickles, dry-ginger sweets, coconut dessert, dried-date bars and multiple-grain flour nutritious laddus (balls) are the power-packed version with balanced proteins, carbohydrates, good fats and many micronutrients. These all-simple recipes are food loaded with nutraceuticals. They need no harsh processing which may lead to nutrient loss. They are chemical free, and preservatives are not chemical but organic and part of the ingredients most of the time. Organic cane sugar, rock salt, oil, ghee and jaggery are used as natural preservatives. These are functional food in Ayurveda.

In geriatric nutritional psychiatry, thus Ayurvedic nutraceuticals and herbal preparation have prospects. Technology in hand with ancient wisdom can promise a wholesome functional food inventory in wellness industry.

Intranasal administration: is a unique effective route due to its immediate access to the skull base. The results and Rasayana properties are achieved sooner with Nasya (nasal instillation of Ayurvedic oil/ghee/herbal juice). For restoration and maintenance of the therapeutic dose in psychological disorders Nasal administration is the most easy and effective way as it surpasses the various stages of digestion and absorption. The nanoparticles in the treated ghee/oil can surpass BBB (blood-brain barrier) easily due to the lipid base. This method is safe, convenient and painless and does not require excess sterile techniques. Nasal cavity's easily accessible, rich vascular plexus permits direct entry of topically administered herbal drugs directly into the blood stream and avoids gastrointestinal destruction as well as hepatic first-pass metabolism [31]. The neural connections between the nasal mucosa and brain provide a unique pathway for noninvasive delivery of therapeutic agents to the CNS. The high permeability, high vasculature and low enzymatic environment of nasal cavity are well suitable for systemic delivery of drug molecules via the nose.

There are many theories to explain how the Nasya acts on the brain or endocrine system.

The olfactory bulb in the brain is directly connected to external environment through the olfactory nerve and its neurons in nasal cavity. (Olfactory bulb and nerve make us able to smell.) The systemic absorption of the medicine used is absorbed through the nerve cells which is transferred to olfactory bulb. Respiratory mucosa in the nasal cavity absorbs the medicines, making it systemic very quickly.

Nootropic herbs like Brahmi (Bacopa Monneri), Shankhapushpi (Convolvulus pleuricaulis), Jatamansi (Nardostachys jatamamsi) and Vacha/Sweet flag (Acorus calamus) are used in Dosha-dominant conditions in psychological disorders and related symptoms. Vacha oil Nasya is used in conditions like depression, decreased cognition due to Kapha Dosha. Psychosis is Vata Pitta-dominant disorders in most of the cases, where Vata Pitta-pacifying herbs like Brahmi (Bacopa monneri), Shankhapushpi (Convolvulus pleuricaulis) and Ashwagandha (Withania somnifera) are used effectively through nasal mucosa. In some cases, plain cow ghee, the purest form of omega-3 fatty acid, is used as Nasya. Where Pitta Dosha is dominant, ghee works as a calming agent on the CNS.

Nasya thus provides a parallel potent administration choice for nutrient administration for brain disorders [33].

Rectal administration/Basti: Ayurveda physicians often encounter an inadequate compliance in 10%–15% patients for oral administration of medicated fats especially in escalating doses. For geriatric patients, this is a very routine obstacle. Fat in the forms of medicine many times is the choice of treatment. These inconveniences can be overcome easily with the administration of aimed oil/ghee rectally. Basti is the word used in Sanskrit in the Ayurvedic text for rectal administration of Ayurvedic medicine in the form of oil/ghee or decoction. Small dose of intended oil/ghee (Anuvasana basti) enema can achieve the desired effects of herbs infused in it. Enteric absorption of herbal molecules in lipid base is easier and quicker than gastric digestion and absorption. Other than desired effects on the psychiatric elements, basti has collateral benefits on old-age gut flora. It decreases flatulence, relives constipation and keeps large intestine lubricated internally reducing Vata Dosha. Just like the stomach and small intestine, colon can also be used as an efficient gateway to absorb some of the nutrients through rich blood vessels and sensitive mucosa.

3. **Ingredients used for nutraceuticals**:

Aging and cognitive deterioration have been suggested to result from an upsurge in the brain neuron loss, which is attributable to continued instability of the brain's oxidant/antioxidant balance. Increased oxidative stress and a concomitant decrease in the brain's antioxidant defense system have been associated with functional aging and organismal maturing. However, nature has configured certain foods to be rich sources of nootropic agents, with research showing that increased consumption of such foods or food ingredients may be protective against aging-related memory decline. This knowledge is becoming increasingly valuable in an era when the boundary that separates food from medicine is becoming blurred. The benefits of food-based antioxidants with nootropic effects and/or food-based nootropic agents in mitigating memory decline and other psychological pathologies have been promisingly proven in many cases and research studies.

There is a vast variety of choices in Ayurvedic diet recommendation in terms of nutraceuticals. A brief overview of some of the food and nootropic nutrients used in Ayurveda will throw light on the potential of Ayurveda dietetics in geriatrics and psychology.

Along with this, few food items need careful diet etiquettes and other food items not for regular consumption are also mentioned [33]. This food list is a classic example of universal list of wholesome therapeutic food. These food items are tactfully used in curing physical and mental disorders successfully. These day to day and globally available food class is an ideal positive diet change among those who are suffering from illnesses. The following is a brief review of nutraceutical perspective of these food classes based on the Ayurveda literature and modern research as well as nutritional science data evidence.

Brown Rice (Shali shashtic, 60-day cropped rice): Among all the diverse varieties of rice (monocotyledon), brown rice is the most wholesome type in Ayurveda. No Pathya diet in any disease completes without red rice. Red rice is cool in nature and easy to digest even with less appetite. It has Pitta-pacifying properties and replenishes a person instantly. Charaka Samhita /Sutrasthana/Chapter 27 mentions various forms of this Shali shashtic rice, and dishes from it such as watery starch, soft liquid rice, soft solid rice and solid rice has therapeutic values with a variety of spices added. Brown rice is called "Laja" in Ayurvedic term. Laja water, laja powder with ghee and milk, and laja snacks are included in the few of the most effective Pathya diets in many diseases. Laja water with organic sugar rock salt, honey is best fluid replenishing in dehydration and nutrient loss in loose motion, Crohn's disease and other malabsorption situations. Brown rice flakes can be easily consumed just like any cereal meal available in market. It does not need any nutrient-compromising process for making. According to nutritional data, brown rice is highly nutritious. It has low calorie and has a high amount of fiber. It is a wonderful resource of magnesium, phosphorus, selenium, thiamine, niacin, vitamin B_6 and manganese. Brown rice and rough rice are rich in vitamins and minerals. Rice bran and husk contain a higher amount of calcium, zinc and iron [34]. The lipid in rice is a decent condition source of linoleic acid and other essential fatty acids [36]. These above nutritional facts support the relevant inclusion of rice in meal in various forms.

Green Mung (Vigna radiata): Interest in mung beans as a functional food is growing recently. Among all the classes of pulses or dicotyledons, mung is considered as the best choice for all in each condition irrespective of health and diseases. It is termed as wholesome (Pathya) food for all ages. Ayurveda states its properties as easy to digest, cool in property Pitta pacifying pulses. Very light and appetizing mung bean soup with medicinal herbs and kitchen spices is the most potent form of mung bean. Apart from this mung curry, mung bean pancake and sweet mung bean dessert (kheer) are some of the Ayurveda recipes.

Mung beans are a rich source of nutrients, including manganese, potassium, magnesium, folate, copper, zinc and various B vitamins. They are also a very satiety-offering food. They have high fiber, protein and resistant starch. Because of their high nutrient density, they are considered useful in defending against several chronic, age-related diseases, including heart diseases, cancers, diabetes and obesity. Current research indicates the efficacy of green mung in protection against Alzheimer's disease. Administration of moong bean sprouts for 15 successive days in different concentrations showed memory enhancement in mice as reflected by reduced transfer latency using elevated plus maze and enhanced in step-down latency in passive avoidance paradigm [35].

Rock salt: Saidhav is a type of rock salt among other five types described in Ayurveda. The group of five salts, viz. Saidhav Lavana, Samudra Lavana, Vida Lavana, Sauvarchala Lavana and Romaka Lavana. Among them, Saidhav Lavana is the best one. Iron sulfide is responsible for the dark violet or purple color of rock salt, whereas sulfur compounds are responsible for the slight savory taste and characteristic smell of the black salt. Saidhav is Rochan (taste bud stimulating), Deepan (stimulates gastric enzymes), Vrushya (good for reproductive organs), Chakshyush (good for eyesight), Avidahi (pH balance) (has lower pH than table salt), Tridoshghna (pacifies Tridoshas) and Sa-Madhur (active presence of sweet sub-taste). Replacing table salt with rock salt adds more nutrients. Rock salt is the purest form of salt which is devoid of environmental pollutants and chemical components. It contains 84 out of the 92 trace elements required by the body including calcium, iron, zinc, potassium, magnesium, copper and so on. Thus, it is available in drug stores and pharmacies in the form of powder, pill supplement or even as a liquid extract in health beverages [36]. Rock salt is beneficial in normalizing the mineralization, stabilizing the pH in tissue and reducing oxidative stress.

Amla: Amla (Emblica officinale) is one of the most recognized herbs from Ayurveda in worldwide research for a number of diseases. Amla is one of the potent Rasayana herbs used for geriatric diseases for thousands of years. Ayurveda texts state amla as Vayasthapak (antiaging), Tridosha pacifying, and favorable to eyesight, skin, hair and immunity. (Charaka Samhita /Sutrasthana/Chapter 27) states that Amalaki possess five tastes as dominant, except saltiness. This rare combination of tastes in single herb increases the medicinal properties of Amalaki. Amalaki is a versatile herb and can be used in many forms (fresh fruit, fresh juice, dry power, decoction, etc.). It is one of the major ingredients in very famous triple-herb combination named as Triphala (Emblica officinale, Terminalia billerica and Terminalia chebula).

Emblica officinalis has high vitamin C content (on average ~600 mg/100 g), and is well recognized as an immunity-boosting food. In addition to vitamin C, it is a rich source of antioxidants, including polyphenols, which confer its free radical-scavenging potential. A study by Carlson et al. revealed that it has an antioxidant content of ~261.5 mmol/100 g, which is substantially higher than numerous other plant-based foods and supplements that were tested using the FRAP assay in the same study. Practical evidence validates the antioxidant and cytoprotective properties of Amalaki in several disease models including Alzheimer's, diabetes, cardiac diseases, inflammatory disorders, hepatic diseases, atherosclerosis, cancer and neuron degeneration.

Yava: Yava is the Sanskrit name of barley, and Ayurveda praises this grain for its light nature and appetite-increasing property. The Ayurvedic literature specifically mentions barley as a potent neuroprotective food. It increases the Medha (intellect). Grasping capacity and memory are preserved and enhanced by the beneficial nutritional properties of barley.

Barley (*Hordeum vulgare* L.) is the fourth most important cereal crop in the world and has the highest dietary fiber content; its malt for functional food is not only the world's largest material for beer, but also often used as one of the 300 species being used in Chinese herbal medicine. Regular consumption of whole-grain barley and its hydroalcoholic extract reduces the risk of chronic diseases (diabetes, cancer, obesity, cardiovascular disease, etc.). Barley grass powder can be consumed as a functional food that provides nutrition and eliminates toxins from cells in human beings. Barley grass is rich in functional ingredients, such as gamma-aminobutyric acid (GABA), flavonoids, saponarin, lutonarin, superoxide dismutase (SOD), K, Ca, Se, tryptophan, chlorophyll, vitamins (A, B1, C and E), dietary fiber, polysaccharide, alkaloid, metallothioneins and polyphenols. Barley promotes sleep; has antidiabetic effect; regulates blood pressure; enhances immunity; protects the liver; has anti-acne/detoxifying and antidepressant effects; improves gastrointestinal function; has anti-cancer, anti-inflammatory, antioxidant, hypolipidemic and antigout effects; reduces hyperuricemia; prevents hypoxia, cardiovascular diseases, fatigue and constipation; alleviates atopic dermatitis; is a calcium supplement; and improves cognition and memory [37].

Yava (barley) is used to prepare Yavagu and Yusha (similar to soup) in many illnesses of Kapha Dosha. It is also used as regular bread flour in various parts of India from ancient times. Inclusion of this high-fiber, low-glycemic-index grain in the western diet in a convenient form will serve as a potent functional food.

Milk: Importance of pure non-adulterated and unprocessed milk is always highlighted from the ancient Vedic era. It is termed as Poorna Anna (complete food) as it can nourish the human body from infancy. Ayurveda has classified various animal milks. These milks with diverse properties can be used wisely in various medical conditions for their nutritional and medicinal effects on the human body. No wonder camel milk is hot-selling milk in some areas for its anti-diabetic property. Usually for common use, buffalo and cow milks are used widely due to their easy availability. Goat milk is also used in some parts of India as a portion of food. Buffalo milk is advised for sleep disorders due to its heavy and cooling properties. Those who have good digestive power are advised to have buffalo milk. Cow milk (organic, hump-bearing cow, unadulterated) is supposedly the best milk used for medicinal and nutritive purposes. Ayurveda states cow milk as a light-to-digest, sweet-taste Pitta Dosha and Vata Dosha pacifying, growth-promoting and immunity-building animal product [38]. It is replenishing and increases luster, reduces tiredness and provides immediate strength.

A2 milk is proving its ability as medicinal food over the A1-type protein milk. Whenever using milk as a therapeutic measure, it is expected from Indian hump-bearing cows. There are many formulations of milk used for the treatment of mental illnesses. Milk here is not just the medium, but it also has its own nutraceutical contribution to curing and nutritive purposes.

Milk and milk products have numerous essential nutrients. In the western societies, consumption of milk has decreased partly due to claimed negative health effects. The content of oleic acid-conjugated linoleic acid, omega-3 fatty acids, short- and medium-chain fatty acids, vitamins, minerals and bioactive compounds may promote positive health effects. Full-fat milk has been shown to increase the mean gastric emptying time compared to half-skimmed milk, thereby increasing the gastrointestinal transit time. Also, the low pH in fermented milk may delay the gastric emptying. Hence, it may be suggested that ingesting full-fat milk or fermented milk might be beneficial for glycemic (and appetite?) regulation. For some persons, milk proteins, fat and milk sugar may be of health concern. The interaction between carbohydrates (both natural milk sugar and added sugar) and proteins in milk while exposed to heat may give products, whose effects on health should be further studied, and the increasing use of sweetened milk products should be questioned. The concentration of several nutrients in milk can be manipulated through feeding regimes. There is no evidence that moderate intake of milk fat gives increased risk of diseases. Ayurvedic therapeutic diet recipes use proper cooking methods to use milk as a functional diet. Ksheerpaka recipe requires also heating of desired herb or food item with milk mixed with water till most of the water evaporates. This slow heating helps maintain the quality and quantity of nutrients. Milk being an integral part of diet can be easily introduced with medicine or other functional food. In geriatric psychiatry, the importance of cow milk always remains above. Many antioxidants and rejuvenating and nootropic medicines can be added to milk as any other milk drink powder to achieve anticipated results.

Honey: Honey is the only insect-derived natural product with therapeutic, traditional, spiritual, nutritional, cosmetic and industrial values. According to Ayurveda, honey is highly nutritive and little heavy to digest. It has healing and constricting properties. It reduces Kapha Dosha and pacifies Pitta Vata. Honey should never be consumed in large quantity or as a large portion of meal. It should not be used as replacement to sugar in meal quantity. Heating honey is contraindicated according to Ayurvedic wisdom as it destroys the delicate bonds in nectars derived from innumerous types of pollens [39]. Modern research too supports this theory. According to the National Center for Biotechnology (NCBI), heating honey is contraindicated as it causes adverse effects. Cooking honey deteriorates its quality and leads to loss of its essential enzymes and nutrients.

Heated honey can produce delirious effects in the body and can be fatal at the same time. Lukewarm water does not change the chemical bonds of honey but hot or boiling water, heating the honey, or using it in cooking does change the original chemical structure of honey. After heating, the molecules of honey form a glue-like sticky form which adheres to the microchannels of the digestive system, resulting in slow digestion and toxic effects after digestion. Recent fancy restaurants are introducing honey-baked ham and honey-cooked steak, which are incompatible if regularly consumed in large quantity. Honey should be consumed raw and in a less quantity. The brilliant medicinal properties of honey are used as catalyst with medicine. Many medicines are mixed with honey to improve its taste and assimilating potency.

The consumption of natural honey as a nutraceutical mediator is related with nutritional benefits and therapeutic possibilities. The composition of honey is mainly sugars and water. In addition, it also comprises several vitamins and minerals, including B. The extra elements of honey are amino acids, antibiotic-rich inhibin, proteins, phenol antioxidants and micronutrients. The sugars in honey are sweeter and give more energy than artificial sweeteners, and the most abundant sugar in honey is fructose. Some of the vitamins found in honey include ascorbic acid, pantothenic acid, niacin and riboflavin, along with minerals such as calcium, copper, iron, magnesium, manganese, phosphorus, potassium and zinc [40].

Raw unadulterated honey possesses anxiolytic, antinociceptive, anticonvulsant and antidepressant effects and improves the oxidative status of the brain. Several honey supplementation studies suggest that honey polyphenols have neuroprotective and nootropic effects. Polyphenol constituents of honey quench biological reactive oxygen species that cause neurotoxicity and aging.

- **Goat meat (Jangal Mans)**: Among all the animal meat and aquatic animals, goat meat and deer meat are praised in Ayurveda. Hunting deer and eating deer meat are impossible and hence excluded from description. Ayurveda discourages the consumption of red meat. Buffalo meat, cow meat and pork are specially termed as heavy-to-digest and Kapha Dosha-increasing types. Eating the above red meat will make the person lazy, obese, ill and will not benefit in long term. Higher levels of myoglobin concentration of cytotoxic lipids produce carcinogens like N-nitroso compounds (NOCs). Heme iron that gives meat its red color may promote carcinogenesis due to its ability to increase cell proliferation in the mucosa. Neu5Gc has been found in high levels in cancerous tissues but isn't produced by the human body, indicating that it comes from our diet. Neu5Gc is naturally produced in most mammals, but humans are the exception. When researchers measured the amount of Neu5Gc in various foods, they found that red meat had especially high levels. Beef, bison meat, pork and lamb had the greatest amounts of the sugar. Poultry, fish (except for caviar), vegetables and fruits lacked Neu5Gc. Among the red meat, goat meat is advocated in Ayurveda texts. Goat meat is more like human flesh and easy to digest and assimilate. It should be used in the form of soup or curry and should not be burnt (barbecuing) or dry roasted. The goat meat soup is a therapeutic choice of diet for people who have compromised immunity and weakness due to chronic diseases, for child growth, and to give strength to old people (Charaka Samhita/Sutrasthana/Chapter 27/ Shloka 61). Goat meat is 50%–65% lower in fat than similarly prepared beef but has a similar protein content. The US Department of Agriculture also has reported that saturated fat in cooked goat meat is 40% less than that of chicken, even with the skin removed [41]. Three ounces of goat meat has about 122 calories, 0.79 g of saturated fat and 3.2 mg of iron, compared to 179 calories, 3 g of saturated fat and 2.9 mg of iron in beef. Goat meat has more iron, equivalent protein and lower levels of saturated fat, calories and cholesterol compared to beef and chicken. Goat meat is superior nutritionally. Comparatively, goat meat also contains higher potassium content with lower sodium levels. Offering more nutritional value and greater health benefits with vitamin B12, it may be next big thing in meat market.

- **Cow ghee**: Ghrita (Ghee) possess Madhura rasa and Prithvi Jala (earth and water) elements in dominance. These elements have Brihana (nourishing and growth promoting) property which is responsible for stability and improves brain functions. Ghrita has appetite increasing, catalyst, Rasayana, Vrishya (aphrodisiac) and Vata Pitta-pacifying effects and overcomes vitiated Kapha Dosha due to processing alteration guna. According to modern science, Ghrita is lipophilic in nature; thus, it diffuses rapidly across the cell membrane which is also composed of bimolecular lipid matrix. Ghrita contains the cholesterol which is responsible for the synthesis of steroid hormones, i.e., estrogen and progesterone. Ayurveda praises many properties of ghee. Ghee promotes memory, intellect and metabolism, and improves and increases the quality of Shukra dhatu (semen, Ojas). It alleviates Vata, Pitta, Visha (poisons), insanity and emaciation. It is the best of all the unctuous substances. Cool in potency, ghee heals internal and external wear and tear. When administered according to the prescribed procedure, it increases thousand times in potency and develops manifold utilities. Ghee properly preserved for longer periods is termed as Puran Ghrita and becomes more potent. Purana ghee is useful in intoxication, epilepsy, fainting, emaciation, schizophrenia, fever, etc. It is best suited for those desiring intellect, memory and intelligence. Ghee.

11.9 Nootropic herbs used in diet and medicine preparation of geriatric psychological management

Ayurveda provides a list of herbs known for nootropic action as well as their multi-dimensional efficiency in various requirements. Medhya Rasayana addressed in Ayurveda under rigorous research have established to be potential precognitive herbs.

Mandukaparni (Centella asiatica Linn.), Yastimadhu (Glycirrhiza glabra Linn.), Guduchi (Tinospora cordifolia), Shankhapushpi (Convolvulus pleuricaulis Chois), Aindri (Bacopa monniera), Jyotishmati (Celastrus panniculata), Kushmanda (Benincasa hispida), Vacha (Acorus calamus) and Jatamamsi (Nardostachys jatamamsi) are rewarding one. The above herbs, alone or in combination with minerals, are proved to show satisfactory results as immune modulator, neuroprotector, free-radical scavengers, memory enhancers, cognition enhancers and hepatoprotectors. The Ayurvedic Medhya Rasayana theory positively holds the prospect of the next big thing in cognitive health management. Preclinical studies on *Medhya Rasayana* (Ayurvedic nootropics) such as Asvagandha, turmeric and Brahmi have demonstrated the ability to clear amyloid-β plaques in neurons that are observed in Alzheimer's disease.

The following is a list of medicinal preparations comprised in functional food. These polyherbal preparations are found in the major Samhitas in Ayurveda like Charaka Samhita, Sushruta Samhita, Vagbhat Samhita, Ashtanga Hridayam, Bhavprakasha, Yogratnakara, Bhaijya Ratnavali, etc. (Table 11.4).

These are few of the most used functional food or Ayurvedic medicinal preparations applied as Pathya nutrition for curing mental illnesses. These formulations contain a lot of Ayurvedic herbs and kitchen spices. It is practically impossible to narrate every single ingredient and its nutraceutical role in the combination in this chapter. In all combinations, one or many herbs are repeated as ingredient. Among all the ingredients, the following are few commonly used herbs with their contribution in brief as potent nutraceutical in geriatrics.

1. **Sesame oil**: For thousands of years, sesame seed oil is used internally and externally to cure a number of health ailments and to maintain health. Sesame seeds are bitter in taste and hot and heavy in nature. It lubricates, soften and penetrates the skin efficiently. It reduces the Kapha Dosha and Vata Dosha and is termed as "Drudhkara" (stabilizing strength). (Charaka Samhita /Sutrasthana/Chapter 27)

   Its oral administration is an excellent method for improving iron level, controlling cholesterol, managing heart diseases and improving strength. Sesame oil is beneficial for the skin. It is an antioxidant as it contains vitamin E and penetrates skin easily. This oil is rich in minerals (copper, calcium, zinc, iron). Calcium and zinc are good for bones and joint health. Copper gives relief in arthritis and gout. Magnesium

Table 11.4 Polyherbal Formulations for Mental Health in Aging Population.

Polyherbal Functional Food	Uses
Maha Kalyanaka Ghrita	Memory loss, schizophrenia, psychosis
Brahmi Ghrita	Depression, fatigue, stress disorders, improves cognition
Panchgavya Ghrita	Psychology disorders, epilepsy
Paishachik Ghrita	
Lashunadi Ghrita	Confusion, convulsions, depression
Chetasa Ghrita	Kapha Dosha-dominant mental disorders
Dadhika Ghrita	Depression, insomnia
Kushmanda Ghrita	Cognitive health enhancer, memory boosting, depression
Siddhartha Ghrita	Psychosis, depression
Mahatiktaka Ghrita	Skin lesion, phobias, complex
Sahacharadi oil	For Nasya in mental disorders
Jyotishmati oil	Antioxidant, for Nasya in sleep disorders, neuron nourishment, depression, etc.
Anu tail	Psychosis, dementia, migraine
Dhanvantaram oil	Externally and internally of intellectual health, psychosis
Mamsyadi oil	Insomnia, mood disorders, dementia, insanity
Chandanadi oil	Insomnia, Pitta Dosha dominant psychosis
Tungbhadradi oil	Convulsions, confusions, mental, depression
Chavanprash	Antiaging, Antioxidant, physical and mental nourishment
Shatavari kalp	Weakness, neural health, general tonic, replenishes pitta, calms mind and promotes digestion
Saraswataarisht syrup	Promotes sleep, used in Stress disorders, mood swings, depression, Psychosis, etc.
Hinguvachadi churnam	Promotes digestion and metabolism, used in kapha Dosha dominant psychological disorders

supports respiratory and vascular health. It increases good cholesterol and decreases bad cholesterol. Sesame oil has a mild purgative action. It relives constipation tendencies in old age. These nutrient-packed seeds are advocated as antiaging and good for teeth and hair in Rasayana description. Chewing black sesame seeds early in the morning is a daily Rasayana practice. Replacing refined and saturated fatty oils with sesame seeds is advisable. Also, the external application of plain or medicated Til oil is highly recommended in aging population to restore the muscular strength, joint health and conditional health. It is a potent antiaging food. Base for most of the medicated oil in Ayurveda is Til (sesame).

2. **Brahmi (Bacopa Monneri):** Ayurvedic and other herbal medications have gained increased acceptance as they are found to be safer than the synthetic counterparts. Indian system of medicine, Ayurveda, in literatures like Sushruta Samhita, Charaka Samhita and Atharva Veda

describe plants which have a Prabhava (specific action) on the intellect and memory as Medhya Rasayana. Brahmi is one of the Medhya Rasayanas. It is bitter in taste, cool in property and has calming effect on Pitta-related mental and physical disorders. Neurotransmitters in Bacopa modify the balance of acetyl choline which is important for memory and cognition. Bacopa has antioxidant effects which enhance cognitive functions. Bacopa extract helps prevent arterial plaque that can lead to heart attack, stroke and other neurodegenerative diseases. Bacopa is used in the form of juice, wet-crushed bolus, extract tablet, powder or capsules. Bacopa has a significant anxiolytic (anti-anxiety) effect. It seems to regulate brain levels of the neurotransmitter serotonin. This influences mood regulation too. Brahmi prash, Brahmi Ghrita and various other Ayurvedic preparations contain Brahmi as the major ingredient.

3. **Vacha (Acorus calamus)**: Vacha is categorized in Sandyasthapana class (anticonvulsant) in Charaka and Sushruta Samhita. Vacha oil is commonly used by Ayurvedic doctors for nasal disorders, headache, migraine and chronic kapha disorders of the nose, head and respiratory system. Vacha is specifically used for Nasya for its quicker absorption quality in respiratory mucosa. Acorus calamus roots have many fatty acids together with palmitic, myristic, stearic, palmitoleic, arachicic, oleic and linoleic. They also contain glucose, fructose and maltose. Vacha roots and leaves are abundant in antioxidants. The oil extraction contains eugenol, calamine, terpenoids, calamenol, camphene and calamenone. Vacha oil is obtained by distillation method and is used for aromatherapy orally or externally. Vacha has the history of its medicinal uses which can be traced back to 4,000 years to the Ayurvedic, Chinese and samurai cultures. Aqueous portion of Acorus calamus shows promising results against oxidative stress and neuroinflammation. It can fight memory loss and can be used as preventive and curative measures in geriatric ailments too [42].

4. **Shatavari (Asparagus racemose)**: Shatavari is cool in property and bitter in taste. Its root has medicinal properties. Shatavari can be used as power food for geriatric population. According to Ayurveda, Shatavari has immediate calming and replenishing action on the very first digestive product called as Rasa Dhatu (lymph). This Ras dhatu being parent dhatu for other subsequent Dhatu/tissue is important. Shatavari is a nerve tonic termed as the friend of women that improves stamina, reduces weakness and acts as a brilliant galactagogue. In geriatric patients, Shatavari can be used to compensate the calorie spill due to less appetite and poor digestion. Shatavari milk powder, Shatavari sweet granules and other forms as soup or sherbet are effective. To correct nutritional error and nutrient deficiencies, Shatavari is proving a potent nutraceutical not only in geriatrics but also in pediatrics, gynecological and other nutritional sciences.

5. **Jatamansi**: *Nardostachys Jatamansi* is an herb known for its potential ability to reduce stress and enhance cognitive function and sleep. Many studies and trials proved fruitful and state that Jatamansi enhanced memory, reduced inflammation and treated insomnia in preclinical studies. Jatamansi is a rare herb found in alpine regions of Himalayas. Its roots are hairy and have a distinct aroma. Jatamansi is used in the form of Phanta sherbet or powder. Nasya with fine powder is stated in some mental illnesses too. Jatamansi is light to digest and assimilate, bitter astringent taste and cool in property. It is termed as Bhutghna (antimicrobial) and is Medhya Rasayana. Nutraceutical preparations like Dhanvantarishtam, Dasahanga Lepa and Sarpgandha Vati contains Jatamansi as an ingredient. The active essential oils and other chemical composition in Jatamansi are proved to be antioxidant, anti-inflammatory, anti-lipogenic and antihypertensive.

6. **Turmeric**: Curcuma longa or turmeric is a kitchen spice used in India from the ancient time for its medicinal uses and exotic aroma in cooking. Curcumin, the prime bioactive compound in turmeric, is responsible for turmeric's color and many of its remarkable health advantages. The role of curcumin is accepted as an analgesic and anti-inflammatory in various diseases, but it is also a standout as a brain enhancer and protector. Curcumin supplements can help lift your mood, control stress and anxiety, and protect your brain against aging and neurodegenerative disease. According to the Ayurvedic text, Haridra (Curcuma longa) is astringent, bitter in taste and excellent in blood purifying and healing through its antimicrobial activity. It is a potent Pitta Dosha purifier and pacifier. It fights against excess Kapha Dosha through taste action. Overall turmeric is one of the most potent immunomodulators and nutraceuticals that can be used without any hassle. Instead of curcumin extract, it is always advisable to use turmeric in cooking and in dishes. Because turmeric has more nutrients than curcumin. Turmeric has more than 300 biological components such as beta-carotene, ascorbic acid (vitamin C), calcium, flavonoids, fiber, iron, niacin, potassium, zinc and other nutrients. Turmeric Latte, Moon Milk, Fresh turmeric root in salad, canned turmeric, turmeric pickle, turmeric curry masala (spice) and jaggery turmeric candies are appetizing forms in food market which are extremely health friendly. Opportunities are endless to use turmeric as a nutraceutical in geriatric psychology too.

7. **Triphala**: Triphala is probably the most used combination of natural herbs applied globally by Ayurveda doctors and common people. Three unexceptionally potent herbs from Ayurveda are combined by the wise sages in the ancient era to come up with Triphala. Triphala is equal combination of Amalaki (Emblica Officinale), Haritaki (Terminalia Chebula) and Bhibhitaka (Terminalia Bellirica). Triphala is tactfully used in geriatric patients to combat with gut dysbiosis, constipation, flatulence, insomnia and overall Rasayana. Various

combinations like with honey, with warm water, with buttermilk and in the form of decoction serve to offer relief in various conditions and symptoms. Triphala is an inexpensive and nontoxic natural product alternative for the prevention and treatment of diseases where vascular endothelial growth factor A–induced angiogenesis is involved. The existence of several polyphenolic combinations enables it with a broad antimicrobial spectrum. It has a very good impact on the cardiac health, skin and eyes, and helps to delay degenerative changes, such as cataracts. Triphala is used as active ingredients in more than 1,500 Ayurvedic classical formulations, and it can be used for several diseases in different forms. Triphala prevents degenerative and metabolic disorders probably through lipid peroxide inhibition and free radical scavenging pathways.

8. **Yashtimadhu**: Yashtimadhu (Glycirrhiza glabra) is herb of choice in hundreds of health conditions. This herb holds tremendous potential as nutraceutical from pediatrics to geriatrics and multiple systemic disorders. Yashtimadhu is highly praised for its Madhur (sweet)-dominant taste, cool nature, and pitta-pacifying, healing, nurturing and tissue regeneration properties in various Ayurvedic literature. Use of Yashtimadhu in geriatric as nutraceutical food has multiple possibilities as ingredient in medicine as well as functional food. Studies have supported the anti-asthmatic, antioxidant, antiulcer, analgesic, anticancer, anti-Alzheimer's, immunomodulation and aphrodisiac nature of Yashtimadhu. Other active constituents of licorice include bioflavonoids, chalcones, coumarins, triterpenoids and sterols, lignans, amino acids, amines, gums and volatile oils which are found to be responsible for its various activities like wound-healing activity, antiulcer activity, memory-enhancing activity, hair growth-promoting activity, antithrombotic effect, hepatoprotective effect, cerebro-protective effect, antidyslipidemic activity, antioxidant activity, etc. Yashtimadhu is naturally sweet and tastes good. It can be easily applied as a functional food in the geriatric field.

9. **Cow urine**: Cow urine is used effectively for its medicinal properties in Ayurveda from the ancient era. Panchgavya is made up of five cow products: milk, curd, ghee, urine and dung, and is also used in many Ayurvedic formulations related to psychological disorders. Panchgavya Ghrita is one of them. The latest discovery linked to cow urine was its active role as a bioenhancer. Distillate cow's urine is an activity enhancer and bioavailability facilitator for bioactive molecules (antibiotic, antifungal and anticancer drugs). Cow urine research studies have satisfactory outputs for its antioxidant, antimicrobial and anticarcinogenic nature. Its effective use in human and animal health and agriculture are being explored from some years. The Ayurveda literature praises cow urine for its mineral contents. Cow urine is strong (Tikshna), has high permeability and is Bhutghna (antibacterial,

antimicrobial). Its bitter astringent taste and hot properties are used for the treatment of skin ailments to mental disorders. The presence of urea, creatinine, swarn kshar (aurum hydroxide), carbolic acid, phenols, calcium and manganese has firmly supported for exposition of the medicinal properties of cow urine [43].

10. **Kushmanda (Benincasa Hispida)**: It is highly cool in property and has healing, nourishing and Pitta-pacifying active roles in metabolism. Kushmanda plays calming, apoptogenic roles in the nerves and brain. Kushmanda Ghrita is choice of medicine in many mental illnesses like depression, insomnia and hypersomnia. It is termed as Medhya. It has Madhura/sweet-dominant taste, is cold in nature and nourishes all the tissues. Kushmanda (white gourd/Petha/Ash gourd) is a rich source of amino acid, mucins, mineral salts, starch, calcium, and vitamins B and C. DSM-IV is used to study the role of ash gourd in many mental illnesses. Within diagnostic criteria of depressive illness, both male and female participants are treated with Kushmanda Ghrita and the results are very convincing after one-month treatment. Kushmanda Ghrita has shown statistically very good results for mental illness symptoms such as sad mood, suicidal tendency, anxiety, lack of confidence, loss of interest, etc.

11. **Jyotishmati**: Jyotishmati is scientifically known as Celastrus paniculatus. This is one of the most significant medicinal herbs in Ayurveda. The plant has shown significant pharmacological activities like anti-arthritic, wound healing, hypolipidemic and antioxidant. Research studies shed light on its activity of balance at neurotransmitter level. Jyotishmati plays a significant action at the acetylcholine level, and it improves cognitive function remarkably. It mainly balances the neurotransmitters like serotonin, epinephrine and dopamine to improve various aspects of cognitive functions of the brain. Jyotishmati is bitter and pungent in taste, and after absorption in blood, the dominant taste remains pungent. It is hot in property. Oil extracted from seeds are extremely beneficial in skin diseases. It is Medhya by its strong piercing nature and is included in Shirovirechana (Dosha-extracting) class by Sushruta and Charaka.

    Antioxidant and neuroprotective: Antioxidants in Jyotishmati drop malondialdehyde in the brain and lessens its negative impacts on neurons, with simultaneous significant increase in the levels of glutathione and catalase. Smritisagar Ras medicine in Ayurveda, which contains Jyotishmati oil, is used in geriatric dementia for memory enhancement and sleep promotion.

Other ingredients also exhibit such extraordinary medicinal properties which can be used in geriatric population for management of psychiatric ailments.

A major challenge in the next century will be to create a health-care system that integrates primary health care and mental health care for older persons.

Influential incumbrances lessen the scope of providing psychological health services within primary care. To increase the effectiveness of treatment for older adults with mental disorders, mental health clinicians may need to make additional efforts to maintain rapport with staff in the primary-care practices that serve these patients. Creating a bridge of mutual understanding across specialties, with advocacy for integration of mental health into a general medical framework, will be a key element in enhancing the overall health and functioning of older persons in the next century. Integrating the multiple aspects of modern medicine and nutritional sciences with the Ayurvedic science can provide the effective possible reach. This approach can provide a comprehensive psychological, social, behavioral and spiritual codes of conduct which can be appropriately tailored and revised to fit the present condition as a social and mental health promotion regimen. The mortality observed in recent decades is reduced. However, in the field of psychiatry, there is a lack of similar population-level initiatives in the prevention of common mental disorders, depression and anxiety. Also, the area of psychiatry is yet not fully opened its arm for the concepts of adapting diet and lifestyle as efficient tools in prevention and management of psychological illnesses. Medicine-oriented approach is yet popular and acquires the major portion of the mental health sector. Integration of the available streams of various sciences such as medicine, nutrition, behavioral therapy, physical therapy, ancient herbal medicine and ancient nutritional theories offers the benefits of multiple choices, custom maid medicine. PPT approach, i.e., prediction, prevention and treatment, is only possible with the help of the above-mentioned interdisciplinary streams and their effective standardized application.

Nutritional psychiatry holds tremendous potential in predicting the health profile and future physical and mental diseases by studying the diet trends, habits, socioeconomical and cultural influence on food choices, etc. Integration of Ayurveda dietetics with the modern nutrition science will increase the horizon of treatment and preventive modalities. Beyond the calculative approach of modern nutrition, Ayurveda dietetics can fulfill the loopholes such as diversity in phenotypes, genotypes, epigenetics and other personalized approach to pinpoint the exact diagnosis, cure and management. Ayurveda offers a wide range of nootropic herbs used as functional food. The theories can be guiding in preventive approach. Organic solution to synthetic drugs will increase the sustainable course of treatment. In all, nutritional psychiatry along with the wisdom of Ayurvedic psychology and dietetics can offer a fundamental integrative foundation in geriatric psychiatry and its management.

References

1. https://www.un.org/en/sections/issues-depth/ageing/.Alth.
2. Murray C, Vos T, Lozano R, et al. The global economic burden of noncommunicable diseases. Program on the Global Demography of Aging. 2012:8712; The Lancet. 2010;380(9859):2197–223. [PubMed] [Google Scholar]

3. https://www.who.int/news-room/fact-sheets/detail/mental-health-of-older-adults.
4. https://www.ncbi.nlm.nih.gov/pmc/articles/PMC3031932/.
5. The Impact of Nutrition and Intestinal Microbiome on Elderly Depression—A Systematic Review Blanca Klimova, Michal Novotny and Martin Valis].
6. https://www.ncbi.nlm.nih.gov/pmc/articles/PMC3046018/#b1-imi-2008-033.
7. Report of the treatment with manganese chloride of 181 cases of schizophrenia, 33 of manic depression, and 16 other defects of psychoses at the Ontario Hospital, Brockville, Ontario. *American Journal of Psychiatry*. 1929;9:569–80.
8. Sydenstricker VP, Cleckley HM. The effect of nicotinic acid in stupor, lethargy, and various other psychiatric disorders. *American Journal of Psychiatry*. 1941;98:83–92.
9. Miller A. The methylation, neurotransmitter, and antioxidant connections between folate and depression. *Alternative Medicine Review*. 2008;13(3):216–26.
10. Simopoulos A. Evolutionary aspects of diet: The omega-6/omega-3 ratio and the brain. *Molecular Neurobiology*. 2011;44:203–15.
11. Nuernberg K, Nuernberg G, Ender K, et al. N-3 fatty acids and conjugated linoleic acids of longissimus muscle in beef cattle. *European Journal of Lipid Science and Technology*. 2002;104(8):463–71.
12. Sandstead HH, Frederickson CJ, Penland JG. History of zinc as related to brain function. *Journal of Nutrition*. 2000;130(2S Suppl):496S–502S.
13. Englard S., Seifter S. The biochemical functions of ascorbic acid. *Annual Review of Nutrition*. 1986;6:365–406. doi:10.1146/annurev.nu.06.070186.002053.
14. Zhang T.Y., Meaney M.J. Epigenetics and the environmental regulation of the genome and its function. *Annual Review of Psychology*. 2010;61:439–466. doi:10.1146/annurev.psych.60.110707.163625. [PubMed]
15. May J.M. Vitamin C transport and its role in the central nervous system. Subcell. *Biochem*. 2012;56:85–103. [PMC free article] [PubMed] [Google Scholar]
16. Berk M., Williams L.J., Jacka F.N., O'Neil A., Pasco J.A., Moylan S., Allen N.B., Stuart A.L., Hayley A.C., Byrne M.L., et al. So depression is an inflammatory disease, but where does the inflammation come from? *BMC Medicine*. 2013;11:200. doi:10.1186/1741-7015-11-200. [PMC free article] [PubMed] [Cross Ref] [Google Scholar]
17. Charaksamhita/ Chikitsasthana /Chapter 1 /Shloka 5, Publication: Chaukhamba Bharati Academy, Varanasi. Authors: Pandit Kashinath Pandey, Dr. Gorakhnath Chaturvedi.
18. Charaka Samhita/ Sutrasthana/Chapter11 shloka 35, Publication: Chaukhamba Bharati Academy, Varanasi. Authors: Pandit Kashinath Pandey, Dr. Gorakhnath Chaturvedi.
19. Charaksamhita /Sutrasthana/Chapter27 /shloka 3 Publication: Chaukhamba Bharati Academy, Varanasi. Authors: Pandit Kashinath Pandey, Dr. Gorakhnath Chaturvedi.
20. Charaka Samhita /Sutrasthana /Chapter26/shloka 102–103 Publication: Chaukhamba Bharati Academy, Varanasi. Authors: Pandit Kashinath Pandey, Dr. Gorakhnath Chaturvedi.
21. Charaka samhita/ Sutrasthana /Chapter26/shloka 38–46 Publication: Chaukhamba Bharati Academy, Varanasi. Authors: Pandit Kashinath Pandey, Dr. Gorakhnath Chaturvedi.
22. https://www.ncbi.nlm.nih.gov/pmc/articles/PMC3402070/.
23. Charaka Samhita /Sutrasthana/Chapter 21 /Shloka 42 to 45 Publication: Chaukhamba Bharati Academy, Varanasi. Authors: Pandit Kashinath Pandey, Dr. Gorakhnath Chaturvedi.
24. Charaka Samhita /Sutrasthana /Chapter 21/Shloka 48, Publication: Chaukhamba Bharati Academy, Varanasi. Authors: Pandit Kashinath Pandey, Dr. Gorakhnath Chaturvedi.
25. https://tools.myfooddata.com/protein-calculator/01003/100g.
26. Charaka Samhita /Chikitsasthana / Chapter 1 /Shloka 3, Publication: Chaukhamba Bharati Academy, Varanasi. Authors: Pandit Kashinath Pandey, Dr. Gorakhnath Chaturvedi.

27. Charaksamhita /Sutrasthana/chapter 5/shloka 113 to149, Publication: Chaukhamba Bharati Academy, Varanasi. Authors: Pandit Kashinath Pandey, Dr. Gorakhnath Chaturvedi.
28. Charaksamhita /Sutrasthana /Chapter 5 / shloka 161, Publication: Chaukhamba Bharati Academy, Varanasi. Authors: Pandit Kashinath Pandey, Dr. Gorakhnath Chaturvedi.
29. Charaksamhita /Sutrasthana /Chapter 5/ shloka,170–172, Publication: Chaukhamba Bharati Academy, Varanasi. Authors: Pandit Kashinath Pandey, Dr. Gorakhnath Chaturvedi.
30. https://www.ncbi.nlm.nih.gov/pmc/articles/PMC4127822/#ref2].
31. http://www.iamj.in/posts/2014/images/upload/607_612.pdf.
32. https://rupalipanse.com/2016/05/18/nasya-the-way-to-brain-through-skull-base/.
33. Charaksamhita /Sutrasthana /Chapter 5 / shloka 105–107 Publication: Chaukhamba Bharati Academy, Varanasi. Authors: Pandit Kashinath Pandey, Dr. Gorakhnath Chaturvedi.
34. https://journalofethnicfoods.biomedcentral.com/articles/10.1186/s42779-019-0017-3.
35. https://www.researchgate.net/publication/303123605_Anti-alzheimer_potential_of_green_moong_bean.
36. https://wjpr.net/admin/assets/article_issue/1480495868.pdf.
37. https://www.ncbi.nlm.nih.gov/pmc/articles/PMC5904770/.
38. Charaka Samhita /Sutrasthana/Chapter 27 /Shloka 218.
39. Charaka Samhita /Sutrasthana/Chapter 27/Shloka 246–248.
40. https://www.ncbi.nlm.nih.gov/pmc/articles/PMC3583289/.
41. https://abga.org/abga-education/nutritional-facts/.
42. https://pubmed.ncbi.nlm.nih.gov/30450168/.
43. https://innovareacademics.in/journal/ijpps/Vol6Issue3/9051.pdf.

12

Skeletomuscular Losses in Aging and Nutraceuticals

Ankita Mehta
Nirma University

Jayvadan Patel
Sankalchand Patel University

Mayur M. Patel and Bhoomika Patel
Nirma University

Contents

DOI: 10.1201/9781003110866-12

12.1 Introduction

Aging or senescence can be defined as the time-related deterioration of the physiological functions necessary for survival and fertility (Gilbert, 2000). Many biologists consider aging as a part of a default process that occurs after the animal has fulfilled the requirements for natural selection rather than calling it a part of a genetic source. Aging can lead to a persistent decrease in survival and reproductive rates. Ultimately, these rates will decline and reach zero at a point where an organism stops living and reproducing (Flatt, 2012). According to evolutionary biologists, aging is not a programmed process; rather, it would be more appropriate to define it as the detritus of selective post-reproductive period of life. Therefore, we could use mechanisms to slower the deleterious effects leading to death (Medawar, 1952; Kirkwood, 1977). Hence, we could say that aging is linked with the sum of deleterious effects and the counteracting and healing mechanisms responding to the injury to the physiological system (Johnson et al, 1999).

Every physiological system of the body gets affected by the normal aging process. It is a steady irreversible process of deterioration of organ functions which rate is reliant on the different organ systems. The rate of aging is equivalent for 45- and 85-year-old men; it's just that the 85-year-old man has mounted up the age-related changes (Boss et al., 1981). Speaking about tissues, in the younger people, healing process is faster in tissues because of the good blood supplies and high metabolic rate of the cells. Extracellular components of the cells play important roles in the aging process, for example, glucose, the most abundant sugar in the body, generates cross-links between adjacent protein molecules irreversibly. With aging, the more cross-link formation will lead to loss of elasticity and stiffening of the tissues. Collagen fibers are increased and lose their quality with the aging process, affecting the strength of the tendon and flexibility of the arterial wall. Elastin, another extracellular component, is responsible for blood vessel and skin elasticity. With the age, it thickens and fragments that will gain more affinity with the calcium which might be associated with atherosclerosis (Tortora and Derrickson, 2009). An overview of the events associated with skeletal muscle losses associated with sarcopenia and osteopenia is provided in Figure 12.1.

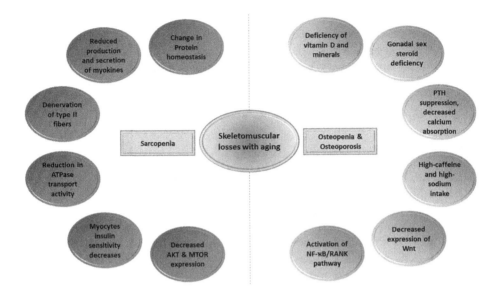

Figure 12.1 *An overview of the events associated with skeletal muscle losses associated with sarcopenia and osteopenia.*

12.2 Skeletal muscle loss with aging (Sarcopenia)

One of the most manifested clinical and functional significances of aging is the loss of muscle mass, called sarcopenia. Sarcopenia was first termed by Rosenburg in 1989 (Rosenberg, 1997). One of the current definitions outlines sarcopenia as "a progressive and generalized skeletal muscle disorder that involves the accelerated loss of muscle mass and function" (Cruz-Jentoft et al., 2019). Skeletal muscle is a crucial muscle involved in maintaining the quality of life as it controls vital functions such as metabolism, movement, posture maintenance, and breathing (Karakelides and Nair, 2005; Marzetti et al., 2009; Sayed et al., 2016). Indicators of sarcopenia include muscle wasting, weakness, falling, slowness, and troubles in carrying out routine activities. Diagnosis is quite straightforward by considering its definition that requires assessing muscle mass, strength, and physical ability (Bruyère et al., 2016). In humans, between the ages of 20 and 80 years, the inevitable loss of muscle mass of about 40% subsidizes to deterioration of muscle strength and its functions (Narici et al., 2004; Roubenoff, 2001; Roubenoff and Hunghes, 2000). Studies suggest the role of hormones, denervation of skeletal muscles, increasing circulating inflammatory mediators, genetics, poor health, nutrition, disuse atrophy, sedentary lifestyle, morbidity, and gender in the development of sarcopenia (Harris, 1997, Gallagher et al., 1997, Baumgartner et al., 1995, Doherty et al., 1993, Tenover, 1997, Bruunsgaard et al., 2003). Smoking has been identified as lowering the muscle mass, whereas malnutrition is not well established in causing loss of muscle mass except in sick and hospitalized aged people (Baumgartner et al., 1995). In fact, studies suggest that muscle wasting is more seen with higher body mass index than the lower, although the other factors such as genetic, morbidity, muscle fiber composition, and ethnicity are not very well established to be affecting muscle mass and strength. There is a necessity to develop newer improved methodologies, epidemiologic studies, and better criteria to measure and predict sarcopenia (Morley et al., 2002, Vittone et al., 1996, Launer et al., 1994).

12.2.1 Gross morphological changes

Sarcopenia can arise from both muscle atrophy (decrease in size of muscle fiber) and hypoplasia (number of muscle fibers) (Larsson et al., 1978; Klitgaard et al., 1990). It can be identified grossly by quantitative measurement of muscle mass and change in muscle performance (Clark and Manini, 2008). Various techniques exist for the diagnosis of sarcopenia including computed tomography, magnetic resonance imaging, dual X-ray absorptiometry, anthropometry or hydrostatic weighing, and the cross-sectional area measurement of muscle mass (Frontera et al., 2000; Van Kan et al., 2011). A decrease in muscle mass is more prevalent after the age of 70 years. After the age of 70 years, muscle mass has been reported to be lost about 0.5%–1.0% per year and per decade, 4.7%, and 3.7% declines in men and women, respectively (Mitchell et al., 2012). Parallel to loss of muscle mass, strength also decays to 10%–15% up to 70 years of age, and it accelerates to 25%–40% afterward for each decade (Goodpaster et al., 2006; Hughes et al., 2001). Revised prevalence estimated with the help of novel DXA technology determines 8.8% and 13.5% during the age of 60–69 years and up to 16% and 29% in the age above 80 years in women and men, respectively (Baumgartner, 2000). Chronic muscle loss affects approximately 30% of people with an age of 60 and above and more than 50% of those with age greater than 80 years (Baumgartner et al., 1998). Decline in skeletal muscle mass progressively with aging leading to weakness is owing to a reduction in maximal voluntary joint power and loss of overall muscle force (Brooks and Faulkner, 1994). Studies have reported that decrease in lean body mass is seen greater in lower limbs which is about 15% than of upper limbs (about 10%) which could be occurring due to a couple of reasons such as constant locomotive activity in lower limbs, detraining effect on lower limbs, more loss of motor units in legs than arms; however, the actual reason for this difference has not been identified (Janssen et al., 2000, Morse et al., 2004). Considering the effect of sarcopenia on different body parts, thigh muscles responsible for locomotor activity lose around 24%–27% of muscle mass (Young et al., 1985).

12.2.2 Physiological changes in sarcopenia

Skeletal muscle is responsible for improving metabolic homeostasis, surge stress resistance, and delay age-associated functional deterioration in the tissues by producing growth factors and cytokines. Reduction in skeletal muscle mass can lead to reduced production and secretion of myokines and deterio-rate physiological and cellular basis in the body leading to a decline in the functional capacity of different organ systems, age-related disorders, and a rise in mortality rate. Physiological changes during sarcopenia are seen in muscle fiber size, muscle strength, function, and performance (Demontis et al., 2013).

As we have mentioned earlier, the production of force and power generation is the most vital function of skeletal muscle to make movement and mobility possible. Several cellular elements that are contributing in so get changed with the aging process leading to weakness in muscles. Multiple studies have been carried out to measure muscle strength, that shows a decline, gain, and no change in muscle strength. These discrepancies could be the result of the level of physical activities, genetic factors, and hormonal levels (Bassey and Harries, 1993; Greig et al., 1993; Padykula and Herman, 1995; Reid et al., 2012). Muscle strength peaks at the age of 30–39 years; afterward, it starts to decline about 1.5% each year starting at the age of 50 years and 3% after the age of 60 (Perna et al., 2016; Emerson et al., 2015). Cross-sectional and longitudinal studies have shown that the strength of the upper and lower limbs reduces 0.5%–1.0% per annum (Frontera et al., 2000; Reid et al., 2014). Muscle strength loss makes day-to-day life activities more challenging which can also lead to dropping independence. Muscle architecture plays an important role in strength differ-ences than muscle size.

Fiber strength is dependent upon fiber characteristics and muscle composition. Fiber characteristics include fiber type, fiber orientation, fiber atrophy, and fiber length. Eighty-five percent of muscle fiber is made up of myofibrillar pro-tein. Based on the expression of myosin heavy chain isoforms, myofibers are classified into two categories: type I myofibers and type II myofibers (Folland and Williams, 2007; Favier et al., 2008). Type I fibers are slow-oxidative and release lesser force than type II fibers which are fast-glycolytic (Pette et al., 1999; de Rezende et al., 2015). Fiber orientation with tendons or connective tissues influences the strength of the muscle. With the advanced age, modifi-cation and denervation of type II fibers and re-innervation of type I fibers lead to a decrease in CSA, and muscle mass (Folland and Williams, 2007). This is due to a reduction in contractile proteins in the muscle that also leads to an increase in contraction/relaxation time, reduction in ATPase transport activ-ity, and muscle strength. The reason behind these changes in muscle fibers is not clear but could be due to apoptotic loss of alfa-motor neurons (Brook et al., 2016; Russ et al., 2012). Also with the age, expression of troponin reduces, expression of desmin used for force transmission and increases post-translational modification increases. These all factors lead to compromised protein functions and therefore weakening the force generation and decreas-ing the strength of the muscle (Russ et al., 2012). The length of the fibers becomes shorter with age which interrupts muscle-specific length-tension and force-velocity relationship (Suetta et al., 2009). A study has shown to be decreased knee extension torque in older people up to 22%–56% compared with adults. Thus, in a more overextended position, older people are unable to generate extension torque in their knees. Muscle quality degrades with the age primarily due to the increasing volume of connective tissues and lipid buildup inside the muscle cells (Melo et al., 2016). Elevation of adipose tissue deposition occurs with the aging of muscle in both intra- and intermuscular sites. This relates to reduced mitochondrial functions. A rise in adipose tissue adversely influences muscle strength, function, and performance (Marcus et al., 2013). These factors affect muscle functions and performance whose restoration requires different rehabilitation procedures including exercise and nutritional supplements.

12.2.3 Changes at the molecular level

Inevitable changes in skeletal muscle due to the aging process leading to muscular atrophy and weakness are important to understand at the cellular and molecular levels. Skeletal muscles are composed of hundreds to thousands of fibers that contain myofibrils which is a linear array of sarcomeres. Sarcomere contains different contractile proteins such as myosin, actin, troponin, and tropomyosin which are important for skeletal muscle functions. With the help of ATP, attachment of myosin and actin leading to contraction of the skeletal muscle. When actin is strongly attached to the myosin chain, force generation takes place. Age-related structural and chemical changes affect this bond leading to decreased force generation for which different molecular changes are responsible (Dreyer and Volpi, 2005; Vandervoort, 2002).

Skeletal muscles are the major reservoir of amino acids, wherein protein homeostasis plays a major role in muscle functions and performance. Protein homeostasis is the maintenance between protein synthesis and proteolysis. Aging is associated with an increased proteolysis process leading to the accumulation of toxic protein aggregates. Also, a decline in protein synthesis has a negative impact on muscle regeneration. Due to changes in the generation of different muscle proteins with aging, muscle protein synthesis gets decreased by the rate of 30%. According to a study, the synthesis rate of myosin heavy chain (MHC) is reduced to 84% from young to middle age of 55 years and 48% from the middle to old age (Balagopal et al., 2001). Accompanied by a decrease in MHC, mitochondrial protein synthesis also falls which subsidizes to decreased muscular strength. Also turnover of other important regulators of muscle functions, calcium-ATPase transporter, and ryanodine receptor decline with aging (Cade and Yarasheski, 2006). Protein homeostasis at the molecular level is regulated with different signaling pathways including IGF-1 binding to tyrosine kinase receptors of myocytes causes intracellular transphosphorylation of the receptor whose activation leads to activation of insulin receptor substrate (IRS-1) and subsequent activation of PI3K and AKT pathway leading to increased protein synthesis and muscular hypertrophy (Philippou et al., 2007). Activation of these pathways works through the inhibition of glycogen synthase kinase-3, activation of mammalian target of rapamycin complex (mTORC-1) leading to phosphorylation of p70S6 kinase, and inhibition of IF-4E-binding protein (4EBF). Despite activation of the PI3K/AKT pathway, IGF-1 furthermore prevents protein degradation of O-type fork headbox (FOXO) that is an important regulator of the cell cycle, apoptosis, and metabolism. FOXO1, FOXO3a, and FOXO4 are expressed in skeletal muscles whose phosphorylation prevents translocation of transcription factors of FOXO into the nucleus resulting in the prevention of proteolytic genes such as muscle atrophy F-BOX and MuRF-1 genes. Insulin is also a critical anabolic factor for myocytes. However, with aging insulin sensitivity of myocytes decreases that endorses muscle mass decline (Philippou et al., 2007). This might be due to increased adipose storage in muscles together with damaged mitochondrial and muscle protein synthesis process. Reduced insulin sensitivity and decreased AKT and MTOR expression can result in reduced PPAR gamma coactivator 1-alpha signaling responsible for mitochondrial biogenesis (Müller et al., 2014).

Protein degradation is induced by hormonal and metabolic stimuli such as glucocorticoids, oxidative stress, and inflammatory cytokines. These changes occur due to pathological conditions in skeletal muscles like denervation, muscle unloading, and malnutrition (Rom and Reznick, 2016). Intracellular protein degradation is regulated mainly by four mechanisms: ubiquitin proteasomal system (chief regulatory mechanism of muscular atrophy), a lysosomal proteolytic system with cathepsin working as main lysosomal protease, calcium-dependent calpains, nonlysosomal protease responsible for cleavage of substrates and the caspases (Pedrozo et al., 2010; Rom and Reznick, 2016). UPS system is responsible for the degradation of 70%–80% of damage, dysfunctional, and misfolded proteins via intracellular proteolytic process to prevent its cytotoxic accumulation. The process of degradation occurs in presence of different co-factors (Jung et al., 2009). E3-ubiquitin ligase is an important determinant of protein substrate specificity of proteolysis mediated through UPS. MAFBx and MuRF-1 are E3-ligases present in skeletal muscles, whose higher expression is associated with muscular atrophy (Bodine et al., 2001). However, there are few controversial results have been published regarding the expression of these proteins and their effects on muscle atrophy, which makes its role unclear (Bodine and Baehr, 2014; Bowen et al., 2015). There have been contradictory outcomes been found for the role of the E-3 ligases in protein turnover (Baehr et al., 2014). In a study, atrophy prompted increase expression of MAFBx and MuRF-1 have been identified and these contradictory results can be explained by the cause of atrophy in skeletal muscle and the time or point of the biopsy of the muscle taken to diagnose the atrophic condition of skeletal muscle (Bodine and Baehr, 2014). A study has shown the time-dependent dynamics of MAFBx and MuRF-1 expression which states that following atrophic trigger, expression of MAFBx and MuRF-1 increases rapidly within 48 hours and subsequent elevation in next 7–10 days after which steady decline to baseline by 14 days (Bodine and Baehr, 2014). Another study revealed that after functional overload, expression of these ligases increases for a short period, and then it decreases for 7–14 days. However, proteasomal activity remains enhanced despite the expression of MAFBx and MuRF-1 came back to normal. Expression of FOXO1 and FOXO3a also acts similarly to MAFBx and MuRF-1 during functional overload (Baehr et al., 2014). These discrepancies lead the UPS out of the attention of sarcopenic molecular studies and there is also a need for studying the individual level of the expression of these markers for a better understanding of their role in proteasomal activity (Wiedmer et al., 2020). In addition to UPS-based protein degradation, lysosomes also play an important role in misfolded and aggregated protein degradation. Unlike UPS, lysosomes are responsible for the degradation of resisting unfolding and long-lived soluble proteins by lysosome fusion (autophagosome) or by chaperone-mediated autophagy (CMA) (Jackson and Hewitt, 2016; Mizushima et al., 2008). The capacity of lysosomal degradation decreases with age that can lead to sarcopenia by impaired protein degradation and subsequent accumulation of damaged and misfolded proteins. Age-associated lysosomal membrane changes lead to a decrease in lysosome-associated membrane protein-2 (LAMP-2A) level that affects CMA activity (Kon and Cuervo, 2010). These disarrangements reduce cell viability and stress response. Concomitantly, it also affects the expression of autophagy-related genes, and the sustained mTORC1 signaling pathway results in the inhibition of autophagy (Jiao and Demontis, 2017). Additionally, autophagy maintains satellite cells of muscles in their quiescent state, which gets into a senescence state with a decline in autophagy leading to the impaired regenerative capacity of muscles with age (García-Prat et al., 2016). Thus, we can say that lysosomal degradation is an essential part of the myocyte functions and fiber integrity. We can conclude that reduced and enhanced autophagy can lead to sarcopenic changes with increasing age and to prevent these it is important to maintain the equilibrium (Masiero et al., 2009).

12.3 Bone loss in aging (osteopenia or osteoporosis)

Osteoporosis and sarcopenia are common in the aging process and are significantly associated with morbidity as well as mortality (Van et al., 2001). Osteopenia is considered as midway to osteoporosis in which bone loss begins and bones starts to get weaker. Patients with osteopenia are at high risk for development of osteoporosis. Osteoporosis is a progressive skeletal disorder that can be defined as a low bone mass with the micro architectural deterioration of bone tissue resulting in increased bone fragility and bone fractures. The term "porous bone" was used to describe osteoporosis at the beginning (Consensus, 1993). Osteoporosis is classified into two main groups: primary osteoporosis and secondary osteoporosis. Primary osteoporosis is further divided into postmenopausal osteoporosis and senile osteoporosis (Cosman et al., 2014). Bone loss is more significant in women than in men after menopause which decreases 2% at 50 years of age and 25% and more after the age of 80. Risk factors for the development of osteoporosis include gender, genetic factors, hormonal changes, lifestyle factors, alcohol consumption, smoking, rheumatoid arthritis, and low body mass index (<21 kg/m^2) (Kanis 2007). In Europe and the US, estimated statistics show that 40% of post-menopausal women and 30% of men will experience osteoporotic fractures in a lifetime (Reginster and Burlet, 2006). According to WHO, criteria for osteoporosis is characterized as bone mineral density lies −2.5 SD or below the average value for healthy young women and for osteopenia score lies between −1.0 and −2.5 SD (Tuzun et al., 2012).

12.3.1 Gross morphological changes

The skeletal system provides mechanical support and protection to other organs. It is responsible for body locomotor and load-bearing ability. With aging, many cellular and physiological changes lead to compromised function of the skeletomuscular system. Bone mass reduction can lead to severe consequences with aging such as an increase in the possibility of bone fractures, decreased load-bearing capacity, decreased bone mineral density, and increased bone fragility (Manolagas, 2010). As for the morphological changes, the geometry of bones gets affected by the aging process. Morphological assessment includes changes in the shape and size of the bones. Changes in the shape of bone can affect several mechanical functions including being able to bear up large forces and energy demands (Jepsen, 2009). With aging, bone shape changes in response to the load, hormones, and growth factors. Shape change can lead to narrowing of bone walls, lengthening of bones, and shift in gravity centers (Woo et al., 1981, Ramanadham et al., 2008). Bone formation and bone resorptions remain balanced in a healthy individual, however, with age, changes in bone geometry significantly affect bone remodeling. In 85-year-old men and women, hip structure and geometry, narrow cortices, decreased bending, and buckling resistance are found very unfavorable study reports have revealed that the older individuals are more prone to fracture risk due to fragile bone structures due to inability to repair the damage and cracks (Goldman et al., 2009; Melton et al., 1996). Aging can lead to reduced toughness in cortical and trabecular bones. For people of more than 85 years' age, the possibility of fracture incidence is 10–15 times higher than that of the 60–65-year age group (Currey et al., 1996).

12.3.2 Physiological changes

There are several factors leading to osteoporotic changes in the elderly including reduced dietary intake, sex hormone deficiency, deficiency of vitamin D and minerals, and many more. Post-menopausal deficiency of estrogen is associated with the onset of rapid bone loss in women (Horton et al., 1966). Due to a decrease in ovarian functions, estrogen secretion reduces which can be prevented with hormone replacement therapy or exogenous administration of estrogen supplements. During the menopausal transition phase, serum levels of 17β-estradiol and estrone decrease up to 85%–90% and 65%–75%, respectively (Lindsay et al., 1976). However, testosterone levels don't reduce much due to its production from ovarian interstitial cells and the adrenal cortex (Khosla et al., 2005). Also, reduced FSH due to diminished inhibin levels also have a role in postmenopausal bone loss (Perrien et al., 2006). Bone resorption increases to 50% in post-menopausal period. In the first 8–10 years after menopause, ratio of bone formation to bone resorption reduces, which contributes to loss of bone mass. Increased bone resorption is an outcome of decreased calcium absorption, increased calcium efflux from bone matrix, suppression of PTH, and prevention of hypercalcemia (Garnero et al., 1996). Osteoporosis mainly affects women, but men also decrease half of the bone mass compared with aging women, and incidents of fractures occurring are one-third to osteoporotic women. However, gonadal sex steroid deficiency is less prominent in men than in women. Few studies have reported hypogonadism as the cause of osteoporosis in men. These studies have marked that, not decreased secretion but decreased bioavailability of gonadal sex steroid levels are associated with osteoporotic changes. Testosterone and estradiol are found in serum as 35%–55% bound with serum albumin, 42%–64% bound with SHBG, and 1%–3% in free form. Only free circulating and bound with albumin forms are bioavailable testosterone and estradiol and can interact with target tissue receptors. Since with age level of SHBC gets doubled, it makes the sex steroids lesser bioavailable to the targeted tissues (Clarke and Khosla, 2009).

Although sex steroid deficiency is the primary cause of bone loss, several other factors that influence age-related bone loss are important to understand. Age-associated decrease in growth hormones can affect bone development. Many growth hormones play an essential part in the differentiation of osteoblast such as growth hormone (GH) and insulin growth hormone (IGF-I). Vitamin D deficiency can also lead to a decrease in bone formation and bone mineral density which is more prevalent in post-menopausal women. Also, age-related reduced physical activity and muscle mass can contribute to bone loss. There are many sporadic means by which age-associated bone loss is seen such as malabsorption, high caffeine and sodium intakes, physical inactivity, glucocorticoid therapy, and anorexia (Clarke and Khosla, 2010). Age-associated muscle loss can contribute to osteoporosis which could be due to reduced loading of muscle on the skeleton. The recent evidence suggests the role of circulating serotonin is capable of maintaining bone mass. A clinical study data has shown serotonin levels to be inversely affecting bone mineral density; however, the mechanism behind this is yet unclear (Mödder et al., 2010). Another factor associated with bone loss during aging is leptin secretion from adipocytes. The action of leptin on bone remodeling is suggested to be happening through the nervous system. In the study, deletion of leptin receptors located on neurons led to increased bone formation and bone resorption, but the same effect was not seen with the deletion of leptin receptors located on osteoclasts. This finding suggests leptin's role in bone remodeling is through the neuronal system (Shi et al., 2088). To summarize, sex steroids, vitamin D, muscle loss, growth hormones, and lifestyle factors are attributed to physiological changes in osteoporosis. In the following section, age-associated cellular and molecular changes in osteoporosis are described.

12.3.3 Changes at the molecular level

There are multiple cellular and molecular signaling pathways that have been identified to affect bone cell differentiation and remodeling. Here we have summarized the pathways which are affected by the aging process. Osteoblast differentiation is regulated by Wnt signaling pathway, and recent findings have suggested its relationship with the aging process. Wnt signaling pathways are classified into two groups as the canonical Wnt pathway dependent on β-catenin and the noncanonical Wnt pathway. Canonical pathway is involved in osteoblast differentiation, mineralization process, production, metabolism, and in the controlling bone formation. Inactivation of the canonical Wnt pathway leads to the reduction in β-catenin. Alteration in Wnt signaling-related protein expression can lead to impaired differentiation of osteoblasts. A preclinical study results from young- and old-aged bone marrow samples of mice showed decreased expression of Wnt with increased bone age (Rauner et al., 2008). In another similar study, researchers have used transgenic mice with overexpression of Wnt 10b and study results revealed beneficial effects of Wnt 10b through prevention of bone loss in aged mice (Bennett et al., 2005). A study carried out in senescence-accelerated mouse (SAM) P6 showed that a protein sFRP-4 responsible for osteoblast differentiation negatively regulates bone formation as well as reduces bone mineral density. These actions were also contributed to inhibition of the Wnt signaling pathway (Nakanishi et al., 2006). One of the recent findings has suggested the role of reactive oxygen species in bone cell aging, also working through the Wnt signaling pathway (Almeida et al., 2007). ROS activates FoxOs which get tied to β-catenin and diminish its concentration in the bone cell leading followed by decreased osteoblast production (Almeida et al., 2007). Activation of PPAR-γ also causes a decrease in the Wnt signaling pathway leading to the reduction in osteoblast production with aging (Manolagas, 2010).

On the other hand, differentiation and production of osteoclast are maintained through the NF-κB/RANK pathway. RANK-L is a member of the TNF superfamily which is vastly expressed in osteoclast cells. It activates osteoclast production by binding with RANK receptors. With age increased, expression of RANK leads to increased osteoclast differentiation. Osteoclasts are responsible for bone resorption and demineralization, and thus increased osteoclast production leads to bone loss (Kim et al., 2016). With the aging process, cytokines such as IL-6 and IL-1β increase and are associated with the increased preosteoclastogenic activity (Gibon et al., 2016). Bone aging is related to a shift in expression of RANK and OPG. Studies have marked increased expression of RANK-L and M-CSF in osteoblasts and stromal cells and decreased

OPG expression in the older population. These changes are associated with increased bone loss and resorption through increased osteoclast formation (Kim et al., 2016). Apoptosis inhibitor protein, connexin 43 responsible for prevention of osteocytes apoptosis, is reduced with aging (Davis et al., 2018). Aged osteoblast has shown decreased sensitivity to growth factors. Aging is associated with decreased levels of IGF-1 and GH together with loss of sensitivity by bone cells. An increase in osteoclast differentiation is also an outcome of increased pro-inflammatory cytokines production (IL-6, TNF-α, and ROS) (Yakar et al., 2018).

12.4 Techniques measurement for muscle and bone loss

Muscles and bones are two interconnected systems responsible for growth and locomotion. The term bone-muscle unit has been established as a part of the strong relationship between muscles and bones responsible for maintenance, development, and correct functioning of the musculoskeletal system. The techniques to identify muscle and bone mass are summarized as follows.

12.4.1 Assessment of body composition

This technique is used to identify muscle mass. Body composition changes as a part of the normal aging process which leads to an increase in ratio of fat mass (FM) to fat-free mass (FFM). Calculating muscle mass is a part of the FFM process. Measurement of body composition can be performed by dividing the body into different compartments at atomic and anatomical levels. Muscle mass can be evaluated through FFM by a five-level compartment model (Woodrow, 2009; Evans et al., 1995). For atomic-level measurement, chief skeletal muscle components such as potassium, oxygen, hydrogen, carbon, and phosphorous are estimated. About 60% of the potassium ions are distributed in the skeletal muscle system (Heymsfield et al., 1990). With the help of total body potassium levels, we can identify whole-body muscle mass. From the cellular levels, the measurement of metabolites of skeletal muscle is useful in identifying muscle mass (Forbes, 1987). Skeletal muscle metabolites include 3-methylhistidine, creatinine, D3-creatinine, and urine creatinine levels (Heymsfield et al., 1983; Lukaski et Al, 1981). However, these can be affected due to many other physiological conditions which makes these techniques quite unreliable and inaccurate for measurement of muscle mass (Rubbieri et al., 2014).

12.4.2 Anthropometry

Anthropometry is simple and easily applicable in clinical practice to identify muscle mass. It is an ancient technique that was established in the 19th century for the measurement of body mass and physiological assessment (Martin et al., 1990). With this technique, a person can identify body fat and limb circumference that is assumed to be reflected in limb muscle and its protein state. However, this does not give an accurate measurement of the muscular mass since it does not involve any visceral fat, only subcutaneous fat is being measured (Britton et al., 2013).

12.4.3 Bioelectrical impedance analysis (BIA)

BIA is a simple and rapid technique for the identification of muscle mass. It works by passing a small AC current through the body that is conducted by the body water (Janssen et al., 2000). As the muscles are highly water-rich components, it allows the measurement of muscle mass. Impedance (flow of charge) is inversely proportional to total body water. However, this method has its limitations as muscle mass can be biased by hydration state and presence of edema (Janssen et al., 2000).

12.4.4 Quantitative imaging techniques for the assessment of osteoporosis and sarcopenia

12.4.4.1 DXA for measurement of osteoporosis and sarcopenia

According to WHO, dual X-ray absorptiometry (DXA) represents the gold standard method to rule out osteoporosis. DXA can differentiate fat mass, non-bone lean mass, and bone mineral content (BMC) with high reproducibility which makes it the most accurate and central method for the study of body composition (Bazzocchi et al., 2014; Bazzocchi et al., 2016). DXA relies on two different energy X-ray beams and the R-value is measured as the ratio of the degree of attenuation of lower and higher energy X-ray beams. By using complex algorithms, it is possible to derive BMC from which we can identify bone mineral density (BMD) as a ratio of BMC/area (g/cm^2) (Bazzocchi et al., 2016; Pietrobelli et al., 1996). DXA is widely available, and the very first test is performed with patients diagnosed with osteoporosis. It has advantages of cost-saving, and minimum radiation exposure (Hawkinson et al., 2007). Other than BMD, parameters such as trabecular bone score (TBS), hip structural analysis (HAS), and advanced hip assessment (AHA) can also be identified with the help of DXA. TBS has been proved to be associated with trabecular, hip, and other major osteoporotic fractures that can be analyzed with DXA, though it does not give a measure of trabecular microarchitecture. HAS and AHA are used for measurement of hip axis length, cross-sectional area, bulking ratio, neck-shaft angle, section modulus, cross-sectional moment of inertia, and outer diameter (Hans et al., 2011; Beck 2007; Bonnick 2007). Quantitative vertebral morphometry can also be obtained from DXA that can be used for vertebral fracture assessment (Genant et al., 1993). For sarcopenia, CT and MRI are considered gold standard methods, but their high cost and complexity limit their use (Erlandson et al., 2016). DXA is also an attractive approach to evaluate age-associated muscle mass loss and represents an alternative method to diagnose sarcopenia for research purposes and clinical use (Bazzocchi et al., 2014). Studies have reported a good level of correlation between CT and MRI results with DXA. DXA evaluates lean mass index, appendicular lean mass, appendicular lean mass index, android/gynoid ratio, and fat mass index. With the age, it is critical to maintaining appendicular lean mass, the most used parameter for evaluation of sarcopenia (Janssen et al., 2002). The major limitation of this technique is that the equipment is not portable limits its use difficult in large epidemiological studies (La Tegola et al., 2018).

12.4.4.2 Computed tomography (CT)

In routine practice, CT is a widely used cross-sectional imagining technique that has been developed quickly and more advanced modalities have been innovated (Erlandson et al., 2016). Quantitative CT scans and peripheral CT scans are designed to assess bone parameters from central and peripheral sites, respectively. Besides these, it can also be used to quantify muscle mass and fat distribution (Krug et al., 2010). High-resolution p-QCT is an advanced technique for investigating muscle and bone at peripheral sites. QCT is primarily used for the identification of volumetric BMD (vBMD) which gives more accuracy than other imaging techniques as it provides true bone density instead of an areal density that was measured by DXA (Genant et al., 1987). Also, it avoids overestimation of BMD that was resulting due to vascular calcification, spinal degeneration, and sclerotic lesions in the surrounding tissues (Engelke et al., 2008). QCT is applied to the lumbar spine, tibia, femur, and forearm. pQCT is used to identify v-BMD, a separate assessment of trabecular and cortical bone parameters, geometric parameters, architectural parameters, detailed bone microarchitecture, and biochemical parameters like a cross-sectional moment of inertia (CSMI) (Stagi et al., 2016). As stated before, CT represents the gold standard to rule out sarcopenia. By calculating the weakening of an X-ray beam going through different tissues, CT can segregate between fat and fat-free mass and can access quantitative and qualitative measurement of muscle mass (Guglielmi et al., 2011). Normal muscle density shows attenuation of X-ray beam range from 31 to 100 HU, while due to aging process, fat infiltration and pathological conditions leading to low-density muscle show 0–30 HU (Ross, 2003). Using a high level of mathematical reconstruction algorithms, a CT scan can be used to quantify skeletal muscle composition and distribution of adipose tissue (Mitsiopoulos et al., 1998). An important limitation of CT scan is homogeneity for image acquisition and analysis together with the high cost and high radiation exposure (Erlandson et al., 2016).

12.4.4.3 Magnetic resonance imaging (MRI)

MRI uses the external magnetic field and radiofrequency energy through hydrogen nuclei to produce diagnostic images. Differences in radiofrequency pulse sequence are used to distinguish between fat-free mass and adipose tissue (Houmard et al., 1995). The most important advantage with MRI over CT scan is the absence of ionizing radiation makes it more suitable to use for a longer period and so can be used to examine disease progression and treatment efficacy (Guglielmi et al., 2011). Recent innovations in MRI have brought significant progress in ruling out the osteoporotic bone. High-resolution MRI allows the determination of trabecular bone density, in vitro as well as in vivo structure with high spatial resolution, and microarchitecture of trabecular bone (Krug et al., 2005). Topology, scale, and orientation can be derived using MRI. Also, cortical parameters can be evaluated by MRI (Krug et al., 2010). Additionally, MRI can quantify marrow adipose tissue (MAT) by H-MRS analysis. For the identification of muscle mass, MRI represents the most fascinating technique (Schellinger et al., 2004). Not only CSA but also comprehensive muscle quality can be identified with MRI. The principal advantage of MRI over other techniques in ruling out sarcopenia is its ability to discover changes in skeletal muscle with aging and disease progression (Mitsiopoulos et al., 1998). Chemical shift-based water-fat separation and two-point Dixon-based technique are two important quantitative MRI technologies used to identify muscle fat content (Fischer et al., 2014; Alizai et al., 2012). Moreover, MRI with diffusion tensor imaging determines muscle microstructure and fatty infiltration (Dixon, 1984). High cost, time consumption, lack of standardized assessment protocol in image analysis, and complexity limit its use (La Tegola et al., 2018; Guerri et al., 2018).

12.4.4.4 Ultrasound

One of the most advantages of ultrasound is the feasibility in clinical practice unlike CT and MRI (Pillen and van Alfen 2011). It uses ultrasound waves in the frequency range of 200 kHz to 1.5 MHz. Interaction between these waves and bone and muscle tissue is used to create an image (Guglielmi et al., 2010). Quantitative US technique allows identification of structural anisotropy of bone and its mechanical properties. It is considered as an alternative approach to other diagnostic technologies to identify bone and muscle mass (Glüer, 1997). Several studies have shown a good correlation of muscle mass measurement with MRI (Sanada et al., 2006). Parameters evaluated by ultrasound are CSA, fascicle length, echo intensity, pennation angle of lower limbs, and muscle thickness. These parameters are important to identify mechanical and contractile properties of skeletal muscle during aging (Narici et al., 2016). Reproducibility is the major concern of this technique and also it is difficult to compare measurements and sometimes can be misleading (Glüer, 1997).

12.5 Nutraceuticals

Aging is an inevitable process that cannot be reversed or stopped, however, few alterations caused due to lack of physical activity, inadequate supply of nutrition, and lack of exercise can lead to a skeletomuscular loss can be managed by geriatric rehabilitation that corrects the age-associated skeleto-muscular impairment (Venturelli et al., 2014; Booth et al., 2011). Many exercise trainings have been identified as significantly effective in skeletomuscular strength, muscle power, and physiological and functional gains (Ryu et al., 2013). In addition to exercise, nutritional supplements can also have positive impact on skeletomuscular system. Studies have also reported that the beneficial effects of nutritional supplements subside even after the intervention has been stopped (Dickinson et al., 2013; Kim et al., 2016). Here we have discussed nutraceutical and their use in skeletomuscular losses.

12.5.1 Nutraceuticals for bone health

Many nutraceuticals have shown affirmative effects on bone health and management of osteoporosis. Nutraceuticals beneficial for bone health and its possible mechanism of actions are summarized in further sections. The following are the categories of different nutraceuticals used for osteoporosis (summarized in Table 12.1).

1. Minerals
2. Herbs and phytochemicals
3. Dairy products
4. Proteins
5. Miscellaneous

12.5.1.1 Minerals
12.5.1.1.1 Calcium

Calcium is the fifth most abundant ion in the body which makes up nearly 1.9% of the bodyweight. Among the total body calcium, 99% remains in bones and teeth, and provides mechanical strength (Matkovic, 1992). During adolescence, it is essential to take an appropriate amount of calcium to prevent osteoporotic changes in the later stage of life. Calcium aids in increasing bone density, and its required intake is about 1,600 mg/day in an adult person (Matkovic, 1992). Calcium-rich food includes cheese, milk, leafy vegetables, soybeans, yogurt, etc. (Lee et al., 1981). A clinical study performed in aging women confirmed that long-term use of 600 mg calcium carbonate twice a day can reduce the possibility of clinical fractures (Prince et al., 2006). Similar studies have been published in which elderly women who were treated with 1 mg/day of calcium citrate showed reduced bone loss and improved turnover, but inconsistency was observed with bone fractures (Reid et al., 2006). Although there are multiple therapeutic interventions available to treat osteoporosis, concomitant administration of calcium supplements is critical for efficient results. For example, bisphosphonates are used to increase bone mass. It works through the inhibition of bone resorption by reducing osteoclast activity and subsequent increase in osteoblast deposition and bone mass, however, adequate calcium supplements are needed for osteoblast to deposit fresh bone minerals. To conclude, calcium becomes an integral part of the interventions for the treatment of osteoporosis (Franklin et al., 2008).

12.5.1.1.2 Magnesium

Around 60% of the total body magnesium is stored in bones working as a source of exchangeable Mg whenever needed to maintain serum levels. It is used for various physiological functions, as a cofactor for enzymes, and stabilization of the cell membrane with its positive charge. Magnesium-rich food includes whole grain, avocados, nuts, banana, dark leafy vegetables, seeds, beans, dark chocolate, etc. (Sojka, 1995). Deficiency in Mg alters the apatite crystal structure leading to larger crystals in bones that cannot bear the normal load. Besides, Mg deficiency can also result in diminished the PTH level. PTH is responsible for homeostasis of calcium and bone growth. Also, it can produce inflammatory cytokines that result in bone loss. Mg protects skeletal from such acidotic conditions and deterioration of bone mass (Castiglioni et al., 2013). In a randomized study, Mg supplements were found to be having a positive effect on bone mass and hip mineral content in the magnesium oxide treated group (Carpenter et al., 2006). If more than the required level of Mg is taken, it can have a negative impact on the osseous metabolism. A study has reported such a consequence wherein women who had maximum Mg intake were more prone to wrist fractures. This can be explained by Mg interference with hydroxyapatite crystal generation due to competing with calcium leading to loss of bone mass (Castiglioni et al., 2013).

12.5.1.1.3 Potassium

Recommended potassium intake for bone growth is 3,500–3,800 mg/day for 1–3 years of age, 3,800 mg/day for 4–8 years of age, 4,500 mg/day for 9–18 years of age, and 4,700 mg/day for 19 years and above. Potassium is amply found in sweet potato, apricot, spinach, avocado, and banana. It helps to preserve bone calcium levels and regulation of the pH by maintaining an alkaline environment. It neutralizes endogenous acids from acid-generating food in the skeletal microenvironment. Thus, it helps in osteoporosis prevention by protecting against the damage (He et al., 2008). For instance, studies have been performed to evaluate its beneficial role. Cross-sectional study performed on menopausal women showed that increased potassium intake significantly increases bone mineral density specific to the femoral neck and lumbar spine (New et al., 1997; Palacios, 2006).

12.5.1.1.4 Boron

Boron helps other elements to work efficiently to improve bone health. It stabilizes vitamin D and estrogen and increases their half-life, and thereby prevents calcium loss and demineralization of bones. Natural sources of boron are prunes, apricots, resins, and avocados. It has been marked that 3 mg/day

Table 12.1 Summary of Nutraceuticals for Bone Health

Nutraceutical Agent	Source	Mechanism	Reference
Minerals			
Calcium	Cheese, milk, leafy vegetables, soybeans, yogurt, etc.	• Inhibition of bone resorption by reducing osteoclast activity • Increase in osteoblast deposition and bone mass	Franklin et al. (2008)
Magnesium	Whole grain, avocados, nuts, banana, dark leafy vegetables, seeds, beans, dark chocolate, etc.	• Protects bones from acidotic conditions and prevents deterioration of bone mass	Castiglioni et al. (2013)
Potassium	Sweet potato, apricot, spinach, avocado, and banana	• Preserves bone calcium levels and regulation of the pH by maintaining an alkaline environment	He et al. (2008)
Boron	Prunes, apricots, resins, and avocados	• Preserves essential bone growth agents by increasing electrolytes and steroid levels, and reduction in calcium and magnesium excretion	Nielsen et al. (1987)
Copper	Shellfish, seeds and nuts, organ meats, wheat-bran cereals, whole-grain products, chocolate	• Antioxidant properties diminish free radical generated by osteoclasts	Mutlu et al. (2007)
Herbs			
Resveratrol	Red wine, grapes, cranberries, and nuts	• Modulation of osteoblast gene expression by its action on Runx2 and Ostrix transcription factors and RANKL expression • Antioxidant and anti-inflammatory properties • Improvement in osteocalcin and alkaline phosphatase levels	Tou (2015) Feng et al. (2014)
Green tea	Camellia sinensis	• Osteoclasts death by activation of caspase-3, suppression of MMP-9 in osteoblast, IL-6 inhibition, and suppression of p44/p42 mitogen-activated protein and Fenton reaction leading to reduced bone resorption • Downregulation of RANKL-induced expression and suppress osteoclast differentiation • Suppression of TNF-alfa and IL-6 and increase in alkaline phosphatase leading to osteoblastogenesis • Increase in osteoblastic activity via Wnt signaling pathway	Ko et al. (2009) Shen et al. (2013)

(Continued)

Table 12.1 (*Continued*) Summary of Nutraceuticals for Bone Health

Nutraceutical Agent	Source	Mechanism	Reference
Onion	Allium cepa L.	• Inhibition of bone resorption and maintenance of mineralization • Alterations in the level of alkaline phosphatase, and free radicals, leading to antioxidant effects and improved BMD	Tsuji et al. (2009) Wong and Rabie (2008) Law et al. (2016)
Berries	Strawberries, blueberries, raspberries, blackberries, and blackcurrant	• Powerful antioxidant and anti-inflammatory activity • Trans-retinoid acid improves osteoblast differentiation in stem cell culture • Flavonoids suppress osteoclastogenesis through inhibition of RNKA-L	Kumar et al. (2012)
Citrus fruits	Oranges, lemons, grapefruits, pomelos, and limes	• Improves bone health by protection from oxidative stress damage	Deyhim et al. (2006)
Red clover	Trifolium pratense L.	• Increases bone mineral density and reduces resorption of bones (structurally similar to estrogen)	Clifton-Bligh et al. (2001) Occhiuto et al. (2007)
Alfalfa	Medicago sativa	• Acts as a mitogen for osteoblasts differentiation • Decreases the activity of different lysosomes in osteoclasts • Ability to potentiate the action of estrogen	Compston (2001)
Horsetail	Equisetum arvense L.	• Important source for bone collagen and calcification • Stimulates osteoblast generation and activate anti-inflammatory pathway • Osteoprotective effects	Bian et al. (2012), Lee et al. (2008)
Plums	P. Domestica	• Increases levels of IGF-1 and alkaline phosphatase • Increases BMD and downregulates osteoclast differentiation, increase in osteoblast synthesis and upregulation of collagen cross-linking	Arjmandi et al. (2002)
Herba Epimedii	Epimedium sagittatum	• Prevention of TNF-α, IL-6, and lipopolysaccharide-induced osteoclastogenesis	Hsieh et al. (2011), Zheng et al. (2012)
Black cohosh	Actaea racemosa L.	• Inhibition of osteoclastogenesis through RANKL or TNF-α inhibition	Qiu et al. (2007)

(Continued)

Table 12.1 (*Continued*) Summary of Nutraceuticals for Bone Health

Nutraceutical Agent	Source	Mechanism	Reference
Dietary products	Milk and milk products	• Proliferation and differentiation of osteoblasts and prevention of osteoclastogenesis and bone resorption • Elevation of serum osteocalcin • Increases BMD and reduces the excretion of Type I collagen in urine • Helps in osteoblastogenesis by stimulating mitogenic activated protein kinase (MAPK) pathway	Cornish et al. (2004) KATO et al. (2000) Uenishi et al. (2006)
Miscellaneous			
Probiotics	Ogurt, kefir, kombucha, sauerkraut, pickles, miso, tempeh, kimchi, sourdough bread and some cheeses	• Increases the trabecular number by production of vitamins D, C, K, and folate • Decrease in PTH through the production of short-chain fatty acids leads to increase in mineral absorption, and antioxidant effects	Parvaneh et al. (2014)
Prebiotics	Chicory root, garlic, onions, leeks, asparagus, bananas, etc.	• Increases the absorption of minerals in bones	Weaver et al. (2011)
Melatonin	Eggs and fish	• Elevates serum corticosteroid levels and increases osteoclast metabolism • Antioxidant properties • Increases procollagen type I c-peptide • Elevates osteoblastic protein, osteoprotegerin and diminish osteoclast differentiation	Satomura et al. (2007) Tresguerres et al. (2014)
Polyunsaturated fatty acids	Salmon, vegetable oils, and some nuts and seeds	• Encourages bone remodeling through calcium absorption, PPAR-gamma pathway, and inflammatory cytokines • Increases calcium absorption in the intestine through increasing calcium ATPase	Maggio et al. (2009)

is associated with an increase in bone mass; however, there are no recommended dosage levels (Devirian and Volpe, 2003). Studies found preventive effects of boron intake on osteoporosis. The study included postmenopausal women who were treated with boron supplements, and there was a significant increase in electrolytes and steroid levels, together with reduced calcium and magnesium excretion by 40% and 33%, respectively, which are essential for bone growth (Nielsen et al., 1987).

12.5.1.1.5 Copper

Copper is a vital element that serves as a cofactor for many antioxidant enzymes used to diminish free radical generated by osteoclasts and thereby, keeping the bone healthy. As a cofactor, it triggers lysyl oxidase and subsequent cross-linking of elastin and collagen with lysine. Copper helps in sustaining the bone matrix. The recommended intake of boron in adults is 0.9 mg/day (Mutlu et al., 2007). A significant deficit in copper with old-age people has more risk for femoral neck fractures (Conlan et al., 1990). A preclinical study in rats indicated that Cu deficiency leads to bone collagen defects and can result in reduced mechanical strength of the bone (Jonas et al., 1993).

12.5.1.2 Herbs and phytochemicals
12.5.1.2.1 Resveratrol

Resveratrol is a polyphenol present in red wine, grapes, cranberries, and nuts and is analogous to diethylstilbestrol. it holds antioxidant and anti-inflammatory properties; in addition to that, it also works through osteoblast gene expression modulation by acting on Runx2 and Ostrix transcription factors and RANKL expression (Tou, 2015). In a preclinical study, resveratrol treatment in ovariectomized rats improved osteocalcin and alkaline phosphatase levels, thereby increasing osteoblastic activity. It also helps improving bone structure (Feng et al., 2014).

12.5.1.2.2 Green tea

Another polyphenol, green tea is a worldwide popular beverage and is made by drying freshly collected leaves of Camellia sinensis at a high temperature to deactivate oxidizing enzymes. Polyphenolic compounds present in tea are important for bone health that includes epigallocatechin gallate, epicatechin, epigallocatechin, and epicatechin gallate (Ko et al., 2009). Epigallocatechin-3-gallate causes osteoclasts death by activation of caspase-3 and fenton reaction that further diminishes bone resorption. Osteoclast reductions also happen due to suppression of MMP-9 in osteoblast, IL-6 inhibition, and suppression of p44/p42 mitogen-activated protein. The polyphenols are also responsible for down-regulation of RANKL-induced expression and suppress osteoclast differentiation. It also prolongs osteoblast survival through suppression of TNF-alfa and IL-6, along with that increase in alkaline phosphatase leads to osteoblastogenesis and increase in osteoblastic activity via Wnt signaling pathway (Shen et al., 2013).

12.5.1.2.3 Onion

Allium cepa L., onion, is widely used for its flavor and health benefits. It is rich in flavonoids quercetin, rutin, and strong antioxidant organo-sulfur conjugates. Several clinical studies have reported onion to be inhibiting resorption of bone and maintaining its mineralization (Tsuji et al., 2009; Wong and Rabie, 2008). An in vitro study confirmed its inhibitory effects on osteoclastogenesis and osteoclast differentiation. In vivo administration of 100 mL of onion juice showed significant alterations in the level of alkaline phosphatase, and free radicals, leading to antioxidant effects and improved BMD (Law et al., 2016).

12.5.1.2.4 Berries

Most commonly used berries are strawberries, blueberries, raspberries, black-berries, and blackcurrant. Berries are fleshy and edible fruits and a rich source of vitamins like A, B9, C, E, and K, carotenoids, minerals, fumaric acid, and citric acid. It has powerful antioxidant and anti-inflammatory activities along with the ability to modulate enzymes, signaling pathways, and gene expressions. Trans-retinoid acid found in raspberry with ketone has been identified to improve osteoblast differentiation in stem cell culture. In addition to these, berries also contain tannins, phenolic acid, stilbenes, and flavonoids. Among these, flavonoids have the means to suppress osteoclastogenesis through inhibition of RNKA-L (Kumar et al., 2012).

12.5.1.2.5 Citrus fruits

Citrus fruits are abundant source of potassium, magnesium, folic acid, flavonoids, vitamin C, and limonoids. Some studies have proven the role of limonoids and flavonoids in improving bone health through antioxidant properties. Oxidative damage has a significant impact on the development of osteoporosis, and by using antioxidants, resorption of bone and demineralization can be prevented. Thus, it is recommended to take dietary citrus fruits to improve bone health and protect from oxidative stress damage (Deyhim et al., 2006).

12.5.1.2.6 Red clover

Red clover (Trifoliumpratense L.) is a source of isoflavones such as genistein, daidzein, biochanin A, and formononetin. It is famous for its use in treating menopausal symptoms. Genistein and daidzein (phytoestrogens) are structurally similar to estrogen, thus, can be used to treat bone loss in post-menopausal women (Occhiuto et al., 2007). Studies have reported a positive impact on BMD which is supported clinically. In a randomized clinical study, it improved bone health by increasing bone mineral density and reducing resorption of bones with negligible side effects compared with hormone replacement therapy (Clifton-Bligh et al., 2001).

12.5.1.2.7 Alfalfa

Isoflavone derivative ipriflavone is an active constituent of the Alfalfa plant, which is reported to be directly inhibiting resorption of bone and increase estrogen activity favoring calcitonin secretion. It also has a proliferative effect on osteoblasts (Alexandersen et al., 2001). Estrogen is known to be inducing gene expression in osteoblasts and acts as a mitogen for osteoblasts differentiation process. It also increases type I collagen and activity of alkaline phosphatase. On the other hand, it decreases the activity of different lysosomes in osteoclasts. Since ipriflavone also has the ability to potentiate the action of estrogen, it helps in improving bone density and bone health (Compston 2001).

12.5.1.2.8 Horsetail

The herb Horsetail is commonly used for the treatment of osteoporosis. Multiple constituents such as silica, flavonoids, and triterpenoids contained in the herb have favorable effects on bone health (Costa-Rodrigues et al., 2012). Silica is an important source for bone collagen and calcification. Flavonoids from horsetail stimulate osteoblast generation and activate anti-inflammatory pathway (Pang et al., 2006), while terpenoids seem to be having osteoprotective effects, elevating differentiation and mineralization of osteoblasts, and promoting osteogenesis (Bian et al., 2012; Lee et al., 2008).

12.5.1.2.9 Plums

Dried plums are a rich source of polyphenols like rutin, chlorogenic acid, and proanthocyanidin carbohydrates, magnesium, potassium, boron, calcium, vitamins A, B, and K, selenium, and dietary fibers (Arjmandi et al., 2002). A clinical study was conducted in postmenopausal women treated with 100 g of plums or 75 g of apple, both having the same caloric value. IGF-1 and bone-specific alkaline phosphatase were analyzed before and after administration of the treatment. Plums intake has shown remarkably higher levels of IGF-1 and alkaline phosphatase compared with the apple regimen (Jabeen and Aslam, 2011). Polyphenol present in plums increases BMD and downregulate osteoclast differentiation, together with an increase in osteoblast synthesis and upregulation of collagen cross-linking (Arjmandi et al., 2002).

12.5.1.2.10 Herba Epimedii

Herba Epimedii is a Chinese medicine used to nourish the bones. The main active ingredient of Herba Epimedii are Icariin, attributor of skeletal benefits. It helps in preventing TNF-α, IL-6 and lipopolysaccharide-induced osteoclastogenesis and thereby, reducing inflammation-induced bone loss and resorption. Moreover, it also decreases osteoclast differentiation and supports osteoblastogenesis (Hsieh et al., 2011; Zheng et al., 2012).

12.5.1.2.11 Black cohosh

Black cohosh (Actaearacemosa L.) belongs to the Ranunculaceae family which is primarily used in treating postmenopausal symptoms (McKenna et al., 2001). Recently, it has been identified to be having a beneficial role in bone health. The active constituent of black cohosh is a triterpenoid glycoside that works by inhibition of osteoclastogenesis through RANKL or TNFα inhibition (Qiu et al., 2007).

12.5.1.3 Dietary products

Dietary products are rich in calcium and thus are useful in preventing osteoporosis. In addition to calcium, milk, and milk products are a rich source of sodium, phosphate, potassium, zinc, vitamins A and B2, proteins, and lipids, and also functional components such as milk basic protein, lactoferrin, and casein phosphopeptide (Uenishi et al., 2006). Growth factors present within the milk protein are responsible for increased proliferation and differentiation of osteoblasts and prevention of osteoclastogenesis and bone resorption. Milk basic protein also contains cystatin C responsible for elevation of serum osteocalcin (chief noncollagenous bone protein) level. A study outcome reported beneficial effects of milk basic protein in post-menopausal women in which it increased BMD by 1.21% after administration of 40 mg/day milk basic protein. Moreover, it also reduced the excretion of Type I collagen in urine (KATO et al., 2000). Lactoferrin, a glycoprotein present in milk has an anabolic effect on the bone and that causes dose-dependent rapid osteoblastogenesis and inhibit of osteoclast differentiation. These effects are the result from stimulation of mitogenic-activated protein kinase (MAPK) leading to rapid mitogenesis of cells (Cornish et al., 2004).

12.5.1.4 Miscellaneous
12.5.1.4.1 Probiotics

Probiotics are comprised of normal intestinal flora that can produce end products of short-chain fatty acids and lactate metabolism. A study carried out in ovariectomized mice fed with *Lactobacillus paracasei and Lactobacillus plantarum* showed a greater trabecular number compared with the control group. Probiotics have positive impact on bone health through various possible mechanisms including production of vitamins D, C, K, and folate essential for bone formation and associated with calcium metabolism, decrease in PTH through the production of short-chain fatty acids leading to increase in mineral absorption, and production of antioxidant effects. These effects can reduce cytokine levels, elevate bone uptake for calcium and minerals, and decrease osteoclast differentiation (Parvaneh et al., 2014).

12.5.1.4.2 Prebiotics

Prebiotics are the food ingredients that are not digested, but they are fermented with the help of intestinal flora and support bacterial growth, which results in positive effects on the host. Nondigestible oligosaccharides are an example of prebiotics. It increases the absorption of minerals that are essential for bone growth and bone mineralization (Scholz-Ahrens et al., 2001). Galactooligosaccharides (GOS) given to Sprague-Dawley rats showed increased absorption of magnesium, increased calcium uptake of the femur, and calcium and magnesium retention in femur and tibia. These effects of GOS have a positive impact in bone health (Weaver et al., 2011).

12.5.1.4.3 Melatonin

Melatonin is secreted through the penial gland specifically at night and produces diurnal variations that have a positive effect on growth hormones (Uslu et al., 2007). It elevates serum corticosteroid levels and increases osteoclast metabolism. It has also been identified as a scavenger of free radicals such as hydroxyl and pyroxyl molecules responsible for its antioxidant properties. Moreover, it increases procollagen type I c-peptide, an essential component in the bone matrix. In addition to this, it also elevates osteoblastic protein, osteoprotegerin which will diminish osteoclast differentiation process (Satomura et al., 2007). A preclinical study report suggested that melatonin-treated rats show higher bone volume with greater modulus bone stiffness compared with the untreated control group (Tresguerres et al., 2014).

12.5.1.4.4 Polyunsaturated fatty acids (PUFA)

PUFA are mainly classified into n-6 and n-3 fatty acids, among which n-6 is present in vegetable oils and derived from linoleic acid, while n-3 is present in fish oil and is derived from eicosapentaenoic acid and docosahexaenoic acid. Several preclinical findings have suggested positive effects of PUFA on bone health. Omega-3 fatty acids encourage bone remodeling through three different pathways including calcium absorption, PPAR-gamma pathway, and inflammatory cytokines. Long-chain PUFA increases calcium absorption in the intestine through increasing calcium ATPase. Dietary intake of n-3 fatty acids replaces n-6 fatty acid in the cell membrane. This change leads to a decrease in IL-1, IL-6, and TNF-alpha levels, whereas PPAR-gamma is a regulator of stem cell differentiation into osteoblast which gets increased and adipogenesis of bone marrow decreases with the presence of n-6 (Maggio et al., 2009).

12.5.2 Nutraceuticals for muscle health

Aging has been associated with decreased food intake together with protein intake which is very essential for muscle strength and functions. As mentioned before protein supplements alone or together with exercise can improve muscle strength and physiological functions. Nutraceuticals reported having a beneficial role in sarcopenia are described in upcoming section with possible mechanism of action (summarized in Table 12.2).

12.5.2.1 Amino acid supplements and its metabolites
12.5.2.1.1 Leucine metabolites

Leucine is a branched-chain amino acid (BCAA) that gets metabolized in muscles. Its metabolites have anabolic properties. A study carried out in pigs showed that infusion of one of the metabolites of leucine, α-ketoisocaproate (α-KIC) increases muscle protein synthesis. However, this effect also could be due to reverse transamination of α-KIC to leucine (Escobar et al., 2010). Many promising results have been published for another distal metabolite of leucine, β-hydroxy-β-methyl butyrate (HMB), formed by cytosolic α-KIC dioxygenase (Nissen et al., 1996). Oral administration of 2.42 g of HMB produced a similar stimulatory effect on muscle synthesis to that of leucine. Anabolic signaling of HMB and leucine was through the rapamycin-mTOR pathway.

Table 12.2 Summary of Nutraceuticals for Health of Muscles

Nutraceutical Agent	Source	Mechanism	Reference
Amino Acid Supplements and Its Metabolites			
Leucine metabolites	Milk, corn, brown rice, cheese, chia seeds, octopus, and pork	• Stimulatory effect on muscle synthesis • Diminishes muscle protein breakdown in an insulin-dependent manner • Increases lean body mass and protein turnover • Maintain the integrity of sarcolemma by participating in de novo cholesterol synthesis	Nissen and Abumrad (1997) Nissen and Abumrad (1997)
Creatine	Fish and meat	• Provides energy to fatigue-susceptible type II fibers • Elevates muscle protein synthesis	Casey et al. (1996) Willoughby and Rosene (2001)
β-Alanine & carnosine	Meat-based food	• Increases muscle capacity by regulation of intracellular buffering capacity and prevents acidotic effects	C. Harris et al. (1998) Hill et al. (2007)
Carnitine	Red meat	• Improves muscle endurance performance and promotes fat oxidation	Stephens et al. (2013)
Micronutrients			
Vitamin D	Oily fish, liver, egg yolks, fortified foods, red meat	• Increase in myotubule size through downregulation of myostatin, upregulation of AKT & sensitization of the mTOR pathway	Deane et al. (2017)
Vitamins C and E	Fruits and vegetables	• Beneficial role in protein homeostasis through free radicals scavenging • Increasing lean body mass	Scott et al. (2010)
Miscellaneous			
N-3 PUFA	Fish oil	• Protein synthesis by increasing phosphorylation of anabolic signaling • Attenuates muscle loss in stress conditions by reducing inflammatory mediators and cytokines	Zhang et al. (2014) Alexander et al. (1986)
Nitrates	Beetroot and lettuce	• Increases nutrient delivery and muscle protein synthesis by NO synthesis	Mitchell et al. (2017)
Ursolic acid	Apple peel	• Increases anabolic activity of muscles through activating p70s6k1 and prolonging mTORc1 activity • Attenuation of murf1 and atrogin-1 atrophy & upregulation of IGF leads to muscle hypertrophy	Sancak et al. (2010) Kunkel et al. (2011)
Phosphatidic acid	Cabbage	• Increases muscle protein synthesis by activation of mTORc1 • Inhibitory effects against atrophy inducing genes	Tanaka et al. (2012) Lehours et al. (2011)

Moreover, HMB also diminished muscle protein breakdown in an insulin-dependent manner (Wilkinson et al., 2013). However, the mechanism of insulin-dependent reduction in protein breakdown effect by HMB remains unclear. A clinical trial studied long term use of HMB in 10 days bed rested healthy older adults, and during the period of muscle disuse, HMB preserved muscle protein (Deutz et al., 2013). In a yearlong study, HMB increased lean body mass and protein turnover in elderly subjects. An increase in lean body mass could be due to the augmentation of muscle protein turnover (Baier et al., 2009). HMB also helps in exercise-induced muscle damage. A study performed in endurance exercise athletes given HMB supplements significantly decreased muscle damage through the reduction in creatine phosphokinase and lactate dehydrogenase. HMB also has been reported to be maintaining the integrity of sarcolemma by participating in de novo cholesterol synthesis (Nissen and Abumrad, 1997).These all effects are associated with improving muscular health.

12.5.2.1.2 Creatine

Creatine is synthesized as a metabolite of arginine, glycine, and methionine endogenously which is mainly located in skeletal muscles. Food such as fish and meat can promote the exogenous synthesis of creatine in the liver and pancreas (Greenhaff et al., 1994). Creatine is taken up by sarcolemma through Na^+/Cl^- transport system and gets phosphorylated intramuscularly to phosphocreatine with the help of creatine kinase. In high energy requirements, it releases phosphate used forming ATP molecules. The ergogenic effect of creatine is due to stored phosphocreatine. Elevation in phosphocreatine storage can be achieved through oral administration of creatine rich foods, that can be used during extensive anaerobic exercise. It provides energy to fatigue-susceptible type II fibers (Casey et al., 1996). Supplemented creatine also improves performance by the increasing rate of recovery after extensive exercise by elevating muscle protein synthesis. Phosphocreatine provides more strength for muscle contraction. Moreover, chronic use of creatine supplements increases muscle mass with 20–30 mg/day for 5 days and subsequent maintenance dose of 5 mg/day of creatine (Volek et al., 1999). When the chronic intake of creatine is given with resistance exercise training, it stimulates accretion of muscle mass that might be the result of enhanced recovery and potentiation of exercise capacity (Willoughby and Rosene, 2001).

12.5.2.1.3 β-Alanine and carnosine

β-Alanine is primarily found in meat-based food and is also produced endogenously in the liver. Carnosine is a product of dipeptide of β-alanine and histidine which has an active impact on the buffering capacity of muscles. β-Alanine supplements increase in levels of carnosine which has an ergogenic effect on muscles. Due to its better bioavailability after oral administration, it can increase carnosine levels up to 40%–65%. Carnosine distribution also depends on the type of fibers, for instance in type II fibers carnosine content is double than type I fibers. By regulation of buffering capacity of muscles, carnosine increases capacity of muscles in resistance exercise. Intensive exercise can increase hydrogen ion concentration and thus decreases intramuscular pH levels. Acidosis generation lowers the ATP generation and increases fatigue. β-Alanine supplements are aimed to prevent acidotic effects during the extensive workout and provide increased performance. Therefore, β-alanine supplements increasing carnosine levels result into improved muscle performance through enhancing intracellular buffering capacity.

12.5.2.1.4 Carnitine

Endogenously carnitine is synthesized from amino acid precursors and can be obtained from red meat exogenously. 95% of the carnitine gets stored in skeletal muscle where it improves muscle endurance performance and promotes fat oxidation while sparing the muscle glycogen content (Stephens et al., 2007). However, carnitine has poor bioavailability after oral administration and fast excretion, which is why it alone does not have an impact on muscular accretion. Several studies have reported insulin-induced muscle carnitine uptake through insulin-induced active transport by organic cation transporter. Carnitine taken together with carbohydrates has shown better muscle uptake and reduce fat gain (Stephens et al., 2013).

12.5.2.2 Micronutrients
12.5.2.2.1 Vitamin D

Vitamins are a very essential part of the metabolic processes. Vitamin D deficiency directly affects muscle wasting and muscle performance which can be due to reduced sun exposure. Vitamin D deficiency is associated with osteoporosis and rickets, and also with a reduction in muscle mass and strength. Muscle tissues have vitamin D receptor (VDR) which brings an interest in its effects on muscle metabolism. Vitamin D intake either through sun exposure or dietary intake will increase the level of vitD-binding protein and vitD complex which then metabolize to 25-hydroxyvitamin D in the lever. Also in the kidney, it gets metabolized to VitD [1,25(OH)2D] that is an active form of vitD. The role of vitD in muscles is proposed to be acting through VDR and downstream signaling pathways. Binding of vitD molecule with VRD caused heterodimerization of the receptor with retinoid X receptor which then binds to VitD response element followed by gene transcription. VitD downregulates myostatin, upregulates AKT, and sensitizes the mTOR pathway leading to an increase in myotubule size. In vitro studies have suggested the anabolic role in skeletal muscles and increase the muscular strength. In elderly people, beneficial effects have been noted with VitD supplements for better muscular functions.

12.5.2.2.2 Vitamins C and E

Vitamins C and E are recognized as potent antioxidants that can scavenge free radicals and have a beneficial role in protein homeostasis (Powers et al, 1999). High levels of reactive oxygen species can disrupt protein homeostasis. Consumption of foods rich in vitamins C and E can neutralize free radicals by adding an electron and thus reduces the chances of protein degradation

(Scott et al., 2010). Fruits and vegetables rich in vitamins C and E are recommended over anti-oxidant supplements (Close et al., 2016). Muscle being a major site for vitamin C storage, it is believed that vitamin C intake can have a beneficial role in increasing lean body mass (Welch, 2014).

12.5.2.3 Miscellaneous
12.5.2.3.1 n-3 Polyunsaturated fatty acids (n-3 PUFA)

n-3 PUFA contains a double bond at the third carbon and is of three types as mentioned before also, α-linoleic acid (ALA), eicosapentaenoic acid (EPA), and docosahexaenoic acid (DHA). Evidence suggests the role of n-3 PUFA in protein synthesis by increasing phosphorylation of anabolic signaling (Alexander et al., 1986). In a preclinical study finding, EPA intake attenuated loss of skeletal muscles by 18% and the possible mechanism proposed was a reduction in prostanoids. Fish oil is rich in EPA and its intake may increase muscle mass and attenuate muscle loss in stress conditions by reducing inflammatory mediators and cytokines. The chronic gain in muscle mass and metabolic flexibility are seen with n-3 PUFA supplements (Zhang et al., 2014).

12.5.2.3.2 Nitrates

Inorganic nitrates containing diets such as beetroot and lettuce are capable of increasing nitric oxide levels (Jones, 2014). Nitric oxide helps in the modulation of muscle-related processes such as contraction, blood flow to the muscle, satellite cell activation, and glucose homeostasis. Nitrates promote anabolism through increasing blood flow to the muscles and thus increasing nutrient delivery and also increases muscle protein synthesis. Dietary arginine is also the principal substrate for nitric oxide synthase leading to NO production. Arginine supplementation also has been reported to have a beneficial role in increasing muscle mass (Mitchell et al., 2017).

12.5.2.3.3 Ursolic acid

Ursolic acid is one of the novel nutraceuticals that has been studied for effects on muscle mass and protein metabolism. It is a natural phytochemical majorly found in apple peel. In a preclinical study, 7% muscle hypertrophy was seen in mice which were proposed to be due to attenuation of MuRF1 and atrogin-1 atrophy inducing genes and upregulation of IGF (Kunkel et al., 2011). Ursolic acid combined with resistance exercise activates p70S6K1 and prolongs the activity of mTORC1, which are essential for anabolic signaling in skeletal muscle (Sancak et al., 2010).

12.5.2.3.4 Phosphatidic acid

Phosphatidic acid is a diacyl-glycerophospholipid and is available both endogenously in the cell membrane and exogenously in cabbage. Phosphatidic acid is believed to be increasing muscle mass and affects protein metabolism

(Mobley et al., 2015). Endogenous phosphatidic acid activates mTORC1 and increase muscle protein synthesis. Moreover, it can also attenuate muscle protein breakdown by inhibiting atrophy-related genes (Tanaka et al., 2012). Exogenous phosphatidic acid has inhibitory effects against atrophy inducing genes in cell culture medium with the presence of TNF-α and dexamethasone (atrophy inducers) (Lehours et al., 2011).

12.6 Conclusion and future direction

The inevitable loss of skeletomuscular system with age has a poor prognosis and reduced quality of life. Management of osteosarcopenia is a part of long-term treatment, and the current pharmacological agents available are having either high cost or adverse effects. This chapter has eluted different nutraceuticals used to either prevent or manage the loss of bones and muscles. A variety of plant-derived natural agents have shown tremendous benefits in age-associated bone and muscle loss. For bone health, calcium and other ions, herbs, and vitamin D are the most important factors, whereas for skeletal muscles, protein, alanine, leucine, carnitine, nitrates, and HMB have shown the most promising results in increasing muscle power and performance. Nutraceuticals should be taken with the proper amount and correct manner to get maximum beneficial effects. By looking at the progress on in vivo and clinical trial studies, there is indeed a need to evaluate pharmacokinetic studies, mechanistic studies, dosage regimens, side effects, off-target effects of the nutraceuticals, and development of formulations. Also, there is a need for comprehensive studies in combination therapies with the available pharmacological treatments that can guide clinicians to recommend nutraceutical agents in the treatment, prevention, and management of skeletomuscular losses.

References

Alexander JW, Saito HI, Trocki O, Ogle CK. The importance of lipid type in the diet after burn injury. *Annals of surgery.* 1986 Jul;204(1):1.

Alexandersen P, Toussaint A, Christiansen C, Devogelaer JP, Roux C, Fechtenbaum J, Gennari C, Reginster JY. Ipriflavone in the treatment of postmenopausal osteoporosis: A randomized controlled trial. *JAMA.* 2001 Mar 21;285(11):1482–8.

Alizai H, Nardo L, Karampinos DC, Joseph GB, Yap SP, Baum T, Krug R, Majumdar S, Link TM. Comparison of clinical semi-quantitative assessment of muscle fat infiltration with quantitative assessment using chemical shift-based water/fat separation in MR studies of the calf of post-menopausal women. *European Radiology.* 2012 Jul 1;22(7):1592–600.

Almeida M, Han L, Martin-Millan M, Plotkin LI, Stewart SA, Roberson PK, Kousteni S, O'Brien CA, Bellido T, Parfitt AM, Weinstein RS. Skeletal involution by age-associated oxidative stress and its acceleration by loss of sex steroids. *Journal of Biological Chemistry.* 2007 Sep 14;282(37):27285–97.

Arjmandi BH, Khalil DA, Lucas EA, Georgis A, Stoecker BJ, Hardin C, Payton ME, Wild RA. Dried plums improve indices of bone formation in postmenopausal women. *Journal of Women's Health & Gender-Based Medicine.* 2002 Jan 1;11(1):61–8.

Baehr LM, Tunzi M, Bodine SC. Muscle hypertrophy is associated with increases in proteasome activity that is independent of MuRF1 and MAFbx expression. *Frontiers in Physiology.* 2014 Feb 21;5:69.

Baier S, Johannsen D, Abumrad N, Rathmacher JA, Nissen S, Flakoll P. Year-long changes in protein metabolism in elderly men and women supplemented with a nutrition cocktail of β-hydroxy-β-methylbutyrate (HMB), L-arginine, and L-lysine. *Journal of Parenteral and Enteral Nutrition.* 2009 Jan;33(1):71–82.

Balagopal P, Schimke JC, Ades P, Adey D, Nair KS. Age effect on transcript levels and synthesis rate of muscle MHC and response to resistance exercise. *American Journal of Physiology-Endocrinology And Metabolism.* 2001 Feb 1;280(2):E203–8.

Bassey EJ, Harries UJ. Normal values for handgrip strength in 920 men and women aged over 65 years, and longitudinal changes over 4 years in 620 survivors. *Clinical Science.* 1993 Mar 1;84(3):331–7.

Baumgartner R. In vivo body composition studies. Ann NY Acad Sci ed. Body composition in healthy aging, ed. WJ Yasumura S, Pierson RN Jr. 2000;904:437–48.

Baumgartner RN, Heymsfield SB, Roche AF. Human body composition and the epidemiology of chronic disease. *Obesity Research.* 1995 Jan;3(1):73–95.

Baumgartner RN, Koehler KM, Gallagher D, Romero L, Heymsfield SB, Ross RR, Garry PJ, Lindeman RD. Epidemiology of sarcopenia among the elderly in New Mexico. *American Journal of Epidemiology.* 1998 Apr 15;147(8):755–63.

Baumgartner RN, Stauber PM, McHugh D, Koehler KM, Garry PJ. Cross-sectional age differences in body composition in persons 60+ years of age. *The Journals of Gerontology Series A: Biological Sciences and Medical Sciences.* 1995 Nov 1;50(6):M307–16.

Bazzocchi A, Diano D, Ponti F, Salizzoni E, Albisinni U, Marchesini G, Battista G. A 360-degree overview of body composition in healthy people: relationships among anthropometry, ultrasonography, and dual-energy x-ray absorptiometry. *Nutrition.* 2014 Jun 1;30(6):696–701.

Bazzocchi A, Ponti F, Albisinni U, Battista G, Guglielmi G. DXA: Technical aspects and application. *European Journal of Radiology.* 2016 Aug 1;85(8):1481–92.

Beck TJ. Extending DXA beyond bone mineral density: Understanding hip structure analysis. *Current Osteoporosis Reports.* 2007 Jun 1;5(2):49–55.

Bennett CN, Longo KA, Wright WS, Suva LJ, Lane TF, Hankenson KD, MacDougald OA. Regulation of osteoblastogenesis and bone mass by Wnt10b. *Proceedings of the National Academy of Sciences.* 2005 Mar 1;102(9):3324–9.

Bian Q, Liu SF, Huang JH, Yang Z, Tang DZ, Zhou Q, Ning Y, Zhao YJ, Lu S, Shen ZY, Wang YJ. Oleanolic acid exerts an osteoprotective effect in ovariectomy-induced osteoporotic rats and stimulates the osteoblastic differentiation of bone mesenchymal stem cells in vitro. *Menopause.* 2012 Feb 1;19(2):225–33.

Bodine SC, Baehr LM. Skeletal muscle atrophy and the E3 ubiquitin ligases MuRF1 and MAFbx/atrogin-1. *American Journal of Physiology-Endocrinology and Metabolism.* 2014 Sep 15;307(6):E469–84.

Bodine SC, Latres E, Baumhueter S, Lai VK, Nunez L, Clarke BA, Poueymirou WT, Panaro FJ, Na E, Dharmarajan K, Pan ZQ. Identification of ubiquitin ligases required for skeletal muscle atrophy. *Science.* 2001 Nov 23;294(5547):1704–8.

Bonnick SL. Hsa: Beyond bmd with dxa. *Bone.* 2007 Jul 1;41(1):S9–12.

Booth FW, Laye MJ, Roberts MD. Lifetime sedentary living accelerates some aspects of secondary aging. *Journal of Applied Physiology.* 2011 Nov;111(5):1497–504.

Boss GR, Seegmiller JE. Age-related physiological changes and their clinical significance. *Western Journal of Medicine.* 1981 Dec;135(6):434.

Bowen TS, Schuler G, Adams V. Skeletal muscle wasting in cachexia and sarcopenia: Molecular pathophysiology and impact of exercise training. *Journal of Cachexia, Sarcopenia and Muscle.* 2015 Sep;6(3):197–207.

Britton KA, Massaro JM, Murabito JM, Kreger BE, Hoffmann U, Fox CS. Body fat distribution, incident cardiovascular disease, cancer, and all-cause mortality. *Journal of the American College of Cardiology.* 2013 Sep 3;62(10):921–5.

Brook MS, Wilkinson DJ, Phillips BE, Perez-Schindler J, Philp A, Smith K, Atherton PJ. Skeletal muscle homeostasis and plasticity in youth and ageing: Impact of nutrition and exercise. *Acta Physiologica.* 2016 Jan;216(1):15–41.

Brooks SV, Faulkner JA. Skeletal muscle weakness in old age: underlying mechanisms. *Medicine and Science in Sports and Exercise.* 1994 Apr 1;26(4):432–9.

Bruyère O, Beaudart C, Reginster JY, Buckinx F, Schoene D, Hirani V, Cooper C, Kanis JA, Rizzoli R, McCloskey E, Cederholm T. Assessment of muscle mass, muscle strength and physical performance in clinical practice: an international survey. *European Geriatric Medicine.* 2016 Jun 1;7(3):243–6.

Cade WT, Yarasheski KE. Metabolic and molecular aspects of sarcopenia. In *Principles of Molecular Medicine* 2006 (pp. 529–534). Humana Press, Totowa, NJ.

Carpenter TO, DeLucia MC, Zhang JH, Bejnerowicz G, Tartamella L, Dziura J, Petersen KF, Befroy D, Cohen D. A randomized controlled study of effects of dietary magnesium oxide supplementation on bone mineral content in healthy girls. *The Journal of Clinical Endocrinology & Metabolism.* 2006 Dec 1;91(12):4866–72.

Casey A, Constantin-Teodosiu D, Howell S, Hultman EG, Greenhaff PL. Creatine ingestion favorably affects performance and muscle metabolism during maximal exercise in humans. *American Journal of Physiology-Endocrinology and Metabolism.* 1996 Jul 1;271(1):E31–7.

Castiglioni S, Cazzaniga A, Albisetti W, Maier JA. Magnesium and osteoporosis: current state of knowledge and future research directions. *Nutrients.* 2013 Aug;5(8):3022–33.

Clark BC, Manini TM. Sarcopenia≠ dynapenia. *The Journals of Gerontology Series A: Biological Sciences and Medical Sciences.* 2008 Aug 1;63(8):829–34.

Clarke BL, Khosla S. Androgens and bone. *Steroids.* 2009 Mar 1;74(3):296–305.

Clarke BL, Khosla S. Physiology of bone loss. *Radiologic Clinics.* 2010 May 1;48(3):483–95.

Clifton-Bligh PB, Baber RJ, Fulcher GR, Nery ML, Moreton T. The effect of isoflavones extracted from red clover (Rimostil) on lipid and bone metabolism. *Menopause.* 2001 Jul 1;8(4):259–65.

Close GL, Hamilton DL, Philp A, Burke LM, Morton J. SPORT TK: RevistaEuroamericana de Ciencias del DeporteReposición del Glucógeno Muscular en la Recuperación del DeportistaP. New strategies in sport nutrition to increase exercise performance. *Free Radical Biology and Medicine.* 2016;98:144–58.

Compston JE. Sex steroids and bone. *Physiological Reviews.* 2001 Jan 1;81(1):419–47.

Conlan D, Korula R, Tallentire D. Serum copper levels in elderly patients with femoral-neck fractures. *Age and Ageing.* 1990 May 1;19(3):212–4.

Consensus A. Consensus development conference: Diagnosis, prophylaxis, and treatment of osteoporosis. *American Journal of Medicine.* 1993;94(6):646–50.

Cornish J, Callon KE, Naot D, Palmano KP, Banovic T, Bava U, Watson M, Lin JM, Tong PC, Chen Q, Chan VA. Lactoferrin is a potent regulator of bone cell activity and increases bone formation in vivo. *Endocrinology.* 2004 Sep 1;145(9):4366–74.

Cosman F, de Beur SJ, LeBoff MS, Lewiecki EM, Tanner B, Randall S, Lindsay R. Clinician's guide to prevention and treatment of osteoporosis. *Osteoporosis International.* 2014 Oct 1;25(10):2359–81.

Costa-Rodrigues J, Carmo SC, Silva JC, Fernandes MH. Inhibition of human in vitro osteoclastogenesis by E quisetumarvense. *Cell Proliferation.* 2012 Dec;45(6):566–76.

Cruz-Jentoft AJ, Bahat G, Bauer J, Boirie Y, Bruyère O, Cederholm T, Cooper C, Landi F, Rolland Y, Sayer AA, Schneider SM. Sarcopenia: Revised European consensus on definition and diagnosis. *Age and Ageing.* 2019 Jan 1;48(1):16–31.

Currey JD, Brear K, Zioupos P. The effects of ageing and changes in mineral content in degrading the toughness of human femora. *Journal of Biomechanics.* 1996 Feb 1;29(2):257–60.

Davis HM, Aref MW, Aguilar-Perez A, Pacheco-Costa R, Allen K, Valdez S, Herrera C, Atkinson EG, Mohammad A, Lopez D, Harris MA. Cx43 overexpression in osteocytes prevents osteocyte apoptosis and preserves cortical bone quality in aging mice. *JBMR Plus.* 2018 Jul;2(4):206–16.

de Rezende Pinto WB, de Souza PV, Oliveira AS. Normal muscle structure, growth, development, and regeneration. *Current Reviews in Musculoskeletal Medicine.* 2015 Jun 1;8(2):176–81.

Demontis F, Piccirillo R, Goldberg AL, Perrimon N. The influence of skeletal muscle on systemic aging and lifespan. *Aging Cell.* 2013 Dec;12(6):943–9.

Deutz NE, Pereira SL, Hays NP, Oliver JS, Edens NK, Evans CM, Wolfe RR. Effect of β-hydroxy-β-methylbutyrate (HMB) on lean body mass during 10 days of bed rest in older adults. *Clinical Nutrition.* 2013 Oct 1;32(5):704–12.

Devirian TA, Volpe SL. The physiological effects of dietary boron. *Critical Reviews in Food Science and Nutrition.* 2003;43:219–231.

Deyhim F, Garica K, Lopez E, Gonzalez J, Ino S, Garcia M, Patil BS. Citrus juice modulates bone strength in male senescent rat model of osteoporosis. *Nutrition.* 2006 May 1;22(5):559–63.

Dickinson JM, Volpi E, Rasmussen BB. Exercise and nutrition to target protein synthesis impairments in aging skeletal muscle. *Exercise and Sport Sciences Reviews.* 2013 Oct;41(4):216.

Dixon WT. Simple proton spectroscopic imaging. *Radiology.* 1984 Oct;153(1):189–94.

Dreyer HC, Volpi E. Role of protein and amino acids in the pathophysiology and treatment of sarcopenia. *Journal of the American College of Nutrition.* 2005 Apr 1;24(2):140S–5S.

Emerson NS, Stout JR, Fukuda DH, Robinson EH, Scanlon TC, Beyer KS, Fragala MS, Hoffman JR. Resistance training improves capacity to delay neuromuscular fatigue in older adults. *Archives of Gerontology and Geriatrics.* 2015 Jul 1;61(1):27–32.

Engelke K, Adams JE, Armbrecht G, Augat P, Bogado CE, Bouxsein ML, Felsenberg D, Ito M, Prevrhal S, Hans DB, Lewiecki EM. Clinical use of quantitative computed tomography and peripheral quantitative computed tomography in the management of osteoporosis in adults: The 2007 ISCD Official Positions. *Journal of Clinical Densitometry.* 2008 Jan 1;11(1):123–62.

Erlandson MC, Lorbergs AL, Mathur S, Cheung AM. Muscle analysis using pQCT, DXA and MRI. *European Journal of Radiology.* 2016 Aug 1;85(8):1505–11.

Escobar J, Frank JW, Suryawan A, Nguyen HV, Van Horn CG, Hutson SM, Davis TA. Leucine and α-ketoisocaproic acid, but not norleucine, stimulate skeletal muscle protein synthesis in neonatal pigs. *Journal of Nutrition.* 2010 Aug 1;140(8):1418–24.

Evans WJ, Heymsfield SB, Gallagher D, Visser M, Nuñez C, Wang ZM. Measurement of skeletal muscle: Laboratory and epidemiological methods. *The Journals of Gerontology Series A: Biological Sciences and Medical Sciences.* 1995 Nov 1;50(Special_Issue):23–9.

Favier FB, Benoit H, Freyssenet D. Cellular and molecular events controlling skeletal muscle mass in response to altered use. *PflügersArchiv-European Journal of Physiology.* 2008 Jun 1;456(3):587–600.

Feng J, Liu S, Ma S, Zhao J, Zhang W, Qi W, Cao P, Wang Z, Lei W. Protective effects of resveratrol on postmenopausal osteoporosis: Regulation of SIRT1-NF-κB signaling pathway. *Acta BiochimBiophys Sin.* 2014 Dec 1;46(12):1024–33.

Fischer MA, Pfirrmann CW, Espinosa N, Raptis DA, Buck FM. Dixon-based MRI for assessment of muscle-fat content in phantoms, healthy volunteers and patients with achillodynia: Comparison to visual assessment of calf muscle quality. *European Radiology.* 2014 Jun 1;24(6):1366–75.

Flatt T. A new definition of aging? *Frontiers in Genetics.* 2012 Aug 23;3:148.

Folland JP, Williams AG. Morphological and neurological contributions to increased strength. *Sports medicine*. 2007 Feb 1;37(2):145–68.

Forbes GB. Lean body mass-body fat interrelationships in humans. *Nutrition Reviews (USA)*. 1987;45:225–31.

Franklin TR, Ehrman R, Lynch KG, Harper D, Sciortino N, O'Brien CP, Childress AR. Menstrual cycle phase at quit date predicts smoking status in an NRT treatment trial: A retrospective analysis. *Journal of Women's Health*. 2008 Mar 1;17(2):287–92.

Frontera WR, Hughes VA, Fielding RA, Fiatarone MA, Evans WJ, Roubenoff R. Aging of skeletal muscle: A 12-yr longitudinal study. *Journal of Applied Physiology*. 2000 Apr 1;88(4):1321–6.

Gallagher D, Visser M, De Meersman RE, Sepúlveda D, Baumgartner RN, Pierson RN, Harris T, Heymsfield SB. Appendicular skeletal muscle mass: Effects of age, gender, and ethnicity. *Journal of Applied Physiology*. 1997 Jul 1;83(1):229–39.

García-Prat L, Martínez-Vicente M, Perdiguero E, Ortet L, Rodríguez-Ubreva J, Rebollo E, Ruiz-Bonilla V, Gutarra S, Ballestar E, Serrano AL, Sandri M. Autophagy maintains stemness by preventing senescence. *Nature*. 2016 Jan;529(7584):37–42.

Garnero P, Sornay-Rendu E, Chapuy MC, Delmas PD. Increased bone turnover in late post-menopausal women is a major determinant of osteoporosis. *Journal of Bone and Mineral Research*. 1996 Mar;11(3):337–49.

Genant HK, Block JE, Steiger P, Glueer CC, Smith R. Quantitative computed tomography in assessment of osteoporosis. *Seminars in Nuclear Medicine*. 1987 Oct 1; 17(4): 316–33.

Genant HK, Wu CY, Van Kuijk C, Nevitt MC. Vertebral fracture assessment using a semi-quantitative technique. *Journal of bone and mineral research*. 1993 Sep;8(9):1137–48.

Gibon E, Lu L, Goodman SB. Aging, inflammation, stem cells, and bone healing. *Stem Cell Research & Therapy*. 2016 Dec;7(1):1–7.

Gilbert SF. *Developmental Biology*. 6th edition. Sunderland, MA: Sinauer Associates; 2000. Aging: The Biology of Senescence. Available from: https://www.ncbi.nlm.nih.gov/books/NBK10041/.

Glüer CC, International Quantitative Ultrasound Consensus Group. Quantitative ultrasound techniques for the assessment of osteoporosis: Expert agreement on current status. *Journal of Bone and Mineral Research*. 1997 Aug;12(8):1280–8.

Goldman HM, McFarlin SC, Cooper DM, Thomas CD, Clement JG. Ontogenetic patterning of cortical bone microstructure and geometry at the human mid-shaft femur. *The Anatomical Record: Advances in Integrative Anatomy and Evolutionary Biology: Advances in Integrative Anatomy and Evolutionary Biology*. 2009 Jan;292(1):48–64.

Goodpaster BH, Park SW, Harris TB, Kritchevsky SB, Nevitt M, Schwartz AV, Simonsick EM, Tylavsky FA, Visser M, Newman AB. The loss of skeletal muscle strength, mass, and quality in older adults: The health, aging and body composition study. *The Journals of Gerontology Series A: Biological Sciences and Medical Sciences*. 2006 Oct 1;61(10):1059–64.

Greenhaff PL, Bodin K, Soderlund K, Hultman E. Effect of oral creatine supplementation on skeletal muscle phosphocreatine resynthesis. *American Journal of Physiology-Endocrinology And Metabolism*. 1994 May 1;266(5):E725–30.

Greig CA, Botella J, Young A. The quadriceps strength of healthy elderly people remeasured after eight years. *Muscle & Nerve: Official Journal of the American Association of Electrodiagnostic Medicine*. 1993 Jan;16(1):6–10.

Guerri S, Mercatelli D, Gómez MP, Napoli A, Battista G, Guglielmi G, Bazzocchi A. Quantitative imaging techniques for the assessment of osteoporosis and sarcopenia. *Quantitative Imaging in Medicine and Surgery*. 2018 Feb;8(1):60.

Guglielmi G, Muscarella S, Bazzocchi A. Integrated imaging approach to osteoporosis: State-of-the-art review and update. *Radiographics*. 2011 Sep;31(5):1343–64.

Guglielmi G, Scalzo G, de Terlizzi F, Peh WC. Quantitative ultrasound in osteoporosis and bone metabolism pathologies. *Radiologic Clinics*. 2010 May 1;48(3):577–88.

Hans D, Barthe N, Boutroy S, Pothuaud L, Winzenrieth R, Krieg MA. Correlations between trabecular bone score, measured using anteroposterior dual-energy X-ray absorptiometry acquisition, and 3-dimensional parameters of bone microarchitecture: an experimental study on human cadaver vertebrae. *Journal of Clinical Densitometry*. 2011 Jul 1;14(3):302–12.

Harris T. Muscle mass and strength: relation to function in population studies. *The Journal of Nutrition*. 1997 May 1;127(5):1004S–6S.

Hawkinson J, Timins J, Angelo D, Shaw M, Takata R, Harshaw F. Technical white paper: Bone densitometry. *Journal of the American College of Radiology*. 2007 May 1;4(5):320–7.

He FJ, MacGregor GA. Beneficial effects of potassium on human health. *Physiologia Plantarum*. 2008 Aug;133(4):725–35.

Heymsfield SB, Arteaga C, McManus C, Smith J, Moffitt S. Measurement of muscle mass in humans: Validity of the 24-hour urinary creatinine method. *The American Journal of Clinical Nutrition*. 1983 Mar 1;37(3):478–94.

Heymsfield SB, Smith R, Aulet M, Bensen B, Lichtman S, Wang JP, Pierson Jr RN. Appendicular skeletal muscle mass: measurement by dual-photon absorptiometry. *The American Journal of Clinical Nutrition*. 1990 Aug 1;52(2):214–8.

Horton R, Romanoff E, Walker J. Androstenedione and testosterone in ovarian venous and peripheral plasma during ovariectomy for breast cancer. *The Journal of Clinical Endocrinology & Metabolism*. 1966 Nov 1;26(11):1267–9.

Houmard JA, Smith RA, Jendrasiak GL. Relationship between MRI relaxation time and muscle fiber composition. *Journal of Applied Physiology*. 1995 Mar 1;78(3):807–9.

Hsieh TP, Sheu SY, Sun JS, Chen MH. Icariin inhibits osteoclast differentiation and bone resorption by suppression of MAPKs/NF-κB regulated HIF-1α and PGE2 synthesis. *Phytomedicine*. 2011 Jan 15;18(2-3):176–85.

Hughes VA, Frontera WR, Wood M, Evans WJ, Dallal GE, Roubenoff R, Singh MA. Longitudinal muscle strength changes in older adults: influence of muscle mass, physical activity, and health. *The Journals of Gerontology Series A: Biological Sciences and Medical Sciences*. 2001 May 1;56(5):B209–17.

Jabeen Q, Aslam N. The pharmacological activities of prunes: The dried plums. *Journal of Medicinal Plants Research*. 2011 May 4;5(9):1508–11.

Jackson MP, Hewitt EW. Cellular proteostasis: Degradation of misfolded proteins by lysosomes. *Essays in Biochemistry*. 2016 Oct 15;60(2):173–80.

Janssen I, Heymsfield SB, Baumgartner RN, Ross R. Estimation of skeletal muscle mass by bioelectrical impedance analysis. *Journal of Applied Physiology*. 2000 Aug 1;89(2):465–71.

Janssen I, Heymsfield SB, Ross R. Low relative skeletal muscle mass (sarcopenia) in older persons is associated with functional impairment and physical disability. *Journal of the American Geriatrics Society*. 2002 May;50(5):889–96.

Janssen I, Heymsfield SB, Wang Z, Ross R. Skeletal muscle mass and distribution in 468 men and women aged 18–88 yr. *Journal of Applied Physiology*. 2000 Jul 1. doi:10.1152/jappl.2000.89.1.81.

Jepsen KJ. Systems analysis of bone. *Wiley Interdisciplinary Reviews: Systems Biology and Medicine*. 2009 Jul;1(1):73–88.

Jiao J, Demontis F. Skeletal muscle autophagy and its role in sarcopenia and organismal aging. *Current Opinion in Pharmacology*. 2017 Jun 1;34:1–6.

Johnson FB, Sinclair DA, Guarente L. Molecular biology of aging. *Cell*. 1999 Jan 22;96(2):291–302.

Jonas J, Burns J, Abel EW, Cresswell MJ, Strain JJ, Paterson CR. Impaired mechanical strength of bone in experimental copper deficiency. *Annals of Nutrition and Metabolism*. 1993;37(5):245–52.

Jones AM. Dietary nitrate supplementation and exercise performance. *Sports Medicine*. 2014 May 1;44(1):35–45.

Jung T, Catalgol B, Grune T. The proteasomal system. *Molecular Aspects of Medicine*. 2009 Aug 1;30(4):191–296.

Kanis JA. Assessment of osteoporosis at the primary health-care level. WHO Collaborating Centre for Metabolic Bone Diseases, University of Sheffield. 2007 May 17.

Karakelides H, Nair KS. Sarcopenia of aging and its metabolic impact. *Current Topics in Developmental Biology*. 2005 Jan 1;68:123–48.

Kato K, Toba Y, Matsuyama H, Yamamura JI, Matsuoka Y, Kawakami H, Itabashi A, Kumegawa M, Aoe S, Takada Y. Milk basic protein enhances the bone strength in ovariectomized rats. *Journal of Food Biochemistry*. 2000 Dec;24(6):467–76.

Khosla S, Riggs BL, Robb RA, Camp JJ, Achenbach SJ, Oberg AL, Rouleau PA, Melton III LJ. Relationship of volumetric bone density and structural parameters at different skeletal sites to sex steroid levels in women. *The Journal of Clinical Endocrinology & Metabolism*. 2005 Sep 1;90(9):5096–103.

Kim H, Suzuki T, Saito K, Kojima N, Hosoi E, Yoshida H. Long-term effects of exercise and amino acid supplementation on muscle mass, physical function and falls in community-dwelling elderly Japanese sarcopenic women: A 4-year follow-up study. *Geriatrics & Gerontology International*. 2016 Feb;16(2):175–81.

Kim HJ, Ohk B, Kang WY, Seong SJ, Suk K, Lim MS, Kim SY, Yoon YR. Deficiency of lipocalin-2 promotes proliferation and differentiation of osteoclast precursors via regulation of c-fms expression and nuclear factor-kappa B activation. *Journal of Bone Metabolism*. 2016 Feb 1;23(1):8–15.

Kirkwood TB. Evolution of ageing. *Nature*. 1977 Nov;270(5635):301–4.

Klitgaard H, Zhou M, Schiaffino S, Betto R, Salviati G, Saltin B. Ageing alters the myosin heavy chain composition of single fibres from human skeletal muscle. *Acta physiologicaScandinavica*. 1990 Sep;140(1):55–62.

Ko CH, Lau KM, Choy WY, Leung PC. Effects of tea catechins, epigallocatechin, gallocatechin, and gallocatechin gallate, on bone metabolism. *Journal of Agricultural and Food Chemistry*. 2009 Aug 26;57(16):7293–7.

Kon M, Cuervo AM. Chaperone-mediated autophagy in health and disease. *FEBS Letters*. 2010 Apr 2;584(7):1399–404.

Krug R, Banerjee S, Han ET, Newitt DC, Link TM, Majumdar S. Feasibility of in vivo structural analysis of high-resolution magnetic resonance images of the proximal femur. *Osteoporosis International*. 2005 Nov 1;16(11):1307–14.

Krug R, Burghardt AJ, Majumdar S, Link TM. High-resolution imaging techniques for the assessment of osteoporosis. *Radiologic Clinics*. 2010 May 1;48(3):601–21.

Kumar A, Bhatnagar S, Paul PK. TWEAK and TRAF6 regulate skeletal muscle atrophy. *Current Opinion in Clinical Nutrition and Metabolic Care*. 2012 May;15(3):233.

Kunkel SD, Suneja M, Ebert SM, Bongers KS, Fox DK, Malmberg SE, Alipour F, Shields RK, Adams CM. mRNA expression signatures of human skeletal muscle atrophy identify a natural compound that increases muscle mass. *Cell Metabolism*. 2011 Jun 8;13(6):627–38.

La Tegola L, Mattera M, Cornacchia S, Cheng X, Guglielmi G. Diagnostic imaging of two related chronic diseases: Sarcopenia and Osteoporosis. *Journal of Frailty, Sarcopenia and Falls*. 2018;3:138–47.

Larsson L, Sjödin B, Karlsson J. Histochemical and biochemical changes in human skeletal muscle with age in sedentary males, age 22–65 years. *Acta PhysiologicaScandinavica*. 1978 May;103(1):31–9.

Launer LJ, Harris T, Rumpel C, Madans J. Body mass index, weight change, and risk of mobility disability in middle-aged and older women: The epidemiologic follow-up study of NHANES I. *JAMA*. 1994 Apr 13;271(14):1093–8.

Law YY, Chiu HF, Lee HH, Shen YC, Venkatakrishnan K, Wang CK. Consumption of onion juice modulates oxidative stress and attenuates the risk of bone disorders in middle-aged and post-menopausal healthy subjects. *Food & Function*. 2016;7(2):902–12.

Lee CJ, Lawler GS, Johnson GH. Effects of supplementation of the diets with calcium and calcium-rich foods on bone density of elderly females with osteoporosis. *The American Journal of Clinical Nutrition*. 1981 May 1;34(5):819–23.

Lee SU, Park SJ, Kwak HB, Oh J, Min YK, Kim SH. Anabolic activity of ursolic acid in bone: Stimulating osteoblast differentiation in vitro and inducing new bone formation in vivo. *Pharmacological Research*. 2008 Nov 1;58(5-6):290–6.

Lehours P, Siffré E, Mégraud F. DPO multiplex PCR as an alternative to culture and susceptibility testing to detect Helicobacter pylori and its resistance to clarithromycin. *BMC Gastroenterology*. 2011 Dec;11(1):1–5.

Lindsay RD, Aitken JM, Anderson LB, Hart DM, MacDonald EB, Clarke AC. Long-term prevention of postmenopausal osteoporosis by oestrogen: evidence for an increased bone mass after delayed onset of oestrogen treatment. *Lancet*. 1976 May 15;307(7968):1038–41.

Lukaski HC, Mendez J, Buskirk ER, Cohn SH. Relationship between endogenous 3-methylhistidine excretion and body composition. *American Journal of Physiology-Endocrinology and Metabolism*. 1981 Mar 1;240(3):E302–7.

Maggio M, Artoni A, Lauretani F, Borghi L, Nouvenne A, Valenti G, Ceda GP. The impact of omega-3 fatty acids on osteoporosis. *Current Pharmaceutical Design*. 2009 Dec 1;15(36):4157–64.

Manolagas SC. From estrogen-centric to aging and oxidative stress: A revised perspective of the pathogenesis of osteoporosis. *Endocrine Reviews*. 2010 Jun 1;31(3):266–300.

Marcus RL, Addison O, LaStayo PC. Intramuscular adipose tissue attenuates gains in muscle quality in older adults at high risk for falling. A brief report. *The Journal of Nutrition, Health & Aging*. 2013 Mar 1;17(3):215–8.

Martin AD, Spenst LF, Drinkwater DT, Clarys JP. Anthropometric estimation of muscle mass in men. *Medicine and Science in Sports and Exercise*. 1990 Oct 1;22(5):729–33.

Marzetti E, Anne Lees H, Eva Wohlgemuth S, Leeuwenburgh C. Sarcopenia of aging: Underlying cellular mechanisms and protection by calorie restriction. *Biofactors*. 2009 Jan;35(1):28–35.

Masiero E, Agatea L, Mammucari C, Blaauw B, Loro E, Komatsu M, Metzger D, Reggiani C, Schiaffino S, Sandri M. Autophagy is required to maintain muscle mass. *Cell Metabolism*. 2009 Dec 2;10(6):507–15.

Matkovic V. Calcium and peak bone mass. *Journal of Internal Medicine*. 1992 Feb;231(2):151–60.

McKenna DJ, Jones K, Humphrey S, Hughes K. Black cohosh: Efficacy, safety, and use in clinical and preclinical applications. *Alternative Therapies in Health and Medicine*. 2001 May 1;7(3):93.

Medawar PB. *An Unsolved Problem in Biology*. 1952. London: HK Lewis. Reprinted.

Melo RC, Takahashi AC, Quitério RJ, Salvini TF, Catai AM. Eccentric torque-producing capacity is influenced by muscle length in older healthy adults. *Journal of Strength & Conditioning Research*. 2016 Jan 1;30(1):259–66.

Melton Iii LJ. Epidemiology of hip fractures: Implications of the exponential increase with age. *Bone*. 1996 Mar 1;18(3):S121–5.

Mitchell WK, Atherton PJ, Williams J, Larvin M, Lund JN, Narici M. Sarcopenia, dynapenia, and the impact of advancing age on human skeletal muscle size and strength; a quantitative review. *Frontiers in Physiology*. 2012 Jul 11;3:260.

Mitchell WK, Phillips BE, Wilkinson DJ, Williams JP, Rankin D, Lund JN, Smith K, Atherton PJ. Supplementing essential amino acids with the nitric oxide precursor, l-arginine, enhances skeletal muscle perfusion without impacting anabolism in older men. *Clinical Nutrition*. 2017 Dec 1;36(6):1573–9.

Mitsiopoulos N, Baumgartner RN, Heymsfield SB, Lyons W, Gallagher D, Ross R. Cadaver validation of skeletal muscle measurement by magnetic resonance imaging and computerized tomography. *Journal of Applied Physiology*. 1998 Jul 1;85(1):115–22.

Mizushima N, Levine B, Cuervo AM, Klionsky DJ. Autophagy fights disease through cellular self-digestion. *Nature.* 2008 Feb;451(7182):1069–75.

Mobley CB, Hornberger TA, Fox CD, Healy JC, Ferguson BS, Lowery RP, McNally RM, Lockwood CM, Stout JR, Kavazis AN, Wilson JM. Effects of oral phosphatidic acid feeding with or without whey protein on muscle protein synthesis and anabolic signaling in rodent skeletal muscle. *Journal of the International Society of Sports Nutrition.* 2015 Dec;12(1):1.

Mödder UI, Achenbach SJ, Amin S, Riggs BL, Melton III LJ, Khosla S. Relation of serum serotonin levels to bone density and structural parameters in women. *Journal of Bone and Mineral Research.* 2010 Feb;25(2):415–22.

Morley JE, Baumgartner RN, Roubenoff R, Mayer J, NAIR KS. From the Chicago meetings. *Journal of Laboratory and Clinical Medicine.* 2001 Apr;137:231–43.

Morse CI, Thom JM, Davis MG, Fox KR, Birch KM, Narici MV. Reduced plantarflexor specific torque in the elderly is associated with a lower activation capacity. *European Journal of Applied Physiology.* 2004 Jun 1;92(1-2):219–26.

Müller MJ, Geisler C, Pourhassan M, Glüer CC, Bosy-Westphal A. Assessment and definition of lean body mass deficiency in the elderly. *European Journal of Clinical Nutrition.* 2014 Nov;68(11):1220–7.

Mutlu M, Argun M, Kilic ES, Saraymen R, Yazar S. Magnesium, zinc and copper status in osteoporotic, osteopenic and normal post-menopausal women. *Journal of International Medical Research.* 2007 Sep;35(5):692–5.

Nakanishi R, Shimizu M, Mori M, Akiyama H, Okudaira S, Otsuki B, Hashimoto M, Higuchi K, Hosokawa M, Tsuboyama T, Nakamura T. Secreted frizzled-related protein 4 is a negative regulator of peak BMD in SAMP6 mice. *Journal of Bone and Mineral Research.* 2006 Nov;21(11):1713–21.

Narici M, Franchi M, Maganaris C. Muscle structural assembly and functional consequences. *Journal of Experimental Biology.* 2016 Jan 1;219(2):276–84.

Narici MV, Reeves ND, Morse CI, Maganaris CN. Muscular adaptations to resistance exercise in the elderly. *Journal of Musculoskeletal and Neuronal Interactions.* 2004;4(2):161–4.

New SA, Bolton-Smith C, Grubb DA, Reid DM. Nutritional influences on bone mineral density: A cross-sectional study in premenopausal women. *American Journal of Clinical Nutrition.* 1997 Jun 1;65(6):1831–9.

Nielsen FH, Hunt CD, Mullen LM, Hunt JR. Effect of dietary boron on mineral, estrogen, and testosterone metabolism in postmenopausal women 1. *FASEB Journal.* 1987 Nov;1(5):394–7.

Nissen S, Sharp R, Ray M, Rathmacher JA, Rice D, Fuller Jr JC, Connelly AS, Abumrad NJ. Effect of leucine metabolite β-hydroxy-β-methylbutyrate on muscle metabolism during resistance-exercise training. *Journal of Applied Physiology.* 1996 Nov 1;81(5):2095–104.

Nissen SL, Abumrad NN. Nutritional role of the leucine metabolite β-hydroxy β-methylbutyrate (HMB). *Journal of Nutritional Biochemistry.* 1997 Jun 1;8(6):300–11.

Occhiuto F, Pasquale RD, Guglielmo G, Palumbo DR, Zangla G, Samperi S, Renzo A, Circosta C. Effects of phytoestrogenic isoflavones from red clover (Trifoliumpratense L.) on experimental osteoporosis. *Phytotherapy Research: An International Journal Devoted to Pharmacological and Toxicological Evaluation of Natural Product Derivatives.* 2007 Feb;21(2): 130–4.

Oursler MJ, Cortese C, Keeting P, Anderson MA, Bonde SK, Riggs BL, Spelsberg TC. Modulation of transforming growth factor-β production in normal human osteoblast-like cells by 17 β-estradiol and parathyroid hormone. *Endocrinology.* 1991 Dec 1;129(6): 3313–20.

Padykula HA, Herman E. The specificity of the histochemical method for adenosine triphosphatas. *Journal of Histochemistry & Cytochemistry.* 1955 May;3(3):170–95.

Palacios C. The role of nutrients in bone health, from A to Z. *Critical Reviews in Food Science and Nutrition.* 2006 Dec 1;46(8):621–8.

Pang JL, Ricupero DA, Huang S, Fatma N, Singh DP, Romero JR, Chattopadhyay N. Differential activity of kaempferol and quercetin in attenuating tumor necrosis factor receptor family signaling in bone cells. *Biochemical Pharmacology*. 2006 Mar 14;71(6):818–26.

Parvaneh K, Jamaluddin R, Karimi G, Erfani R. Effect of probiotics supplementation on bone mineral content and bone mass density. *Scientific World Journal*. 2014;2014:595962.

Pedrozo Z, Sánchez G, Torrealba N, Valenzuela R, Fernández C, Hidalgo C, Lavandero S, Donoso P. Calpains and proteasomes mediate degradation of ryanodine receptors in a model of cardiac ischemic reperfusion. *Biochimica et Biophysica Acta (BBA)-Molecular Basis of Disease*. 2010 Mar 1;1802(3):356–62.

Perna FM, Coa K, Troiano RP, Lawman HG, Wang CY, Li Y, Moser RP, Ciccolo JT, Comstock BA, Kraemer WJ. Muscular grip strength estimates of the US population from the national health and nutrition examination survey 2011–2012. *Journal of Strength and Conditioning Research*. 2016 Mar;30(3):867.

Perrien DS, Achenbach SJ, Bledsoe SE, Walser B, Suva LJ, Khosla S, Gaddy D. Bone turnover across the menopause transition: Correlations with inhibins and follicle-stimulating hormone. *Journal of Clinical Endocrinology & Metabolism*. 2006 May 1;91(5):1848–54.

Pette D, Peuker H, Staron RS. The impact of biochemical methods for single muscle fibre analysis. *Acta PhysiologicaScandinavica*. 1999 Aug;166(4):261–77.

Philippou A, Halapas A, Maridaki M, Koutsilieris M. Type I insulin-like growth factor receptor signaling in skeletal muscle regeneration and hypertrophy. *Journal of Musculoskeletal and Neuronal Interactions*. 2007 Jul;7(3):208–18.

Pietrobelli AN, Formica CA, Wang ZI, Heymsfield SB. Dual-energy X-ray absorptiometry body composition model: review of physical concepts. *American Journal of Physiology-Endocrinology And Metabolism*. 1996 Dec 1;271(6):E941–51.

Pillen S, van Alfen N. Skeletal muscle ultrasound. *Neurological Research*. 2011 Dec 1;33(10):1016–24.

Powers SK, Ji LL, Leeuwenburgh CH. Exercise training-induced alterations in skeletal muscle antioxidant capacity: A brief review. *Medicine and Science in Sports and Exercise*. 1999 Jul;31(7):987–97.

Prince RL, Devine A, Dhaliwal SS, Dick IM. Effects of calcium supplementation on clinical fracture and bone structure: results of a 5-year, double-blind, placebo-controlled trial in elderly women. *Archives of Internal Medicine*. 2006 Apr 24;166(8):869–75.

Qiu SX, Dan C, Ding LS, Peng S, Chen SN, Farnsworth NR, Nolta J, Gross ML, Zhou P. A triterpene glycoside from black cohosh that inhibits osteoclastogenesis by modulating RANKL and TNFα signaling pathways. *Chemistry & Biology*. 2007 Jul 30;14(7):860–9.

Ramanadham S, Yarasheski KE, Silva MJ, Wohltmann M, Novack DV, Christiansen B, Tu X, Zhang S, Lei X, Turk J. Age-related changes in bone morphology are accelerated in group VIA phospholipase A2 (iPLA2β)-null mice. *The American Journal of Pathology*. 2008 Apr 1;172(4):868–81.

Rauner M, Sipos W, Pietschmann P. Age-dependent Wnt gene expression in bone and during the course of osteoblast differentiation. *Age*. 2008 Dec 1;30(4):273–82.

Reginster JY, Burlet N. Osteoporosis: a still increasing prevalence. *Bone*. 2006 Feb 1;38(2):4–9.

Reid IR, Mason B, Horne A, Ames R, Reid HE, Bava U, Bolland MJ, Gamble GD. Randomized controlled trial of calcium in healthy older women. *The American Journal of Medicine*. 2006 Sep 1;119(9):777–85.

Reid KF, Doros G, Clark DJ, Patten C, Carabello RJ, Cloutier GJ, Phillips EM, Krivickas LS, Frontera WR, Fielding RA. Muscle power failure in mobility-limited older adults: Preserved single fiber function despite lower whole muscle size, quality and rate of neuromuscular activation. *European Journal of Applied Physiology*. 2012 Jun 1;112(6):2289–301.

Reid KF, Pasha E, Doros G, Clark DJ, Patten C, Phillips EM, Frontera WR, Fielding RA. Longitudinal decline of lower extremity muscle power in healthy and mobility-limited older adults: Influence of muscle mass, strength, composition, neuromuscular activation and single fiber contractile properties. *European Journal of Applied Physiology.* 2014 Jan 1;114(1):29–39.

Rom O, Reznick AZ. The role of E3 ubiquitin-ligases MuRF-1 and MAFbx in loss of skeletal muscle mass. *Free Radical Biology and Medicine.* 2016 Sep 1;98:218–30.

Rosenberg IH. Sarcopenia: origins and clinical relevance. *The Journal of Nutrition.* 1997 May 1;127(5):990S–1S.

Ross R. Advances in the application of imaging methods in applied and clinical physiology. *Acta Diabetologica.* 2003 Oct 1;40(1):s45–50.

Roubenoff R. Origins and clinical relevance of sarcopenia. *Canadian Journal of Applied Physiology.* 2001;26:78–89.

Roubenoff R, Hughes VA. Sarcopenia: Current concepts. *The Journals of Gerontology Series A: Biological Sciences and Medical Sciences.* 2000 Dec 1;55(12):M716–24.

Rubbieri G, Mossello E, Di Bari M. Techniques for the diagnosis of sarcopenia. *Clinical Cases in Mineral and Bone Metabolism.* 2014 Sep;11(3):181.

Russ DW, Gregg-Cornell K, Conaway MJ, Clark BC. Evolving concepts on the age-related changes in "muscle quality". *Journal of Cachexia, Sarcopenia and Muscle.* 2012 Jun 1;3(2):95–109.

Ryu M, Jo J, Lee Y, Chung YS, Kim KM, Baek WC. Association of physical activity with sarcopenia and sarcopenic obesity in community-dwelling older adults: the Fourth Korea National Health and Nutrition Examination Survey. *Age and Ageing.* 2013 Nov 1;42(6):734–40.

Sanada K, Kearns CF, Midorikawa T, Abe T. Prediction and validation of total and regional skeletal muscle mass by ultrasound in Japanese adults. *European Journal of Applied Physiology.* 2006 Jan 1;96(1):24–31.

Sancak Y, Bar-Peled L, Zoncu R, Markhard AL, Nada S, Sabatini DM. Ragulator-Rag complex targets mTORC1 to the lysosomal surface and is necessary for its activation by amino acids. *Cell.* 2010 Apr 16;141(2):290–303.

Satomura K, Tobiume S, Tokuyama R, Yamasaki Y, Kudoh K, Maeda E, Nagayama M. Melatonin at pharmacological doses enhances human osteoblastic differentiation in vitro and promotes mouse cortical bone formation in vivo. *Journal of Pineal Research.* 2007 Apr;42(3):231–9.

Sayed RK, de Leonardis EC, Guerrero-Martínez JA, Rahim I, Mokhtar DM, Saleh AM, Abdalla KE, Pozo MJ, Escames G, López LC, Acuña-Castroviejo D. Identification of morphological markers of sarcopenia at early stage of aging in skeletal muscle of mice. *Experimental Gerontology.* 2016 Oct 1;83:22–30.

Schellinger D, Lin CS, Lim J, Hatipoglu HG, Pezzullo JC, Singer AJ. Bone marrow fat and bone mineral density on proton MR spectroscopy and dual-energy X-ray absorptiometry: Their ratio as a new indicator of bone weakening. *American Journal of Roentgenology.* 2004 Dec;183(6):1761–5.

Scholz-Ahrens KE, Schaafsma G, van den Heuvel EG, Schrezenmeir J. Effects of prebiotics on mineral metabolism. *American Journal of Clinical Nutrition.* 2001 Feb 1;73(2):459s–64s.

Scott D, Blizzard L, Fell J, Giles G, Jones G. Associations between dietary nutrient intake and muscle mass and strength in community-dwelling older adults: The Tasmanian Older Adult Cohort study. *Journal of the American Geriatrics Society.* 2010 Nov;58(11):2129–34.

Shen CL, Chyu MC, Wang JS. Tea and bone health: Steps forward in translational nutrition. *American Journal of Clinical Nutrition.* 2013 Dec 1;98(6):1694S–9S.

Shi Y, Yadav VK, Suda N, Liu XS, Guo XE, Myers MG, Karsenty G. Dissociation of the neuronal regulation of bone mass and energy metabolism by leptin in vivo. *Proceedings of the National Academy of Sciences.* 2008 Dec 23;105(51):20529–33.

Sojka JE. Magnesium supplementation and osteoporosis. *Nutrition Reviews*. 1995 Mar 1;53(3):71–4.

Stagi S, Cavalli L, Cavalli T, de Martino M, Brandi ML. Peripheral quantitative computed tomography (pQCT) for the assessment of bone strength in most of bone affecting conditions in developmental age: A review. *Italian Journal of Pediatrics*. 2016 Dec 1;42(1):88.

Stephens FB, Constantin-Teodosiu D, Greenhaff PL. New insights concerning the role of carnitine in the regulation of fuel metabolism in skeletal muscle. *Journal of Physiology*. 2007 Jun 1;581(2):431–44.

Stephens FB, Wall BT, Marimuthu K, Shannon CE, Constantin-Teodosiu D, Macdonald IA, Greenhaff PL. Skeletal muscle carnitine loading increases energy expenditure, modulates fuel metabolism gene networks and prevents body fat accumulation in humans. *Journal of Physiology*. 2013 Sep;591(18):4655–66.

Suetta C, Hvid LG, Justesen L, Christensen U, Neergaard K, Simonsen L, Ortenblad N, Magnusson SP, Kjaer M, Aagaard P. Effects of aging on human skeletal muscle after immobilization and retraining. *Journal of Applied Physiology*. 2009 Oct;107(4):1172–80.

Tanaka T, Kassai A, Ohmoto M, Morito K, Kashiwada Y, Takaishi Y, Urikura M, Morishige JI, Satouchi K, Tokumura A. Quantification of phosphatidic acid in foodstuffs using a thin-layer-chromatography-imaging technique. *Journal of Agricultural and Food Chemistry*. 2012 Apr 25;60(16):4156–61.

Tortora GJ, Derrickson BH. *Principles of Anatomy and Physiology*. John Wiley & Sons; 12th Edition, 2009, p. 141.

Tou JC. Resveratrol supplementation affects bone acquisition and osteoporosis: Pre-clinical evidence toward translational diet therapy. *Biochimica et Biophysica Acta (BBA)-Molecular Basis of Disease*. 2015 Jun 1;1852(6):1186–94.

Tresguerres IF, Tamimi F, Eimar H, Barralet JE, Prieto S, Torres J, Calvo-Guirado JL, Tresguerres JA. Melatonin dietary supplement as an anti-aging therapy for age-related bone loss. *Rejuvenation Research*. 2014 Aug 1;17(4):341–6.

Tsuji M, Yamamoto H, Sato T, Mizuha Y, Kawai Y, Taketani Y, Kato S, Terao J, Inakuma T, Takeda E. Dietary quercetin inhibits bone loss without effect on the uterus in ovariectomized mice. *Journal of Bone and Mineral Metabolism*. 2009 Nov 1;27(6):673–81.

Tuzun S, Eskiyurt N, Akarirmak U, Saridogan M, Senocak M, Johansson H, Kanis JA. Incidence of hip fracture and prevalence of osteoporosis in Turkey: The FRACTURK study. *Osteoporosis International*. 2012 Mar 1;23(3):949–55.

Uenishi K. Prevention of osteoporosis by foods and dietary supplements. Prevention of osteoporosis by milk and dairy products. *Clinical Calcium*. 2006 Oct 1;16(10):1606–4.

Uslu S, Uysal A, Oktem G, Yurtseven M, Tanyalcin T, Basdemir G. Constructive effect of exogenous melatonin against osteoporosis after ovariectomy in rats. *Analytical and Quantitative Cytology and Histology*. 2007 Oct 1;29(5):317–25.

Van Kan GA, Cedarbaum JM, Cesari M, Dahinden P, Fariello RG, Fielding RA, Goodpaster BH, Hettwer S, Isaac M, Laurent D, Morley JE. Sarcopenia: biomarkers and imaging (International Conference on Sarcopenia research). *Journal of Nutrition, Health & Aging*. 2011 Dec 1;15(10):834–46.

Van Staa TP, Dennison EM, Leufkens HA, Cooper C. Epidemiology of fractures in England and Wales. *Bone*. 2001 Dec 1;29(6):517–22.

Vandervoort AA. Aging of the human neuromuscular system. *Muscle & Nerve: Official Journal of the American Association of Electrodiagnostic Medicine*. 2002 Jan;25(1):17–25.

Venturelli M, Morgan GR, Donato AJ, Reese V, Bottura R, Tarperi C, Milanese C, Schena F, Reggiani C, Naro F, Cawthon RM. Cellular aging of skeletal muscle: Telomeric and free radical evidence that physical inactivity is responsible and not age. *Clinical Science*. 2014 Sep 1;127(6):415–21.

Vittone JL, Ballor DL, Sreekumaran Nair K. Muscle wasting in the elderly. *Age & Nutrition (Paris)*. 1996;7(2):96–105.

Volek JS, Duncan ND, Mazzetti SA, Staron RS, Putukian MA, Gomez AL, Pearson DR, Fink WJ, Kraemer WJ. Performance and muscle fiber adaptations to creatine supplementation and heavy resistance training. *Medicine and Science in Sports and Exercise.* 1999 Aug 1;31(8):1147–56.

Weaver CM, Martin BR, Nakatsu CH, Armstrong AP, Clavijo A, McCabe LD, McCabe GP, Duignan S, Schoterman MH, van den Heuvel EG. Galactooligosaccharides improve mineral absorption and bone properties in growing rats through gut fermentation. *Journal of Agricultural and Food Chemistry.* 2011 Jun 22;59(12):6501–10.

Welch AA. Nutritional influences on age-related skeletal muscle loss. *Proceedings of the Nutrition Society.* 2014 Feb;73(1):16–33.

Wiedmer P, Jung T, Castro JP, Pomatto LC, Sun PY, Davies KJ, Grune T. Sarcopenia–molecular mechanisms and open questions. *Ageing Research Reviews.* 2020 Oct 29;65:101200.

Wilkinson DJ, Hossain T, Hill DS, Phillips BE, Crossland H, Williams J, Loughna P, Churchward-Venne TA, Breen L, Phillips SM, Etheridge T. Effects of leucine and its metabolite β-hydroxy-β-methylbutyrate on human skeletal muscle protein metabolism. *Journal of Physiology.* 2013 Jun 1;591(11):2911–23.

Willoughby D, Rosene J. Effects of oral creatine and resistance training on myosin heavy chain expression. *Medicine & Science in Sports & Exercise.* 2001 Oct;33(10):1674–81.

Wong RW, Rabie AB. Effect of quercetin on preosteoblasts and bone defects. *Open Orthopaedics Journal.* 2008;2:27.

Woo SL, Kuei SC, Amiel D, Gomez MA, Hayes WC, White FC, Akeson WH. The effect of prolonged physical training on the properties of long bone: A study of Wolff's Law. *JBJS.* 1981 Jun 1;63(5):780–7.

Woodrow G. Body composition analysis techniques in the aged adult: Indications and limitations. *Current Opinion in Clinical Nutrition & Metabolic Care.* 2009 Jan 1;12(1):8–14.

Yakar S, Werner H, Rosen CJ. Insulin-like growth factors: Actions on the skeleton. *Journal of Molecular Endocrinology.* 2018 Jul;61(1):T115.

Young A, Stokes M, Crowe M. The size and strength of the quadriceps muscles of old and young men. *Clinical Physiology (Oxford, England).* 1985 Apr 1;5(2):145–54.

Zhang S, Hulver MW, McMillan RP, Cline MA, Gilbert ER. The pivotal role of pyruvate dehydrogenase kinases in metabolic flexibility. *Nutrition & Metabolism.* 2014 Dec;11(1):1–9.

Zheng D, Peng S, Yang SH, Shao ZW, Yang C, Feng Y, Wu W, Zhen WX. The beneficial effect of Icariin on bone is diminished in osteoprotegerin-deficient mice. *Bone.* 2012 Jul 1;51(1):85–92.

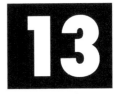

Nutritional Psychiatry in Aging
Leads from Ayurveda with Clinical Evidence

Asmita Wele and Swati Gadgil
Bharati Vidyapeeth (Deemed to be University)

Contents

13.1 Introduction

'Aging is a disease which is treatable and healthy longevity is the aim of human life' is the fundamental concept well elaborated in Ayurvedic science, the traditional medicine system of India. *Vayasthapana* meaning arresting aging or maintaining youth is the central theme of the medicine section of *Charaksamhita* [1]. After years of experience, a set of 10 herbs termed *Vayasthapana gana* is put together as the best anti-aging medicines [2]. Various Ayurvedic texts have discussed the concept of *jaranashana* meaning eliminating old age and also the therapies and formulations termed *rasayana* (immunomodulation) which help achieving longevity [3]. The function of the living body which starts deteriorating at an early age but exists till the last

DOI: 10.1201/9781003110866-13

breath is cognition. Loss of consciousness and cognition confirms death of the brain [4]. A lot of scientific literature has shown that loss of cognitive skills is associated with aging. Similarly, Ayurvedic texts are replete with a variety of substances that act on the cognitive function. In this chapter, we discuss some theories of aging, the foods and nutraceuticals reported for their effects on aging and cognition which are practiced in Ayurveda.

13.2 Process of cognition

Learning is the process of acquisition of information and skills, while subsequent retention of that information is called memory. Learning and memory together are called cognition. Principally, the memory process consists of registration, consolidation and retrieval. Registration is the process of sensory perception and the ability to act on the information perceived (known as behavioral response), which involves a change in electrical or electrochemical brain activity and referred to as short-term memory. Consolidation is the process of conversion of registered short-term information to a long-term memory trace, where physicochemical changes in neuronal networks happen. The sorted information is made accessible by the process known as retrieval [5].

Ayurveda explains the process of knowledge acquisition and roles of entities involved in a very subtle and clear manner. When the conscious desires for knowledge or material object, it stimulates the mind. Mind instructs the particular sense organ/s which pass on the instruction to motor organs. Motor organs perform action and send a return signal via the same route of senses, mind and finally to conscious. Thereby, the desire is fulfilled. This process of knowledge acquisition explained in *Charaksamhita* explicitly marks the importance of the role of mind in coordination [6]. It is a powerful entity having dual role of controlling the outgoing and incoming signals (Figure 13.1).

13.3 Prakriti (constitution) and features associated with mental aging

Similar to *doshaj prakriti* (physical constitution), psyche types have been discussed in detail in *Sushrutasamhita*. The broad classification of mental constitution based on *Triguna* is *Satvik*, *Rajas* and *Tamas* each having specific features and many subtypes [7]. Signs of aging like greying of hair and

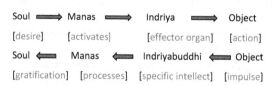

Figure 13.1 *Role of psyche in the process of knowledge acquisition (Charaksamhita).*

formation of wrinkles in a *kapha*-predominant *doshaj prakriti* and *satva*-predominant *manas prakriti* person appear in later decades. On the contrary, the persons of *pitta*- or *vata*-dominant *dosha prakriti* associated with *rajas* and or *tamas manas prakriti* are likely to age early.

The parameters to diagnose age-related loss of cognition or mental aging are explained as the decline of *grahana* (power of understanding), *dharana* (retention), *smarana* (recall memory), *vidnyan* (power of analysis), *utsaha* (enthusiasm/self-motivation), *pourush* (daring/valor), *bala* (mental strength), *oja* (reduced immunity), and *kriya-asamrthata* (nonperformance) [8]. Each of the subjective parameters can be assessed by using a variety of scales (observational studies) or by associated biomarkers using experimental designs. Just like chronological and biological/physiological age, cognitive age can also be determined.

13.4 Nutritional beginning of psyche development

Humans are composed of physical body, sensory organs, motor organs, mind, and consciousness (*Sharir indriya satva atma samyogodhari jeevitam*) [1]. Perfect coordination of the functions of the body depends on the meaningful interaction between the consciousness and mind. Any psychological dysfunction in adulthood has some linkage to the intrauterine life of the individual. Embryonic development of mind completes in the fifth month, whereas that of intellect happens in the sixth month of pregnancy. The distinctive functions of intellect and mind are also clearly listed in *Charaksamhita* (Figure 13.2). To fulfil nutritional requirements of organs and mind, from the first month fresh organic cow milk, cultured butter, and ghee made from cultured butter are included in the diet of a pregnant woman [9]. The herbs specifically added during pregnancy for health promotion are *Yashtimadhu* (*Glycyrrhiza*

Mind	Intellect: buddhi/pragya/medha
Chintan : thinking stimulus to do/not	Dhee: Nischaya : Decision making
Vichar: usefull /useless	Dhruti: retention ability
Uhya : various possibilities	Smriti: memory [all types]
Dhyeya: goal setting	
Sankalpa: determination to achieve the goal	
Indriya abhigraha : stimulates sensory motor apparatus and back	
Svanigraha: controls [bad desires, anger, obsessions, cheating, lying]	

Figure 13.2 Functions of mind and intellect.

glabra, Linn.), *Gokshura* (*Tribulus terrestris*, Linn.), *Brahmi* (*Bacopa monnieri*, Linn.), *Aindri* (*Centella asiatica*), *Shatavari* (*Asparagus racemosus*, Willd.), *Sahashravirya* (*Cynodon dactylon*, Linn.), *Amogha* (*Stereospermum suaveolens*, Roxb.), *Vayastha* (*Tinospora cordifolia*, Willd), *Shiva* (*Terminalia chebula*, Retz.), *Arishta* (*Picrorhiza kurroa*, Royal ex Benth.), *Vatyapushpi* (*Sida cordifolia*, Linn), and *Vishwasenkanta* (*Callicarpa macrophylla*, Vahl.). These are boiled with milk and administered with ghee and honey [10]. Each of these herbs is known to have psychotropic effect [11]. Cow milk is reported to contain saturated fatty acids (SFA), particularly C14:0 and C16:0, and small amounts of monounsaturated fatty acids (MUFA), poly unsaturated fatty acids (PUFA) and omega-3 fatty acids. The ghee prepared from cultured butter consists of long chain omega-3 fatty acids and DHA which are components of brain tissue [12]. Wild multifloral honey has been reported to possess various neurological effects like antinociceptive, anxiolytic, excitatory and many more [13]. Unifloral honey collected from cultivated plantation having particular biological effects have been in market. Agastache rugosa (Fisch. et Mey, O. Kuntze) is reported to possess antifungal, antimicrobial and wound healing activities [14–16].

Undoubtedly, the psychological health of a living being begins before the birth and continues during the lifetime keeping in tune with the environment, seasonally and daily. The code of conduct including exercise, yoga and meditation as daily routine takes care of influences on physiological health and psyche balance. The etiology of diseases where mind is a risk factor is explained as *pradnyaparadh* [6]. Therefore, it is very essential to learn about the substances and their dietary amounts which positively prevent or reverse the age-associated psychological derangements.

13.5 Food and cognition

The brain is always working, even during sleep. It takes care of thoughts and movements, breathing and heartbeat and also of the senses. It means that the brain requires a constant supply of fuel which comes from the foods that one consumes. The types of food directly affect the structure and function of the brain and, ultimately, mood [17].

This very fact has been explained in Ayurveda precisely. Food or diet (*Ahara*) is the foremost among three pillars of life; the other two being sleep (*nidra*) and regulated sexual life (*brahmacharya*[1]). Primary classification of food is made on its appropriateness to body and mental constitution which is based on the five elements and the *tridosa* theories [18]. Also, individual's nutritional needs vary according to age, seasonal and diurnal changes, etc. Consumption of inappropriate diet which is further categorized into incompatible food articles, food that generates toxins in the body, and food consumed without

---

[1] Conventionally Brahmacharya is celibacy. But its contextual meaning for *grihasthashrama* (married adult life) is experiencing bodily pleasures as per the code of conduct

Table 13.1 Life Span Division and Associated Decline from *Sharangdhar Samhita*

Decades of Life	Specification in Decline
0–10	*Balya* (childhood)
10–20	*Vriddhi* (physical growth)
20–30	*Chavi* (complexion)
30–40	*Medha* (knowledge retention power)
40–50	*Twak* (tone and luster of skin)
50–60	*Drishti* (vision)
60–70	*Shukra* (sexual vigor)
70–80	*Vikram* (overall physical and mental vigor)
80–90	*Buddhi* (intellect)
90–100	*Karmendriya* (motor skills and power)

following hygiene is one of the causative factors of psychic disorders which are described under the umbrella term *Unmad* and *Apasmar* [19]. It is a clear indication of the role of diet in maintenance of mental wellbeing. Adaptation of personalized diet patterns and appropriate food articles is very valuable because it has been associated with the loss of cognitive functions, mental vigor and decision-making power, at an early age than expected.

From conception to death, the human body undergoes subtle changes every moment. During the average lifespan of 100 years, the first part is of growth, while the latter is of loss. It is also termed as progressive deterioration. The decade-wise milestones measuring life faculties based on losing a particular characteristic are highlighted in *Sharangdharasamhita* (Table 13.1) [20]. According to this hypothesis, a person's *medha* means intellect starts declining in the fourth decade of life while *buddhi* means cognitive ability starts declining in the decade of the nineties. The measures to prolong the loss of specific characteristics are discussed under various topics such as *rasayana*, *dincharya* (daily regimen) *ritucharya* (seasonal regimen) and *garbhinipa-richarya* (antenatal care). Remedial changes should be practiced from the beginning of that decade using dietary substances, medicinal herbs and formulations, and lifestyle consisting of exercise and yoga.

13.6 Dietary products or nutritional supplement

Ayurveda classifies substances in two categories termed as dietary and medicinal (*aharadravya, aushadhadravya*) where dietary substances are dominant in taste (*rasa*) and medicinal herbs are dominant in potency (*virya*). The class of spices known as *aharyogi dravya* is on the borderline of food and drug. Spices enhance the flavor, preserve food article, bring out visual appeal and also balance the *doshas*. The influence of food, spices and herbal medicines is in an increasing order [21]. Also, the category of foods advised to patients popularly known as *pathya*, during and after the panchakarma procedure (*samsarjana krama*), is an intelligent combination of foods and spices. They are *manda*, *peya*, *vilepee*, *yavagu*, *yusha* and *krishara* (Table 13.2).

Grains are the base of these preparations, and spices are added to get specific pharmacological effect like appetizing, carminative, antiflatulence, stimulating, soothing, etc. Spices are known to modulate eicosanoid or prostanoids which are lipid-soluble compounds, produced by almost every cell which is responsible for proper function [22]. Spices are also available in capsules and tablet forms as nutritional supplement across the globe.

The three sources of substances herbal, animal and mineral are effectively used as supplements by mixing with daily foods or converting those into drinks,

Table 13.2 Food Articles During Recovery Period of a Disease

Sr. No.		Base and Spices	Preparation Method	Dose	Therapeutic Effect
1.	Manda	Cereal (brown rice), rock salt, dry ginger powder and ghee 1 teaspoon. (Wheat or millet can be used instead of rice according to the native food habits)	Boil of 1 portion of rice/cereal with 14 portions of water. Strain and leave aside solid. Add salt, pinch of ginger powder and ghee to the warm liquid	The filtrate is to be consumed 200–300 mL at a time	Appetizer, carminative
2.	Peya	Cereal, dry ginger powder, rock salt, ghee	Boil of 1 portion of rice/cereal with 14 portions of water. Add garnishes when warm.	Whole soupy portion is to be consumed.	Digestive, facilitates tissue nourishment.
3.	Vilepi	Cereal, rock salt, cumin powder, coriander/black pepper powder and ghee	Cook 1 portion rice with 4 portions of water to make porridge. Add garnishes	Whole thick portion to be consumed	Relieves weakness, gives satiety and strength, and is also diuretic
4.	Yavagu	Cereal, black pepper, cumin, rock salt, ghee	Cook 1 part of any grain with 6 portions of water, add the garnishes	Whole portion should be consumed	Nourishes tissues, strengthens
5.	Yusha	Legumes/pulses (dal) e.g., de-husked green gram/lentil/dolichos, etc. (vegetable protein source), ghee, spices	Shallow fry 1 portion of green gram, add 16 portions of water and cook to make thick soup. Garnish with spices	1 portion as a complete meal	Fulfilling, digestive, strengthening yet light to digest
6.	Krishara	Mixture of cereal and pulses (dal) in the proportion of 2:1, oil, mustard/cumin seeds curry leaves, curcuma, asafetida, rock salt, coriander, celery	Heat the oil and add mustard/cumin seeds, curcuma and asafetida powder pinch, curry leaves and then add washed mixture of rice and dal. For 1 portion, add 2 portions of water. Cook till it gets soft	1 portion with buttermilk	Nourishes, gives energy, yet light to digest. Buttermilk replenishes gut flora

chutneys, smoothies, milkshakes and medicated ghee. Various cognitive issues during aging can be effectively managed by adding the Ayurveda natural products to the daily or periodic regime of elderly population. The substances having activity on CNS or psyche from the three groups are listed below. These, together with *manda, peya*, etc., make simple yet effective neuroprotective foods.

1. **The Herbs**: Brahmi (*Bacopa monnieri* Linn), Mandukparni (*Centella asiatica* Urbn.), Kushmanda (*Benincasa hispida* Thunb.), Shankhapushpi (*Convolvulus pluricaulis* Choisy), Guduchi (*Tinospora cordifolia* Willd-Mierss), Jyotishmati (*Celastrus panniculatus* Willd), Jatamanasi (*Nordostachys jatamansi* DC), Vacha (*Acorus calamus*), Haritaki (*Terminalia chebula* Retz.), Amalaki (*Emblica officinalis*), garlic (*Allium sativum*), ginger (*Zinzibar officinalis*), turmeric (*Curcuma longa*) and a few more (Table 13.3).
2. **The minerals**: Natural minerals like Shilajit (Ozokerite), calcium from mineral and marine source, and elements or metals like iron (Fe), copper (Cu), gold (Au), silver (Ag), and zinc (Zn) have direct and indirect actions on cognition related to aging.
3. **The animal produce**: Various dairy products like curd, whey, butter, ghee, honey and the famous combination *panchamrita* have been proved for their efficacy in neuropsychological disorders.

Generally the herbal and dairy products should be made fresh because they have limited shelf life. Now-a-days owing to advanced preservation and packaging techniques some of the above mentioned products with longer shelf life are also available in supermarkets. Most of the products are administered with either honey, milk or ghee. Various evidences for some of the herbs, minerals and elements are mentioned here (Table 13.3).

Table 13.3 List of Herbs with Specific Action on Aging and Cognition

Serial No.	Botanical Name	Sanskrit Name	Uses
1.	*Centella asiatica* Urbn.	*Mandookparni*	Utilized as a traditional herbal medicine in Malaysia and all other regions of Asia including India and China [23]. This plant functions as an herb, spice, vegetable, and juice as well as in nutraceutical and cosmetic products [24]. Used as a memory enhancer, brain tonic, useful in the treatment of mental disorders. Neuroprotective and brain growth promoter. Possess anti-aging, antioxidant and antidepressant activities. Showed significant increase in both general ability and behavioral pattern of mentally retarded children. Showed significant increase in the dendritic length (intersections) and dendritic branching points in rat brain [25].
2.	*Tinospora cordifolia* Willd-Mierss	*Guduchi*	Possess antioxidant activity, immunomodulatory effect, antidepressant property and enhance cognitive power [25].

(Continued)

Serial No.	Botanical Name	Sanskrit Name	Uses
3.	*Glycerrhiza glabra* Linn.	*Yashtimadhu*	Possess antioxidant property, anxiolytic effect memory enhancing activity [25].
4.	*Convolvulus pluricaulis Chois*	*Shankhapushpi*	Possess antioxidant activity, memory enhancer and anxiolytic effect [25].
	Evolvulus alsinoides Linn		It is a natural tranquilizer that promotes deep and revitalizing sleep. Recommended where the mind becomes overactive, agitated and restless. It is a rejuvenative herb with anti-aging properties. May also help in preventing changes in the neuron cell bodies in specific brain areas [26]. Alcohol extract of both the species showed nootropic activity in animal models [27].
5.	*Bacopa monniera* Linn.	*Brahmi*	It is a perennial, creeping herb found in warm wetlands and native to India and Australia and found growing in the United States and East Asia. Brahmi demonstrates massive potential in the amelioration of various neuropharmacological conditions, depressions, inflammation, and other disorders [28].
			Bacopa monnieri Linn is one among the most praised medhya rasayana drugs—class of herb taken to sharpen intellect and attenuate mental deficits. Brahmi is attributed with properties like lifespan and cognition enhancer, voice quality, luster and complexion promoter, antiaging. Clinically brahmi is known for safely enhancing the cognitive performance in elderly and in individuals with already high cognitive abilities [29].
			It provides neuroprotection against dementia, amnesia, memory dysfunction, Parkinson's disease (PD), Alzheimer's disease (AD), epileptic seizures and schizophrenia, It has sedative, anti-inflammatory, calcium antagonistic, anticonvulsant, anti-aging, cognitive enhancive activities [30].
6.	*Asparagus racemosus* Willd	*Shatawari*	Commonly seen in Asia and Africa, possess antidepressant, antiamnesic, antianxiety, hypolipidemic, antidiabetic, anticonvulsant, immunoadjuvant, and antioxidant effects [31].
7.	*Nordostachys Jatamansi, DC*	*Jatamansi*	Neuroprotective, antioxidant and stress relieving herb. Possess nootropic, antidepressant, anticonvulsant and cardioprotective activities [32].
8.	*Punica granatum* Linn.	*Dadimphala*	Possess antiatherogenic, antioxidant, anti-carcinogenic, anti-inflammatory, antidiabetic, gastroprotective, hepatoprotective and nephroprotective, anti-inflammatory activities [33].
9.	*Terminalia chebula* Retz.	*Haritaki*	Possess antibacterial, antifungal, antiviral, antidiabetic, antimutagenic, antioxidant, antiulcer and wound healing properties, cytoprotective and antiaging activities [34]. Have antioxidant, free radical scavenging, anticarcinogenic, antimutagenic, radioprotective and chemopreventive, hepatoprotective, cardioprotective, cytoprotective, antidiabetic and renoprotective, antifungal, antiviral, antiprotozoal, anti-inflammatory and anti-arthritic, anti-allergic, adaptogenic and antianaphylactic, hypolipidemic and hypocholesterolemic, gastrointestinal motility improving and anti-ulcerogenic, antispasmodic, anticaries, wound healing, and immunomodulatory activities. Possess purgative property [35].

(Continued)

Serial No.	Botanical Name	Sanskrit Name	Uses
10.	*Acorus calamus* Linn.	*Vacha*	Possess anticonvulsant, antidepressant, antihypertensive, anti-inflammatory, immunomodulatory, neuroprotective, cardioprotective and anti-obesity effects [36].
11.	*Piper longum*	*Pippali*	Possess anti-stress and nootropic activities [37]. Piperine, a main active alkaloid in fruit of *Piper nigrum* improves memory impairment and neurodegeneration in hippocampus [38] piperine possesses anti-depression like activity and cognitive enhancing effect [39].
12.	*Celastrus paniculatus* Wild	*Jyotishmati*	Jyotishmati sidhha ghrita found effective in performance intelligence quotient in school children [40]. Jyotishmati oil nasya along with brahmi ghrita is found effective in ameliorating the symptoms of cognitive deficit (Borderline mental retardation) in school children [41].
13.	*Allium sativum*	*Rasona*	Garlic extract showed decrease in body weight, visceral fat, plasma cholesterol, and MDA levels and improvement in cognitive function and brain mitochondrial function [42]. Garlic extract proved as a natural memory protectant and people taking garlic in their food as nutrient might slow the onset and/or progression neurodegenerative diseases [43].
14.	*Semecarpus anacardium*	*Bhallataka*	Possess anti-inflammatory, antioxidant activity, memory-enhancing effects [44]. Phytochemicals in bhallataka have proved to possess anti-inflammatory and neuroprotective therapeutics and the bioactive compounds in the nut showed positive changes at neuronal, behavioral and cellular level in treated animals [45].
15.	*Cuminum cyminum* Linn	*Jeeraka*	The cumin plant and its essential part is one of the most common aromatics in the Mediterranean kitchen. It is one of the popular spices regularly used as a flavoring agent. According to the nutritional profile, cumin had a carbohydrate, protein, fat and soluble dietary fibers along with vitamins such as thiamine, riboflavin and niacin. It is also a rich source of iron and minerals, having $Fe2+$ (6.0) and $Zn2+$ (6.5) (mg/100 g) that is useful to generate energy, immune systems and for skin disorders [46]. It's a proven anxiolytic spice [47].
16.	*Gmelina arborea* Roxb.	*Kashmari*	The whole plant is medicinally very important. It promotes digestive power, improves memory, overcomes giddiness, and acts as a rasayana (rejuvinetor), balya and brimhana (muscle strengthening & nourishment), hridya (cardiac tonic) [48].

13.7 Food articles: Soups, salads, *yavagu (base of Rice) and yusha (base of legumes)*

Centella is commonly eaten fresh as a vegetable in Malaysia and Indonesia region. The fresh plants are blended to make drink and juice. Cooked *Centella* is served as soup which act as an appetizer. The salads are eaten together with the main meal or as a main vegetable along with fresh coconut or sweet potato or potatoes. In Thailand, it is used as vegetable and tonic, drunk as a tea and juice. In India, it is one of the constituents of the Indian summer drinks *Thandayi* and praised as brain tonic. *Centella* products are available in many forms such as powder, infusion, soluble and extract of fresh and dried plants. By using response surface methodology (RSM) model, the formulation of the *Centella* herbal noodles was developed. The introduction of this product will enhance the multi-functional properties of *Centella* in food applications and an alternative consumption of natural products such as in cakes, ice-creams, desserts and puddings [24,49,50].

The soupy formulations termed as *yavagu* made with the base of rice and *yusha* made from *dal* are mixed with various medicinal herbs and served as meal portions after panchakarma procedure, and during recovery period of any disease like viral fevers, diarrhea, diabetes, polycystic ovarian disease, liver diseases and many more.

Rice cooked in *panchakol siddha jala* (*panchkol* comprising *Pippali* (*Piper longum*), *Pippalimula* (root of *Piper longum*), *Chavya* (*Piper chaba Hunter*), *Chitraka* (*Plumbago zelynica*) and *Nagara* (*Zingiber officinale*) in equal proportion processed in sixty four parts of water reduced to half) was administered to a group of patients of *agnimandya* (loss of appetite). At the end of the 7-day study, *Panchakola Siddha Yavagu* group shows highly significant results ($P < 0.001$) as against the control group who were having only cooked rice yavagu [51].

The *Panchmushtika yush* comprising barley, jujube, horse gram, green gram, and Indian gooseberry is prescribed in pittaj cough with malaise. *Kulathapancha yusha* made using horse gram, black gram, flat bean, green gram, and pigeon pea is prescribed as lubricative [52]. *Dadima-amalaka yusha* having pomegranate and Indian gooseberry as ingredients is part of daily diet for epilepsy and hallucinations [6]. However, these practices are yet to be studied and validated in scientific manner.

13.8 Extracts

Powdered garlic capsule (400 mg) was administered to 20 healthy volunteers for a period of 5 weeks to evaluate its effects on visual memory, verbal memory, attention and executive function. Statistically significant difference ($p < 0.05$) was found in several parameters of visual memory and attention due to Allium Sativum ingestion; however, there was no significant change on verbal memory and executive function [53].

Curcuma capsules or curcuma-piperine combination tablets or capsules in varying doses of 400–500 mg have been proved helpful in post-traumatic stress disorder (PTSD), obsessive-compulsive disorder (OCD), bipolar disorder, psychotic disorders, and autism in different clinical trials and also metanalysis of the trials [54,55].

Ginger has been studied in different trials for its neuroprotective effects in age-related degeneration and associated diseases [56].

13.9 *Ksheerpaka*: herbal milk/latte

Milk is universally accepted as a complete meal owing to its nutritive value. It is *tridoshshamak, saptadhatuvardhak, medhya* and *ojovardhak.*[2] It should be consumed every day by the person who desires longevity. Milk sourced from animals like goat, camel, sheep, and horse is used for various purposes, yet cow milk is the most praised and utilized variety due to its qualitative superiority. Cow milk has *madhur rasa* (sweet taste), *madhur vipaka* (post-digestive effect), shita veerya (cold potency), snigdha ([3]~creamy/oily) guna, sara (~attribute contributing to the effective elimination of bodily wastes), jiivaniya (~revitalization), rasaayana (rejuvenation), medhya (~enhancing the intellect), balya (~imparting physical strength), and stanyakara (~galactogouge) functions. The attributes of cow milk render it as a best medium for herbal extraction. The powders or fresh pastes of the drug/s, milk and water are mixed in the proportion of 1:8:32. The mixture is then boiled until water evaporates. It is then strained, and medicated *ksheerpaka* is collected. The famous golden milk or turmeric latte is made in this way. Saffron milk, Ashwagandha and Shatavari milk are also available as health drinks.

The nuts of *S. anacardium*, Linn. extracted with milk when tested for its locomotor and nootropic activities using animals showed positive results [57,58]. A case study by Akhila M suggests that menopausal syndrome can be successfully managed through Ayurvedic treatment of *basti* (medicated enema) of *ksheerapaka* formulation along with oral medication for 8 days. A case report by Suprabha K indicates that in conditions of IUGR, administration of *Shatavaryadi Ksheerapaka Basti* proves beneficial for fetal growth and maternal wellbeing. In geriatric age group, *ksheerapaka* of drugs of *jeevaniya gana* or *medhya* like *shatavari, yashti, shankhapushpi, brahmi* may prove a good nutraceutical source for maintenance cognitive function.

13.10 Siddha ghrita

The well-known desi cow ghee of India is not only a fatty substance, but it is a powerhouse of complete nutrition. The Components, flavour compounds, different types of manufacturing methods of ghee including the desi (boiling of milk -fermentation using culture - separation of butter- heating of butter to make ghee), effect of heat, keeping quality, etc. are explicitly discussed in many research papers. Comparison of compounds of cow ghee and buffalo, goat and camel ghee is also made [59].

Ghrita or ghee enhances *smriti, buddhi, agni, shukra, oja, kapha,* and *meda* and pacifies aggravated *vata, pitta, visha,* and useful in *unmad, shosha,* and *jwara.* The specific function or unique attribute of Ghrita called *Sanskarasyanuvartana*

---

[2] *Oja/ojas*: It is the vitality or vigor or life force of each individual perceived by self and others. The energy of a person is expressed as *Oja.*

[3] The sign "~" indicates congruent/equivalent term but not exact translation.

is highlighted in Ayurveda. Due to it, ghee imbibes and enhances the properties of herbs or minerals which are processed with it, without losing its own qualities. This group of products is termed as *siddha ghrita* (medicated ghee formulations). Also it is stable on shelf for about 2 years unlike herbal powders. That is why it serves as a base for herbals having short shelf life. Nutritionally, ghee works best for *pitta dosha*-predominant individuals, and ghee formulations are prescribed to treat diseases of pitta-vata vitiation. Siddha ghrita is prepared using paste of herbs (sometimes minerals are also added), ghee and liquids like water, decoction, juice, milk, urine, etc. with a general ratio of 1:4:16. The mixture is heated on a constant low flame till achievement of the testing criteria. Many studies have reported the efficacy of siddha ghrita for various conditions.

Administration of *Jyotishmati Ghrita* to school going children for a period of 3 months at a dose of 10 mL/day showed improvement in Backward Digit Span Test [40].

Oral administration of Brahmi Ghrita in a dose of 10 g twice daily along with nasal drops of *Jyotishmati Tail* in the dose of two drops in each nostril twice daily for 12 weeks were found effective in alleviating the symptoms of cognitive deficit (Borderline Mental Retardation) with no adverse effects [41].

Hingwadi Ghrita is a well-studied medicated ghee. The ingredients of Hingwadi Ghrita are *Hingu, Sunthi, Maricha, Pippali, Souvarchal lavan*, cow urine (gomutra) and cow ghee. The herbal drugs are predominant in kaṭu rasa (pungent taste) and uṣṇa vīrya (hot potency). Ghrita and lavan opens the channels and hydrate the tissues. The formulation pacifies vāta and kapha doṣa, clears obstructions in srotas (channels), and sharpen senses. Ghee enhances memory, *Hiṅgu* is a stimulant and anticonvulsant, *Śuṇṭhi* is an antidepressant, *Mārīca* is sedative and anti-convulsant and *Pippalī* is a CNS stimulant. *Sauvarcala lavaṇa* and *Gomūtra* have physiological roles. The sodium ions present in *Sauvarcala lavaṇa* are most required for initializing nerve cell activity by generation of action potential. Influx of sodium ions generates electric charges and triggers excitatory neurotransmitters. This stimulation is crucial to start the thought process [60].

Vachadi Ghrita (VG) is another formulation studied for anxiety and depression. It comprises *Vacha (Acorus calamus), Guduchi (Tinospora cordifolia), Shathi (Hedychium spicatum), Haritaki (Terminalia chebula), Shankhapushpi (Convolvulius pluricaulis), Vidanga (Embelia ribes), Shunti (Zingiber officinale), Apamarga (Achyranthes aspera)* and *Go-ghrita* (cow ghee). The antidepressant, antipsychotic, anti-stress antioxidant, memory enhancer, and anticonvulsant activities of the ingredients are reported. Nootropic and antipsychotic activities of VG are also proven in Morris water maze ($p \leq 0.001$) and 5 HTP-induced head twitches ($p \leq 0.001$) mice models, respectively [61].

Panchagavya Ghrita (PGG) contains five cow products: cow ghee, cow milk, cow urine, cow dung juice and cow curd. Nootropic activity of PGG at 5 and 3.5 g/kg is determined in Diazepam-induced amnesia and Morris water maze models, respectively [62].

A formulation titled Brahmi ghrita from Charaksamhita is also studied for analytical profile and scopolamine-induced amnesia in a dose of 400 and 800 mg/kg, p.o. in Charles Foster rats using elevated plus maze, passive avoidance, and active avoidance tests and compared with standard drug Piracetam where Brahmi Ghrita proved to be equally effective [63,64].

Open-label nonrandomized exploratory clinical studies on *Vachadi*, *Hingwadi*, *Panchagavya* and *Brahmyadi ghrita* ($p < 0.005$) used as an adjuvant in patients of mild to moderate depression showed statistically significant reduction in HAMD scores ($p < 0.05$) displaying their therapeutic potential for the same in a dose of 10 g/ twice a day for 60 days duration. All the drugs showed beneficial effects on patients' appetite and bowel clearance. *Panchagavya* ghrita showed beneficial effects on insomnia as well [65–69].

Brahmyadi Ghrita comprising *Brahmi*, *Siddharthak* (*Brassica juncea* Linn.), *Vacha*, *Sariva*, *Kushtha*, *Pippali* and *Saindhav* processed in cow ghee is advised especially for various CNS conditions of children in the text *Ashtanghridayam*. This formulation and Vachadi ghrita (10 g/day; 30 days) proved effective in improving the learning and memory ability of school children [70].

In a nonrandomized positive-controlled clinical trial, *Vachadi* and *Brahmyadi ghrita* (10 g twice daily; 30 days) showed a statistically significant improvement in PGI memory scores of healthy individuals in 40–50 years age group [71].

Medhyarasayana ghrita (10 g twice daily; 90 days) along with Vachadi ghrita nasya (2 drops/nostril twice a day; 90 days) proved efficacious in senile dementia gauged using batteries like Hamilton Anxiety Rating Scale, Hamilton Depression Rating Scale, and Brief Psychiatry Rating Scale [72].

The medicated ghee formulations can be prescribed to elderly population in the dose of 5/10 g (1–2 teaspoons) to improve or maintain learning, memory and general cognition. The challenge of palatability for a few individuals may be overcome by developing soft-gel capsules.

13.11 Herbo-minerals drugs

Ayurveda uses a lot of mineral and metal substances after specific processes known as *shodhan* and *maran*. The processes are carried out using various herbs like Aloe, Curcuma, Amalaki, *Triphala* and animal products such as cow urine, cow milk, etc. The most widely used supplements from this group are Shilajit, *loha bhasma* (herbomineral iron) *kukkutandtwak bhasma* (hen eggshell), and *Calcipral* (proprietary calcium supplement consisting of various seashells). Many brands containing these are available as nutraceuticals.

Shilajit is a natural product comprising humic and fulvic acids along with 84 elements in trace amounts. It has been studied for processing, and its use in India and Nepal is protected by 5 and 6 patents, respectively [73]. Its protective and precognition activities in neurodegenerative disorders like Alzheimer's, osteoporosis, impaired cognition, etc. associated with aging have been explored [74–76].

Though iron, calcium and zinc are known to facilitate cognitive function by various mechanisms, there is no direct reference of such experimental or clinical studies on Ayurvedic bhasmas. Suvarna bhasma has been very well studied to be effective for cognition, stress management, and mental vigor [77,78]. Some mercurial and arsenical formulations like *Unmadgajkesari* have been proved to show antiepileptic and antipsychotic effects; however, they cannot be used as nutraceuticals [79,80]. They are prescription medicines only.

13.12 Challenges and future scope

Identification of the *manasprakriti* psychological constitution of an individual is equally important yet grossly overlooked area of research. Comprehensive mapping of physical and mental constitution of a person will give a better idea regarding personalized foods and daily regime including the best suitable work pattern for that person. For example, the ability of performing higher intellectual functions of *vanaspatya* subtype of *Tamas* prakriti group is comparatively low, and they lack self-motivation. It is likely that these individuals may suffer from dementia earlier than other constitution types. Some of the above-mentioned measures may delay the onset of dementia.

A variety of beverages can be infused with nootropic herbs after trials in human participants.

Palatability of ghee formulation is a big challenge. Dosage form development like nano ghee capsules based on its clinically effective dose is another area for research. Ghee is a very Indian-Asian product, and its availability in other parts of the world is very limited and export-dependent. It is a potential nutraceutical product for global market. New aspects will provide useful leads for research in cognitive nutrition.

13.13 Summary

Nutrition is the basis for healthy aging and active senses. Incorporation of some herbs and minerals in daily diets may take care of cognitive impairments associated with healthy aging.

The theories of aging and associated neuropsychological milestones from Ayurveda provide a structure to understand the time points of nutritional interventions for optimum cognition.

The plants acting on aging and cognition both can be incorporated in the diet, in various suitable forms. *Pippali*, *Kashmari fruit*, *Vacha*, *Bhallataka* and

Guduchi can be used to make flavored latte. Similar to black pepper, long pepper powder can be used as a seasoning for *yusha*, soups, pasta, etc. *Chutny/dips/spreads* of *fresh Brahmi, Mandukparni, Shankhapushpi*, and *Rasona* would make interesting accompaniment of various breads. Pomegranate should be used as fresh fruit or juice or its dry powder can be added in cordials like lemonade that is made from Dates. *Shatawari* roots can be processed into multiple food articles like soups, *ksheerapaka*, medicated ghee, nutri-bar, and some more; *Jyotishmati, Bhallataka*, and *Pippali* in the form of medicated ghee and *Jatamansi* in the form of cold or hot infusion or tea. *Haritaki* can also be infused in the form of dry powder with different savory dishes.

Herbs acting on cognition can be categorized into two classes based on two types of activities. The first group consists of *Haritaki, Vacha, Shankhapushpi, Pippali, Jeeraka, Jyotishmati, Rasona, Bhallataka, Kashmari, Vishnukranta*, etc. with predominant *kaṭu rasa, katu vipaka* and *uṣṇa vīrya*. These herbs pacify *vāta* and *kapha doṣhas*; clear obstructions within the *srotas* (channels) facilitate nutrient transport to the brain and also alert or sharpen the senses. The second group of herbs consisting of *Brahmi, Yashtimadhu, Shatawari, Dadimphala*, and *Jatamansi* having predominant *sheeta virya* nourish the brain and act as immunomodulators.

Minerals like rock salt and elements like iron, calcium, zinc and gold when treated with herbs are biologically active inorganics which are essential to carry out many physiological functions. Bhasmas/bio-inorganic supplements from Ayurveda may open up a new dimension of neuropsychiatric applications. Some of them can be fortified into ready-to-cook foods for increasing nutritive value and support cognitive health of aging population.

Well-planned prospective clinical and experimental studies on different Ayurvedic nutraceuticals, *yavgu, yusha*, milk and ghee covered in this chapter would certainly bring conclusive evidence regarding the age-related cognitive disorders.

References

1. Devi D, Srivastava R, Dwivedi B. A critical review of concept of aging in Ayurveda. *AYU (An Int Q J Res Ayurveda)* 2010;31:516. doi:10.4103/0974-8520.82030.
2. Rajoriya R, Nathani S. Importance of vayasthapana-mahakashaya drugs WSR to its potential uses in geriatric care. n.d.
3. Ray S. Medhya rasayanas in brain function and disease. *Med Chem (Los Angeles)* 2015;5. doi:10.4172/2161-0444.1000309.
4. Dhanwate A. Brainstem death: A comprehensive review in Indian perspective. *Indian J Crit Care Med* 2014;18:596–605. doi:10.4103/0972-5229.140151.
5. Nille G. Introduction to sudha varga (pharmaceutico-therapeutic approach), 2020.
6. Sharma, RK, Dash B. Charaka samhita-text with English translation and critical exposition based on Chakrapani Datta's Ayurveda dipika. Chaukhambha Orientalia, Varanasi; 2003.
7. Purvya M, Meena M. A review on role of prakriti in aging. *AYU (An Int Q J Res Ayurveda)* 2011;32:20. doi:10.4103/0974-8520.85719.

8. Rao PS. Ashtang Samgraha vol. 1 and 2. Varanasi: Choukhamba Krishnadas Academy, Varanasi, India; 2005.

9. Koppikar S. Garbhini Paricharya (Regimen for the pregnant woman) n.d.:37–9.

10. Rasane S, Bhangale K. Garbhini Paricharya according to various Samhita. *MedPulse Int J Ayurveda* 2016;10:5–8.

11. Khare CP, Katiyar CK. *The Modern Ayurveda: Milestones Beyond the Classical Age.* Taylor & Francis, Boca Raton, Florida; 2012.

12. Joshi KS. Docosahexaenoic acid content is significantly higher in ghrita prepared by traditional Ayurvedic method. *J Ayurveda Integr Med* 2014;5:85–8. doi:10.4103/0975-9476.131730.

13. Mijanur Rahman M, Gan SH, Khalil MI. Neurological Effects of Honey: Current and Future Prospects. *Evidence-Based Complement Altern Med* 2014;2014:1–13. doi:10.1155/2014/958721.

14. Anand S, Deighton M, Livanos G, Pang ECK, Mantri N. Agastache honey has superior antifungal activity in comparison with important commercial honeys. *Sci Rep* 2019;9:18197. doi:10.1038/s41598-019-54679–w.

15. Anand S, Deighton M, Livanos G, Morrison PD, Pang ECK, Mantri N. Antimicrobial activity of agastache honey and characterization of its bioactive compounds in comparison with important commercial honeys. *Front Microbiol* 2019;10:263.

16. Anand S, Pang E, Livanos G, Mantri N. Characterization of physico-chemical properties and antioxidant capacities of bioactive honey produced from australian grown agastache rugosa and its correlation with colour and poly-phenol content. *Mol* 2018;23. doi:10.3390/molecules23010108.

17. Adan RAH, van der Beek EM, Buitelaar JK, Cryan JF, Hebebrand J, Higgs S, et al. Nutritional psychiatry: Towards improving mental health by what you eat. *Eur Neuropsychopharmacol* 2019;29:1321–32. doi:10.1016/j.euroneuro.2019.10.011.

18. Payyappallimana U, Venkatasubramanian P. Exploring ayurvedic knowledge on food and health for providing innovative solutions to contemporary healthcare. *Front Public Heal* 2016;4. doi:10.3389/fpubh.2016.00057.

19. Pandey MM, Rastogi S, Rawat AKS. Indian traditional ayurvedic system of medicine and nutritional supplementation. *Evidence-Based Complement Altern Med* 2013;2013:1–12. doi:10.1155/2013/376327.

20. Vidyasagar PS, editor. *Sharangadhar Samhita with Adhamalla's Dipika and Kashirama's Gudhartha-Dipika Commentary.* Edition 4. Varanasi: Chaukhambha Orientalia, Varanasi; 2000.

21. Kumar S, Dobos GJ, Rampp T. The significance of ayurvedic medicinal plants. *J Evid Based Complementary Altern Med* 2017;22:494–501. doi:10.1177/2156587216671392.

22. Srivastava KC, Mustafa T. Pharmacological effects of spices: Eicosanoid modulating activities and their significance in human health. *Biomed Rev* 1993;2:15. doi:10.14748/bmr.v2.208.

23. Centella asiatica: from folk remedy to the medicinal biotechnology – A state revision. *Int J Biosci* 2013;3:49–67. doi:10.12692/ijb/3.6.49-67.

24. Puttarak P, Dilokthornsakul P, Saokaew S, Dhippayom T, Kongkaew C, Sruamsiri R, et al. Effects of Centella asiatica (L.) Urb. on cognitive function and mood related outcomes: A systematic review and meta-analysis. *Sci Rep* 2017;7. doi:10.1038/s41598-017-09823-9.

25. Kilmer PD. Review article: Review article. *J Theory Pract Crit* 2010;11:369–73. doi:10.1177/1461444810365020.

26. Alam Khan Q, Ali Khan A, Jabeen A, Ansari S. Sankhaholi evolvulus alsinoides linn: A review. *Innov J Health Sci* 2016;4:1–3.

27. Kothiyal P, Rawat MSM. Comparative nootropic effect of evolvulus alsinoides and convolvulus pluricaulis. *Int J Pharma Bio Sci* 2011;2:616–21.

28. Rai K, Gupta N, Dharamdasani L, Nair P, Bodhankar P. Bacopa monnieri: A wonder drug changing fortune of people. *Int J Appl Sci Biotechnol* 2017;5:127. doi:10.3126/ijasbt.v5i2.16952.

29. Gadgil SS, Wele AA, Sharma VR PM. Comparative efficacy of Ekapākī (1x) and Daśapākī (10x) Brāhmī ghṛta in chronic unpredictable mild stress induced behavioral alterations in rats. *Anc Sci Life* 2018;37:141–7.

30. Sukumaran NP, Amalraj A, Gopi S. Complementary therapies in medicine neuropharmacological and cognitive e ff ects of Bacopa monnieri (L.) Wettst – A review on its mechanistic aspects. *Comple Ther Med* 2019;44:68–82. doi:10.1016/j.ctim.2019.03.016.

31. Sciences M. A comprehensive review of the pharmacological actions of asparagus racemosus. *Am J Pharmatech Res* 2017;7:1–20.

32. Sahu R, Dhongade HJ, Pandey A, Sahu P, Sahu V, Patel D, et al. Medicinal properties of nardostachys jatamansi (A review). *Orient J Chem* 2016;32:859–66. doi:10.13005/ojc/320211.

33. Sharma R, Garg N, Verma D, Rathi P, Sharma V, Kuca K, Prajapati P. K. Indian medicinal plants as drug leads in neurodegenerative disorders. In: *Nutraceuticals in Brain Health and Beyond*, Elsevier, 2021, pp. 31–45.

34. Gupta PC. Biological and pharmacological properties of Terminalia chebula Retz. (haritaki)- an overview. *Int J Pharm Pharm Sci* 2012;4:62–8.

35. Meher SK, Panda P, Das B, Bhuyan GC, Rath KK. Pharmacological Profile of Terminalia chebula Retz. and Willd. (Haritaki) in Ayurveda with Evidences. *Res J Pharmacol Pharmacodyn* 2018;10:115. doi:10.5958/2321-5836.2018.00023.x.

36. Rajput SB, Tonge MB, Karuppayil SM. An overview on traditional uses and pharmacological profile of Acorus calamus Linn. (Sweet flag) and other Acorus species. *Phytomedicine* 2014;21:268–76. doi:10.1016/j.phymed.2013.09.020.

37. Kilari EK, Sudeepthi L, Rao N, Sreemanthula S, Kola PK. Anti-stress and nootropic activity of aqueous extract of Piper longum fruit, estimated by noninvasive biomarkers and Y-maze test in rodents. *Environ Exp Biol* 2015;13:25–31.

38. Chonpathompikunlert P, Wattanathorn J, Muchimapura S. Piperine, the main alkaloid of Thai black pepper, protects against neurodegeneration and cognitive impairment in animal model of cognitive deficit like condition of Alzheimer's disease. *Food Chem Toxicol* 2010;48:798–802. doi:10.1016/j.fct.2009.12.009.

39. Wattanathorn J, Chonpathompikunlert P, Muchimapura S, Priprem A, Tankamnerdthai O. Piperine, the potential functional food for mood and cognitive disorders. *Food Chem Toxicol* 2008;46:3106–10. doi:10.1016/j.fct.2008.06.014.

40. Dhodapkar S, Kale A, Swami T, Rana A. Efficacy of Jyotishmati Siddha Ghrita on Intelligence Quotient and Memory of School going children. *J Res Tradit Med* 2018;4:97. doi:10.5455/jrtm.2018/6777.

41. Kute A, Ojha N, Abhimanyu K. A study on improvement of IQ level in borderline mentally retarded children by. *Int J Ayurveda* 2017;5:1–9.

42. Development of a guided inquiry-based e-module on respiratory system content based on research results of the potential single garlic extract (allium sativum) to improve student creative thinking skills and cognitive learning outcome. *J Pendidik Sains Indones (Indonesian J Sci Educ)* 2020;8:228–40. doi:10.24815/jpsi. v8i2.17065.

43. Tasnim S, Haque PS, Bari MS, Hossain MM, Islam SMA, Shahriar M, et al. Allium sativum L. improves visual memory and attention in healthy human volunteers. *Evidence-Based Complement Altern Med* 2015;2015. doi:10.1155/2015/103416.

44. Farooq SM, Alla TR, Venkat Rao N, Prasad K, Shalam, Nandakumar K, et al. A study on CNS effects of milk extract of nuts of Semecarpus anacardium. Linn, (Anacardiaceae). *Pharmacologyonline* 2007;1:49–63. https://manipal.pure.elsevier. com/en/publications/a-study-on-cns-effects-of-milk-extract-of-nuts-of-semecarpus-anac (accessed March 21, 2021).

45. Sawale S., Pandey S. A short overview of 'Marking nut' – Semecarpus anacardium linn. *GPG J Sci Educ* 2020;1: 35–45.

46. Gangadharappa H V., Mruthunjaya K, Singh RP. Cuminum cyminum – A popular spice: An updated review. *Pharmacogn J* 2017;9:292–301. doi:10.5530/pj.2017.3.51.

47. Harpreet K, Rajmeet S, Sumeet G, Jaswinder K, Jasvir K. Anxiolytic activity of ethanolic extract of seeds of cuminum cyminum linn in albino wistar rats. *Available Online WwwIjtprCom Int J Toxicol Pharmacol Res* 2016;8.

48. Karalam SB, Pillai NS. International journal of ayurveda and pharma research a critical review on Avaleha Kalpana. *Int J Ayur Pharma Res* 2017;5:12.

49. Tsoukalas D, Fragkiadaki P, Docea AO, Alegakis AK, Sarandi E, Thanasoula M, et al. Discovery of potent telomerase activators: Unfolding new therapeutic and anti-aging perspectives. *Mol Med Rep* 2019;20:3701–8. doi:10.3892/mmr.2019.10614.

50. Hashim P. MiniReview Centella asiatica in food and beverage applications and its potential antioxidant and neuroprotective effect. vol. 18. 2011.

51. More S, Dwivedi R. A clinical study of Panchakola Siddha Yavagu in the management of Agnimandya. *AYU (An Int Q J Res Ayurveda)* 2011;32:70. doi:10.4103/0974–8520.85733.

52. Sharma PV. *Kaiyadeva Nighantu*. Varanasi,UP: Chaukambha Orientalia; 2013.

53. Tasnim S, Haque PS, Bari MS, Hossain MM, Islam SMA, Shahriar M, et al. Allium sativum L. improves visual memory and attention in healthy human volunteers. *Evidence-Based Complement Altern Med* 2015;2015. doi:10.1155/2015/103416.

54. Lopresti AL. Curcumin for neuropsychiatric disorders: A review of in vitro, animal and human studies. *J Psychopharmacol* 2017;31:287–302. doi:10.1177/0269881116686883.

55. Al-Karawi D, Al Mamoori DA, Tayyar Y. The role of curcumin administration in patients with major depressive disorder: Mini meta-analysis of clinical trials. *Phyther Res* 2016;30:175–83. doi:10.1002/ptr.5524.

56. Mohd Sahardi NFN, Makpol S. Ginger (Zingiber officinale Roscoe) in the prevention of ageing and degenerative diseases: Review of current evidence. *Evidence-Based Complement Altern Med* 2019;2019:1–13. doi:10.1155/2019/5054395.

57. Farooq, SM, Alla T, Rao V, N P, K S, Nandakumar K, et al. A study on CNS effects of milk extract of nuts of Semecarpus anacardium. Linn, (Anacardiaceae). *Pharmacologyonline* 2007;1:49–63.

58. Joseph JP, Raval SK, Sadariya KA, Jhala M, Kumar P. Anti cancerous efficacy of Ayurvedic milk extract of Semecarpus anacardium nuts on hepatocellular carcinoma in Wistar rats. *African J Tradit Complement Altern Med AJTCAM* 2013;10:299–304.

59. Sserunjogi ML, Abrahamsen RK, Narvhus J. A review paper: Current knowledge of ghee and related products. *Int Dairy J* 1998;8:677–88. doi:10.1016/S0958-6946(98)00106-X.

60. Gupte PA, Dawane J, Wele AA. Experimental evaluation of Hiṅgvādi Ghṛta in behavioral despair using animal models. *Anc Sci Life* 2016;36:84.

61. Pawar Madhuri S, Kunal G, Yogita K, Asmita W. Assessment of nootropic activity of Vachadi Ghrita, a medicated ghee formulation using animal models. 2015.

62. Pandey A, Pawar MS. Assessment of nootropic activity of Panchagavya Ghrita in animal models. *Nternational J Sci Res Publ* 2015;5:1–5.

63. Agarwal A, Yadav K, Reddy KC. Preliminary physico-chemical profile of Brahmi Ghrita. *AYU (An Int Q J Res Ayurveda)* 2013;34:294. doi:10.4103/0974-8520.123130.

64. Reddy KRC, Kumar V, Yadav K. Study of Brāhmī Ghṛta and piracetam in amnesia. *Anc Sci Life* 2012;32:11. doi:10.4103/0257-7941.113791.

65. Madhuri P, Asmita W. Comparative assessment of therapeutic potential of Vachadi and hingwadi ghrita in patients of mild to moderate depression. *Asian J Pharm Clin Res* 2017;10:59–62. doi:10.22159/ajpcr.2017.v10i12.20263.

66. Viraj Shreekant B, Swati G, Vidyapeeth B. Evaluation of antidepressant potential of an ayurvedic formulation panchgavya ghrita as an adjuvant in patients of depression. 2017.

67. Rashmi K, Madhuri P. Evaluation of therapeutic effect of vachadi ghrita in patients of mild to moderate depression. *Int J Res Ayurveda Pharm* n.d.;8:2017. doi:10.7897/2277-4343.083185.

68. Pawar M, Magdum P. Clinical study of assessment of therapeutic potential of Vachadi Ghrita, a medicated ghee formulation on healthy individual's cognition. *Int J Pharm Sci Res* 2018;9:3408. doi:10.13040/IJPSR.0975-8232.9(8).3408-13.

69. Pusadkar S, Rathi B, Topare S. Medhya activity of brahmyadi ghrita. *Res Artcile* 2020;9:2–17. doi:10.20959/wjpps20205-16062.
70. Patki P., A clinical study of the effect of vachadi ghrita on memory in healthy subjects, M.D. Dissertation of Dept. of RSBK, Bharati Vidyapeeth DU, Pune, 2016.
71. Rasal S., A clinical study to evaluate memory enhancing effect of brahmyadi ghrita in healthy individuals, M.D. dissertation of Dept. of RSBK, Bharati Vidyapeeth DU, Pune, 2016.
72. Mudiyanselage S, Samarakoon S, Chandola H. Clinical evaluation of Medhyarasayana Ghrita along with Vachadi Ghrita Nasya (Pratimarsha) on Senile Dementia. vol. 3. n.d.
73. Mishra T, Sircar D, Dhaliwal HS, Singh N. Spectroscopic and chromatographic characterization of crude natural shilajit from Himachal Pradesh, India. *Nat Prod J* 2020;10:244–56. doi:10.2174/2210315509666190112111808.
74. Carrasco-Gallardo C, Guzmán L, MacCioni RB. Shilajit: A natural phytocomplex with potential procognitive activity. *Int J Alzheimers Dis* 2012;2012. doi:10.1155/2012/674142.
75. Das A, S. El Masry M, Gnyawali SC, Ghatak S, Singh K, Stewart R, et al. Skin transcriptome of middle-aged women supplemented with natural herbo-mineral shilajit shows induction of microvascular and extracellular matrix mechanisms. *J Am Coll Nutr* 2019;38:526–36. doi:10.1080/07315724.2018.1564088.
76. Carrasco-Gallardo C, Farías GA, Fuentes P, Crespo F, Maccioni RB. Can nutraceuticals prevent Alzheimer's disease? Potential therapeutic role of a formulation containing shilajit and complex B vitamins. *Arch Med Res* 2012;43:699–704. doi:10.1016/j.arcmed.2012.10.010.
77. Shah ZA, Gilani RA, Sharma P, Vohora SB. Attenuation of stress-elicited brain catecholamines, serotonin and plasma corticosterone levels by calcined gold preparations used in Indian system of medicine. *Basic Clin Pharmacol Toxicol* 2005;96:469–74. doi:10.1111/j.1742-7843.2005.pto_10.x.
78. Shah ZAZA, Vohora SBSB. Antioxidant/restorative effects of calcined gold preparations used in Indian systems of medicine against global and focal models of ischaemia. *Pharmacol Toxicol* 2002;90:254–9. doi:10.1034/j.1600-0773.2002.900505.x.
79. Joseph R. Evaluation of multitargeted antipsychotic activity of unmadgajakesari – A herbomineral formulation – An animal experimental study. 2019;10:2852–60. doi:10.13040/IJPSR.0975-8232.10(6).2852-60.
80. Joseph R, Pandit V, Wele A, Deshmane G. Antiepileptic activity of unmadgajakesari – A herbomineral formulation: An experimental evaluation. *Int J Phytomedicine* 2015;7:106–11.

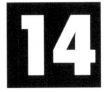

Epigenetics and Aging

Kavita Trimal and Siddhesh Solanke
Department of Technology, Savitribai Phule Pune University

Kalpana Joshi
Department of Biotechnology, Sinhgad College of Engineering,
Affiliated to Savitribai Phule Pune University

Contents

DOI: 10.1201/9781003110866-14

14.1 Introduction

Aging is a complex and irreversible biological process characterized by the time-dependent functional decline of many physiological processes that result in deterioration of vital body functions such as regeneration and capacity of reproduction [1,2]. Aging is associated with increased susceptibility to many chronic diseases such as cancer, cardiovascular disorders, and metabolic disorders, like diabetes and neurodegenerative diseases [3–5], ultimately leading to mortality risk [6]. Aging population and associated morbidity and mortality risk have emerged as a major public health burden in India [7,8]. The process of aging results from complex interaction of genetic, epigenetic, environmental, and stochastic factors during development, growth, maturity, and older stages [9]. In 2013, López-Otín, C. and co-workers attempted to identify and categorize the cellular and molecular hallmarks of aging [2]. Among them, epigenetic alteration plays a crucial role in determining physiological changes associated with the progression of aging and age-related diseases.

Epigenetics is the study of heritable changes in gene expression and function without sequence variation in the DNA [10]. Epigenetics mainly involves mechanisms like DNA methylation, histone modification, and noncoding RNAs which regulate many cellular and nuclear processes. Dysregulation of these epigenetic patterns affects gene expression and silencing, replication, recombination and repair of DNA, progression of cell cycle and structure and function of telomere and centromere [11]. Several human and animal studies provided strong evidence of trans-generational inheritance that suggests that certain types of epigenetic alteration can produce stable epigenetic effect that can be transmitted from parents to offspring [12]; however, they can also change dynamically throughout life time in response to nutritional or environmental stimuli [13–15]. Epigenetics is a link between genotype and phenotype; change in phenotype is a cause of post-translational modification or histone modifications in genome without altering genome sequence [16]. The reversible nature of epigenetic alterations provides promising future for development of therapeutic intervention strategies to delay aging and age-related diseases.

Epigenetic alterations caused during the aging process can be controlled by caloric restrictions and nutraceutical. Caloric restriction (CR) involves the reduction of total caloric intake by 20%–40% without malnutrition. CR is the most studied and effective intervention for extending lifespan in animal models by modulating nutrient signaling pathways including insulin/IGF1-like signaling, mTOR and sirtuin activity [17–23]. Even though caloric restriction plays a pivotal role in aging, a variety of nutraceutical can mimic the same effect and further reduce the risk associated with caloric and dietary restriction side effects. Anti-aging properties of nutraceutical can provide healthy and slow aging. Nutraceuticals include bioactive compounds derived from food or herbal products and microorganisms. Numerous pieces of evidence have reported that the natural compounds such as polyphenols, flavonoids, stillbenoids, isoflavonoids, isothyocyanates, and short-chain fatty acids play a crucial role to achieve control against epigenetic alterations involved in aging and related diseases [24–28].

The purpose of this chapter is to highlight the involvement of epigenetic modifications in progression of aging and age-related diseases and necessity of development of nutraceutical intervention strategies intended to reverse epigenetic alterations accompanying aging and provide insights into advances being made with respect to nutraceutical interventions, which will help in delaying of aging and prevention of age-related disease.

14.2 The role of epigenetics in aging

The term epigenetics was first introduced in 1942 by C. H. Waddington. Epigenetics is the study of all mitotically and in certain cases meiotically heritable changes in gene expression without affecting the primary DNA sequence [29]. These modifications collectively form the epigenome, which mainly includes DNA methylation, histone modification and noncoding RNAs. Dysregulation of theses heritable epigenetic remarks results in decline in molecular and cellular functions and cause of diseases.

Since the late 1980s, epigenetic alterations are connected with aging [30]. Epigenetics has the potential to explain many features of aging and numerous reports have demonstrated epigenetic alterations as a major contributor of aging phenotype [31,32]. Aging is associated with lifestyle factors (For example: diet, obesity, smoking and stress) and epigenetic alterations that can be modified by nutrition, lifestyle, and environmental stimuli [33]. López-Otín, C. and co-workers have identified and categorized major hallmarks of aging, which involves genomic instability, telomere attritions, epigenetic alterations, loss of proteolysis, deregulated nutrient sensing, mitochondrial dysfunction, cellular senescence, stem cell exhaustion, and altered intercellular communication [2]. This classification highlights the crucial role of epigenetic alterations in determining physiological changes associated with the progression of aging. The reversible character of epigenetics provides opportunity for development of effective intervention strategies targeting epigenetic alteration underlying during progression of aging which will promote anti-aging or slow aging effect.

14.2.1 DNA methylation in aging

DNA modification is one of the most important and extensively studied epigenetic modifications. The most commonly studied DNA modifications are methylation and hydroxymethylation of cytosine bases. DNA methylation plays a crucial role in expression and imprinting of genes, inhibitions of recombination, defense against viral sequences and assembly of heterochromatin structure [34]. DNA methylation is a covalent and post-replicative phenomenon which consists of the addition of methyl group at the 5-carbon cytosine (5 mC). The enzymes responsible for transfer of methyl group from donor S-adenosylmethionine (SAM) to cytosine base are called DNA methyltransferases (DNMTs). In mammals, three active DNMTs have been identified: DNMT1, DNMT3A, and DNMT3B [35,36]. DNMT1 is responsible for maintaining methylation patterns during cell division. DNMT3A and DNMT3B are responsible for *de novo* DNA methylation during development. Decreased expression of DNMT genes is associated with aging [37].

DNA methylations play very important roles in regulation of gene transcription mechanism and show dynamic reprograming with age [38,39]. Several lines of evidence indicated that a global hypomethylation at the repetitive regions of genome and site specific hypermethylation of certain gene promoters are associated with aging [40,41].

Interestingly, DNA methylation patterns are found to be gene and tissue specific [42,43]. They are mainly important during developmental stage, during various stages of development it shows dynamic reprograming to ensure normal cell differentiations and embryogenesis. Different lines of evidence have shown that a gradual loss of methylated cytosine with aging occurs in lots of vertebrate tissues including humans [44]. Similarly, some recent studies have highlighted the distinctive role of DNA methylation in aging [45,46]. In addition to its effects on the aging process, DNA methylations can also predict aging status by acting as a biomarker of aging and enable accurate age estimation for any tissue across the lifespan [47]. Correlation of DNA methylation change with age is explained by two phenomena, epigenetic clock, and epigenetic drift. Epigenetic clock refers to a specific site in the genome showing DNA methylation changes with age that are common across individuals, whereas epigenetic drift is defined as DNA methylation changes that are distinct in each individual, which results in intra- and interindividual variabilities with age [48]. Accumulating evidence specifies that dietary bioactive compounds could have an important role in anti-aging nutraceutical intervention therapy by targeting DNA methylation.

14.2.2 Histone modifications in aging

The level of histone acetylation depends on the activity of two enzymes, namely, histone acetyltransferases (HATs) and histone deacetylases (HDACs). The balance between activities of these two enzymes is a major contributing factor in the aging process [49]. Aberrant expression of HATs and HDACs has been reported in many aging-related studies [49–52]. Similarly, increased histone acetylation has been shown to cause age-associated phenotype [53–55]. Collectively these results suggest that bioactive compounds could have an important role in the development of intervention strategies for reversibility of acetylation by targeting HATs or/and HDACs activities. Just like histone acetylation, methylation is also another important epigenetic modification. The level of histone methylation depends on the activity of two enzymes, namely, histone methyltransferases (HMTs) and histone demethylases (HDMs). Several pieces of evidence have indicated the role histone methylation in longevity and aging phenotypes and revealed the correlation of HMTs and HDMs, with increasing lifespan [56].

14.2.3 Noncoding RNA in aging

Another class of epigenetic mechanism involves noncoding RNAs (ncRNAs). ncRNAs are the diverse group of RNAs that are not translated into proteins but has regulatory functions in chromatin remodeling and gene expression by controlling transcriptional or post-transcriptional gene silencing [57]. Many studies have investigated the regulatory role of microRNA (miRNA) and long ncRNA (lncRNA) in aging and aging-related complications [58–61].

14.3 The role of epigenetics in age-related diseases

Aging is characterized by a progressive decline of several physiological processes which lead to functional deterioration of cells and increased susceptibility to diseases. Growing evidence suggests that dysregulation of epigenetic patterns during aging is a major risk factor for numerous age-related diseases such as cancer, cardiovascular disease, neurodegenerative disease and metabolic diseases such as type 2 diabetes mellitus. Here will discuss the evidence of the role epigenetic mechanisms in biological pathways underlying age-related diseases.

Cancer is a disease, caused due to accumulation of genetic mutations and epigenetic alterations during aging which results in increased proliferation of cells and genomic instability. Aging is a major risk factor for most cancers. The first indication of association of cancer with altered DNA methylation pattern was reported by Feinberg, A.P. and Vogelstein, B. in 1983. After that, several studies emphasized the fundamental role of epigenetics in the onset of cancer and mainly focused on canonical epigenetic mechanisms such as DNA methylation and histone modifications [62]. Cancer is characterized by genome-wide hypomethylation and site-specific promoter hypermethylation [62]. Global hypomethylation at repeat sequences leads to increase in genomic instability and aberrant activation of proto-oncogenes that plays a major role in cancer development and progression [63,64]. Conversely, site-specific hypermethylation of CpG islands in the promoter region of tumor suppressor gene causes transcriptional silencing which leads to tumor suppressor inactivation. In addition, DNA hypermethylation also contribute to inactivation of additional classes of genes by silencing transcription factors and DNA repair genes [65–67]. Moreover, alterations in histone modifications also contribute to development of cancer [68]. Global loss of H4K16ac and overexpression of HDACs are often found in various types of cancers [69–71], which leads to silencing of tumor suppressor genes. Similarly, dysregulation of activity of several HATs found to be responsible for gene expression changes underlying carcinogenesis [72–74]. In addition to these histone acetylation, alteration of histone methylation pattern such as decreased levels of H4K20me3 and H3K9me3 is also associated with aberrant gene silencing in cancer [69,75]. HMTs and HDMs play pivotal roles in maintaining global histone methylation patterns, and dysregulation of these enzymes has been involved in progression of various types of cancers [76–79]. Furthermore, numerous studies have indicated widespread changes in miRNA expression profiles during tumorigenesis [80]. Evidence suggests that many tumor suppressor miRNAs which target growth-promoting genes are downregulated and oncogenic miRNAs that target growth inhibitory pathways are often upregulated in cancer [81–86].

Cardiovascular disease is another age-related disease which leads to heart failure and increased risk of death. Several lines of evidence have shown correlation of aberrant epigenetic modification during aging with cardiovascular pathologies such as atherosclerosis, myocardial infarction, cardiac hypertrophy and heart failure [87–89]. DNA methylation and histone modification play major roles in modulating smooth muscle cells (SMCs) and endothelial cells (ECs) homeostasis, which leads to development of atherosclerosis [88]. Global DNA hypomethylation has been present in atherosclerotic lesions [90]. In addition, other studies carried out in cardiovascular disease have also reported altered pattern of global DNA methylation [91,92]. The balance between two enzymes HAT and HDAC plays a crucial role in regulating gene expression and dysregulation of this balance is implicated in development of cardiovascular diseases [93]. HDACs have a significant role in maintaining vascular homeostasis and dysregulation of it could result in development of atherosclerotic lesions [94]. miRNAs are key players in regulating different cellular functions involved in atherosclerosis such as cholesterol metabolism, oxidative stress and endothelial dysfunction [95]. Thus, dysregulation of miRNA has been found to be associated with cardiovascular diseases, lipid metabolism and endothelial function [90,96,97]. Likewise, several lncRNAs have been reported to play important regulatory roles in various cardiovascular pathologies [98]. Collectively, these results have indicated the role of epigenetics in cardiovascular aging and in the onset of cardiovascular disease.

Neurodegenerative diseases such as Alzheimer's disease (AD) are strongly associated with changes in epigenetic modification during aging and characterized by accumulation of amyloid β peptides and abnormally phosphorylated tau proteins [99,100]. Growing evidence suggests that epigenetic mechanisms play a pivotal role in various age-related neurodegenerative processes [101]. AD is the most common type of age-related neurodegenerative diseases and known to be associated with several specific alterations in epigenetic processes [3]. Decreased levels of DNA methylation and DNMTs in the AD patients suggested the association of global DNA hypomethylation with AD [102]. Another study carried out in frontal cortex of AD patients has demonstrated hypomethylation of promoter region of trans-membrane protein 59 which is involved in post-translational processing of amyloid-β precursor [103]. Other studies have also reported the alteration in methylation pattern of transcription factor binding sites of tau promoter [104]. In addition to aberrant DNA methylation, changes in histone modification such as decrease in histone acetylation and increase in histone methylation have been also reported in AD [105,106]. Dysregulation of various ncRNAs such as miRNA and lncRNA have also been associated with AD [107–109]. Taken together, these results showed the involvement of the epigenetic mechanisms in age-related neurodegenerative diseases.

Metabolic diseases such as type 2 diabetes mellitus (T2DM) is an age-related disease, and aging represents a major risk factor. Aging is associated with a decline in insulin sensitivity and skeletal muscle mass, which increases the risk of T2DM [110]. It has been reported that age-related promoter hypermethylation of COX7A1 gene, which is important in the metabolism of glucose is associated with increased risk of T2DM [111]. Furthermore, numerous studies have reported alterations of DNA methylation in different tissues such as pancreatic islets, skeletal muscle, adipose tissue and the liver of diabetic patients, indicating the role of epigenetics in the pathogenesis of T2DM [112–114]. In addition to DNA methylation, histone modifications have also been involved in pathogenesis of T2DM [115]. miRNAs play a significant role in the regulation of genes involved in insulin secretion, fat metabolism, cholesterol biosynthesis and adipogenesis which are crucial pathways in pathogenesis of T2DM [116,117]. Further, it has been reported that change in miRNA levels that occurs during aging affects the pancreatic beta cell function which may result in the development of T2DM [118].

Collectively, these results suggest that biological pathways involved in age-related diseases are associated with epigenetic dysregulation. Development of therapeutic interventions strategies targeting these epigenetic marks can enable to prevent the onset of age-related diseases and promote healthy aging.

14.4 Cellular, animal and insect models to get insights of epigenetics in aging

In order to fully appreciate the role of epigenetic mechanisms in progression of aging, there is need to understand the complex interplay between individual epigenetic mechanisms, and their interaction and influence of nutritional factors. Data obtained from various cell lines and organismal experiments allow us to uncover the complex interplay between the epigenome and nutritional impact in a highly controlled manner. However, the use of model system is essential in order to completely understand how the impact of nutritional factors can modulate epigenetic marks and how these modifications can manifest them in terms of healthy aging or lifespan extension. Till date, many researchers have studied these model systems and provided valuable information regarding the progression of aging, associated epigenetic marks and their modification in response to nutritional factors. Here we will discuss the evidence obtained from model systems which was helpful in explaining the epigenetic modifications underlying aging and age-related diseases and modulatory role of nutrition on them.

From last many years, researchers have used invertebrate model systems as a valuable tool to explore the underlying mechanism of aging. Fruit flies, nematodes, and budding yeast are the most frequently used model organisms in aging research due to their short lifespan and ease of genetic manipulation [119–122]. *Saccharomyces cerevisiae* (*S. cerevisiae*) has appeared as a simple and potent model organism for aging research and played very crucial role in revealing the epigenetic mechanisms associated with aging. Aging of *S. cerevisiae* can be modeled in two different ways, replicative or chronological. Phenotypes linked with replicative lifespan and chronological lifespan provide the understanding of stem cells (dividing) and post-mitotic cells (nondividing) aging, respectively [123]. The studies conducted on silent information regulator 2 (SIR2) in *S. cerevisiae* was the first evidence implying the role of sirtuins (SIRT1, SIRT2, SIRT6 and SIRT7) in aging. Sirtuins are mammalian orthologs of histone deacetylase SIR2 and the best example of epigenetic changes associated with cause of aged phenotypes [124]. Simultaneously, over the years, the studies on invertebrate models such as *Drosophila melanogaster* (*D. melanogaster*) and *Caenorhabditis elegans* (*C. elegans*) and vertebrate models such as mice and rats provided valuable information for a deeper understanding of the process of aging and the influence of epigenetic mechanisms on its outcome [119,125].

C. elegans is a very powerful model in studying epigenetics in aging research due to its short lifespan. The first indications that ncRNAs play an important role in the aging process came from studies carried out on *C. elegans* [126–128] where miRNA lin-4 had been shown to control developmental timing in *C. elegans* by decreasing the levels of its target mRNA of protein lin-14 [126,129]. The impact of mechanism of miRNA regulation on global gene expressions and phenotypic outcomes of aging was demonstrated by the *C. elegans* aging model [130]. Further a large number of studies investigating the role of miRNA in the aging process was carried out on *C. elegans* which provided a deeper understanding of dynamic changes of miRNA expression during aging and influence of miRNA regulation on the process of aging in other organisms. In the case of histone modification, a causative role of the H3K36me3 marking in modulating age-dependent gene expression stability and longevity was revealed by the study conducted on *C. elegans* and *D. melanogaster* [131].

The first evidence of trans-generational epigenetic inheritance of longevity was provided by study performed on *C. elegans* [132] where it was reported that deficiencies in the H3K4mc3 chromatin modifiers ASH-2, WDR-5, or SET-2 in the parental generation extend the lifespan of descendants up until the third generation. These findings suggest that manipulation of specific chromatin modifiers only in parents can induce an epigenetic memory of longevity in offspring. The study carried out to identify DNA methylation in *C. elegans* revealed the presence of N6 adenine methylation (6mA) and suggested the high possibility that 6mA may be a carrier of heritable epigenetic information in eukaryotes [133]. However, further studies are required to determine the significance of N6 adenine methylation (6mA) in the mammalian aging process and epigenetic inheritance to validate these findings.

Insect model systems are the valuable tools to study epigenetic inheritance and lifespan determinants mainly due to their phenotypic plasticity. Their phenotype and lifespan significantly differ in response to environmental stimuli, despite constant genotype [134]. The example of honeybee (*Apis mellifera*) shows the impact of nutrition after birth and its influence on phenotype via epigenetic mechanisms in aging. The diet decides the development of female larvae in the two different types such as long-living queens and short-living worker bees due to DNA methylation changes caused by the type of diet they consume. The HDAC inhibitor phenyl butyrate, one of the components of royal jelly, has been shown responsible for the development of the queen by increasing net histone acetylation [135–137]. Further, *D. melanogaster* is a well-known model organism to study genetics as well as epigenetics modification associated with the aging process especially for unravelling of histone modifications. *D. melanogaster* using as a model organism possesses several advantages like having homologues to more than 75% of human disease genes, and 50% of *D. melanogaster* genes are homologues to human genes [138]. The study carried out in *D. melanogaster* revealed that moderate reduction of H3K27me3 histone methylation complex can extend life span and stress resistance [139]. The study in the *D. melanogaster* model also revealed the correlation of methionine metabolic enzymes and histone modifiers in regulating histone methylation [140]. Furthermore, the significant role of HAT:HDAC balance on gene transcriptional regulation during development and diseases was demonstrated using the insect host model of greater wax moth (*Galleria mellonella*) by the use of specific inhibitors of HAT and HDAC enzyme activities [141].

Despite the great insights provided by the use of invertebrate animal models in aging epigenetics, many efforts have been made to assess whether these fundamental mechanisms are also shared by mammalian model systems. In this regard, mouse models have become valuable tools in the aging research due to their relatively short lifespan and feasibility to genetic modulations. Several lines of evidence reported that the epigenetic modifications play an important role in the aging process by studies performed on mice which allowed a fascinating characterization of the molecular and functional changes that adult stem cells undergo over time and consequently uncovered many factors that transform stem cell behavior with age [142,143]. Additionally, models have also demonstrated that stem cell rejuvenation can slow down the aging process [144,145]. Epigenetic aging signatures can be delayed by longevity-promoting interventions such as caloric restrictions and rapamycin treatment also demonstrated using mice models [146]. Another study carried out in mice reported the intergenerational effect of aging on conserved longevity regulatory pathway, life span and aging-associated phenotypes [147]. Recently, researchers have also used mouse models to explore causative epimutations in various epigenetic diseases by the generation of epigenome-edited mice [148]. This suggests that model organisms are powerful tools to understand the epigenetics in human aging and develop therapeutic intervention strategies to alleviate the diseases that are associated with aging.

14.5 Effect of nutrition on epigenetic alteration and aging

Nutrition is a major environmental factor that influences aging phenotype via epigenetic modifications [149]. Growing evidence suggests that specific nutrients can change epigenetic patterns and thereby alter gene expression of critical genes involved various physiological and pathological process [150]. Nutrients can act as a potential modulator of epigenetic mechanisms either directly by inhibition of enzymes involved in DNA methylation, histone modification or indirectly by altering the availability of substrates or cofactors required for those enzymatic reactions [150]. There are many key enzymes involved in the formation and maintenance of epigenetic marks such as in the case of DNA methylation – DNMT1, DNMT3A and DNMT3B – and histone modifications are regulated by HDAC, HATs, HMTs and HDMs enzymes.

Bioactive compounds, also referred to as nutraceuticals (the term coined in 1989 by Stephen L. DeFelice), are the essential or nonessential compounds derived from food or herbal products that can be beneficial to health [151]. There are a variety of bioactive compounds reported that have the ability to influence the efficacy. These enzymes therefore have the capacity to alter epigenetic patterns associated with physiological and pathological processes such as aging and age-related diseases [152]. These bioactive natural compounds could be classified into different groups depending on their chemical nature such as flavonoids (curcumin, quercetin and apigenin), polyphenol catechins from tea (epigallocatechin gallate (EGCG)), stillbenoids (resveratrol and pterostilbene), isoflavonoids (genistein), isothyocyanates (sulforaphane) and short-chain fatty acids (butyrate).

In addition to influencing the key enzymes involved in epigenetic modifications, various nutrients including folate, vitamin B12, vitamin B6, choline, methionine, zinc and selenium can act as substrates or co-factors to enzymes involved in the one-carbon metabolism. One-carbon metabolism is a well-defined pathway that influences the methylation of both DNA and histone by formation of S-adenosylmethionine (SAM). B vitamins act as coenzymes in one-carbon metabolism, which suggests that nutrients are involved in the regulation of epigenetic reaction [153]. The amino acid methionine gets converted into SAM and acts as a methyl donor for many biological methylation reactions including DNA and histone methylation [150]. Folate and choline provide the methyl group for remethylation of homocysteine to methionine. In addition, the availability of zinc may affect the activity of zinc metalloenzymes betaine-homocysteine S-methyltransferease (BHMT) and cystathionine β synthase (CBS) and therefore may alter the homocysteine levels [154].

Selenium is a trace element; it is an essential component of antioxidant selenoproteins such as glutathione peroxidase [155]. Selenium plays an important role in the transsulfuration pathway in one-carbon metabolism, and thus affects the conversion of homocysteine to cysteine and ultimately glutathione [156]. It has been found that selenium inhibits the activity of DNMT enzyme and influence the plasma homocysteine levels and SAM:SAH ratio [157,158]. Another study also reported that the selenium is associated with reduced DNMT expression, which would be expected to decrease DNA methylation [159]. It was reported that selenium reduces the availability of homocysteine for methionine cycle by converting homocysteine into selenohomocysteine, cystathionine, selenocystathionine, glutathione and selenocysteine, which eventually leads to reduction of global DNA methylation [160]. Moreover, selenite inhibits the binding of the activator protein 1 (AP-1) transcription factors to DNA, which reduces the ability of DNMT1 binding to DNA and eventually reduces the DNA methylation [161]. These findings collectively indicate that selenium can alter one-carbon metabolism leading to both genomic and gene-specific alterations in DNA methylation pattern.

14.5.1 Flavonoids

Flavonoids are a class of polyphenolic secondary metabolites of plants. A great number of studies have reported that dietary intake of flavonoids exert anti-aging effects via epigenetic alterations [164,165,170,171,180]. Flavonoids affect the expression or activity of enzymes involved in epigenetic modifications. The most investigated flavonoids in aging and age-related disease treatments are curcumin, quercetin, and apigenin.

14.5.1.1 Curcumin

Curcumin, a polyphenolic component of *Curcuma longa*, shows various beneficial activities such as anti-inflammatory, anti-oxidative, and anticancer [162]. Curcumin is primarily known for its anti-oxidative properties which affect replicative and chronological aging [163]. Studies in rats have elucidated the anti-aging properties of curcumin in the perspective of adipose tissue-derived mesenchymal stem cell aging through TERT gene expression [164]. Another study also reported the beneficial effect of curcumin supplementation on muscle characteristics in aging rats [165]. Furthermore, curcumin has inhibitory activity against HAT and HDAC, and especially shows a strong inhibition of HAT in cancer models [166,167]. Reports have also showed the possible therapeutic potential of curcumin with increased apoptosis in cancer cells and promoted neuronal differentiation of stem cells [168].

14.5.1.2 Quercetin

Quercetin is an antioxidant flavonoid mainly found in fruits and vegetables and is actively responsible for maintaining cellular reactive oxygen species (ROS) levels. Quercetin shows poor water solubility and relatively low bioavailability [169]. Studies carried out in different organisms reported that quercetin plays a crucial role in extending the lifespan of different organisms. Administration of quercetin in *Podospora anserine* induced extension of lifespan and demonstrated the role of S-adenosylmethionine-dependent O-methyltransferase PaMTH1 [170]. Another study reported that quercetin treatment in mice delays post-ovulatory aging of oocytes by modulating SIRT expression and activity of maturation-promoting factors (MPF). Furthermore, quercetin treatment during postovulatory aging also enhanced the early development of embryo [171].

14.5.1.3 Apigenin

Apigenin is a plant flavonoid present in common vegetables and fruits such as parsley, onions, wheat sprouts, tea, oranges and chamomile [172]. Numerous studies have demonstrated that apigenin has anti-inflammatory, antioxidant, anticancer and anti-mutagenic properties, which indicates the protective effect of apigenin on aging-related diseases such as skin cancer, colon cancer and many others [173–179]. A study determined the protective effect of apigenin administration in mouse model for delaying the aging process and showed anti-senescent effect of apigenin by activating the Nrf2 pathway which is responsible for slow aging [180]. Another study investigated the effect of apigenin on the skin and found that the apigenin-containing cream increased elasticity and dermal density of the skin with reduced fine wrinkle length and also found improvement in skin moisture content, evenness and transepidermal water loss. These findings clearly suggested cellular and clinical efficacy of apigenin in anti-aging treatment [181]. However, another study reported the effect of apigenin in epigenetic-related enzyme DNMT, and the treatment of apigenin showed a marked decrease in DNMT activity in an in vitro study [182].

14.5.2 Polyphenol catechins
14.5.2.1 Epigallocatechingallate (EGCG)

Epigallocatechingallate (EGCG) is a major polyphenol component of green tea, which shows very promising results in various lung cancer, leukemia, breast cancer and neurodegenerative diseases by its demethylating properties that inhibit DNMT enzyme [183–185]. It has been reported that EGCG from green tea inhibits DNMT1 directly by fitting to the binging pocket of DNMT1 which results in reducing its ability to methylate DNA [186,187]. Furthermore, EGCG along with reduced availability of dietary methyl donor has been reported to inhibit HMT enzyme [188,189]. Other studies that investigated the effect of EGCG treatment showed decreased 5mC, mRNA and protein expressions of DNMT1, DNMT3A and DNMT3B in human cancer cell lines and also reported decreased histone deacetylase activity with increased levels of H3-Lys 9 and 14 [190]. Similarly, another study carried out in human cancer cell lines revealed that EGCG can inhibit DNMT activity in a dose-dependent manner and reactivate methylation-silenced genes in cancer cells which indicate the potential use of EGCG for the prevention or reversal of related gene-silencing in anti-cancer activity [186]. In addition to the direct inhibition of DNMT1 activity, it was also stated that polyphenol consumption could increase the formation of SAH, which suggests another mechanism inhibiting DNA methylation by EGCG activity [187]. In line with these results, animal studies also reported that the consumption of EGCG through drinking water could moderately decrease intestinal levels of SAM [182]. Collectively these observations clearly conveyed the inhibitory effect of EGCG on DNMT1 activity which is indirectly correlated to one-carbon metabolism.

14.5.3 Stillbenoids

14.5.3.1 Resveratrol

Resveratrol is a phytoalexin polyphenol found in grapes, cranberries, blueberries, almond and peanuts [191]. Anti-inflammatory, anti-oxidative and anti-cancer effects of resveratrol have been demonstrated in a variety of in vitro and in vivo studies. Resveratrol also possesses anti-diabetogenic and anti-aging properties. However, various organismal models showed the effect of resveratrol on lifespan; when given to organisms such as yeast, flies, honeybees and worms, it resulted in lifespan extension [192–195]. Studies conducted in mice have reported that a low dose of resveratrol limited the effect of caloric restriction and delayed some aspects of aging by inhibiting gene expression associated with cardiac and skeletal muscle aging and also prevented age-related cardiac dysfunction [196]. Another study carried out in middle-aged mice showed that resveratrol along with a high-calorie diet improves health and survival by influencing mechanisms associated with extended lifespan which includes increased insulin sensitivity, increased AMP-activated protein kinase (AMPK) and peroxisome proliferator-activated receptor-γ coactivator 1α (PGC-1α) activity, increased mitochondrial number and reduced insulin-like growth factor-1 (IGF-I) levels [197]. With respect to epigenetic mechanisms, resveratrol has been shown to decrease the expression of DNMT1 and DNMT3B genes and reactivation of tumor suppressor by demethylation of promoter region in breast cancer [198].

14.5.3.2 Pterostilbene

Besides resveratrol, pterostilbene is another phytoalexin compound produced by plants as part of their defense system, commonly found in grapes, peanut and berries. Pterostilbene exhibits pharmacokinetic and pharmacodynamics properties. A study conducted in human prostate cancer showed that the administration of pterostilbene decreases cell proliferation and increases apoptosis and angiogenesis by inhibiting epigenetic modifier metastasis-associated protein 1 (MTA1) [199]. Another study reported antioxidant and cardiomyocyte protection effects of pterostilbene in mouse and cell lines [200]. In addition, synergic effect of resveratrol and pterostilbene was investigated in triple-negative breast cancer (TNBC) study showed that combination of resveratrol and pterostilbene alters DNA damage response by affecting SIRT1 and DNMT enzyme expression and subsequently inhibits TNBC [201]. These observations suggest that the administration of pterostilbene alone or in combination with resveratrol may serve as a therapeutic target for various age-related diseases such as cancer.

14.5.4 Isoflavonoids
14.5.4.1 Genistein

Genistein is an isoflavone mainly found in soybeans, fava beans and olives. It has been demonstrated that genistein showed a great potential to regulate the epigenetic mechanisms and possesses photoprotective and wound-healing properties [202]. The first evidence of *in utero* effect of dietary genistein was reported by [203], and a study carried out in mouse showed that dietary genistein affects gene expression and alters susceptibility of offspring to obesity in adulthood by permanently altering the epigenome. Another study in mouse embryonic stem cells reported that genistein altered the methylation pattern of differentiated embryonic stem cells after *de novo* methylation [204]. Furthermore, Fang MZ et al. found that genistein can reactivate methylation silence genes partially through a direct inhibition of DNMT, which suggests the potential of genistein in epigenetic mechanisms [182,205]. Additionally, the photoprotective effect of genistein in combination with daidzein on UVB-induced DNA was investigated [206]. Inhibitory effect of genistein on H3 deacetylation and DNMT1-DNMT3A activity has been demonstrated in an animal study carried out in the mouse model [207]. These results collectively suggest that genistein administration in a dose-dependent manner could help in aging-related diseases through epigenetic alterations.

14.5.5 Isothiocyanates
14.5.5.1 Sulforaphane

Sulforaphane is isothiocyanate mainly found in cruciferous vegetables, such as cauliflower and broccoli, which shows anticancer and antioxidant effects [208].

Numerous studies have reported that sulforaphane has the potential to modulate several epigenetic modifications such as DNA methylation and histone modification by inhibiting the activities of enzymes HDAC and DNMT [202,209,210]. Furthermore, sulforaphane has been demonstrated as a key inducer of the antioxidant protective response during aging [211,212]. Administration of sulforaphane along with other bioactive compounds such as EGCG can positively modulate the epigenome, these changes in the epigenome aid in the prevention of cancer and potentiate the longevity effects of caloric restrictions [213]. Furthermore, several studies have demonstrated the protective effect of sulforaphane against ultraviolet-induced skin damage by reducing oxidative stress and other cellular mechanisms of action [214] and maintaining collagen levels during photo-aging by inhibiting AP-1 activation [215]. The effect of sulforaphane on longevity was reported by a study carried out in red flour beetle (*Tribolium castaneum*) where dietary supplementation of lyophilized broccoli resulted in significant increase in the life span by regulation of key stress-resistant factors such as Nrf-2, Jnk-1 and Foxo-1 [216]. These findings showed the potential of sulforaphane administration in prevention of cancer and improvement of cellular lifespan and health span.

14.5.6 Short-chain fatty acids

14.5.6.1 Butyrate

Butyrate is a short-chain fatty acid produced during the fermentation of dietary fiber in the large intestine [202]. Butyrate is known as a HDAC inhibitor due to its ability to increase histone acetylation [217,218]. It also plays an important role in free fatty acid receptor signaling and metabolic regulation, and promotes the expression of neurotrophic and anti-inflammatory genes [218]. Even though maximum numbers of studies on butyrate have focused on its effects on histone acetylation, evidence has shown that butyrate can also modulate DNA methylation patterns [219–221]. A study carried out in mice showed that butyrate treatment increases the levels of prolongevity hormone fibroblast growth factor 21 (FGF21), which suggests the correlation of butyrate with prolongevity phenotype [222]. Another study carried out in mice reported that butyrate has a potential to improve metabolism and reduce muscle atrophy during aging [223]. Administration of butyrate along with dietary soluble fiber results in improvement of neuroinflammation associated with aging in mice [224].

Aging is an inevitable and complex biological process that is associated with various age-related diseases. Many studies have provided evidence that epigenetic mechanisms are responsible for the progression of aging. Several nutritional and dietary factors have the potential to modulate or reverse the epigenetic marks associated with aging, and this indicates that even though aging is inevitable, there are still opportunities for delaying and prevention of aging and age-related diseases, respectively.

14.6 Conclusion

Several studies have provided understanding of the modulatory role of diet and nutrition in epigenetic mechanisms underlying aging and age-related diseases which is described by nutritional epigenetics which elucidate the gene-diet interactions. The growing interest in nutritional epigenetics in aging in recent years is largely due to the reversible nature of epigenetic mechanisms that may be targeted by nutritional interventions. However, the impact of nutritional influence on epigenetic modifications is highly dependent on a number of factors including the nutrient dose, interaction of nutrient with other dietary components, target tissue or organ of interest, target epigenetic modification under investigation, the period and duration of exposure, and additionally interaction with genetic, lifestyle and environmental stimuli. Therefore, further research is warranted to understand cell-tissue specificity, optimal dosage and temporal association of dietary treatment and its influence on epigenetic modifications. Better understanding of the impact of dietary and nutritional treatment on the epigenome and the consequences on health and diseases may support the development of significant public heath recommendations to promote healthy aging and prevent age-related complications.

Acknowledgments

We are grateful to Dr. Bhushan Patwardhan for his continuous guidance. We thank Dr. Aditya S. Abhyankar, Dean and Head, Department of Technology, Savitribai Phule Pune University, Pune and Dr. S.D. Lokhande, Principal, Sinhgad College of Engineering, SPPU, Pune for support.

References

1. Berdasco M, Esteller M. Hot topics in epigenetic mechanisms of aging: 2011. *Aging cell*. 2012 Apr;11(2):181–6.
2. López-Otín C, Blasco MA, Partridge L, Serrano M, Kroemer G. The hallmarks of aging. *Cell*. 2013 Jun 6;153(6):1194–217.
3. Calvanese V, Lara E, Kahn A, Fraga MF. The role of epigenetics in aging and age-related diseases. *Ageing Research Reviews*. 2009 Oct 1;8(4):268–76.
4. Niccoli T, Partridge L. Ageing as a risk factor for disease. *Current biology*. 2012 Sep 11;22(17):R741–52.
5. Rowbotham DA, Marshall EA, Vucic EA, Kennett JY, Lam WL, Martinez VD. Epigenetic changes in aging and Age-related disease. *Journal of Aging Science*. 2015 Jan 22;2015.
6. Fransquet PD, Wrigglesworth J, Woods RL, Ernst ME, Ryan J. The epigenetic clock as a predictor of disease and mortality risk: A systematic review and meta-analysis. *Clinical Epigenetics*. 2019 Dec 1;11(1):62.
7. Dey S, Nambiar D, Lakshmi JK, Sheikh K, Reddy KS. Aging in Asia: Findings from new and emerging data initiatives. ed. Majmundar M Smith JP, *Chapter Markers and Drivers: Cardiovascular Health of Middle-Aged and Older Indians*. National Academies Press (US). 2012.

8. Agarwal A, Lubet A, Mitgang E, Mohanty S, Bloom DE. Population aging in India: Facts, issues, and options. In *Population Change and Impacts in Asia and the Pacific* 2020 (pp. 289–311). Springer, Singapore.

9. Montesanto A, Dato S, Bellizzi D, Rose G, Passarino G. Epidemiological, genetic and epigenetic aspects of the research on healthy ageing and longevity. *Immunity & Ageing.* 2012 Dec;9(1):1–2.

10. Dupont C, Armant DR, Brenner CA. Epigenetics: Definition, mechanisms and clinical perspective. InSeminars in reproductive medicine 2009 Sep (Vol. 27, No. 5, p. 351). NIH Public Access.

11. Gonzalo S. Epigenetic alterations in aging. *Journal of Applied Physiology.* 2010 Aug;109(2):586–97.

12. Xavier MJ, Roman SD, Aitken RJ, Nixon B. Transgenerational inheritance: How impacts to the epigenetic and genetic information of parents affect offspring health. *Human Reproduction Update.* 2019 Sep 11;25(5):519–41.

13. Abdul QA, Yu BP, Chung HY, Jung HA, Choi JS. Epigenetic modifications of gene expression by lifestyle and environment. *Archives of Pharmacal Research.* 2017 Nov 1;40(11):1219–37.

14. Vaiserman A. Developmental tuning of epigenetic clock. *Frontiers in Genetics.* 2018 Nov 22;9:584.

15. Xiao FH, Wang HT, Kong QP. Dynamic DNA methylation during aging: A "prophet" of age-related outcomes. *Frontiers in Genetics.* 2019 Feb 18;10:107.

16. Goldberg AD, Allis CD, Bernstein E. Epigenetics: A landscape takes shape. *Cell.* 2007 Feb 23;128(4):635–8.

17. McCay CM, Crowell MF, Maynard LA. The effect of retarded growth upon the length of life span and upon the ultimate body size: One figure. *The journal of Nutrition.* 1935 Jul 1;10(1):63–79.

18. Omodei D, Fontana L. Calorie restriction and prevention of age-associated chronic disease. *FEBS letters.* 2011 Jun 6;585(11):1537–42.

19. Larson-Meyer DE, Newcomer BR, Heilbronn LK, et al.. Effect of 6-month calorie restriction and exercise on serum and liver lipids and markers of liver function. *Obesity.* 2008 Jun;16(6):1355–62.

20. Heilbronn LK, De Jonge L, Frisard MI, et al. Effect of 6-month calorie restriction on biomarkers of longevity, metabolic adaptation, and oxidative stress in overweight individuals: A randomized controlled trial. *JAMA.* 2006 Apr 5;295(13):1539–48.

21. Colman RJ, Anderson RM, Johnson SC, et al. Caloric restriction delays disease onset and mortality in rhesus monkeys. *Science.* 2009 Jul 10;325(5937):201–4.

22. Mattison JA, Roth GS, Beasley TM, et al. Impact of caloric restriction on health and survival in rhesus monkeys from the NIA study. *Nature.* 2012 Sep;489(7415):318–21.

23. Bacalini MG, Friso S, Olivieri F, et al. Present and future of anti-ageing epigenetic diets. *Mechanisms of Ageing and Development.* 2014 Mar 1;136:101–15.

24. Akone SH, Ntie-Kang F, Stuhldreier F, et al. Natural products impacting DNA Methyltransferases and histone deacetylases. *Frontiers in Pharmacology.* 2020;11.

25. Gensous N, Garagnani P, Santoro A, et al. One-year Mediterranean diet promotes epigenetic rejuvenation with country-and sex-specific effects: A pilot study from the NU-AGE project. *GeroScience.* 2020 Jan 24:1–5.

26. Maiti P, Dunbar GL. Use of curcumin, a natural polyphenol for targeting molecular pathways in treating age-related neurodegenerative diseases. *International Journal of Molecular Sciences.* 2018 Jun;19(6):1637.

27. Simioni C, Zauli G, Martelli AM, et al. Oxidative stress: Role of physical exercise and antioxidant nutraceuticals in adulthood and aging. *Oncotarget.* 2018 Mar 30;9(24):17181.

28. Zhong J, Karlsson O, Wang G, et al. B vitamins attenuate the epigenetic effects of ambient fine particles in a pilot human intervention trial. *Proceedings of the National Academy of Sciences.* 2017 Mar 28;114(13):3503–8.

29. Egger G, Liang G, Aparicio A, Jones PA. Epigenetics in human disease and prospects for epigenetic therapy. *Nature.* 2004 May;429(6990):457–63.
30. Holliday R. The inheritance of epigenetic defects. *Science.* 1987 Oct 9;238(4824):163–70.
31. Fraga MF, Ballestar E, Paz MF, et al. Epigenetic differences arise during the lifetime of monozygotic twins. *Proceedings of the National Academy of Sciences.* 2005 Jul 26;102(30):10604–9.
32. Hannum G, Guinney J, Zhao L, et al. Genome-wide methylation profiles reveal quantitative views of human aging rates. *Molecular cell.* 2013 Jan 24;49(2):359–67.
33. Pagiatakis C, Musolino E, Gornati R, Bernardini G, Papait R. Epigenetics of aging and disease: A brief overview. *Aging Clinical and Experimental Research.* 2019 Dec 6:1–9.
34. Bird A. DNA methylation patterns and epigenetic memory. *Genes & Development.* 2002 Jan 1;16(1):6–21.
35. Okano M, Xie S, Li E. Cloning and characterization of a family of novel mammalian DNA (cytosine-5) methyltransferases. *Nature Genetics.* 1998 Jul;19(3):219–20.
36. Okano M, Bell DW, Haber DA, Li E. DNA methyltransferases Dnmt3a and Dnmt3b are essential for de novo methylation and mammalian development. *Cell.* 1999 Oct 29;99(3):247–57.
37. Ciccarone F, Malavolta M, Calabrese R, et al. Age-dependent expression of DNMT 1 and DNMT 3B in PBMC s from a large European population enrolled in the MARK-AGE study. *Aging Cell.* 2016 Aug;15(4):755–65.
38. Zampieri M, Ciccarone F, Calabrese R, Franceschi C, Bürkle A, Caiafa P. Reconfiguration of DNA methylation in aging. *Mechanisms of Ageing and Development.* 2015 Nov 1;151:60–70.
39. Petkovich DA, Podolskiy DI, Lobanov AV, Lee SG, Miller RA, Gladyshev VN. Using DNA methylation profiling to evaluate biological age and longevity interventions. *Cell Metabolism.* 2017 Apr 4;25(4):954–60.
40. Pal S, Tyler JK. Epigenetics and aging. *Science Advances.* 2016 Jul 1;2(7):e1600584.
41. Sen P, Shah PP, Nativio R, Berger SL. Epigenetic mechanisms of longevity and aging. *Cell.* 2016 Aug 11;166(4):822–39.
42. Day K, Waite LL, Thalacker-Mercer A, et al. Differential DNA methylation with age displays both common and dynamic features across human tissues that are influenced by CpG landscape. *Genome Biology.* 2013 Sep 1;14(9):R102.
43. Guarasci F, D'Aquila P, Mandalà M, et al. Aging and nutrition induce tissue-specific changes on global DNA methylation status in rats. *Mechanisms of Ageing and Development.* 2018 Sep 1;174:47–54.
44. Richardson B. Impact of aging on DNA methylation. *Ageing Research Reviews.* 2003 Jul 1;2(3):245–61.
45. Li X, Wang J, Wang L, et al. Impaired lipid metabolism by age-dependent DNA methylation alterations accelerates aging. *Proceedings of the National Academy of Sciences.* 2020 Feb 25;117(8): 4328–36.
46. Gensous N, Bacalini MG, Pirazzini C, Marasco E, Giuliani C, Ravaioli F, Mengozzi G, Bertarelli C, Palmas MG, Franceschi C, Garagnani P. The epigenetic landscape of age-related diseases: The geroscience perspective. *Biogerontology.* 2017 Aug 1;18(4):549–59.
47. Jiang S, Guo Y. Epigenetic Clock: DNA Methylation in Aging. *Stem Cells International.* 2020 Jul 8;2020.
48. Jones MJ, Goodman SJ, Kobor MS. DNA methylation and healthy human aging. *Aging Cell.* 2015 Dec;14(6):924–32.
49. Saha RN, Pahan K. HATs and HDACs in neurodegeneration: A tale of disconcerted acetylation homeostasis. *Cell Death & Differentiation.* 2006 Apr;13(4):539–50.
50. Boutillier AL, Trinh E, Loeffler JP. Selective E2F-dependent gene transcription is controlled by histone deacetylase activity during neuronal apoptosis. *Journal of Neurochemistry.* 2003 Feb;84(4):814–28.

51. Rouaux C, Jokic N, Mbebi C, Boutillier S, Loeffler JP, Boutillier AL. Critical loss of CBP/p300 histone acetylase activity by caspase-6 during neurodegeneration. *The EMBO Journal.* 2003 Dec 15;22(24):6537–49.

52. Toussirot E, Abbas W, Khan KA, et al. Imbalance between HAT and HDAC activities in the PBMCs of patients with ankylosing spondylitis or rheumatoid arthritis and influence of HDAC inhibitors on TNF alpha production. *PLoS One.* 2013 Aug 15;8(8):e70939.

53. Dang W, Steffen KK, Perry R, et al. Histone H4 lysine 16 acetylation regulates cellular lifespan. *Nature.* 2009 Jun;459(7248):802–7.

54. Kawahara TL, Michishita E, Adler AS, et al. SIRT6 links histone H3 lysine 9 deacetylation to NF-κB-dependent gene expression and organismal life span. *Cell.* 2009 Jan 9;136(1):62–74.

55. Lee S, Jung JW, Park SB, et al. Histone deacetylase regulates high mobility group A2-targeting microRNAs in human cord blood-derived multipotent stem cell aging. *Cellular and Molecular Life Sciences.* 2011 Jan 1;68(2):325–36.

56. McCauley BS, Dang W. Histone methylation and aging: Lessons learned from model systems. *BiochimicaetBiophysicaActa (BBA)-Gene Regulatory Mechanisms.* 2014 Dec 1;1839(12):1454–62.

57. Kaikkonen MU, Lam MT, Glass CK. Non-coding RNAs as regulators of gene expression and epigenetics. *Cardiovascular Research.* 2011 Jun 1;90(3):430–40.

58. Jin L, Song Q, Zhang W, Geng B, Cai J. Roles of long noncoding RNAs in aging and aging complications. *BiochimicaetBiophysicaActa (BBA)-Molecular Basis of Disease.* 2019 Jul 1;1865(7):1763–71.

59. Cao Q, Wu J, Wang X, Song C. Noncoding RNAs in vascular aging. *Oxidative Medicine and Cellular Longevity.* 2020 Jan 4;2020.

60. Trembinski DJ, Bink DI, Theodorou K, et al. Aging-regulated anti-apoptotic long non-coding RNA Sarrah augments recovery from acute myocardial infarction. *Nature Communications.* 2020 Apr 27;11(1): 1–4.

61. He J, Tu C, Liu Y. Role of lncRNAs in aging and age-related diseases. *Aging Medicine.* 2018 Sep;1(2):158–75.

62. Jones PA, Baylin SB. The fundamental role of epigenetic events in cancer. *Nature Reviews Genetics.* 2002 Jun;3(6):415–28.

63. Rodriguez J, Frigola J, Vendrell E, et al. Chromosomal instability correlates with genome-wide DNA demethylation in human primary colorectal cancers. *Cancer Research.* 2006 Sep 1;66(17):8462–9468.

64. Eden A, Gaudet F, Waghmare A, Jaenisch R. Chromosomal instability and tumors promoted by DNA hypomethylation. *Science.* 2003 Apr 18;300(5618):455.

65. Di Croce L, Raker VA, Corsaro M, et al. Methyltransferase recruitment and DNA hypermethylation of target promoters by an oncogenic transcription factor. *Science.* 2002 Feb 8;295(5557):1079–82.

66. Jones PA, Baylin SB. The epigenomics of cancer. *Cell.* 2007 Feb 23;128(4):683–92.

67. Baylin SB. DNA methylation and gene silencing in cancer. *Nature Clinical Practice Oncology.* 2005 Dec;2(1):S4–11.

68. Wang GG, Allis CD, Chi P. Chromatin remodeling and cancer, Part I: Covalent histone modifications. *Trends in Molecular Medicine.* 2007 Sep 1;13(9):363–72.

69. Fraga MF, Ballestar E, Villar-Garea A, et al. Loss of acetylation at Lys16 and trimethylation at Lys20 of histone H4 is a common hallmark of human cancer. *Nature Genetics.* 2005 Apr;37(4):391–400.

70. Halkidou K, Gaughan L, Cook S, Leung HY, Neal DE, Robson CN. Upregulation and nuclear recruitment of HDAC1 in hormone refractory prostate cancer. *The Prostate.* 2004 May 1;59(2):177–89.

71. Song J, Noh JH, Lee JH, et al. Increased expression of histone deacetylase 2 is found in human gastric cancer. *Apmis.* 2005 Apr;113(4):264–8.

72. Chen J, Luo Q, Yuan Y, et al. Pygo2 associates with MLL2 histone methyltransferase and GCN5 histone acetyltransferase complexes to augment Wnt target gene expression and breast cancer stem-like cell expansion. *Molecular and Cellular Biology*. 2010 Dec 15;30(24):5621–35.

73. Yang XJ, Ullah M. MOZ and MORF, two large MYSTic HATs in normal and cancer stem cells. *Oncogene*. 2007 Aug;26(37):5408–19.

74. Tillinghast GW, Partee J, Albert P, Kelley JM, Burtow KH, Kelly K. Analysis of genetic stability at the EP300 and CREBBP loci in a panel of cancer cell lines. *Genes, Chromosomes and Cancer*. 2003 Jun;37(2):121–31.

75. Nguyen CT, Weisenberger DJ, Velicescu M, et al. Histone H3-lysine 9 methylation is associated with aberrant gene silencing in cancer cells and is rapidly reversed by 5-aza-2′-deoxycytidine. *Cancer Research*. 2002 Nov 15;62(22):6456–61.

76. Varambally S, Dhanasekaran SM, Zhou M, Barrette TR, Kumar-Sinha C, Sanda MG, Ghosh D, Pienta KJ, Sewalt RG, Otte AP, Rubin MA. The polycomb group protein EZH2 is involved in progression of prostate cancer. *Nature*. 2002 Oct;419(6907):624–9.

77. Agger K, Cloos PA, Rudkjær L, et al. The H3K27me3 demethylase JMJD3 contributes to the activation of the INK4A–ARF locus in response to oncogene-and stress-induced senescence. *Genes & Development*. 2009 May 15;23(10):1171–6.

78. Chen MW, Hua KT, Kao HJ, et al. H3K9 histone methyltransferase G9a promotes lung cancer invasion and metastasis by silencing the cell adhesion molecule Ep-CAM. *Cancer Research*. 2010 Oct 15;70(20):7830–40.

79. Dong C, Wu Y, Yao J, Wang Y, Yu Y, Rychahou PG, Evers BM, Zhou BP. G9a interacts with Snail and is critical for Snail-mediated E-cadherin repression in human breast cancer. *The Journal of Clinical Investigation*. 2012 Apr 2;122(4):1469–86.

80. Lu J, Getz G, Miska EA, et al. MicroRNA expression profiles classify human cancers. *Nature*. 2005 Jun;435(7043):834–8.

81. Zhang B, Pan X, Cobb GP, Anderson TA. microRNAs as oncogenes and tumor suppressors. *Developmental Biology*. 2007 Feb 1;302(1):1–2.

82. Ventura A, Jacks T. MicroRNAs and cancer: Short RNAs go a long way. *Cell*. 2009 Feb 20;136(4):586–91.

83. Friedman JM, Liang G, Liu CC, et al. The putative tumor suppressor microRNA-101 modulates the cancer epigenome by repressing the polycomb group protein EZH2. *Cancer Research*. 2009 Mar 15;69(6):2623–9.

84. Chan JA, Krichevsky AM, Kosik KS. MicroRNA-21 is an antiapoptotic factor in human glioblastoma cells. *Cancer Research*. 2005 Jul 15;65(14):6029–33.

85. Dorsett Y, McBride KM, Jankovic M, et al. MicroRNA-155 suppresses activation-induced cytidinedeaminase-mediated Myc-Igh translocation. *Immunity*. 2008 May 16;28(5):630–8.

86. Mendell JT. miRiad roles for the miR-17–92 cluster in development and disease. *Cell*. 2008 Apr 18;133(2):217–22.

87. Gentilini D, Garagnani P, Pisoni S, et al. Stochastic epigenetic mutations (DNA methylation) increase exponentially in human aging and correlate with X chromosome inactivation skewing in females. *Aging (Albany NY)*. 2015 Aug;7(8):568.

88. Zhang W, Song M, Qu J, Liu GH. Epigenetic modifications in cardiovascular aging and diseases. *Circulation Research*. 2018 Sep 14;123(7):773–86.

89. Lind L, Ingelsson E, Sundström J, Siegbahn A, Lampa E. Methylation-based estimated biological age and cardiovascular disease. *European Journal of Clinical Investigation*. 2018 Feb;48(2):e12872.

90. Udali S, Guarini P, Moruzzi S, Choi SW, Friso S. Cardiovascular epigenetics: From DNA methylation to microRNAs. *Molecular Aspects of Medicine*. 2013 Jul 1;34(4):883–901.

91. Sharma P, Kumar J, Garg G, et al. Detection of altered global DNA methylation in coronary artery disease patients. *DNA and Cell Biology*. 2008 Jul 1;27(7):357–65.

92. Castro R, Rivera I, Blom HJ, Jakobs C, De Almeida IT. Homocysteine metabolism, hyperhomocysteinaemia and vascular disease: An overview. *Journal of Inherited Metabolic Disease: Official Journal of the Society for the Study of Inborn Errors of Metabolism.* 2006 Feb;29(1):3–20.

93. Yang J, Xu WW, Hu SJ. Heart failure: Advanced development in genetics and epigenetics. *BioMed Research International.* 2015 Jan 1;2015.

94. Williams SM, Golden-Mason L, Ferguson BS, et al. Class I HDACs regulate angiotensin II-dependent cardiac fibrosis via fibroblasts and circulating fibrocytes. *Journal of Molecular and Cellular Cardiology.* 2014 Feb 1;67:112–25.

95. Schober A, Weber C. Mechanisms of microRNAs in atherosclerosis. *Annual Review of Pathology: Mechanisms of Disease.* 2016 May 23;11:583–616.

96. Oyama Y, Marie Bartman C, Gile J, Eckle T. Circadian MicroRNAs in cardioprotection. *Current Pharmaceutical Design.* 2017 Jul 1;23(25):3723–30.

97. Ordovás JM, Smith CE. Epigenetics and cardiovascular disease. *Nature Reviews Cardiology.* 2010 Sep;7(9):510.

98. Prasher D, Greenway SC, Singh RB. The impact of epigenetics on cardiovascular disease. *Biochemistry and Cell Biology.* 2020;98(1):12–22.

99. Bennett DA, Yu L, Yang J, Klein HU, De Jager PL. Epigenomics of Alzheimer's disease. In *Translating Epigenetics to the Clinic* 2017 Jan 1 (pp. 227–278). Academic Press.

100. Li L, Zhang C, Zi X, Tu Q, Guo K. Epigenetic modulation of Cdk5 contributes to memory deficiency induced by amyloid fibrils. *Experimental Brain Research.* 2015 Jan 1;233(1):165–73.

101. Lardenoije R, Iatrou A, Kenis G, et al. The epigenetics of aging and neurodegeneration. *Progress in Neurobiology.* 2015 Aug 1;131:21–64.

102. Chouliaras L, Mastroeni D, Delvaux E, et al. Consistent decrease in global DNA methylation and hydroxymethylation in the hippocampus of Alzheimer's disease patients. *Neurobiology of Aging.* 2013 Sep 1;34(9):2091–9.

103. Bakulski KM, Dolinoy DC, Sartor MA, et al. Genome-wide DNA methylation differences between late-onset Alzheimer's disease and cognitively normal controls in human frontal cortex. *Journal of Alzheimer's Disease.* 2012 Jan 1;29(3):571–88.

104. Wang J, Yu JT, Tan MS, Jiang T, Tan L. Epigenetic mechanisms in Alzheimer's disease: Implications for pathogenesis and therapy. *Ageing Research Reviews.* 2013 Sep 1;12(4):1024–41.

105. Francis YI, Fa M, Ashraf H, Zhang H, Staniszewski A, Latchman DS, Arancio O. Dysregulation of histone acetylation in the APP/PS1 mouse model of Alzheimer's disease. *Journal of Alzheimer's Disease.* 2009 Jan 1;18(1):131–9.

106. Rao JS, Keleshian VL, Klein S, Rapoport SI. Epigenetic modifications in frontal cortex from Alzheimer's disease and bipolar disorder patients. *Translational Psychiatry.* 2012 Jul;2(7):e132.

107. Lukiw WJ. Micro-RNA speciation in fetal, adult and Alzheimer's disease hippocampus. *Neuroreport.* 2007 Feb 12;18(3):297–300.

108. Sethi P, Lukiw WJ. Micro-RNA abundance and stability in human brain: Specific alterations in Alzheimer's disease temporal lobe neocortex. *Neuroscience Letters.* 2009 Aug 7;459(2):100–4.

109. Holden T, Nguyen A, Lin E, et al. Exploratory bioinformatics study of lncRNAs in Alzheimer's disease mRNA sequences with application to drug development. *Computational and Mathematical Methods in Medicine.* 2013 Oct;2013.

110. Sakuma K, Aoi W, Yamaguchi A. The intriguing regulators of muscle mass in sarcopenia and muscular dystrophy. *Frontiers in Aging Neuroscience.* 2014 Aug 29; 6:230.

111. Rönn T, Poulsen P, Hansson O, et al. Age influences DNA methylation and gene expression of COX7A1 in human skeletal muscle. *Diabetologia.* 2008 Jul 1;51(7):1159.

112. Davegårdh C, García-Calzón S, Bacos K, Ling C. DNA methylation in the pathogenesis of type 2 diabetes in humans. *Molecular Metabolism.* 2018 Aug 1;14:12–25.

113. Willmer T, Johnson R, Louw J, Pheiffer C. Blood-based DNA methylation biomarkers for type 2 diabetes: Potential for clinical applications. *Frontiers in Endocrinology.* 2018 Dec 4;9:744.

114. Zhou Z, Sun B, Li X, Zhu C. DNA methylation landscapes in the pathogenesis of type 2 diabetes mellitus. *Nutrition & Metabolism.* 2018 Dec 1;15(1):47.

115. Singh R, Chandel S, Dey D, Ghosh A, Roy S, Ravichandiran V, Ghosh D. Epigenetic modification and therapeutic targets of diabetes mellitus. *Bioscience Reports.* 2020 Sep 30;40(9).

116. Poy MN, Eliasson L, Krutzfeldt J, et al. A pancreatic islet-specific microRNA regulates insulin secretion. *Nature.* 2004 Nov;432(7014):226–30.

117. Poy MN, Spranger M, Stoffel M. microRNAs and the regulation of glucose and lipid metabolism. *Diabetes, Obesity and Metabolism.* 2007 Nov;9:67–73.

118. Tugay K, Guay C, Marques AC, Allagnat F, Locke JM, Harries LW, Rutter GA, Regazzi R. Role of microRNAs in the age-associated decline of pancreatic beta cell function in rat islets. *Diabetologia.* 2016 Jan 1;59(1):161–9.

119. Guarente L, Kenyon C. Genetic pathways that regulate ageing in model organisms. *Nature.* 2000 Nov;408(6809):255–62.

120. Ram JL, Costa II AJ. Invertebrates as model organisms for research on aging biology. In *Conn's Handbook of Models for Human Aging* 2018 Jan 1 (pp. 445–452). Academic Press.

121. Vanhooren V, Libert C. The mouse as a model organism in aging research: Usefulness, pitfalls and possibilities. *Ageing Research Reviews.* 2013 Jan 1;12(1):8–21.

122. Pun PB, Gruber J, Tang SY, Schaffer S, Ong RL, Fong S, Ng LF, Cheah I, Halliwell B. Ageing in nematodes: Do antioxidants extend lifespan in Caenorhabditiselegans? *Biogerontology.* 2010 Feb 1;11(1):17–30.

123. Dahiya R, Mohammad T, Alajmi MF, Rehman M, Hasan GM, Hussain A, Hassan M. Insights into the Conserved Regulatory Mechanisms of Human and Yeast Aging. *Biomolecules.* 2020 Jun;10(6):882.

124. Wierman MB, Smith JS. Yeast sirtuins and the regulation of aging. *FEMS Yeast Research.* 2014 Feb 1;14(1):73–88.

125. Harel I, Benayoun BA, Machado B, et al. A platform for rapid exploration of aging and diseases in a naturally short-lived vertebrate. *Cell.* 2015 Feb 26;160(5):1013–26.

126. Boehm M, Slack F. A developmental timing microRNA and its target regulate life span in C. elegans. *Science.* 2005 Dec 23;310(5756):1954–7.

127. Kato M, Chen X, Inukai S, Zhao H, Slack FJ. Age-associated changes in expression of small, noncoding RNAs, including microRNAs, in C. elegans. *RNA.* 2011 Oct 1;17(10):1804–20.

128. Kato M, Slack FJ. Ageing and the small, non-coding RNA world. *Ageing Research Reviews.* 2013 Jan 1;12(1):429–35.

129. Lee RC, Feinbaum RL, Ambros V. The C. elegansheterochronic gene lin-4 encodes small RNAs with antisense complementarity to lin-14. *cell.* 1993 Dec 3;75(5): 843–54.

130. Inukai S, Pincus Z, De Lencastre A, Slack FJ. A microRNA feedback loop regulates global microRNA abundance during aging. *RNA.* 2018 Feb 1;24(2):159–72.

131. Pu M, Ni Z, Wang M, et al. Trimethylation of Lys36 on H3 restricts gene expression change during aging and impacts life span. *Genes & Development.* 2015 Apr 1;29(7):718–31.

132. Greer EL, Maures TJ, Ucar D, et al. Transgenerational epigenetic inheritance of longevity in Caenorhabditiselegans. *Nature.* 2011 Nov;479(7373):365–71.

133. Greer EL, Blanco MA, Gu L, et al. DNA methylation on N6-adenine in C. elegans. *Cell.* 2015 May 7;161(4):868–78.

134. Srinivasan DG, Brisson JA. Aphids: A model for polyphenism and epigenetics. *Genetics Research International.* 2012;2012.

135. Kucharski R, Maleszka J, Foret S, Maleszka R. Nutritional control of reproductive status in honeybees via DNA methylation. *Science.* 2008 Mar 28;319(5871):1827–30.

136. Kamakura M. Royalactin induces queen differentiation in honeybees. *Nature.* 2011 May;473(7348):478–83.
137. Lyko F, Foret S, Kucharski R, Wolf S, Falckenhayn C, Maleszka R. The honey bee epigenomes: Differential methylation of brain DNA in queens and workers. *PLoS Biol.* 2010 Nov 2;8(11):e1000506.
138. Halim MA, Tan FH, Azlan A, et al. Ageing, Drosophila melanogaster and Epigenetics. *The Malaysian Journal of Medical Sciences: MJMS.* 2020 May;27(3):7.
139. Siebold AP, Banerjee R, Tie F, Kiss DL, Moskowitz J, Harte PJ. Polycomb Repressive Complex 2 and Trithorax modulate Drosophila longevity and stress resistance. *Proceedings of the National Academy of Sciences.* 2010 Jan 5;107(1):169–74.
140. Liu M, Barnes VL, Pile LA. Disruption of methionine metabolism in Drosophila melanogaster impacts histone methylation and results in loss of viability. *G3: Genes, Genomes, Genetics.* 2016 Jan 1;6(1): 121–32.
141. Mukherjee K, Fischer R, Vilcinskas A. Histone acetylation mediates epigenetic regulation of transcriptional reprogramming in insects during metamorphosis, wounding and infection. *Frontiers in Zoology.* 2012 Dec 1;9(1):25.
142. Liu B, Wang Z, Zhang L, Ghosh S, Zheng H, Zhou Z. Depleting the methyltransferase Suv39h1 improves DNA repair and extends lifespan in a progeria mouse model. *Nature Communications.* 2013 May 21;4(1):1–2.
143. Ocampo A, Reddy P, Martinez-Redondo P, et al. In vivo amelioration of age-associated hallmarks by partial reprogramming. *Cell.* 2016 Dec 15;167(7):1719–33.
144. Pollina EA, Brunet A. Epigenetic regulation of aging stem cells. *Oncogene.* 2011 Jul;30(28):3105–26.
145. Neves J, Sousa-Victor P, Jasper H. Rejuvenating strategies for stem cell-based therapies in aging. *Cell Stem Cell.* 2017 Feb 2;20(2):161–75.
146. Wang T, Tsui B, Kreisberg JF, et al. Epigenetic aging signatures in mice livers are slowed by dwarfism, calorie restriction and rapamycin treatment. *Genome Biology.* 2017 Dec 1;18(1):57.
147. Xie K, Ryan DP, Pearson BL, et al. Epigenetic alterations in longevity regulators, reduced life span, and exacerbated aging-related pathology in old father offspring mice. *Proceedings of the National Academy of Sciences.* 2018 Mar 6;115(10): E2348–57.
148. Horii T, Morita S, Hino S, et al. Successful generation of epigenetic disease model mice by targeted demethylation of the epigenome. *Genome Biology.* 2020 Dec;21: 1–7.
149. Rakyan VK, Down TA, Balding DJ, Beck S. Epigenome-wide association studies for common human diseases. *Nature Reviews Genetics.* 2011 Aug;12(8):529–41.
150. Choi SW, Friso S. Epigenetics: A new bridge between nutrition and health. *Advances in Nutrition.* 2010 Nov;1(1):8–16.
151. Biesalski HK, Dragsted LO, Elmadfa I, et al. Bioactive compounds: Definition and assessment of activity. *Nutrition.* 2009 Nov 1;25(11–12):1202–5.
152. Davis CD, Ross SA. Dietary components impact histone modifications and cancer risk. *Nutrition Reviews.* 2007 Feb 1;65(2):88–94.
153. Friso S, Choi SW. Gene-nutrient interactions and DNA methylation. *The Journal of Nutrition.* 2002 Aug 1;132(8):2382S–7S.
154. Mathers JC, Ford D. Nutrition, epigenetics and aging. *Nutrients and Epigenetics.* 2009 May 7:175–205.
155. Jackson-Rosario SE, Self WT. Targeting selenium metabolism and selenoproteins: Novel avenues for drug discovery. *Metallomics.* 2010;2(2):112–6.
156. Davis CD, Uthus EO. Dietary folate and selenium affect dimethylhydrazine-induced aberrant crypt formation, global DNA methylation and one-carbon metabolism in rats. *The Journal of Nutrition.* 2003 Sep 1;133(9):2907–14.
157. Uthus EO, Yokoi K, Davis CD. Selenium deficiency in Fisher-344 rats decreases plasma and tissue homocysteine concentrations and alters plasma homocysteine and cysteine redox status. *The Journal of Nutrition.* 2002 Jun 1;132(6):1122–8.

158. Uthus EO, Ross SA. Dietary selenium affects homocysteine metabolism differently in Fisher-344 rats and CD-1 mice. *The Journal of Nutrition.* 2007 May 1;137(5):1132–6.

159. Xiang N, Zhao R, Song G, Zhong W. Selenite reactivates silenced genes by modifying DNA methylation and histones in prostate cancer cells. *Carcinogenesis.* 2008 Nov 1;29(11):2175–81.

160. Davis CD, Uthus EO, Finley JW. Dietary selenium and arsenic affect DNA methylation in vitro in Caco-2 cells and in vivo in rat liver and colon. *The Journal of Nutrition.* 2000 Dec 1;130(12):2903–9.

161. Spyrou G, Björnstedt M, Kumar S, Holmgren A. AP-1 DNA-binding activity is inhibited by selenite and selenodiglutathione. *FEBS Letters.* 1995 Jul 10;368(1):59–63.

162. Boyanapalli SS, Kong AN. "Curcumin, the king of spices": Epigenetic regulatory mechanisms in the prevention of cancer, neurological, and inflammatory diseases. *Current Pharmacology Reports.* 2015 Apr 1;1(2):129–39.

163. Stępień K, Wojdyła D, Nowak K, Młoń M. Impact of curcumin on replicative and chronological aging in the Saccharomyces cerevisiae yeast. *Biogerontology.* 2020 Feb 1;21(1): 109–23.

164. Pirmoradi S, Fathi E, Farahzadi R, Pilehvar-Soltanahmadi Y, Zarghami N. Curcumin affects adipose tissue-derived mesenchymal stem cell aging through TERT gene expression. *Drug Research.* 2018 Apr;68(04):213–21.

165. Receno CN, Liang C, Korol DL, DeRuisseau KC. Curcumin supplementation effects on aging skeletal muscle. *The FASEB Journal.* 2017 Apr;31(1_supplement):1021–22.

166. Goel A, Aggarwal BB. Curcumin, the golden spice from Indian saffron, is a chemosensitizer and radiosensitizer for tumors and chemoprotector and radioprotector for normal organs. *Nutrition and Cancer.* 2010 Sep 23;62(7):919–30.

167. Marcu MG, Jung YJ, Lee S, Chung EJ, Lee MJ, Trepel J, Neckers L. Curcumin is an inhibitor of p300 histone acetylatransferase. *Medicinal Chemistry.* 2006 Mar 1;2(2):169–74.

168. Kang SK, Cha SH, Jeon HG. Curcumin-induced histone hypoacetylation enhances caspase-3-dependent glioma cell death and neurogenesis of neural progenitor cells. *Stem cells and Development.* 2006 Apr 1;15(2):165–74.

169. Sak K. Site-specific anticancer effects of dietary flavonoid quercetin. *Nutrition and Cancer.* 2014 Feb 1;66(2):177–93.

170. Warnsmann V, Hainbuch S, Osiewacz HD. Quercetin-induced lifespan extension in Podosporaanserina requires methylation of the flavonoid by the O-methyltransferase PaMTH1. *Frontiers in Genetics.* 2018 May 4;9:160.

171. Wang H, Jo YJ, Oh JS, Kim NH. Quercetin delays postovulatory aging of mouse oocytes by regulating SIRT expression and MPF activity. *Oncotarget.* 2017 Jun 13; 8(24):38631.

172. Patel D, Shukla S, Gupta S. Apigenin and cancer chemoprevention: Progress, potential and promise. *International Journal of Oncology.* 2007 Jan 1;30(1):233–45.

173. Birt DF, Hendrich S, Wang W. Dietary agents in cancer prevention: Flavonoids and isoflavonoids. *Pharmacology & Therapeutics.* 2001 May 1;90(2–3):157–77.

174. Surh YJ. Cancer chemoprevention with dietary phytochemicals. *Nature Reviews Cancer.* 2003 Dec;3(10):768–80.

175. Manach C, Scalbert A, Morand C, Rémésy C, Jiménez L. Polyphenols: Food sources and bioavailability. *The American Journal of Clinical Nutrition.* 2004 May 1;79(5):727–47.

176. Birt DF, Walker B, Tibbels MG, Bresnick E. Anti-mutagenesis and anti-promotion by apigenin, robinetin and indole-3-carbinol. *Carcinogenesis.* 1986 Jun 1;7(6):959–63.

177. Wei H, Tye L, Bresnick E, Birt DF. Inhibitory effect of apigenin, a plant flavonoid, on epidermal ornithine decarboxylase and skin tumor promotion in mice. *Cancer Research.* 1990 Feb 1;50(3):499–502.

178. Choi JS, Islam MN, Ali MY, Kim EJ, Kim YM, Jung HA. Effects of C-glycosylation on anti-diabetic, anti-Alzheimer's disease and anti-inflammatory potential of apigenin. *Food and Chemical Toxicology.* 2014 Feb 1;64:27–33.

179. Banerjee K, Mandal M. Oxidative stress triggered by naturally occurring flavone apigenin results in senescence and chemotherapeutic effect in human colorectal cancer cells. *Redox Biology*. 2015 Aug 1;5:153–62.

180. Sang Y, Zhang F, Wang H, et al. Apigenin exhibits protective effects in a mouse model of d-galactose-induced aging via activating the Nrf2 pathway. *Food & Function*. 2017;8(6):2331–40.

181. Choi S, Youn J, Kim K, et al. Apigenin inhibits UVA-induced cytotoxicity in vitro and prevents signs of skin aging in vivo. *International Journal of Molecular Medicine*. 2016 Aug 1;38(2):627–34.

182. Fang M, Chen D, Yang CS. Dietary polyphenols may affect DNA methylation. *The Journal of Nutrition*. 2007 Jan 1;137(1):223S–8S.

183. Zhang Y, Wang X, Han L, Zhou Y, Sun S. Green tea polyphenol EGCG reverse cisplatin resistance of A549/DDP cell line through candidate genes demethylation. *Biomedicine & Pharmacotherapy*. 2015 Feb 1;69:285–90.

184. Berletch JB, Liu C, Love WK, Andrews LG, Katiyar SK, Tollefsbol TO. Epigenetic and genetic mechanisms contribute to telomerase inhibition by EGCG. *Journal of Cellular Biochemistry*. 2008 Feb 1;103(2):509–19.

185. Wang Y, Li M, Xu X, Song M, Tao H, Bai Y. Green tea epigallocatechin-3-gallate (EGCG) promotes neural progenitor cell proliferation and sonic hedgehog pathway activation during adult hippocampal neurogenesis. *Molecular Nutrition & Food Research*. 2012 Aug;56(8):1292–303.

186. Fang MZ, Wang Y, Ai N, Hou Z, Sun Y, Lu H, Welsh W, Yang CS. Tea polyphenol (–)-epigallocatechin-3-gallate inhibits DNA methyltransferase and reactivates methylation-silenced genes in cancer cell lines. *Cancer Research*. 2003 Nov 15;63(22):7563–70.

187. Lee WJ, Shim JY, Zhu BT. Mechanisms for the inhibition of DNA methyltransferases by tea catechins and bioflavonoids. *Molecular Pharmacology*. 2005 Oct 1;68(4):1018–30.

188. Balasubramanyam K, Altaf M, Varier RA, et al. Polyisoprenylatedbenzophenone, garcinol, a natural histone acetyltransferase inhibitor, represses chromatin transcription and alters global gene expression. *Journal of Biological Chemistry*. 2004 Aug 6;279(32):33716–26.

189. Pogribny IP, Tryndyak VP, Muskhelishvili L, Rusyn I, Ross SA. Methyl deficiency, alterations in global histone modifications, and carcinogenesis. *The Journal of Nutrition*. 2007 Jan 1;137(1):216S–22S.

190. Nandakumar V, Vaid M, Katiyar SK. (–)-Epigallocatechin-3-gallate reactivates silenced tumor suppressor genes, Cip1/p21 and p 16 INK4a, by reducing DNA methylation and increasing histones acetylation in human skin cancer cells. *Carcinogenesis*. 2011 Apr 1;32(4):537–44.

191. Hardy TM, Tollefsbol TO. Epigenetic diet: Impact on the epigenome and cancer. *Epigenomics*. 2011 Aug;3(4):503–18.

192. Bauer JH, Goupil S, Garber GB, Helfand SL. An accelerated assay for the identification of lifespan-extending interventions in Drosophila melanogaster. *Proceedings of the National Academy of Sciences*. 2004 Aug 31;101(35):12980–5.

193. Jarolim S, Millen J, Heeren G, Laun P, Goldfarb DS, Breitenbach M. A novel assay for replicative lifespan in Saccharomyces cerevisiae. *FEMS Yeast Research*. 2004 Nov 1;5(2):169–77.

194. Agarwal B, Baur JA. Resveratrol and life extension. *Annals of the New York Academy of Sciences*. 2011 Jan;1215(1):138–43.

195. Rascón B, Hubbard BP, Sinclair DA, Amdam GV. The lifespan extension effects of resveratrol are conserved in the honey bee and may be driven by a mechanism related to caloric restriction. *Aging (Albany NY)*. 2012 Jul;4(7):499.

196. Barger JL, Kayo T, Vann JM, et al. A low dose of dietary resveratrol partially mimics caloric restriction and retards aging parameters in mice. *PLoS One*. 2008 Jun 4;3(6):e2264.

197. Baur JA, Pearson KJ, Price NL, et al. Resveratrol improves health and survival of mice on a high-calorie diet. *Nature*. 2006 Nov;444(7117):337–42.
198. Qin W, Zhang K, Clarke K, Weiland T, Sauter ER. Methylation and miRNA effects of resveratrol on mammary tumors vs. normal tissue. *Nutrition and Cancer*. 2014 Feb 1;66(2):270–7.
199. Dhar S, Kumar A, Zhang L, et al. Dietary pterostilbene is a novel MTA1-targeted chemopreventive and therapeutic agent in prostate cancer. *Oncotarget*. 2016 Apr 5;7(14):18469.
200. Liu D, Ma Z, Xu L, Zhang X, Qiao S, Yuan J. PGC1α activation by pterostilbene ameliorates acute doxorubicin cardiotoxicity by reducing oxidative stress via enhancing AMPK and SIRT1 cascades. *Aging (Albany NY)*. 2019 Nov 30;11(22):10061.
201. Kala R, Shah HN, Martin SL, Tollefsbol TO. Epigenetic-based combinatorial resveratrol and pterostilbene alters DNA damage response by affecting SIRT1 and DNMT enzyme expression, including SIRT1-dependent γ-H2AX and telomerase regulation in triple-negative breast cancer. *BMC Cancer*. 2015 Dec;15(1):1–8.
202. Meeran SM, Ahmed A, Tollefsbol TO. Epigenetic targets of bioactive dietary components for cancer prevention and therapy. *Clinical Epigenetics*. 2010 Dec 1;1(3–4): 101–16.
203. Dolinoy DC, Weidman JR, Waterland RA, Jirtle RL. Maternal genistein alters coat color and protects Avy mouse offspring from obesity by modifying the fetal epigenome. *Environmental Health Perspectives*. 2006 Apr;114(4):567–72.
204. Sato N, Yamakawa N, Masuda M, Sudo K, Hatada I, Muramatsu M. Genome-wide DNA methylation analysis reveals phytoestrogen modification of promoter methylation patterns during embryonic stem cell differentiation. *PLoS One*. 2011 Apr 29; 6(4):e19278.
205. Fang MZ, Chen D, Sun Y, Jin Z, Christman JK, Yang CS. Reversal of hypermethylation and reactivation of p16INK4a, RARβ, and MGMT genes by genistein and other isoflavones from soy. *Clinical Cancer Research*. 2005 Oct 1;11(19):7033–41.
206. Iovine B, Iannella ML, Gasparri F, Monfrecola G, Bevilacqua MA. Synergic effect of genistein and daidzein on UVB-induced DNA damage: An effective photoprotective combination. *Journal of Biomedicine and Biotechnology*. 2011 Jan 1;2011.
207. Li Y, Chen F, Wei A, Bi F, Zhu X, Yin S, Lin W, Cao W. Klotho recovery by genistein via promoter histone acetylation and DNA demethylation mitigates renal fibrosis in mice. *Journal of Molecular Medicine*. 2019 Apr 12;97(4):541–52.
208. Tuorkey MJ. Cancer therapy with phytochemicals: Present and future perspectives. *Biomedical and Environmental Sciences*. 2015 Nov 1;28(11):808–19.
209. Myzak MC, Tong P, Dashwood WM, Dashwood RH, Ho E. Sulforaphane retards the growth of human PC-3 xenografts and inhibits HDAC activity in human subjects. *Experimental Biology and Medicine*. 2007 Feb;232(2):227–34.
210. Tortorella SM, Royce SG, Licciardi PV, Karagiannis TC. Dietary sulforaphane in cancer chemoprevention: The role of epigenetic regulation and HDAC inhibition. *Antioxidants & Redox Signaling*. 2015 Jun 1;22(16):1382–424.
211. Kubo E, Chhunchha B, Singh P, Sasaki H, Singh DP. Sulforaphane reactivates cellular antioxidant defense by inducing Nrf2/ARE/Prdx6 activity during aging and oxidative stress. *Scientific Reports*. 2017 Oct 26;7(1):1–7.
212. Greco T, Shafer J, Fiskum G. Sulforaphane inhibits mitochondrial permeability transition and oxidative stress. *Free Radical Biology and Medicine*. 2011 Dec 15;51(12):2164–71.
213. Daniel M, Tollefsbol TO. Epigenetic linkage of aging, cancer and nutrition. *Journal of Experimental Biology*. 2015 Jan 1;218(1):59–70.
214. Talalay P, Fahey JW, Healy ZR, et al. Sulforaphane mobilizes cellular defenses that protect skin against damage by UV radiation. *Proceedings of the National Academy of Sciences*. 2007 Oct 30;104(44):17500–5.

215. Zhu M, Zhang Y, Cooper S, Sikorski E, Rohwer J, Bowden GT. Phase II enzyme inducer, sulforaphane, inhibits UVB-induced AP-1 activation in human keratinocytes by a novel mechanism. *Molecular Carcinogenesis: Published in Cooperation with the University of Texas MD Anderson Cancer Center.* 2004 Nov;41(3):179–86.

216. Grünwald S, Stellzig J, Adam IV, Weber K, Binger S, Boll M, Knorr E, Twyman RM, Vilcinskas A, Wenzel U. Longevity in the red flour beetle Triboliumcastaneum is enhanced by broccoli and depends on nrf-2, jnk-1 and foxo-1 homologous genes. *Genes & Nutrition.* 2013 Sep;8(5):439–48.

217. Riggs MG, Whittaker RG, Neumann JR, Ingram VM. n-Butyrate causes histone modification in HeLa and Friend erythroleukaemia cells. *Nature.* 1977 Aug;268(5619):462–4.

218. Huuskonen J, Suuronen T, Nuutinen T, Kyrylenko S, Salminen A. Regulation of microglial inflammatory response by sodium butyrate and short-chain fatty acids. *British Journal of Pharmacology.* 2004 Mar;141(5):874–80.

219. Sarkar S, Abujamra AL, Loew JE, Forman LW, Perrine SP, Faller DV. Histone deacetylase inhibitors reverse CpG methylation by regulating DNMT1 through ERK signaling. *Anticancer Research.* 2011 Sep 1;31(9):2723–32.

220. Shin H, Kim JH, Lee YS, Lee YC. Change in gene expression profiles of secreted frizzled-related proteins (SFRPs) by sodium butyrate in gastric cancers: Induction of promoter demethylation and histone modification causing inhibition of Wntsignaling. *International Journal of Oncology.* 2012 May 1;40(5):1533–42.

221. Wei YB, Melas PA, Wegener G, Mathé AA, Lavebratt C. Antidepressant-like effect of sodium butyrate is associated with an increase in TET1 and in 5-hydroxymethylation levels in the Bdnf gene. *International Journal of Neuropsychopharmacology.* 2015 Feb 1;18(2).

222. Kundu P, Lee HU, Garcia-Perez I, et al. Neurogenesis and prolongevitysignaling in young germ-free mice transplanted with the gut microbiota of old mice. *Science Translational Medicine.* 2019 Nov 13;11(518).

223. Walsh ME, Bhattacharya A, Sataranatarajan K, Qaisar R, Sloane L, Rahman MM, Kinter M, Van Remmen H. The histone deacetylase inhibitor butyrate improves metabolism and reduces muscle atrophy during aging. *Aging Cell.* 2015 Dec;14(6):957–70.

224. Matt SM, Allen JM, Lawson MA, Mailing LJ, Woods JA, Johnson RW. Butyrate and dietary soluble fiber improve neuroinflammation associated with aging in mice. *Frontiers in Immunology.* 2018 Aug 14;9:1832.

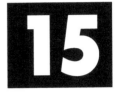

Cancer during Aging and Nutraceuticals for Prevention and Mitigation

Shruti U. Rawal
Nirma University

Jayvadan Patel
Sankalchand Patel University

Mayur M. Patel
Nirma University

Contents

DOI: 10.1201/9781003110866-15

15.1 Introduction

Cancer demographics suggest the population of the age group >50 years to be at higher risk of developing cancer [1]. The fact is backed by statistical data that demonstrate the population group aged 50 years to contribute to higher incidence rates (~90% of the total cancer cases recorded in the USA) [1,2]. Advanced medical interventions have increased life expectancies of the human population by an average of two to three decades. Consequently, the prevalence of age-related diseases like cancer has increased immensely. The scientists express grave concern over the globally advancing oncological scenario and implore a unified approach to mitigate its spread. Still worse, the current lifestyle and nutritional deficit have resulted in the early onset of aging and related diseases like cancer, obesity and diabetes [3]. The scientific explorations to date have astonishingly revealed immense etiological similarity between aging and cancer. However, relating clinical oncology with biogerontology is still defied by the complexity of cellular senescence, mutational and malignant transformations, lack of clinical data from the aged population, and diversity in molecular, microenvironmental and mutational landscapes [1,2,4]. While the scientists still struggle with ambiguities relating to these processes, there is growing epidemiological evidence that conveys the explicit role of nutraceuticals and dietary interventions in the prevention as well as treatment of cancer. The recent clinical and epigenetic evidence on the preventive and mitigative roles of nutraceuticals in numerous malignancies like prostate, breast and colorectal cancer has opened new grounds for researchers and oncologists.

Nutraceuticals offer an enormous repertoire of chemopreventive and anticancer agents that can substantially prevent and mitigate several types of cancers and can be used safely in the aged population. Unlike the currently used anticancer therapeutics, the nutraceuticals have been observed to exert chemopreventive activity in addition to their anticancer activity. Other overwhelming advantages of employing a nutraceutical-based approach over other approaches for cancer are no severe side-effects, maintenance of positive energy-balance, prevention and treatment of cancer cachexia, more economical and multi-modal therapeutic activity, and usable over a long duration. Nutraceuticals belonging to a diverse class of bioactives such as terpenoids, phenolics, indoles, organo-sulfur compounds, isothiocyanates, fatty acids (mono- and poly-unsaturated fatty acids), allyl compounds, vitamins, minerals and prebiotics have been reported to have immense anticancer potential [5–7]. Nutraceuticals have been reported to influence various cellular and physiological processes such as cel-lular senescence, DNA methylation and repair, cellular growth and differentia-tion, oxidative stress, mitochondrial functions, apoptosis, inflammation, etc. [8–11].

Nutraceuticals have congregated enough evidence to favor their utilization as a futuristic approach for healthy aging and better longevity. This can be attributed to their potential to relegate mutational phenotypic selection upon evolving cellular and microenvironmental landscapes, a major malefactor in tumorigenesis as well as aging [2]. The present chapter recapitulates the theo-ries relating aging to carcinogenesis, nutraceuticals employed for the preven-tion and mitigation of cancer, molecular targets of their anticancer activity, novel approaches for enhancing their anticancer potential, and perspectives. Recent updates and supportive and critical arguments germane to the claims of nutraceuticals as anti-aging and anticancer complementary medicine have been incorporated to address the interest of readers of the rapidly advancing segments like biogerontology and oncology.

15.2 Aging: a high-risk factor for cancer

Aging has not only been associated with higher cancer susceptibility but also with higher resultant mortality. Most of the cancer-associated deaths have been reported in patients aged >65 years [12]. "Aging" and "cancer" are among the most difficult domains to be that await to be explored beyond the extant perimeters. Despite tremendous scientific and medical advances, the complex oncogeraitric co-ordination is still surrounded by ambiguities.

There is no unanimous theory that adequately describes the process of aging. According to a theory, aging is "persistent physiological deterioration and resultant degradation of an organism's fitness components" [13]. While aging is an evolutionary trait, carcinogenesis is not. Numerous posits attempt to link carcinogenesis with aging and try to explain the dynamic alterations in cellular and physiological microenvironmental and mutational settings. Table 15.1 correlates the physiological and cellular alterations between can-cer and aging.

The interplay of numerous intrinsic and extrinsic factors has been associ-ated with higher oncological incidences and deaths. Although there is limited knowledge in this regard, some of the well-evidenced contributive factors that correlate aging and cancer have been summarized as follows.

Table 15.1 Altered Physiological, Epigenetic and Cellular Features Upon Aging and in Cancer

Aging	Cancer
Increased genomic instability	Increased genomic instability
Global DNA hypomethylation	Hypermethylation of tumor suppressor gene Hypomethylation of oncogenic complexes
miR-17–92 downregulation	miR-17–92 upregulation
Impaired chaperoning	Augmented chaperoning
Proteosomal activity and autophagy-lysosome activity	Proteosomal activity and autophagy-lysosome activity
Insulin inhibition and mTOR lifespan increment	Inhibition of insulin and antineoplastic mTOR signaling
Increased cell senescence	Senescence observed in premalignant condition but evaded in fully malignant tumors
Exhausted stem cell	Tumorigenesis through potential nidus

15.2.1 Intrinsic, extrinsic, or inherited mutations, genetic instability and epigenetic alterations

Alteration(s) in the DNA sequence is termed as "mutation". Mutations may be inherited or may have a sporadic origin. Aging has been identified to dictate the process of somatic evolution by governing tissue microenvironmental alterations [2]. There are numerous intrinsic (cell division), inherited (MMR mutation, BRCA1/BRCA2 mutations) and extrinsic (excessive alcohol consumption, smoking, etc.) assaults that increase the chances of cancer upon aging. These risk factors give rise to phenotypic evolutions as a part of the process of adaptive somatic evolution, some of which may result in oncogenic mutations and eventually, carcinogenesis. Mutations in tumor suppressor genes, free radical-associated DNA damage and impaired DNA repair result in phenotypic tissue evolution such as higher preneoplastic cell population, insufficient purging of dysfunctional cells and consequently higher chances of oncogenesis.

Besides these, epigenetic alterations (altered genetic expression without change in DNA sequence) like noncoding DNA, chromatin remodeling, DNA methylation and histone modifications have also been associated well with cancer and neoplastic proliferation [14].

15.2.2 Dysregulated "Hayflick limit", senescence and telomere shortening

It was established long back in 1960 by Hayflick and Moorhead that the cells undergo finite divisions before they approach the stage of growth arrest. The effect termed as "Hayflick limit" refers to a physiological response that prevents genomic instability and cumulation of DNA damage through the process of telomere shortening upon every cell division. The phenomenon is now referred to as "replicative senescence." However, any insult like metabolic, oncogenic, or genotoxic stress can induce accelerated senescence response, also termed as "stress-induced premature senescence (SIPS)" that progresses without the telomere shortening process. Cellular senescence is associated with the deteriorated physiological performance of tissues and accumulation upon aging and has also been associated with pathologies. Senescence is one of the most important phenomena that play a central role in various phases of tumorigenesis like initiation, proliferation, progression and escape. The complex role and mechanisms of senescence in cancer upon aging has been explained succinctly in the review by Calcinotto [4]. Several nutraceutical agents participate directly or indirectly in the process of senescence. Some of the well-evidenced nutraceuticals that exert anticancer activity through their senolytic properties are piperlongumine, nicotinamide riboside, quercetin and fisetin.

A strong association of mortality to telomere length has also been established. Shorter telomere lengths have been well associated with higher age-related morbidity and mortality. Telomere length has been evidenced to be inherited. Upregulated human telomerase reverse transcriptase (hTERT) is a well-identified hallmark of cancer. The cells with upregulated telomerase expression dodge the Hayflick limit and do not undergo apoptosis, leading to telomere attrition and a higher risk of carcinogenesis [14].

15.2.3 Compromised immunity

Compromised immunity upon aging is one of the most important factors that contribute to cancer development. It has been established that the immunoregulation process is adversely affected upon aging. Aging has been associated with a remarkable reduction in T-cell function and proliferation, which eventually results in a reduced population of the naïve T-cells and accumulation of the memory cells. B-cell colony formation has also been reported to be reduced upon aging. "Paraproteinemia" characterized by monoclonal gammopathy of undetermined significance has been well correlated with declination in life expectancy by almost 2 years as compared to the age-matched unaffected control group subjects. At least 15%–30% of the individuals with benign monoclonal gammopathy develop myeloma over 30 years. Declined T-cell functions, altered cytokines, reduced IL-2 levels, and increased IL-6 levels are important hallmarks of age-related diseases like Alzheimer's disease, osteoporosis and myeloma [1].

15.2.4 Dysregulated proteostasis and Autophagy malfunction

Proteome homeostasis (proteostasis) has been identified to play a central role in several age-related diseases including cancer. Proteostasis mechanisms encompass processes like chaperone (heat shock protein HSPs)-mediated protein folding, proteasomal degradation and lysosome-mediated autophagy. Disturbed proteostasis and the resultant cumulation of misfolded and proteo-toxic components have been associated with compromised cell vitality and functioning.

Small chemical motifs/molecules involved in folding or refolding of the polypeptide to proteins and degradation of misfolded/unfolded polypeptide are termed as chaperones orco-chaperones. They play important evolutionary roles in cell differentiation, genetic expression, replication of DNA, cellular signaling and transduction, immune system regulation, senescence, apoptosis and carcinogenesis. Proteostasis targeted drugs have been recognized as potential anticancer agents in preclinical and clinical trials also.

Two of the main proteolytic mechanisms include ubiquitin-proteasome and autophagy-lysosomal pathways. There has been an indirect relationship between aging and proteasome activation. Proteosome activators like dietary fatty acids, spices, pollens and several other synthetic agents have been reported to aid in healthy aging and reduced carcinogenesis. Lysosome-mediated autophagy is one of the major degradation pathways that facilitate cytoplasmic delivery of the materials and disposition of intracellular pathogens, misfolded/unfolded proteins and damaged cell organelles. Autophagy has been established to play a dual role in carcinogenesis. While it promotes tumor growth by some mechanisms, it exerts tumor-suppressive effects otherwise. Malfunctioned autophagy has been associated with malignant transformation of tumors to benign oncocytomas due to the accumulation of defective mitochondria. Dietary intervention that restricts calorie intake is one of the most potent ways to inhibit oncogenesis and tumor proliferation through several signaling pathways like upregulation of sirtuin and inhibition of mTOR, involved in autophagy. Nutraceuticals like spermidine and resveratrol have been well-established to increase lifespan, enhance autophagy and improve prognosis [14].

15.2.5 Dysfunctional cell purging and cell competition

The cellular and tissue landscapes are maintained by several mechanisms that involve quality control of the healthy tissues through efficient purging and elimination of dysfunctional or abnormal cells. Apoptotic and senescent mechanisms are the major intrinsic mechanisms that govern the changing mutational and adaptive landscapes of cells and tissues. It has been reported that with advancing age, there is a considerable reduction in cell functionality and purging due to impaired feedforward loop. The higher the damaged cells, the less efficient the purging, the higher the damaged cell accumulation and tissue decline. The declined ability of cellular resilience to respond and recover from acute environmental perturbations is typical of aging and is considered to be one of the contributive factors for carcinogenesis [2].

15.2.6 Decontrolled nutrient sensing and mitochondrial malfunction

Aging is most often associated with higher visceral fat, insulin resistance, reduced lean muscle mass and increased muscle red fibers with defective mitochondria, featuring in most of the age-related morbidities including cancer.

Insulin and IGF signaling has been evidenced to constrain cell apoptosis and stimulate cell division and cell proliferation of genetically modified cells, thereby increasing the risk of prostate cancer, colorectal cancer and breast cancer. Higher circulating levels of insulin-like growth factor-binding protein 3 (IGFBP3) and insulin-like growth factor (IGF1) have been evidenced to have various implications in the development, progression and differentiation of various cancers including prostate cancer, breast cancer and colorectal cancer. Nutrient sensing pathways like mTOR (a member of the phosphatidylinositol 3-kinase-related kinase family of protein kinases) and AMP kinase pathways have been well associated with cellular growth, metabolism, proliferation and longevity. Downregulation of mTOR pathways has been well evidenced to significantly extend the longevity in mammals [14].

15.2.7 Age-related frailty

Frailty refers to a syndrome that develops as a result of different age-interactive mechanisms like chronic inflammation, comorbidity, sarcopenia and dysregulated multiple physiology. Frailty develops chronically and has both environmental and inherited causes. Frailty also refers to the degree of susceptibility to stress and has been well correlated with cancer prognosis and survival. Frailty is often assessed as one of the most important comprehensive geriatric assessment (CGA) tools in terms of the frailty index (FI). FI is one of the true determinants of physiological age and is a term that refers to degrees of personally accumulated functional deficits. Lower the frailty, higher the prognosis and lower the risk of cancer upon aging. Frailty is a factor that can be best managed with nutraceuticals and dietary interventions [12].

15.3 Common mechanisms and molecular targets of chemopreventive and anticancer nutraceuticals

Some of the pathways through which nutraceuticals exert chemopreventive and anticancer activity while promoting healthy aging have been summarized in this section.

15.3.1 Oxidative stress regulation

One of the well-accepted mechanisms of carcinogenesis upon aging is high oxidative stress and compromised xenobiotic defense. Free radicals like superoxide ion, peroxy and hydroxyl radical and singlet oxygen often referred to as reactive oxygen species (ROS) are often evidenced to contribute to higher oxidative stress, cell damage and mutations, cumulatively leading to a higher risk of carcinogenesis. ROS cause DNA strand and base cleavage and have also been established manipulators of cellular signaling, affecting expression and/or activation of numerous kinases/transcription factors, thereby leading to diminished, reversed, or annulled antioxidant activity. Several nutraceuticals exert their chemopreventive action by preventing cellular damage and DNA mutation through a potent antioxidant and free radical scavenging activity [15].

15.3.2 Cytoprotective enzyme activation and defense mechanisms

The agents that inhibit carcinogenesis through interrupting the DNA-carcinogen adduct formation are termed as blocking agents. These agents exhibit chemopreventive action and inhibit tumor growth and differentiation through manipulation of the enzymes that are pivotal in the metabolism and activation of pro-carcinogens. Ascorbic acid has been established to prevent carcinogen uptake through inhibition of phase-I metabolizing enzymes and induction of phase-II metabolizing enzymes, respectively. Similarly, S-allyl cysteine and diallyl sulfides have been reported to reduce benzopyrene-DNA adduct formation *in-vitro* [16].

15.3.2.1 Inhibition of phase I metabolizing enzymes

Enzymes of cytochrome P450 (CYP450) family (also termed as phase I metabolizing enzymes) play a central role in cancer initiation through the metabolism of extrinsic pro-carcinogens to reactive biomolecular adducts through the bioactivation process. Curcumin has been well evidenced to exhibit chemopreventive action through inhibition of the phase I metabolizing enzymes like CYP 450 isoforms and the CYP 450 reductase upon exposure to toxins or pro-carcinogen metabolites (reactive intermediates/ electrophiles) [17].

15.3.2.2 Induction of phase II metabolizing enzymes

Phase II enzymes lower the toxicity, increase the water solubility and aid in the elimination of the intermediates formed upon phase-I metabolism of the pro-carcinogens [18]. The phase II enzymes often form conjugates of the drug with glucuronic acid or glutathione (GSH) to facilitate the same.

Nutraceuticals derived from *Moringa Oleifera* have been reported to detoxify the carcinogens through induction of phase II metabolizing enzymes and through E2 related factor 2 (NrF2) mediated cell defense pathways, and it will be discussed in the forthcoming section [19].

15.3.3 Modulation in signal transduction

There are several mechanisms by which the body maintains homeostasis and defends against extrinsic and intrinsic carcinogens like electrophiles and oxidants [20]. Several signaling pathways have been reported to get involved upon being subjected to oxidative and electrophilic stress. One of the most important signaling pathways that have been established to play a centralized role in the process of carcinogencsis, inflammation, and the oxidative and toxin-induced stress response is the Keap1-Nrf2-ARE signaling pathway [21]. Upon exposure to such stress, the antioxidant response elements abbreviated as AREs induce upstream signaling that is present on the responsive gene in multiple or single replicates. Thereafter, the Nrf2 binds to the AREs to facilitate the expression of the genes regulated by the AREs [21]. The NrF2 activity is closely regulated by its retention in the cell cytoplasm upon binding with repressor protein Keap1 and consequent proteasomal degradation. Nutraceuticals like some terpenoids, certain flavonoids [21], isothiocyanates, chlorophyllin, glucosinolates [22], etc. have been reported to induce the chemoprotective and detoxifying enzymes. Sulphoraphanes have been established to induce gene expression upon direct interaction with Keap1 [23]. Some of the phytoconstituents that are most prominent chemoprotective enzyme inducers include lycopene, carotenoids, triterpenoids, genistein, coumarins, flavonoids, capsaicin, allicin, resveratrol and epigallocatechin-3-gallate (EGCG) [21].

Growth receptor-mediated signal modulation is yet another transduction mechanism that operates through the activation of the mitogen-activated protein kinase (MAPK) pathway, upregulating the tyrosine kinase receptors. MAPK activation results in platelet-derived or epidermal growth factors (PDGFs and EGFs)-mediated activation of extracellular-regulated kinases (ERK1 and ERK2), leading to cell proliferation and differentiation upon stimulation. Yet another important signaling pathway that plays a central role in tumorigenesis is the pathway regulated by the NF-κB/Rel transcription factor family. Numerous nutraceutical inhibitors of this pathway have been well reported to induce apoptosis, regulate cell responses like inflammation, proliferation, etc., and inhibit tumorigenesis [24,25]. EGCG has been reported to inhibit extracellular ERK1/2 phosphorylation and suppress the p38 MAPK pathway in the human fibroblast HT1080 cells [26].

Upon exposure to pro-inflammatory cytokine tumor necrosis factor-a (TNF-a), the cells express inflammatory genes through activation of NF-kB. TNF is one of the well-established growth factors for inflammation and tumorigenesis. Inflammatory mediators derived from arachidonic acid metabolism through COX and the LOX pathways such as IL-8, iNOS and platelet-activating factor have been well correlated with higher tumorigenic potential and carcinogenesis. Nutraceuticals that intervene in the expression and stimulation of these inflammatory mediators are proven chemopreventive agents [15]. Peroxidase activity of COX has been well correlated to activate pro-carcinogens to carcinogens. Cysteine protease, cathepsin B, produced through. LOX-produced 12(S)-hydroxyeicosatetraenoic acids activation results in reduced surface integrin receptor expression, leading to lower cell adhesion, consequently tumor metastasis and higher cell invasion [27,28].

15.3.4 Cell apoptosis

Programmed cell death, also termed apoptosis involves death receptor-mediated (extrinsic) as well as mitochondrial (intrinsic) pathways. Some nutraceuticals natural ligands to death receptors like Fas (overexpressed over cell surfaces), lead to receptor clustering and forming death-inducing Signaling Complex (DISC). The complex has been known to recruit procaspase-8 and activate caspase-8 to cleave it further to caspase-3 and lead to cell apoptosis.

Release of cytochrome c upon being subjected to cellular stress or due to lack of survival factors cause activation of caspase-9 mediated pathway and consequently caspase-3 activation. Caspase-3 has been associated with the cleavage of numerous cellular processes and signaling transduction. Gingerols derived from ginger rhizomes are well-reported apoptosis inducers [29].

15.3.5 Senolytic and anti-senescence activity

Nutraceuticals like tocotrienols, quercetin and piperlongumine have been reported to exert senolytic properties while nutraceuticals like curcumin, quercetin naringenin, apigenin, kaempferol, EGCG, genistein, resveratrol, pterostilbene, vitamin B 3 complex and NAD+ have been associated with anti-SASP activity. Some other nutraceuticals that have been reported for their anti-senescence activity include phloroglucinol, ginsenosides, oleacin, oleuopein, spermedine and urolithins [10]. The mode of action by which nutraceuticals regulate senescence-associated with aging and cancer has been schematically described in Figure 15.1.

15.4 Nutraceuticals for prevention, treatment and mitigation of cancer in the geriatric population

Several nutraceuticals have phytoconstituents that help in healthy aging and have immense chemopreventive and anticancer activities. Some of the dietary nutraceuticals with well-established chemopreventive and anticancer activity include are derived from food sources like tomatoes (lycopene), capsicum and green chilies (capsaicin), turmeric (curcuminoids), garlic and onion (allicin, diallyl sulfide), fennel and other umbelliferae fruits (anethole and other terpenoids), carrots (ß-carotene), rhododendron cinnabarium (quercetin), grapes (resveratrol), cabbage, cauliflower (sulphoraphane, indole-3-carbinol, apigenin), propolis (caffeic acid phenylester), ginger (gingerol), green tea (epigallocatechin gallate), citrus fruits (tangeretin), silymarin (silibinin) and soya beans (daidzein, genistein) [7].

15.4.1 Polyphenols

Polyphenolic compounds are one of the most prevalent phytoconstituents present in fruits, leaves, seeds, flowers and barks of several plants and herbs.

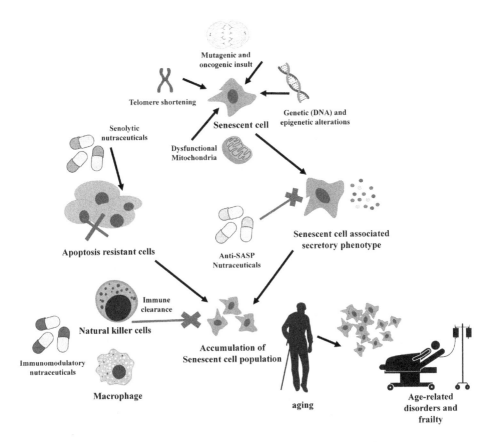

Figure 15.1 Impact of nutraceuticals on senescence in cancer and aging.

Polyphenolic agents encompass wide range of compounds like flavonoids, lignans, stilbenes and curcuminoids, with molecular weights ranging from 100 to 30,000 Da [30].

a. **Flavonoids**:

Polyphenolic compounds that bear flavan (2-phenyl-1,4-benzopyrone) nucleus with galloyl, methoxy, hydroxyl or glycoside substitutions are classified as flavonoids. With approximately 5050 well identified structures, the flavanoids constitute more than 60% of the dietary polyphenolic intake. Some of the most widely researched flavonoids with strong chemopreventive and anticancer activity are: anthocyanins (cyanidin, apigenidin), flavan-3-ols like (+) catechin, (−) epigallocatechin gallate (EGCG), flavanones (naringenin, taxifolin, hesperidin), flavones (gingerols, naringenin, taxifolin, hesperidin, Rutin, luteolin, apigenin, chrysin), flavonols (quercetin, myricetin) and isoflavonoids (soy isoflavones like genistein and daidzein), flavonolignans (silymarin) and phenolic acids (gallic acid, caffeic acid, capsaicin) [31].

Various flavonoids have been reported for their anti-aging, anticancer and chemopreventive actions in several forms of cancers including the lung, colorectal, prostate, breast and pancreatic cancers [32–34]. Proposed modes of action of these flavonoids are: ROS and nitrogen free radical scavenging activity, inhibition of ROS-generating enzymes, redox-reactive metal chelation and cytoprotective gene induction. Flavonoids are mechanistically blocking agents that prevent DNA damage through ROS mediated insults through antioxidant, redox-interactions and regulation of the expression of NFκB and Nrf2 genes [31,35].

b. **Lignans**:

These fiber-associated phenolic dimers are mostly present in their glycosidic forms in minor quantities in several herbs, plants and functional foods like nuts, grains, wine, vegetables, tea and coffee. Linseed/flax seeds have highest amount of lignin known as secoisolariciresinol diglucoside. Some of the common lignans like matairesinol, lariciresinol, sesamin and pinoresinol are some other dietary lignans. The lignan metabolites produced upon their metabolism by intestinal metabolism like enterolactone, enterodiol and enterolignans have been well reported to prevent the risk of colorectal cancer. The lignan metabolites reduce cancer risk due to their antioxidant and free radical scavenging properties. Also, they have been reported to induce NADPH: quinone reductase detoxification enzymes and hence prevent colon cancer. Wheat bran lignans have also been shown to inhibit intestinal neoplasia due to their apoptotic and cytostatic properties. Furofuran lignans derived from sesame have been associated with the suppression of NF-Kb [36].

c. **Stilbenes**:

Stilbenes are chemically phytoalexins with diarylethene nucleus that is synthesized by almost 70 plant species upon pathogenic stress. Resveratrol and pterostilbene are two of the most established anti-aging, chemopreventive and anticancer agents. Resveratrol (3,5,4′-trihydroxy-*trans*-stilbene) is one of the most potent anticancer agents present in the skin of red grapes, red wine, peanuts and berries. Anticancer and chemopreventive activities of resveratrol can be attributed to its ability to activate sirtuin (SIRT)-1, a histone deacetylase (HDAC) enzyme with various pharmacological roles. Activation of SIRT-1 prevents carcinogenic molecular aberrations, aids in DNA repair, regulates cell cycle, cell survival, apoptosis and inflammatory response [37]. Resveratrol has been reported to reduce preneoplastic lesions, tumor multiplicity and tumor incidences in several cancer cell lines, preclinical and clinical models of prostate, breast, colorectal and skin cancer [38–40]. However, further studies are in need to suffice clinical evidence of its tumor suppressive, apoptotic and anti-inflammatory activities. The problem of bioavailability and lack of supporting evidence to determine its influence on oncological pathways mediated by Bcl-2, NFκB, growth factor receptor, Nrf2 and PI3K/Akt/mTOR undermines realization of this otherwise potent molecule [7].

d. **Curcuminoids**:

Curcuma longa rhizomes, traditionally named as turmeric or golden spice is the source of three distinct polyphenolic phytoconstituents collectively termed as "curcuminoids". Curcuminoids comprise of diarylheptanoids or diferuloylmethane derivatives such as curcumin, tetrahydrocurcumin, turmerones, bisdemethoxycurcumin and demethoxycurcumin. Among these, curcumin is one of the most extensively explored phytoconstituent that exhibits several health benefits besides its chemopreventive, anticancer and anti-aging actions. Curcumin exerts its chemopreventive and anticancer activity through multiple molecular interventions encompassing a wide range of molecular targets such as carcinogen blocking, free-radical scavenging ability, antioxidant activity, growth factor regulation, pro-apoptotic and apoptotic action, inhibition of tumor proliferation, epigenetic enzyme modifying ability, redox state-modulating ability, immunomodulatory activity, anti-inflammatory activity and transcription factor regulatory action [41–43]. Curcumin has been observed to exhibit anticancer activity against breast cancer, prostate cancer, lung cancer, skin cancer, colorectal cancer, ovarian cancer, oral cancer and several other forms of cancers [44–46].

15.4.2 Terpenoids (terpenes)

Terpenoids are secondary isoprenoid phytometabolites that are present in several plants and herbs. Terpenoids have been classified according to their chemical structure into six different classes such asmono-, di-, tri-, tetra- and poly-terpenes. Several anticancer terpenoids have been reported to exert anticancer activity by several mechanisms like suppression of tumorigenesis, tumor invasion, proliferation, tumor progression and tumor metastasis in addition to apoptotic, anti-angiogenic activity. Some of the most explored anticancer terpenoids include: (i) monoterpenoids like carvacrol (thyme oil), carvone (caraway oil), thymol (thyme oil), thymoquinone (black cumin seeds), limonene (citrus oils), linalool (cinnamon and coarander leaf oils), menthol (peppermint oil), myrcene (verbena oil and bay laurel oil), perrillyl alcohol (grapefruit, bergamot, dill, spearmint, etc.), 1–8-cineole (eucalyptus and rosemary oil), α-β pinene (*Pinus* species) and terpinen-4-ol (tea tree oil, mandarins, lemonwood tree); (ii) sesquiterpenoids like Artemisinin (sweet wormwood) and parthenolide (feverfew); (iii) diterpenoids like Acanthoic acid (*Acanthopanax koreanum*), carnosol (sage), ginkgolides (*Ginkgo biloba*), Tanshinone II A (Danshen) and Taxol (Pacific yew); (iv) triterpenoids like lupeol (aloe, tomato, olives), ursolic acid (holy basil, bilberry), ginsenosides (Asian ginseng) and glycyrrhizin (licorice); and (v) tetraterpenoids like lycopene (tomato), lutein (spinach) and β carotene (carrot). These phytoconstituents have been observed to exhibit anticancer and chemopreventive activity against breast, colorectal, cervical, skin, prostate, hepatic, lung, ovarian cancer, leukemia and neuroma [47].

15.4.3 Alkaloids

A diverse group of phytoconstituents, constituted by ~2,500 compounds with basic nitrogen moiety, present in almost 150 plant species are alkaloids. Some of the most potent anticancer agents such as vincristine, vinblastine (alkaloids from *Vinca rosea* and *Catharanthus roseus*), Camptothecin (*Camptotheca acuminate*), Cryptolepine and Neocryptolepine (*Cryptolepis sanguinolenta*), Sanguinarine (greater *celandine*), Berberine (*Rhizoma coptidis*), Harmaline, tryptoline and harmalol (*Harmina harmane*), Piperine (*Piper nigrum*), Vincamine (*Ambelania occidentalis*), Tylophorinine and Tylophorine (*Tylophora indica*) are some of the most widely explored alkaloids that have been explored against their chemopreventive action against several forms of cancers by several mechanisms of action [48,49].

15.4.4 Organosulphur compounds

Organosulfur compounds from garlic and onion such as allin, allicin, sulfenic acid, diallyl trisulfides and tetrasuslfides have been reported to inhibit tumor cell proliferation selectively. These compounds act by several mechanisms like alteration of nitrosamine formation, antioxidant activity, inhibition of carcinogenic bioactivation, selective cell cycle inhibition, modulation of histone hyper-acetylation and reactivation of tumor suppressor genes through inhibition of cell proliferation [50,51].

Glucosinolates are major organosulfur compounds present in most of the cruciferous vegetables like cabbage, cauliflower, broccoli, watercress, Brussels srpouts and bok choy. Glucosinolates are further of four sub-types such as (i) sulforaphanes; (ii) indole-3-carbinol; (iii) benzyl isothiocyanate, allyl isothiocyanate, allyl thiocyanate and allyl isocyanate; and (iv) glucoiberin, sinigrin and progoitrin. Upon subjecting plants containing these phytoconstituents to mechanical stress, their hydrolysis is initiated due to release of the enzyme myrosinase from their cell walls. In case of thermal inactivation of the myrosinase enzyme, hydrolysis of these compounds occurs by gut bacterial enzymes to release Indoles and isothiocyanates. The sulphoraphanes exert anticancer and chemopreventive action by induction of apoptosis, attenuation of AKT and NFκB signaling pathways, and activation of the Nrf2 pathway. While glucoiberin, sinigrin and progoitrin are chemosuppressive agents that prevent carcinogenesis through induction of Phase II metabolizing enzymes and inhibition of phase I enzymes. The glucosinolates of benzyl iosthiocyanate and indole-3-carbinol class have been reported to be chemopreventive. However, the mechanism of their action is not yet established [51].

15.4.5 Vitamins, micronutrients and minerals

Several vitamins, micronutrients and minerals have been well established for their anti-aging and chemopreventive actions. Higher dietary calcium and vitamin D3 intake has been associated with reduced risks of cancer development [52]. The anticancer role of other vitamins and minerals have been summarized in Table 15.2. Ubiquinone (coenzyme Q 10) is a unique biochemical moiety that plays pivotal role in cellular respiration and generation of ATP. It is a potent antioxidant. Lower levels of this coenzyme have been associated with higher risks of breast cancer and geriatric bipolar disorders [53]. Zinc has been associated with involved in thymic functions, immune functions, DNA synthesis, cellular proliferation and differentiation. Its chemopreventive action has been linked with antioxidant and immunosenescent activity [54].

15.4.6 Probiotics and prebiotics

Probiotics are the microflora of *Lactobacillus* and *Bifidobacterium* species, while prebiotics are chiefly nondigestible oligosaccharides that promote the growth of the further. Probiotics and prebiotics are important to maintain health and homoeostasis. Their imbalance (dysbiosis) has been associated with higher risks of GI disorders and colon cancer. They not only help in preventing colorectal cancer, but also prevent emergence of health conditions like lactose intolerance, malnutrition, constipation and calcium absorption. Mechanistically, colon cancer prevention of these agents may be attributed to their immunomodulatory, detoxification of procarcinogens, anti-inflammatory, pro-apoptotic, antiproliferative and intestinal barrier functions [55,56].

Table 15.2 Role of Micronutrients, Vitamins and Minerals in the Treatment of Several forms of Cancers

Nutraceutical	Mechanism of Action	Cancer
Vitamin A		
Vitamin B complex	Phosphorylation and redox modulation	All cancers
Vitamin D	1,25-dihydroxycholecalciferol	All cancers
Vitamin E (α tocopherol)	Antiproliferative, antioxidant	Breast cancer, prostate cancer, colon cancer
Folic acid	5-Mehthyltetrehydrofolate	All cancers
Copper	Anti-angiogenic, catalase inhibition	All cancers
Zinc	Zn-endopeptidase (MMP) inhibition	All cancers
Calcium	Calmodulin, Ca^{+2} channel modulation	All cancers
Selenium	cdk2, PKC, G1/S DNA breaks	Breast, colon, gastric, pancreatic, intestinal and prostate cancer

15.4.7 Oryzanol

Chemopreventive activity of gamma oryzanol (rice bran oil) has been well established against prostate, breast and intestinal carcinoma. However, the phytochemical still needs to be evaluated for its anticancer activity [57].

15.5 Recent novel approaches for enhanced nutraceutical efficacy

Some novel nutraceutical approaches have been recently explored for enhanced anticancer and chemopreventive efficacy. Some of the promising approaches that have gained significant attention of the scientific community are as follows:

a. **Combination nutraceuticals**:

   Many of the nutraceuticals have been reported to exhibit synergistic anticancer and chemopreventive activity. The fact that the nutraceutical combination exhibits synergism was realized upon observation of anticancer activity only in certain nutraceutical combinations and the absence of such activity upon the individual component analysis. However, the intricacies and logical explanation need to suffice FDA approval for the combination nutraceuticals [58]. Several nutraceutical combinations that have been reported for anticancer efficacy against various types of cancers have been illustrated in Figure 15.2. Curcumin (CUR) in combination with paclitaxel, xanthorrhizol, docosahexenic acid, genistein, sulphinosine, celecoxib, resveratrol and epigallocatechin gallate (EGCG) has been reported to exert excellent anticancer activity against breast, lung and colorectal cancers. Quercetin chalcone (QC) in combination with apigenin, baicalein and genistein, pH-modified citrus pectin (MCP) and EGCG has displayed excellent anticancer activity against breast, colorectal and prostate cancer respectively. The combination of resveratrol (RSV) with estrogen (E2), quercetin and catechin, cyclophosphamide, genistein, 5-fuorouracil and n-butyrate has also been reported to exert anticancer activity against breast, prostate and colon cancer respectively. Combination of sulforaphane with genistein, benzylisothiocyanite, apigenin, 3,3- diindolylmethane (DIM) and dibenzoymethane (DMB) has been reported to exert chemopreventive and anticancer activity against esophagus, colon and pancreas, respectively. Combination of Coltect and 5-aminosalicylic acid (ASA) and the combination of soy, sencha leaves, turmeric, yucca roots, saw palmetto, chamomile flowers and gingko were reported to have anticancer activity against prostate cancer, D-limonene+docetaxcel, tomato powder+broccoli powder, lycopene+ketosamine (fructose/amino acid Fru/His), lycopene and docetaxel was employed for anticancer activity against prostate cancer cells [6].

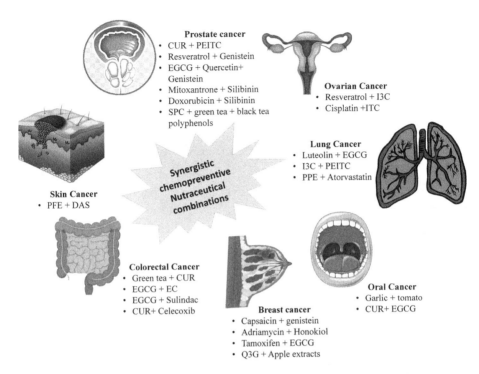

Figure 15.2 *Synergistic nutraceutical combinations in the treatment of various cancers.*

b. **Mucus diffusion enhancers and absorption enhancers**:

   One of the major issues confronted in nutraceuticals is insufficient oral absorption and bioavailability. Considering the fact, a Nutraceutical Bioavailability Classification System (NuBACS) has been devised to classify the nutraceuticals based on issues faced in their oral bioavailability. The parameters such as bioaccessibility, absorption and transformations are taken into consideration for NuBACS-based classification of the nutraceuticals (Figure 15.3) [59]. Considering the criticality of absorption in the oral bioavailability of the nutraceuticals, various approaches like intestinal permeation enhancers, employing protease inhibitor excipients, mucolytics, prodrug formation and encapsulation in delivery vehicles such as nanoparticles have gained popularity [59].

c. **Food matrix design (excipient foods)**:

   Some nutraceutical bioactives have poor bioavailability due to reasons like poor liberation from food matrix poor solubility in the GI environment, poor intestinal permeability and absorption, metabolic instability, etc. Modulation of the food matrix or the addition of some agents that may enhance their liberation, solubility, transport, absorption and transformation can significantly enhance the

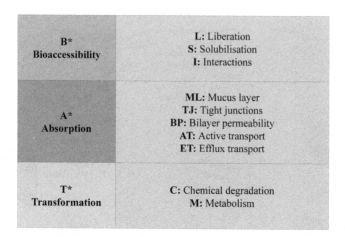

Figure 15.3 *NuBACS classification for nutraceuticals.*

oral bioavailability of nutraceuticals. Excipient food is defined as a food or liquid beverage with constituents that enhance the bioavailability of nutraceuticals or drugs upon co-ingestion. Some of the commonly employed examples of excipient foods are yogurt (probiotics, vitamins, etc.), dessert (phytosterols), salad dressings (carotenoids), beverages, sauces (conjugated linoleic acid, carotenoids, omega-3 and -6 fatty acids, flavonoids, vitamins, etc.), dips, soups (flavonoids, vitamins, minerals, etc.), baked products, candies and spreads (phytosterols, vitamins, etc.). The food matrix containing bio-enhancers like piperine, gingerols, curcumin and quercetin also play a pivotal role in enhancing the absorption of various anticancer phytoconstituents [60].

d. **Nanonutraceuticals:**

Nanotechnology has expanded its application to several sectors including pharmaceutical and nutraceutical delivery. Nanocarriers of several types have been employed to enhance the bioabsorption and bioavailability of nutraceuticals. Some of the nutraceuticals have several issues that render them less efficacious despite being potent anticancer agents when evaluated *in-vitro*. This can be attributed to absorption and metabolism issues mainly. Encapsulation of such nutraceuticals in nanocarrier delivery cargoes can safely deliver such nutraceuticals and enhance their efficacy significantly. Some of the most explored nanocarriers include liposomes, nanoemulsions, niosomes, solid lipid nanoparticles, nanostructured lipid carriers, biopolymeric nanoparticles, polyelectrolyte complexes, protein-carbohydrate (self-assembly structures), nanocapsules and nanocomposite hydrogels [61,62]. Novel nanonutraceutical nanocarriers devised from food matrices have been exemplified in reference [59].

15.6 Outlook

Novel nutraceutical interventions can not only prevent cancer-causing mutations but also preserve cell integrity, maintain physiological homeostasis and slow down the process of aging. Nutraceuticals provide a safe, effective, economical and convenient means to tackle aging, cancer in addition to several other physiological conditions. Despite limited knowledge of the use of nutraceuticals in the allopathic era, several pieces of evidence from traditional and alternative therapies support their safe clinical consumption. Research directed toward understanding the molecular mechanism of action of these nutraceuticals may not only help faster approval of the nutraceuticals as chemopreventive agents but also suggest novel targets for cancer therapy. Novel and traditional nutraceutical bioavailability enhancing approaches, backed with strong preclinical efficacy and safety studies need to be paced toward clinical studies for faster commercialization. Coordination of the global regulatory agencies and the agencies for traditional and alternative medicines across the globe can help gain significant momentum in the race against cancer. Dietary Supplement Health and Education Act (DSHEA) impedes the FDA from regulating dietary supplements due to the unclear delineation of rules for the creation and evaluation of drugs and dietary supplements. Standardization of the rules and standards for manufacture and evaluation of the nutraceuticals and dietary supplements can help the jeopardized, aged population toward healthy and cancer-free life.

Acknowledgment

The authors are grateful to Nirma University for providing the necessary facilities.

References

1. W.B. Ershler, D.L. Longo, Aging and cancer: Issues of basic and clinical science, *J. Natl. Cancer Inst.* 89 (1997) 1489–1497. doi:10.1093/jnci/89.20.1489.
2. E. Laconi, F. Marongiu, J. DeGregori, Cancer as a disease of old age: Changing mutational and microenvironmental landscapes, *Br. J. Cancer.* 122 (2020) 943–952. doi:10.1038/s41416-019-0721–1.
3. G. Carruba, L. Cocciadiferro, A. Di Cristina, O.M. Granata, C. Dolcemascolo, I. Campisi, M. Zarcone, M. Cinquegrani, A. Traina, Nutrition, aging and cancer: Lessons from dietary intervention studies, *Immun. Ageing.* 13 (2016) 1–9. doi:10.1186/s12979-016-0069-9.
4. A. Calcinotto, J. Kohli, E. Zagato, L. Pellegrini, M. Demaria, A. Alimonti, Cellular senescence: Aging, cancer, and injury, *Physiol. Rev.* 99 (2019) 1047–1078. doi:10.1152/physrev.00020.2018.
5. B. Villeponteau, R. Cockrell, J. Feng, Nutraceutical interventions may delay aging and the age-related diseases, *Exp. Gerontol.* 35 (2000) 1405–1417. doi:10.1016/S0531-5565(00)00182-0.

6. S.N. Saldanha, T.O. Tollefsbol, The role of nutraceuticals in chemoprevention and chemotherapy and their clinical outcomes, *J. Oncol.* 2012 (2012). doi:10.1155/2012/192464.
7. D. Bagchi, H.G. Preuss, A. Swaroop, Nutraceuticals and functional foods in human health and disease prevention, 2015. doi:10.1201/b19308.
8. K.H. Kwon, A. Barve, S. Yu, M.T. Huang, A.N.T. Kong, Cancer chemoprevention by phytochemicals: Potential molecular targets, biomarkers and animal models, *Acta Pharmacol. Sin.* 28 (2007) 1409–1421. doi:10.1111/j.1745-7254.2007.00694.x.
9. M. Wargovich, Nutraceutical use in late-stage cancer, *Cancer Metastasis.* 29 (2010) 503–510. doi:10.1007/s10555-010-9240-5.
10. F. Gurău, S. Baldoni, F. Prattichizzo, E. Espinosa, F. Amenta, A.D. Procopio, M.C. Albertini, M. Bonafè, F. Olivieri, Anti-senescence compounds: A potential nutraceutical approach to healthy aging, *Ageing Res. Rev.* 46 (2018) 14–31. doi:10.1016/j.arr.2018.05.001.
11. D. Vranesic-Bender, The role of nutraceuticals in anti-aging medicine, *Acta Clin. Croat.* 49 (2010) 537–544. doi:10.1016/j.ucl.2013.08.003.
12. M. Extermann, Cancer and aging from bench to clinics, in: T. Fulop (Ed.), *Interdiscip. Top. Gerontol.*, Karger, Basel, 2013.
13. A. Galloway, The evolutionary biology of aging., *Am. J. Phys. Anthropol.* 91 (1993) 260–262. doi:10.1002/ajpa.1330910217.
14. J.R. Aunan, W.C. Cho, K. Søreide, The biology of aging and cancer: A brief overview of shared and divergent molecular hallmarks, *Aging Dis.* 8 (2017) 628–642. doi:10.14336/AD.2017.0103.
15. V.J. Bhatia, S.S. Nair, Nutraceuticals as potential chemopreventive agents: A review, *Nat. Prod. J.* 8 (2018) 3–13. doi: 10.2174/2210315507666170613101649.
16. H.L. Nicastro, S.A. Ross, J.A. Milner, Garlic and onions: their cancer prevention properties., *Cancer Prev. Res. (Phila).* 8 (2015) 181–189. doi:10.1158/1940-6207.CAPR-14-0172.
17. M. Imran, A. Ullah, F. Saeed, M. Nadeem, M.U. Arshad, H.A.R. Suleria, Cucurmin, anticancer, & antitumor perspectives: A comprehensive review, *Crit. Rev. Food Sci. Nutr.* 58 (2018) 1271–1293. doi:10.1080/10408398.2016.1252711.
18. X.-L. Tan, S. Spivack, Dietary chemoprevention strategies for induction of phase II xenobiotic-metabolizing enzymes in lung carcinogenesis: A review, *Lung Cancer.* 65 (2009) 129–137. doi:10.1016/j.lungcan.2009.01.002.Dietary.
19. N.A. Abd Karim, M.D. Ibrahim, S.B. Kntayya, Y. Rukayadi, H.A. Hamid, A.F.A. Razis, Moringa oleifera Lam: Targeting chemoprevention, *Asian Pacific J. Cancer Prev.* 17 (2016) 3675–3686. doi:10.14456/apjcp.2016.155/APJCP.2016.17.8.3675.
20. M. Margaret Pratt, A.P. Reddy, J.D. Hendricks, C. Pereira, T.W. Kensler, G.S. Bailey, The importance of carcinogen dose in chemoprevention studies: Quantitative interrelationships between, dibenzo[a,l]pyrene dose, chlorophyllin dose, target organ DNA adduct biomarkers and final tumor outcome, *Carcinogenesis.* 28 (2007) 611–624. doi:10.1093/carcin/bgl174.
21. J. Fahey, T. Kensler, Role of dietary supplements/nutraceuticals in chemoprevention through induction of cytoprotective enzymes, *Chem. Res. Toxicol.* 20 (2007) 572–576. doi:10.1021/tx7000450.
22. JW Fahey, KL Wade, KK Stephenson, et al. Bioavailability of sulforaphane following ingestion of glucoraphanin-rich broccoli sprout and seed extracts with active myrosinase: A pilot study of the effects of proton pump inhibitor administration. *Nutrients.* 2019 Jun;11(7). DOI: 10.3390/ nu11071489. PMID: 31261930; PMCID: PMC6682992.
23. F. Hong, M.L. Freeman, D.C. Liebler, Identification of sensor cysteines in human Keap1 modified by the cancer chemopreventive agent sulforaphane, *Chem. Res. Toxicol.* 18 (2005) 1917–1926. doi:10.1021/tx0502138.
24. Y.-J. Surh, J.K. Kundu, H.-K. Na, J.-S. Lee, Redox-sensitive transcription factors as prime targets for chemoprevention with anti-inflammatory and antioxidative phytochemicals, *J. Nutr.* 135 (2005) 2993S–3001S. doi:10.1093/jn/135.12.2993S.

25. H.A.R. Suleria, M.S. Butt, N. Khalid, S. Sultan, A. Raza, M. Aleem, M. Abbas, Garlic (Allium sativum): Diet based therapy of 21st century – A review, *Asian Pacific J. Trop. Dis.* 5 (2015) 271–278. doi:10.1016/S2222-1808(14)60782-9.

26. L. Chen, H.-Y. Zhang, Cancer preventive mechanisms of the green tea polyphenol (-)-epigallocatechin-3-gallate, *Molecules.* 12 (2007) 946–957. doi:10.3390/12050946.

27. V.E. Steele, Current mechanistic approaches to the chemoprevention of cancer, *J. Biochem. Mol. Biol.* 36 (2003) 78–81. doi:10.5483/bmbrep.2003.36.1.078.

28. V.E. Steele, E.T. Hawk, J.L. Viner, R.A. Lubet, Mechanisms and applications of non-steroidal anti-inflammatory drugs in the chemoprevention of cancer, *Mutat. Res. Mol. Mech. Mutagen.* 523–524 (2003) 137–144. doi:https://doi.org/10.1016/S0027-5107(02)00329-9.

29. S. Abdullah, S.A.Z. Abidin, N. Morad, S. Makpol, W.Z.W. Ngah, Y. Mohd Yusof, Ginger extract (Zingiber officinale) triggers apoptosis and G0/G1 cells arrest in HCT 116 and HT 29 colon cancer cell lines, *Afr J Biochem Res.* 4 (2010) 134–142.

30. A. Crozier, I.B. Jaganath, M.N. Clifford, Dietary phenolics: Chemistry, bioavailability and effects on health, *Nat. Prod. Rep.* 26 (2009) 1001–1043. doi:10.1039/b802662a.

31. K. Heim, Natural polyphenol and flavonoid polymers, in: Antioxid. Polym. Synth. Prop. Appl., 2012. doi:10.1002/9781118445440.ch2.

32. Y. Cui, H. Morgenstern, S. Greenland, Dietary flavonoid intake and lung cancer – A population based case control study, *Cancer.* 112 (2008) 2241–2248. doi:10.1117/12.2549369. Hyperspectral.

33. D. Romagnolo, O. Selmin, Flavonoids and cancer prevention: A review of the evidence, *J. Nutr. Gerontol. Geriatr.* 31 (2012) 206–238. doi:10.1080/21551197.2012.702534.

34. H. Amawi, C.R. Ashby, A.K. Tiwari, Cancer chemoprevention through dietary flavonoids: What's limiting? *Chin. J. Cancer.* 36 (2017) 1–13. doi:10.1186/s40880-017-0217-4.

35. W. BORS, C. MICHEL, Chemistry of the antioxidant effect of polyphenols, *Ann. N. Y. Acad. Sci.* 957 (2002) 57–69. doi:10.1111/j.1749-6632.2002.tb02905.x.

36. S.C. Yoder, S.M. Lancaster, M.A.J. Hullar, J.W. Lampe, Chapter 7- gut microbial metabolism of plant lignans: Influence on human health, in: K. Tuohy, D. Del Rio (Eds.), *Diet-Microbe Interact. Gut*, Academic Press, San Diego, 2015: pp. 103–117. doi:10.1016/B978-0-12-407825-3.00007-1.

37. M.C. Haigis, D.A. Sinclair, Mammalian sirtuins: Biological insights and disease relevance, *Annu. Rev. Pathol. Mech. Dis.* 5 (2010) 253–295. doi:10.1146/annurev.pathol.4.110807.092250.

38. M. Calvani, A. Pasha, C. Favre, Nutraceutical boom in cancer: Inside the labyrinth of reactive oxygen species, *Int. J. Mol. Sci.* 21 (2020). doi:10.3390/ijms21061936.

39. X.Y. Mao, M.Z. Jin, J.F. Chen, H.H. Zhou, W.L. Jin, Live or let die: Neuroprotective and anti-cancer effects of nutraceutical antioxidants, *Pharmacol. Ther.* 183 (2018) 137–151. doi:10.1016/j.pharmthera.2017.10.012.

40. J.A. McCubrey, K. Lertpiriyapong, L.S. Steelman, S.L. Abrams, L. V. Yang, R.M. Murata, P.L. Rosalen, A. Scalisi, L.M. Neri, L. Cocco, S. Ratti, A.M. Martelli, P. Laidler, J. Dulinska-Litewka, D. Rakus, A. Gizak, P. Lombardi, F. Nicoletti, S. Candido, M. Libra, G. Montalto, M. Cervello, Effects of resveratrol, curcumin, berberine and other nutraceuticals on aging, cancer development, cancer stem cells and microRNAs, *Aging (Albany. NY).* 9 (2017) 1477–1536. doi:10.18632/aging.101250.

41. B. Aggrawal, M. Kuiken, L. Iyer, K. Harikumar, S. Bokyung, Molecular Targets of nutraceuticals derived from dietary spices: Potential role in suppression of inflammation and tumorigenesis, *Exp. Biol Med.* 234 (2009) 825–849. doi:10.3181/0902-MR-78.

42. S. Park, D.H. Cho, L. Andera, N. Suh, I. Kim, Curcumin enhances TRAIL-induced apoptosis of breast cancer cells by regulating apoptosis-related proteins, *Mol. Cell. Biochem.* 383 (2013) 39–48. doi:10.1007/s11010-013-1752-1.

43. N.G. Vallianou, A. Evangelopoulos, N. Schizas, C. Kazazis, Curcumin and Sp-1, *Anticancer Res.* 652 (2015) 645–651.

44. S. Prasad, S.C. Gupta, A.K. Tyagi, B.B. Aggarwal, Curcumin, a component of golden spice: From bedside to bench and back, *Biotechnol. Adv.* 32 (2014) 1053–1064. doi:10.1016/j.biotechadv.2014.04.004.

45. A. Goel, B.B. Aggarwal, Curcumin, the golden spice from Indian saffron, is a chemosensitizer and radiosensitizer for tumors and chemoprotector and radioprotector for normal organs, *Nutr. Cancer.* 62 (2010) 919–930. doi:10.1080/01635581.2010.509835.

46. H.J. Mehta, V. Patel, R.T. Sadikot, Curcumin and lung cancer – A review, *Target. Oncol.* 9 (2014) 295–310. doi:10.1007/s11523-014-0321-1.

47. M.S. Akhtar, H.C. Practices, Natural bio-active compounds, 2019. doi:10.1007/978-981-13-7205-6.

48. S. Khattak, H. Khan, Anti-cancer potential of phyto-alkaloids: A prospective review, *Curr. Cancer Ther. Rev.* 12 (2016) 66–75. doi:10.2174/1573394712666160617081638.

49. K. Mohan, R. Jeyachandran, Alkaloids as anticancer agents, *Ann. Phytomedicine.* 1 (2012) 46–53.

50. J.A. Milner, Mechanisms By Which Garlic and Allyl Sulfur Compounds Suppress Garlic : Its Historical Usage and Current, (1997).

51. N. Mi ekus, K. Marszałek, M. Podlacha, A. Iqbal, C. Puchalski, A.H. Swiergiel, Health benefits of plant-derived sulfur compounds, glucosinolates, and organosulfur compounds, *Molecules.* 25 (2020). doi:10.3390/molecules25173804.

52. M. Meehan, S. Penckofer, The role of vitamin D in the aging adult, *J. Aging Gerontol.* 2 (2014) 60–71. doi:10.12974/2309-6128.2014.02.02.1.

53. T.Y. Wu, C.P. Chen, T.R. Jinn, Traditional Chinese medicines and Alzheimer's disease, *Taiwan. J. Obstet. Gynecol.* 50 (2011) 131–135. doi:10.1016/j.tjog.2011.04.004.

54. H. Haase, L. Rink, The immune system and the impact of zinc during aging, *Immun. Ageing.* 6 (2009) 1–17. doi:10.1186/1742–4933–6–9.

55. D.M. Patel, S. Rawal, J. Patel, Nutraceutical's role in proliferation and prevention of colorectal cancer, in: 2019: pp. 61–114. doi:10.1201/9780429489129-4.

56. P. Ambalam, M. Raman, R.K. Purama, M. Doble, Probiotics, prebiotics and colorectal cancer prevention, *Best Pract. Res. Clin. Gastroenterol.* 30 (2016) 119–131. doi:10.1016/j.bpg.2016.02.009.

57. R.D. Verschoyle, P. Greaves, H. Cai, R.E. Edwards, W.P. Steward, A.J. Gescher, Evaluation of the cancer chemopreventive efficacy of rice bran in genetic mouse models of breast, prostate and intestinal carcinogenesis, *Br. J. Cancer.* 96 (2007) 248–254. doi:10.1038/sj.bjc.6603539.

58. Y. Shukla, J. George, Combinatorial strategies employing nutraceuticals for cancer development, *Ann. N. Y. Acad. Sci.* 1229 (2011) 162–175. doi:10.1111/j.1749-6632.2011.06104.x.

59. J.P. Gleeson, S.M. Ryan, D.J. Brayden, Oral delivery strategies for nutraceuticals: Delivery vehicles and absorption enhancers, *Trends Food Sci. Technol.* 53 (2016) 90–101. doi:10.1016/j.tifs.2016.05.007.

60. D.J. McClements, H. Xiao, Excipient foods: Designing food matrices that improve the oral bioavailability of pharmaceuticals and nutraceuticals, *Food Funct.* 5 (2014) 1320–1333. doi:10.1039/c4fo00100a.

61. P.K. Singh, H. Singh, *Challenges in the Development of Functional Foods: Role of Nanotechnology*, CRC Press, Boca Raton, 2017.

62. A.M. Grumezescu, (Nanotechnology in the agri-food industry (ScienceDirect (Firm)) volume 4) Alexandru Grumezescu-Nutraceuticals. Nanotechnology in the Agri-Food Industry Volume 4-Academic Press (2016), n.d.

16

Gastrointestinal Tract and Digestion Challenges in Aging and Nutraceuticals

Rajiv Dahiya
The University of the West Indies

Sunita Dahiya
University of Puerto Rico

Contents

DOI: 10.1201/9781003110866-16

16.1 Introduction

Aging is a multidimensional biological process characterized by temporal continuity and heterogeneity at cellular, somatic and molecular levels. The ability of being modulated during the aging process is marked by diverse physical, social and physiological modifications during the pathway of the life [1]. The age of the elderly or the senior citizens varies globally. The 'elderly' are the persons aged 60 years or above according to the 'National Policy on Older', whereas a country is said to be 'aging' if 7% of population reaches the age of above 65 years [2]. Early alterations in gene expression and cumulative cell damage are the basis of some aging theories [3]. Aging influences various physical, physiological and cognitive functions in the human body. In normal aging, all physiological processes face irreversible changes which progress with age. The speed of the functional weakening differs with the organ system, yet nearly consistent within a given system [3]. A crucial step for the treatment of the elderly is that the regular age-associated functional weakening occurring within all persons are critically differentiated with the functional loss marked by the beginning of various pathological changes occurring due to diseased pathology in the older persons [4].

This chapter discusses the functional weakening of the aging gastrointestinal tract (GIT) and the consequences of malnutrition on the health status of the elderly. The alternations in the aging GIT including the mechanical disintegration and swallowing of food, gastrointestinal motility and food digestion which may cause various gastrointestinal disorders as well as nutraceuticals which are beneficial to the aging GIT are discussed.

16.2 The aging GIT

16.2.1 Effect of aging on gastrointestinal motor functions

16.2.1.1 Esophageal motility

The primary reason for age-related changes in esophageal functions is disturbed esophageal motility which includes reduced peristaltic response, increased nonperistaltic response, slow transit time or diminished relaxation of the lower sphincter while swallowing [5]. The decreased peristalsis and delayed transit may cause swallowing difficulties (dysphagia), which may cause an intentionally decreased food intake and reduced caloric consumption. The lower two-third region of the esophagus shows nonperistaltic contractions, leading to a rare esophageal motility disorder in the distal esophagus (corkscrew esophagus) [6]. In the elderly, a reduced relaxation of the lower esophageal sphincter upon swallowing is a common cause of achalasia [7]. Overall esophageal function is well-preserved in older adults; however, disturbances in the function of the lower esophageal sphincter are common [8]. Lower esophageal sphincter pressure is characteristically elevated in the elderly with dysphagia, leading to the swallow-induced incomplete relaxation [9]. High resolution manometry was used to characterize motor dysfunctions of the swallowing mechanism, paying specific attention on motility of lower esophageal sphincter [10]. The studies revealed that healthy older people possessed a reduced percentage of swallows with complete lower esophageal sphincter relaxation as compared to the young adults and demonstrated a higher integrated relaxation pressure [11]. The decreased amplitude of the peristaltic waves reduces clearance of the esophageal contents and lengthens the reflux episodes leading to not only dysphagia but also to the gastroesophageal reflux diseases (GERD) which are commonly exacerbated by nondigestive disease [12].

16.2.1.2 Gastric emptying and small intestinal transit

The consequences of aging on gastrointestinal motility are still controversial [13]. The gamma camera technique was employed to determine the gastric emptying and small intestine transit rates in the elderly of mean age above 80 years. The gastric emptying, small intestinal transit and postprandial frequency of antral contractions remained unaffected with aging [14]. However, radio labelled liquids or digestible solids were found to be emptied at slower rates from the stomach of the elderly as compared to that of younger patients.

The electrogastrography and the (13)C-acetate breath test were used to study the gastric motility of active and inactive elderly [15]. The studies revealed the reduced post-prandial peristalsis and gastric contractile force in the elderly; however, the decrease was greater in the inactive group than in the active group of the elderly [16]. Moreover, the lipid was found to cause a slowdown in gastric motor function and gastric motility in healthy elderly persons. It was found that the lipid-based delay in gastric motility is increased in the elderly; however, the lipase administration promotes the emptying of lipid from the stomach [17]. In rodent species, the aging enteric nervous system caused age-related neurodegeneration of the enteric nervous system [18]. However, such study results have been conflicting, keeping the mechanisms of slower gastric emptying in the elderly still ill-understood [18].

16.2.1.3 Colonic transit

The tendency of a longer colonic transit time in the elderly was evidenced from a study on healthy elderly of age greater than 80 years. It was indicated that the regular aging process tends to decrease the propellant efficiency of the colon [13,19], which might be assigned to age-related changes in neurons and receptors of the enteric nervous system [19]. It is suggested that the decline in the colonic enteric neurons starts relatively early in the human life. This creates significant decreases in submucosal and myenteric plexuses which in turn leads to a reduced release of neurotransmitters, making only fewer neurons available to respond to the signals [20]. In addition, researchers proposed the role of decreased neuronal nitric oxide synthase (NOS) expression with simultaneous reduction in synthesis of NO in the aging colon [21]. In old rat colonic preparations, a 50% reduced release of acetylcholine was reported in response to electrical stimulation. Modifications in colonic functioning and persistent constipation are outcomes of the regular aging process. It is also found that the colonic tissues of the older animals exhibited reduced secretory responses to nicotinic agonists as compared to that of younger animals [22].

16.2.2 Effect of aging on gastrointestinal histology

Aging affects gastrointestinal histology by changing the structural features of the gastrointestinal layers. Aging also affects motor functions of the GIT due to the activities of muscles present in different layers of the GIT. For instance, the muscles of the digestive apparatus assure proper chewing and disintegration of the food in the mouth, swallowing of the food contents, digestion of the food and intestinal wall functionality for movement of luminal contents through the digestive tract as well as elimination of undigested food wastes from the body. Aging brings about changes in the GIT including the gastrointestinal mucosal growth, carcinogenesis, gastrointestinal secretions and transit, bacterial growth and small bowel changes as well as malnutrition.

16.2.2.1 Gastrointestinal mucosal growth control

The constant cell renewal process maintains the structural and the functional integrity of the GIT mucosa [23]. The aging was found to be associated with increased mucosal proliferative activity of the GIT of Fischer-344 rats, while the functional properties were found to be either decreased or remain unchanged with aging [23]. Also, basal gastric acid, pepsin and gastrin secretions declined, while antral gastrin levels and mucosal histidine decarboxylase activity increased during aging [24]. The age-associated reduction in gastrin secretion could be partially contributed by elevated somatostatin to gastrin cells ratio in the antral mucosa but not to the mucosal proliferative activity of either gastrin or bombesin [25]. Contrarily, epidermal growth factor (EGF) and transforming growth factor-alpha (TGF-alpha) regulated mucosal growth during aging due to (i) higher levels of membrane-bound TGF-alpha precursors followed by increased activation EGFR signaling processes; (ii) higher sensitivity of mucosal EGFR to EGF and TGF-alpha, requiring lower levels of these peptides to activate EGFR; and (iii) loss of ERRP (EGFR-related protein) which are 'negative regulator' of EGFR [26,27].

Additionally, growth and biological development of gastrointestinal tissues get disturbed in the presence of injury, starvation or refeeding which is regulated by nutritional factors [28]. A restricted caloric intake in aging rats was related to higher apoptotic index in the jejunum and colon, indicating that the aging affects nutritional modulation of mucosal cell growth [29]. Moreover, age-related modifications in gastrointestinal mucosal cell growth are also influenced by hormonal imbalances in the gastric mucosa. It was found that the response of the gastric mucosa to the changes in different peptides (such as gastrin, bombesin and EGF) occurs at different life stages [30,31]. In addition, a continuous loss of gastric mucosal responsiveness such as acid secretory and growth-promoting actions of gastrin occurs due to the age-related functional loss of gastrin receptors. Elevated serum gastrin concentrations are caused by certain conditions such as hypochlorhydria or gastrinomas due to autoimmune or *H. pylori*-induced chronic atrophic gastritis or use of acid suppressing drugs and gastrin producing tumors, respectively [32].

16.2.2.2 Gastrointestinal carcinogenesis

The elderly show an increased risk of gastric and colorectal cancers due to altered carcinogen metabolism and continuous exposure of cancer-causing agents [33]. Carcinogenesis results via mutations taking place during the course of development of normal epithelium to carcinoma [34]. In colon cancer, the inactivation of the tumor suppressor gene adenomatous polyposis coli (APC) leads to genomic instability causing phenotype adenoma. This phenotypic adenoma furthers modifications in tumor suppressor oncogenes such as 'p53' and 'deleted in colon carcinoma (DCC)', which eventually develops adenomatous polyp, and then a carcinoma [34]. The gastric mucosa of the older person is at a higher incidence of mutations of several tumor suppressor genes, specifically APC, p53 and DCC, making them more susceptible to carcinogenesis [35].

16.2.2.3 Gastric changes

There has been a controversial conclusion based on the studies conducted in the 20th and 21st centuries about the changes that occur during aging. The studies conducted between 1920 and 1980 were retrospective and did not consider possible gastric atrophic lesions, concluding a considerable decrease in secretion of gastric acid with aging. In an important study enrolling patients with 80 years or more, normal gastric acid secretion was reported in 90% of older patients without gastric atrophic lesions [36]. It was shown that gastric acid secretion in *Helicobacter pylori*-negative patients was unaffected by aging, while the acid secretion reduced with age in *H. pylori*-positive patients. In addition, the decreased secretions were dependent on the increased prevalence of fundic atrophic gastritis and inflammatory cytokines (IL-1), which inhibits parietal cells [37]. Moreover, both atrophic gastritis and intestinal metaplasia were found to be associated largely with *H. pylori* infection, and not with aging [38]. The decreased acid secretion due to atrophic gastritis may lead to overgrowth of bacteria within the proximal intestinal tract as well as malabsorption. When the small bowel overgrowth of bacteria in the elderly was determined by hydrogen breath test using abdominal complaints and nutritional intake data, a 15.6% prevalence of bacterial overgrowth was found. The intake of gastric acid production inhibitors contributed significantly to the high incidence of a positive breath test in the elderly, which was related to the low body weight, low body mass index, low plasma albumin concentration as well as high prevalence of diarrhea [39].

One of the clinical consequences of bacterial overgrowth is malnutrition. The use of antibiotics in such patients helps to improve patients' anthropometric parameters including height, weight, body mass index (BMI), body circumferences (waist, hip and limbs) and skinfold thickness [40]. In addition, gastric malabsorption may be another result of decreased acid gastric secretion [41]. Malabsorption of food-bound cobalamin may occur due to decreased gastric acid production in elderly patients, combined with bacterial overgrowth [42]. Subsequently, decreased gastric acid production may lead to reduced release of free vitamin B12 from food protein [42]. Conditions like hypochlorhydria cause intestinal bacterial overgrowth, which interferes with vitamin B12 absorption [39]. The effect of atrophic gastritis on vitamin B12 in the elderly patients has remained contradictory. No significant difference was found in vitamin B12 absorption between subjects of median age 75 years [42]. In contrast, a reduction in dietary vitamin B12 absorption occurred with increasing age which was related to elevated serum gastrin levels, indicating hypochlorhydria [43]. Moreover, one study reported the *H. pylori* as the causative agent of vitamin B12 deficiency in 56% of the *H. pylori*-positive patients. The eradication of *H. pylori* was able to improve anemia and low serum vitamin B12 levels in 40% of patients [44]. Also, atrophic gastritis was found to affect calcium absorption in the elderly. It was suggested to use relatively insoluble salt (such as calcium carbonate) along with meals, as well as the increased use of highly soluble calcium source (such as calcium citrate and milk) for the better absorption of the calcium in the elderly patients with the gastritis [45].

16.2.2.4 Small bowel changes

The small intestinal structures including surface areas, crypt depth, villous height, crypt-to-villus ratio, enterocytes, brush border and Brunner glands remained unaffected with advancing age [46]. A decreased absorption of D-xylose in aging humans was subjected to poor renal function and bacterial overgrowth [39], whereas the *D*-xylose excretion was liable to renal function, which is usually declined with aging. The elderly patients with normal renal function showed only a moderate decrease in D-xylose absorption [47]. Another study in the elderly demonstrated higher time required for the absorption of fat, as well as lower levels of post-prandial serum bile acid. Also, the elderly showing the delayed fat absorption demonstrated 'post-prandial satiety' which is fullness or prolonged persistence of food after the meals, resulting in decreased overall food intake [48]. Thus, the functional intestinal reserve of the elderly patients may be declined, with eventual rapid undernourishment during acute hospitalizations, causing reduced adaptive responses and requiring longer intensive nutritional monitoring [49].

16.3 Malnutrition and the aging GIT

16.3.1 Causes of malnutrition in the elderly

Malnutrition in the elderly is generally underestimated while treating the gastrointestinal disorders. The major causes of malnutrition in the elderly are presented in Figure 16.1.

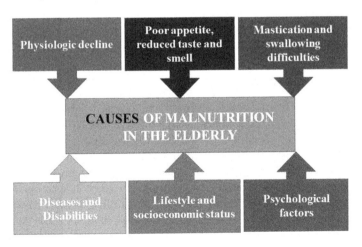

Figure 16.1 *Causes of malnutrition in the elderly.*

16.3.1.1 Physiological decline

The elderly population shows a physiologic decline in food intake even in the absence of chronic diseases, which may be subjected to physiologic changes that decrease food intake, known as 'the anorexia of aging' [49]. The age-related physiological changes involve alterations in neurotransmitters and hormones which affect the central and peripheral feeding regulation of food and satiation. This leads to decreased lean body mass and basal metabolic rate affecting the appetite and food intake [50].

16.3.1.2 Appetite

The major cause of malnutrition in the elderly is poor appetite (anorexia), which is mediated by different factors [51]. In general, the energy intake decreases with age which leads to micronutrient deficiencies [52]. A difference in the mechanisms for the control of food intake was found between old and young men. During an ad libitum feeding experiment, both young and old men lost weight after underfeeding. However, the young men were able to regain the lost weight rapidly after the ad libitum period, while the old men were unable to regain their lost weight. The studies concluded the aging-associated impairment to regulate the food intake [53]. In addition, it was found that the impaired ability might be related to an insufficiency of the elderly to reduce their energy expenditure during the ad libitum period [54]. This causes serious consequences in the anorexia-suffering elderly during the diseased state or enforced post-surgery fasting conditions, since it requires more time to regain the weight lost during such conditions, eventually leading to greater risks of getting malnutrition-associated problems. There are several endogenous substances which regulate appetite. This includes gut peptide hormones including ghrelin, cholecystokinin, peptide-YY, glucagon-like peptide 1, oxyntomodulin and pancreatic polypeptide, cytokines, glucocorticoids, catecholamines, decreased growth hormone and sex hormones which increase the TNFα, IL1, IL6 and serotonin levels causing anorexia [55].

16.3.1.3 Taste and smell

The elderly suffers from declined sensory response for both smell and taste, resulting in decreased food enjoyment, which leads to decrease in dietary variety. This sensory decline is compensated by increased use of salt and sugar in diet [56]. The commonly occurring loss of taste and smell in the elderly is due to declined olfactory functions, which can be aggravated by the presence of diseased conditions and use of drugs. It was shown that the elderly persons with one or more diseases and taking three or more medications on an average need 11 times more salt and 3 times more sugar to find salty and sweet tastes in foods as compared to the younger people [51,57]. The exact cause of taste loss is not fully clear; however, it could be assigned to a decreased number of taste buds or declined functioning of the cell membrane receptors involved in the taste sensation. For example, taste sensation receptors like Toll-like receptors (TLR) and interferon (IFN) function together to recognize pathogens and mediate inflammatory responses in taste tissue [58]. Certain categories of drugs like lipid lowering agents, antihistamines, antibiotics, anti-inflammatory agents, bronchodilators and other antiasthmatic agents, antihypertensives, anti-Parkinson's agents and antidepressants can change the taste and smell of food [51]. The study results showed that improving the flavor of the foods can improve both food intake and body weight of not only hospitalized patients but also of the healthy elderly, whereas dietary restrictions of sugar, salt and fat may make the food unpalatable in the elderly [59].

16.3.1.4 Mastication and swallowing

Oral health decline is usual in the elderly which significantly affects their food intake [60]. Most of the elderly have less of their own teeth and edentate older persons face more difficulty while eating certain food types such as fruits and vegetables due to problems in mastication or swallowing difficulties (dysphagia) [61]. Lower energy intake and lower levels of micronutrients such as calcium, iron, vitamins A, C and E, and some B vitamins, fiber and protein are commonly found in the edentate elderly [62]. It was found that in the presence of dysphagia and without instigating tube feeding, daily intake might be as low as 275 kcal which is only 14.5% of estimated energy requirements (EER) in the elderly [63]. High-protein oral supplementation and complementary enteral nutrition can improve the clinical status of certain under- or malnourished elderly subjects, whereas rehabilitation therapy and nutritional assistance can improve the functional independence of the elderly patients [64].

16.3.1.5 Diseases and disabilities

Various types of diseases including endocrine diseases like hypothyroidism, cardiovascular diseases and respiratory diseases often lead to unintentional weight loss due to hypermetabolism, decreased appetite and low caloric intake [65]. The treatment of certain chronic diseases and conditions including diabetes, hypertension, congestive heart failure and coronary artery disease includes dietary restrictions, along with the use of medicines which affect appetite. Certain drugs induce side effects like anorexia, delayed gastric emptying, dry mouth, malabsorption, nausea, diarrhea and changed taste sensitivity through altered nutrient absorption, metabolism and excretion which may lead to malnutrition [65]. Neurological diseases like Parkinson's disease or Alzheimer's disease or factors such as dementia, accidents, infections like urinary tract or chest infections, etc. are contributing factors toward malnutrition [49]. Physical disability such as arthritis and poor mobility, dependency and neglect, drug interactions among digoxin, metformin, antibiotics, etc. or the presence of other diseases like cancer significantly reduce food intake leading to malnutrition [51].

16.3.1.6 Psychological factors

In the elderly, depression, anxiety or stress show negative effects on eating behavior and nutrient intake, which commonly causes loss of weight and malnutrition [51]. For example, low mood and emotion such as anger or joy may change the food intake behavior, whereas anxiety may decrease food intake [66]. However, emotional stress experiences like interpersonal conflict, loss of loved ones and unemployment have been found challenging to some variations in their response to stress depending on eating and fasting or acute and chronic anxiety [67].

16.3.1.7 Lifestyle and socioeconomic status

Lifestyle and low socioeconomic status relate to several health-associated conditions in the elderly [68]. The living cost of housing and medication often leads to struggle for the food expenditure [49]. In addition, physical and cognitive decline affect a person's ability to access the food in terms of buying, preparing and cooking of food [69]. Loss of contributory skills related to day-to-day living activities such as shopping, transportation, housework, meal preparation, medication administration, financial management, use of the telephone or other modern equipment, etc. leads to dependency on others. In addition, lack of interactions with others at mealtime, feeling of loneliness and poor social support networks cause social detachment, which commonly leads to lethargy for food and decreased overall intake [49].

16.3.2 Malnutrition aftereffects on the health status of the elderly

Malnutrition shows a detrimental effect on the health and nutritional status of the elderly due to its negative effects on the functions and recovery of every organ system including liver, gut and renal functions [49,51]. Malnutrition delays wound healing and causes depression, apathy, as well as decreased immunity, muscle strength and cardiac output [51] (Figure 16.2). Malnutrition may be subjected to increased mortality irrespective of weight loss or body mass index in the elderly of 60 years and above. In addition, malnutrition may cause extended hospital stays, hospital re-admission and increased need of health care services. Malnutrition also leads to an increased risk of long-term disability such as frailty, development of sarcopenia and dementia. Earlier research efforts targeted the declined cognitive functions including attention, working and procedural memory, perception, speech and language and decision-making with advancing age [70]. Although GIT is crucial for the release and absorption of the dietary nutrients, the adequate research on the GIT events which take place with advancing age and impact on malnutrition on these events is inadequately explored. The malnutrition aftereffects could ultimately lead to an impaired quality of life in the elderly [71]. Thus, malnutrition is a serious issue which should be intervened for management and treatment of gastrointestinal disorders in the elderly, failure to which may cause serious aftereffects which negatively impact the health status of the elderly.

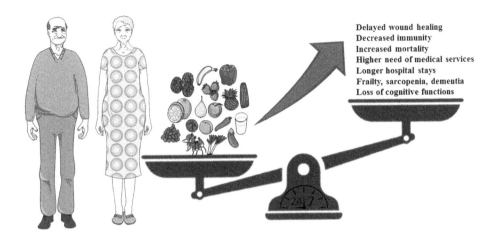

Figure 16.2 *Malnutrition aftereffects negatively impact the health status of the elderly.*

16.4 GIT disorders in the elderly

The GIT is composed of a muscular tube (alimentary tube), which extends from the mouth to the anus including adjunct digestive organs such as liver, gallbladder and pancreas. The functionality of these organs is subjected to dimensional changes, indicating the importance of biomechanical properties of a particular function [72]. This alimentary tube is approximately 23 feet long and comprised of the esophagus, stomach, small and large intestines, liver, gallbladder and pancreas. The complex structure of the GIT relies on the coordination of the organs, sphincters, hormones, as well as intestinal, nervous, lymphatic and circulatory systems to bring about its primary responsibility of imparting nutrients to the body [73]. Digestion, absorption, excretion and immune defense are major tasks of the gastrointestinal system. For digestion of nutrients and medications, a sequence of mechanical and chemical processes take place, which finally decreases the particles to the molecular sizes that are absorbable into the systemic circulation, as well as removal of the nonabsorbable particles through the colon. The lymph nodules containing the lymphocytes are present inside the gastrointestinal mucosa, which show immunologic response to the bacteria that are capable of crossing the epithelial tissues. The liver sinusoids contain biggest accumulation of tissue macrophages or phagocytic cells including Kupffer cells which are not only bactericidal but also crucial for the hereditary immunity. The frequently occurring GIT disorders in the elderly can be divided as oral cavity diseases, upper GIT diseases and lower GIT diseases (Figure 16.3). The GIT is impacted by the aging process, leading to functional or structural disorders [74]. The major functional and structural GIT in the elderly along with their etiology and clinical symptoms are summarized in Table 16.1.

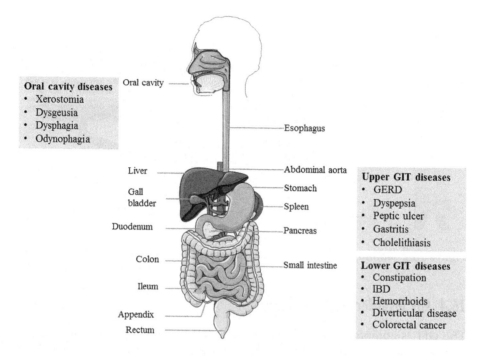

Oral cavity diseases
- Xerostomia
- Dysgeusia
- Dysphagia
- Odynophagia

Oral cavity

Esophagus

Liver

Gall bladder

Duodenum

Colon

Ileum

Appendix

Rectum

Abdominal aorta

Stomach

Spleen

Pancreas

Small intestine

Upper GIT diseases
- GERD
- Dyspepsia
- Peptic ulcer
- Gastritis
- Cholelithiasis

Lower GIT diseases
- Constipation
- IBD
- Hemorrhoids
- Diverticular disease
- Colorectal cancer

Figure 16.3 *Commonly occurring gastrointestinal diseases in the elderly.*

16.4.1 Functional gastrointestinal disorders

The main purpose of the GIT is to mechanically disintegrate as well as chemically and enzymatically digest the food, perform the absorption of water and nutrients, protect the body from microbial attack and remove the undigested wastes [74]. As soon as the food enters the mouth, its mechanical and enzymatic digestion occurs, followed by propelling the food down to the stomach where the digestion process continues [75]. From the stomach, the food passes through the small intestine, where its further digestion and absorption occur with the help of the enzymes secreted by the small intestine, liver and pancreas. Further, most of the water absorption and feces formation take place in the large intestine, which is then temporarily stored in the rectum and removed *via* defecation through the anus [76]. Functional disorders of GIT have persistent or recurring symptoms like pain and bloating, which are diagnosed by techniques such as endoscopies, blood tests and diagnostic imaging to confirm the absence of any structural abnormalities [77]. In functional disorders, the functions of GIT such as motility, sensation and brain-gut function are affected. If the GI motility is disturbed, the GI muscle spasms occur causing pain. If GI sensation is disturbed, the GI nerves are unable to respond normally to different stimuli like digestion causing pain. If GIT's brain-gut function is disturbed, the GIT cannot communicate normally [78].

Table 16.1 Summary of Etiology and Clinical Symptoms of Gastrointestinal Diseases in the Elderly

Gastrointestinal Disease	Etiology	Clinical Symptoms
Dysphagia	Neuromuscular disorders; multiple sclerosis; pharyngeal cancer	Difficulty in swallowing
Odynophagia	Infections; malignancies	Painful swallowing
Atrophic gastritis	Increased *Helicobacter pylori* and decreased secretion of intrinsic factor which is essential for vitamin B12 absorption in the small intestines	Burning ache or pain due to indigestion; nausea or vomiting that is not attributed to diet
Functional dyspepsia	Motility disorders; sensorimotor dysfunction; immune activation or elevated mucosal permeability in the proximal small intestine; disorders of the autonomic and enteric nervous systems	Epigastric pain and/or burning, postprandial fullness and early satiety
Peptic ulcer disease	*Helicobacter pylori* infection; polypharmacy	Epigastric pain with burning sensation after the meals; feeling of fullness or bloating
Constipation	Intrinsic problems of colonic or anorectal function; organic disease, systemic disease or medications	Hard, dry or infrequent stools; need for excessive straining to evacuate; incomplete evacuation
Inflammatory bowel disease (IBD)	Defective immune system which responds abnormally to environmental triggers	Abdominal pain, diarrhea and anemia
Hemorrhoids	Increased pressure and subsequent engorgement of the arteriovenous plexuses, which is believed to interfere with venous return	Bleeding during and after bowel movements; itching, pain, discomfort or burning in the anus; anal leakage of fluid; and swelling and painful lumps in the anal region
Diverticular disease	Age-related alterations within the colon wall; disordered colonic motility; and dietary deficiencies of fibers	Abdominal pain, changes in bowel habits, constipation, fever and nausea
Colorectal cancer	Colon or rectum cells' DNA mutation causing uncontrollable	Persistent changes in bowel habits or a change in the consistency of stool; rectal bleeding or bloody stool; persistent abdominal discomfort
Cholelithiasis	Over-accumulation of cholesterol in the bile that is stored in the gallbladder. The cholesterol may harden to form stone-like substances	Severe biliary colic, right upper quadrant pain

16.4.1.1 Xerostomia and dysgeusia

These are disorders of oral cavity in the elderly due to conditions caused by systemic diseases, local trauma or medication side effects [79]. It was reported that the oral sensorial complaints were prevalent in the elderly of more than

65 years where 50% of elderly possessed at least one of the oral sensorial complaints. The prevalence of oral sensorial complaints was higher in the elderly taking the prescription medications [80]. Xerostomia is defined as dryness in mouth which is associated with decreased salivary secretion or changes in composition of saliva. Among the several causes of xerostomia are systemic diseases like Sjogren's syndrome, neurological disorders, glandular diseases and radiotherapy of the head and neck, or medication-related side effects with the use of tricyclic antidepressants, atropine and antiparkinsonian drugs [81]. Permanent xerostomia occurs due to destruction of the salivary glands after the chemotherapy of head and neck cancer. Medication-induced xerostomia can often be reversed upon discontinuation of the upsetting medications. Permanent xerostomia is treated by salivary supplements. Dysgeusia is the distortion of the taste sensitivity, whereas ageusia is the complete lack of taste [79]. Medication-related side effects with the use of lithium, metronidazole, levodopa, glipizide, captopril and clarithromycin can cause these disorders in the elderly. Malnourished elderly with deficiency of zinc shows dysgeusia, whereas the peripheral nervous system disorder such as Bell's palsy is commonly associated with the taste disorders [74].

16.4.1.2 Dysphagia and odynophagia

Dysphagia is an oropharyngeal disorder which causes difficulty in swallowing. It can result from alterations that affect the complex neuromuscular mechanism for coordinating the tongue, pharynx and upper esophageal sphincter [82]. Oropharyngeal dysphagia commonly occurs due to neuromuscular disorders including muscular dystrophy, stroke, myasthenia gravis, Parkinson's disease, multiple sclerosis or local mechanical causes such as pharyngeal cancers [83]. Dysphagia and odynophagia (painful swallowing) particularly occur in patients with head and neck cancers, whereas swallowing disorders may also occur in patients with other types of cancers [84]. Neurologic disorders like cerebrovascular accident which is caused by sensorimotor disability of the oral and pharyngeal swallowing phases or dementia often result in decreased oropharyngeal [85]. Dysphagia creates either problems or inability to swallow certain foods or liquids causing coughing or sticking in the throat when eating or drinking or bringing the food back through the nose [86]. Oropharyngeal dysphagia affects up to 13% elderly of 65 and plus to 50% of in-patients [86]. Dysphagia is diagnosed by physical examination and swallowing tests, detailed history or fluoroscopic examination [8]. Odynophagia is painful swallowing in which pain can be experienced in mouth, throat, or esophagus when drinking or eating [74]. The most common infections include those caused by *Candida*, herpes simplex virus and cytomegalovirus in low-immunity patients as well as different types of malignancies [87]. As reported by several studies, the elderly patients possess a greater pain sensation threshold as compared to younger persons because of age-associated decline in myenteric neurons, due to which the elderly seek help at an advanced stage of their disease [86].

16.4.1.3 Gastroesophageal Reflux Disease (GERD)

GERD occurs due to mucosal damage produced by the abnormal reflux of gastric contents into the esophagus, causing troublesome symptoms [88]. The reflux of gastric acid, pepsin or duodenogastric reflux of bile can damage the esophagus. The pathogenesis of GERD involves a defective anti-reflux barrier, abnormal esophageal clearance, decreased salivary production, altered esophageal mucosal resistance and delayed gastric emptying [89]. In addition, the presence of diseases such as diabetes and neurologic disorders or drug-related adverse effects can aggravate GERD symptoms by triggering the reflux of stomach contents back into the esophagus [12]. The clinical symptoms of GERD include acid reflux, stomach pain and hunger pain in the belly, dyspepsia, nausea, bloating and burping along with anorexia, weight loss, vomiting, dysphagia, coughing, wheezing, chest pain and dental erosion [74,88]. Many patients show similar reflux-associated symptoms that overlap with non-GERD conditions like gastroparesis, dyspepsia and hypersensitive esophagus in patients who do not respond to an acid-suppressive therapy. In such patients, usually GERD is not the cause for the symptoms, and a search for non-GERD conditions which are responsible for the overlapping symptoms must be carefully diagnosed [90]. Techniques such as proton pump inhibitor trial, esophageal pH monitoring, upper endoscopy, barium esophagram or esophageal manometry are used for the diagnosis of the GERD [91].

16.4.1.4 Atrophic gastritis

The elderly are prone to atrophic gastritis, which is chronic inflammation of the mucous membrane of the stomach linings [92]. Atrophic gastritis is related to the increased *H. pylori* and decreased secretion of intrinsic factor which is required for the absorption of vitamin B12 in the small intestines [42]. Clinical symptoms of gastritis include dyspeptic symptoms, burning ache or pain due to indigestion, nausea or vomiting that is not attributed to diet, which may be persistent for more than 6 months. Gastritis is diagnosed by endoscopy and is treated by identifying the underlying etiological causes such as *H. pylori* eradication or vitamin B12 replacement [93]. The elderly patients of gastritis should be treated by *H. pylori* eradication or vitamin B12 deficiency and also advised to avoid nonsteroidal anti-inflammatory drugs to prevent relapse of gastritis in future [74].

16.4.1.5 Functional dyspepsia

Functional dyspepsia includes persistent or recurrent upper abdominal symptoms such as epigastric pain and burning, postprandial satiety, as well as early satiety, which occurs from heterogeneous and multifactorial causes [94]. Various systematic pathophysiological studies reported functional dyspepsia as an organic disorder, which is associated with motility and sensorimotor dysfunction, immune activation, higher proximal small intestinal mucosal permeability, autonomic nervous system disorders as well as enteric nervous system disorders [95]. Dyspepsia shows complaints of bloating, flatulence, heartburn and diarrhea. Dysphagia can be treated by using prokinetic agents, dietary management and less frequently by treatment of depression, which is related to the dyspepsia [94]. In addition, causes of secondary forms of dyspepsia such as medications, organic disease of the digestive tract such as atrophic gastritis, peptic ulcer disease, tumors and gallstones, vascular and neurological disorders, consumption of high-fat large size meals, strong alcoholic drinks or carbonated beverages and smoking are required to be identified and treated. Moreover, the damage to the gastric mucosa caused by duodenogastric reflux and bile salts present in the stomach is treated by prokinetic drugs [74]. First-line treatment of dyspepsia is carried out by acid suppression treatment with antacids, H2 receptor antagonist proton pump inhibitors as well as over-the-counter antacids composed of alumina, magnesium, calcium carbonate or simethicone [94]. Recent studies showed the decreased dominance of dyspepsia in the elderly; however, investigations must confirm its diagnosis by upper gastrointestinal endoscopy which excludes organic diseases such as ulcers associated with nonsteroidal anti-inflammatory drugs, *H. pylori* pathologies, cancer, coeliac disease and autoimmune gastritis [96].

16.4.1.6 Peptic ulcer disease

Peptic ulcer disease covers injury of stomach or duodenum mucosal lining which leads to painful ulcers. The higher occurrence of gastric ulcers in the elderly is associated with higher prevalence *H. pylori* infection and polypharmacy involving the use of aspirin and nonsteroidal anti-inflammatory drugs as well as anticoagulants, selective serotonin reuptake inhibitors (SSRI) such as antidepressants and oral steroids [97]. The elderly show age-related physiologic changes that add up to ulcers by causing reduced blood flow through the gastrointestinal system as well as decreased secretion of bicarbonates, mucin and prostaglandins which are the major components of gastrointestinal protective mechanisms [74]. Both the *H. pylori*-associated alterations in gut microbiota and atrophic gastritis lead to hypochlorhydria (lower level of stomach acid), causing a reduced gastric acid secretion in the elderly [98]. Peptic ulcer is characterized by epigastric pain with burning sensation which occurs after the meals and feeling of fullness or bloating. Peptic ulcer can be diagnosed by a breath test which detects *H. pylori*, a blood or stool test, aggressive endoscopy or sometimes using imaging tests such as X-rays and CT scans to detect ulcers [99]. According to a recent report, the general population have shown reduced incidence of peptic ulcers. However, hospitalization and mortality have remained very high among the elderly patients with the peptic ulcer disease [100]. The essential treatment of the peptic ulcer disease includes suppression of the gastric acid with antisecretory drugs, and the eradication of *H. pylori* infection.

16.4.1.7 Constipation

Constipation refers to the difficulties that patients experience with their bowel movements. Constipation is manifested by hard, dry or infrequent stools, abdominal cramping or bloating, need for over-straining to evacuate, incomplete evacuation, excess time required for evacuation or failure to evacuate. Constipation is the most commonly encountered condition in the elderly, which is related to the decreased intestinal transit rates in the large intestine [101]. The primary causes of constipation relate to the inherent colonic or anorectal function problems, whereas secondary causes of constipation relate to organic disease, systemic disease or medications. In addition, the elderly show constipation associated with decline in chewing ability, gastric acid secretion, fluid and fiber intake and physical activity [102]. Constipation may also be a result of endocrine and metabolic diseases such as diabetes and hypothyroidism, neurologic cerebrovascular diseases, multiple sclerosis, myopathy or Parkinson disease, psychiatric disorders like depression and anxiety, organic colorectal disease caused by tumors such as stenosis, Crohn's disease or hemorrhoids, fissures and rectal prolapse [100–102]. Constipation can also be induced by different categories of medications such as anticholinergics, antidepressants, antihistamines, antihypertensives, opioids, hypnotics and antacids [101]. Constipation is diagnosed by certain medical tests such as lab tests including blood, stool or urine test or endoscopy to look inside anus, rectum and colon. Constipation can be treated by consuming adequate fluid intake, fiber-rich diet, physical activity and use of laxatives such as vegetable and mineral oil, liquid paraffin, docusate sodium and osmotic hydrating agents like magnesium hydroxide, magnesium sulfate, magnesium citrate and sodium biphosphate [103].

16.4.2 Structural gastrointestinal disorders

A structural gastrointestinal disorder occurs when an organ or other internal structure becomes abnormal and does not work properly resulting in organ malfunction [78]. The intestinal epithelial barrier is one of the most important structures of the gastrointestinal system that allows transport of contents between blood and intestinal lumen, while preventing the entry of the toxic contents in the blood [104]. The structural gastrointestinal disorders are typically diagnosed by endoscopic techniques. The structural abnormality may be removed by surgical procedures if required. The structural gastrointestinal disorders include inflammatory bowel disease, hemorrhoids, diverticular disease, colorectal cancer and cholelithiasis.

16.4.2.1 Inflammatory Bowel Disease (IBD)

IBD is a chronic idiopathic disease characterized by chronic inflammation of the GIT which is comprised of two conditions: firstly, the Crohn's disease, which usually occurs in small intestine but may also occur in any part of the GIT from mouth to anus, and secondly, the ulcerative colitis, which occurs in the large intestine [105]. Although the specific IBD etiology is unclear, it is known to result from a defective immune system which responds abnormally to environmental triggers, causing inflammation of the GIT. This process can be stimulated by the genetic susceptibility of the individual toward these triggers, leading to complex etiological interactions among the genetic, microbial or environmental factors with the immune responses [106]. Hence, a person with a family history of IBD is more prone to develop such an inappropriate immune response. The elderly IBD patients experience abdominal pain, diarrhea and anemia less frequently; however, they often show weight loss, bleeding, fever and paradoxical constipation with distal ulcerative colitis [107]. IBD is diagnosed using endoscopy (for Crohn's disease), colonoscopy (for ulcerative colitis) and imaging studies (contrast radiography, MRI or CT scan) or combination techniques. IBD can be treated by several types of medications including aminosalicylates, corticosteroids such as prednisone and immunomodulators [108]. In addition, several vaccinations can be recommended to prevent infections in the elderly IBD patients. IBD is quite different with irritable bowel syndrome (IBS); however, people with IBS may experience some similar symptoms to IBD. Unlike IBD, IBS is commonly found in patients with psychological conditions such as depression and anxiety rather than inflammation or damage of the bowel tissues. However, IBS patients experience abdominal pain and altered bowel habits without having specific organic pathology [105,109].

16.4.2.2 Hemorrhoids

Hemorrhoids, also called piles, is a common anorectal condition characterized by engorgement of the venous tissue in the anal region and lower rectum [110]. It is more common in the elderly suffering from bowel conditions such as constipation. The studies reported an increasing number of surgical procedures in the elderly within the past few decades. In addition, the elderly undergoing the surgery are at higher risk of mortality due to the presence of comorbidities, malnutrition and impaired reserve functions in comparison to the younger patients. It was found that the hemorrhoids due to liver and kidney impairment dominated in elderly patients, negating aging alone as a risk factor for post-surgery complications [111]. Although there is little evidence that exists to relate hemorrhoids etiology, low-fiber diets resulting in increased straining during defecation or constipation can cause increased pressure, and subsequent engorgement of the arteriovenous plexuses, which is believed to interfere with venous return. Aging causes weakening of the support structures, facilitating the prolapse which gets worse by prolonged sitting due to venous return problem in the perianal area. The symptoms of hemorrhoids include bleeding during and after bowel movements, itching, pain, discomfort or burning in the anus, anal leakage of fluid, as well as painful swelling and lumps in the anal region. Hemorrhoids can be diagnosed by digital examination to find unusual growths or by visual examination of the lower colon and rectum. Hemorrhoids can be treated by medical, surgical and conservative measures [112]. Moreover, the elderly patients are advised to avoid activities that require straining, for instance, lifting of heavy weights or putting strain to defecate. The medications which increase the risk of constipation should be properly reviewed and managed [113].

16.4.2.3 Diverticular disease

Diverticular disease of the colon is a symptomatic and asymptomatic disease prevalent in Western society as a result of lack of fiber in the diet. Diverticulosis is described by two conditions, namely diverticulosis and diverticulitis. Diverticulosis is the formation of bulges, pouches or pockets (diverticula) in the walls of digestive tract, and diverticulitis is an infection or inflammation of pouches characterized by fever, pain and leukocytosis (increased number of white blood cells) [114]. It may occur mainly in distal colon in the elderly as a consequence of age-associated alterations within the large intestinal wall such as elevated intraluminal colonic pressure in the muscular wall, disordered colonic motility and very low intake of dietary fibers [114]. The aging colon is prone to the oncogenic effects of growth factors and carcinogens, whereas digestive products accumulate in the pockets of the colon due to its sharp curvature [115]. The most common clinical complication of diverticular disease is diverticulitis, which affects 10%–25% of patients with diverticula and is also a major cause of frequent visits to clinic and hospitalization. Most of the hospitalized patients with acute diverticulitis respond to traditional treatment including intake of high-fiber diet and/or fiber supplementation or use of probiotics; however, 15%–30% of the patients require surgery [115]. Diverticulosis symptoms vary among patients and are usually diagnosed by colonoscopy or computed tomography. The most common symptoms of diverticulosis include pain in lower left or sometimes right side of the abdomen, changes in bowel habits, constipation, fever and nausea. Diverticulosis can be treated by fiber, antibiotics and probiotics [116].

16.4.2.4 Colorectal cancer

The occurrence of colorectal cancer is increasing among the older patients. It is the world's fourth most fatal cancer with about 900,000 deaths annually [117]. Almost 60% of patients with colorectal cancer are of more than 70 years of age at the time of diagnosis, and 43% are more than 75 years of age [118]. Since colorectal cancer is usually asymptomatic, its screening for prevention is significant for its early diagnosis and treatment. Colorectal cancer begins with an unknown growth over the epithelial wall of the colon, which is known as polyps. Although polyp is usually a kind of noncancerous growth, it can be developed into cancer and invade the colonic wall if left untreated [119]. Colorectal cancer forms when the cell DNA of colon or rectum mutates, causing them to grow uncontrollably. These mutated cells are either attacked by the immune system or die or escape from the immune system and grow uncontrollable, forming a tumor in the colon or rectum. Although the exact cause of colorectal cancer is unknown, associated high risk factors include the presence of diseases, quality of diet, the use of tobacco, smoking and heavy alcohol, advancing age as well as family history or hereditary factors. Although invasive, tedious and expensive, colonoscopy is a commonly used diagnostic tool for colorectal cancer [119]. The symptoms of colorectal cancer include long-lasting changes in the bowel habits such as diarrhea or constipation or altered stool consistency, rectal bleeding or bloody stool, as well as persistent abdominal discomfort, including cramps, gas or pain. Approaches for treatment of colorectal cancer include surgery, adjuvant therapy and targeted therapies [119].

16.4.2.5 Cholelithiasis

Cholelithiasis (calculi or gallstones) is the presence of one or more stony deposits that form in the biliary tract inside the gallbladder which cause inflammation or infection of the gallbladder in older adults [120]. Three main pathways of gallstone formation are (i) cholesterol supersaturation, (ii) excess bilirubin and (iii) gallbladder hypomotility or impaired contractility [121]. Cholelithiasis is the result of over-accumulation of cholesterol in the bile which is stored within the gallbladder. The cholesterol may harden to form stone-like deposits of various sizes. The increased levels of cholesterol in the bile can be linked to increased body weight and older age. The elderly patients with cholelithiasis may be asymptomatic or show severe pain originating from the gall bladder and radiating to the back, which may last for 30 minutes to 12 hours with or without fever, nausea or vomiting [122]. Cholelithiasis can be diagnosed by ultrasound. Surgical intervention is sought in case of severe biliary pain or obstruction, which is required to be removed from the gallbladder to relieve the biliary symptoms. Both the symptomatic and complicated gallstones can be treated by laparoscopic cholecystectomy as the surgical choice [123].

16.5 Nutraceuticals in gastrointestinal disorders

'Nutraceuticals', derived from 'nutrition' and 'pharmaceutical', are dietary components naturally present in foods and believed to possess medical or health benefits [124]. The global nutraceutical market was valued at US$ 252,535.4 million in 2018 and is estimated to reach US$ 465,709.8 million by 2027, at a compound annual growth rate (CAGR) of 7.1% during the projection period of 2019–2027 [125]. Since ancient times, herbs are being used for various ailments in Ayurveda and traditional Chinese medicine; however, less of them have scientific evidence. Moreover, it is a quite general approach to consider the treatment of a disease along with a protective fiber-rich diet or supplementation with specifically beneficial bioactive compounds, like omega-3-fatty acids, as well as use of complementary medicines as supportive therapies.

In this milieu, nutraceuticals may play the major, additive or synergistic role in the treatment of various gastrointestinal disorders in the elderly [78]. The major nutraceuticals with beneficial effects in preventing, treating or enhancing gastrointestinal health of the elderly are summarized in Table 16.2 and presented in Figure 16.4.

16.5.1 Dietary fiber

Dietary fibers are carbohydrate polymers with more than 10 monomeric units from the food or plant material which are neither digested nor absorbed by digestive enzymatic hydrolysis in the GIT but are digested through fermentation by bacterial microflora in the gut [126]. Dietary fibers are sourced from barley, whole grains, oatmeals, beans, nuts, fruits and vegetables. Dietary fibers mainly include resistant nonstarch polysaccharides which are not hydrolyzed, digested or absorbed in the small intestine. Examples of dietary fibers include celluloses, hemicelluloses, gums and pectins, lignin, resistant dextrins and resistant starches [127]. Based on water solubility, dietary fibers can be divided into two forms: (i) insoluble dietary fiber such as celluloses, certain hemicelluloses and lignins which can be fermented to a limited extend in the colon and (ii) soluble dietary fiber such as β-glucans, pectins, gums, mucilages and other hemicelluloses which are readily fermented in the colon [128]. The soluble components of dietary fiber possess bulking capabilities which delay the gastric emptying of the stomach. This effect improves both the digestion rate and the nutrients uptake, creating a feeling of fullness for longer time [129]. Dietary fibers also increase the stool weight, decrease the colonic transit time and aid in water-retention in the colon, which together results in less dry stools that can be easily evacuated [130]. Due to their high water retention capacity, dietary fibers have become an essential element of a healthy diet for the normal bowel movement, which helps to prevent and treat digestive disorders such as constipation [130]. In addition, the fermentation of soluble fiber causes increased fecal bacterial mass, promoting the growth of gut Bifidobacteria [129]. Persons consuming adequate amounts of dietary fiber are at lower risk of certain gastrointestinal disorders as compared to those with minimal fiber intake [131]. Increased fiber intake benefits a number of gastrointestinal disorders including the following: GERD, duodenal ulcer, diverticulitis, constipation and hemorrhoids [131]. Dietary fibers may retard the absorption of vitamins, minerals, proteins and calories [129].

16.5.2 Herbs and spices

The traditional history of herbs and spices to impart sensory qualities to foods is thousands of years old. The consumption of a variety of spices in different amounts is common in the tropical countries with the purposes to impart characteristic aroma, flavor and color to the foods, which stimulates appetite and modifies the food texture [129]. Dietary spices in small quantities have a

Table 16.2 Major Nutraceutical or Natural Constituents Effective in Gastrointestinal Disorders

Nutraceutical Constituent	Potential Sources	Effects or Functions	Conditions
Dietary fiber	Barley; whole grains; oatmeal; beans; nuts; fruits; vegetables	High water retention agent; bulking agent; promotes the growth of Bifidobacteria in the gut	Constipation; hemorrhoids; GERD[a], duodenal ulcer, diverticulitis
Herbs and spices	Common herbs and spices such as turmeric (curcumin); ginger; cumin; ajowan; fennel; coriander; onion; garlic	Impart flavor, taste and color to food; antioxidative, chemopreventive, antimutagenic, anti-inflammatory, immunomodulatory effects	Digestive disorders
Antioxidant nutrients (vitamins A, C, E, betacarotenoids and selenium)	Fruits and vegetables; Vitamin E is sourced from vegetable oil; nuts and seeds; selenium is sourced from Brazil nuts, sea foods and organ meat	Free-radical scavenging and antioxidant effects	Colorectal cancer
Fat-soluble vitamins (vitamins D and A)	Vitamin D is sourced from sunlight; vitamin A from liver, fish, meat, dairy, carrots, tomatoes and green leafy vegetables	Vitamin D has TNF-α gene suppression activity; vitamin A has tumor regression effect	IBD[b]; colorectal cancer
Probiotics, prebiotics, synbiotics	Probiotics are sourced from various species of genus Lactobacillus or Bifidobacterium; prebiotics from chicory roots, banana, tomato, alliums, beans and peas	Increases host-friendly bacteria and reduces the evading pathogenic organisms; eradicate *H. pylori* infection	IBD
Polyphenols: (i) EGCG (ii) Curcumin (iii) Anthocyanins	Fresh tea leaves; apples; blackberries, broad beans; cherries, black grapes; pears; raspberries Turmeric (*Curcuma longa*) Pigmented fruits and vegetables like black and blueberries; grapes and eggplants	Inhibition of cancer stem cells Anti-inflammatory and anti-cancer effects in treatment of cytotoxic effect on colon cancer cells Free-radical scavenging and antioxidant capacities; cytokine-induced inflammatory response	Colorectal cancer IBD; colorectal cancer IBD
Polyunsaturated fatty acids (PUFA)	Canola; soybeans and flaxseeds; fish oil; salmon, trout and blue fin tuna	Anti-inflammatory	IBD
Phytosterols	Vegetables; nuts; fruits and seeds	Anti-inflammatory and antioxidant effects; mucosal healing; regulation of gut microflora	IBD; Intestinal inflammation; gastroprotection

(*Continued*)

Table 16.2 (*Continued*) Major Nutraceutical or Natural Constituents Effective in Gastrointestinal Disorders

Nutraceutical Constituent	Potential Sources	Effects or Functions	Conditions
Anthraquinone glycosides	Dried leaflets of *Cassia senna*; dried bark of *Cascara sagrada*	Alteration of motility patterns and increase of colonic fluid volume; apoptosis of colonic epithelial cells	Constipation
Psyllium husk	Isabgol	Excessive water absorption	Constipation
Aloe vera	Gel of the plant aloe vera	Hepatoprotective, anti-inflammatory and anti-ulcerative benefits	IBS[c]
Bael	Ripe or unripe fruit of *Aegle marmelos*	Anti-inflammatory effect	IBD
Garlic	Bulbs of *Alliun sativum*	Antioxidant, anti-inflammatory, anticancer, hepatoprotective and digestive system protective	Gastroprotectant
Honey	Liquid that is prepared by different species of honeybees from the nectar of flowers	Stimulation of tissue growth; inhibition of growth of *H. pylori*	Gastric ulcers
Amla	Fruits of *Emblica officinalis*	Antioxidant and hepatoprotective effect	Gastric ulcers
Glycyrrhizin	Licorice (roots of *Glycyrrhiza glabra*)	Antioxidant effect; apoptotic effect on tumor cells for colon cancer	Gastrointestinal ulcers

[a] Gastroesophageal Reflux Disease;
[b] Inflammatory Bowel Disease
[c] ntestinal Bowel Syndrome.

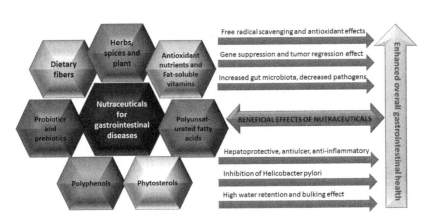

Figure 16.4 *Nutraceuticals and their beneficial effects which enhance gastrointestinal health of the elderly.*

vital effect on the human health due to their antioxidative, chemopreventive, antimutagenic, anti-inflammatory or immunomodulatory effects on cells. Also, spices are known to impart a wide array of favorable effects on human health due to their beneficial actions on gastrointestinal, cardiovascular, respiratory, metabolic, reproductive, neural and other systems [129]. Herbs and spices such as turmeric (curcumin), ginger, cumin, ajowan, fennel, coriander, onion and garlic exert digestive stimulant action [132]. The active herbal constituents like curcumin and capsaicin cause dissolution of cholesterol gallstones, whereas turmeric/curcumin, garlic and asafetida show antimicrobial action. Several herbs and spices contain terpenes and other components of essential oils as their active constituents, which have been found be effective in their raw forms [132]. Mostly, the use of spices as food components is harmless. However, when used as medication, the doses or possible interaction of spices with other medications must be carefully considered. The excessive consumption of garlic was found to cause anemia, weight loss and heart, liver and kidney toxicity in rats [133] as well as dermatological problems [134]. High doses of onion (500 mg/kg) caused lung and tissue damage in rats [135]. The herbs and spices have been considered 'generally recognized as safe' (GRAS) for human consumption by the US Code of Federal Regulations [129].

16.5.3 Antioxidant nutrients

Vitamins A, C, E, carotenoids and selenium are the major antioxidants, among which vitamin C, vitamin E and carotenoids are antioxidant vitamins that prevent oxidative reactions responsible for several degenerative diseases like cancer, cardiovascular diseases, cataracts, etc., when used either singly or synergistically [136]. These vitamins exert protective action by free-radical scavenging mechanisms and are abundant in many fruits and vegetables [129]. Tocopherols and tocotrienols (known as tocochromanols) are amphiphilic antioxidants and belong to the vitamin E family, which are found in vegetable oil like sunflower, soybean and wheat germ, nuts like almonds, peanuts and hazelnuts, seeds like sunflower seeds and green leafy vegetables like spinach and broccoli. Vitamin E is particularly involved in transfer of hydrogen atom and scavenging singlet oxygen and other reactive species [137]. Antioxidants are potential chemopreventive agents due to their direct scavenging effect on reactive oxygen species (ROS), thus reducing oxidative damage to DNA [138]. An inverse association between the intake of dietary beta carotene and the risk of colorectal adenomas was found [139]. Carotenoids, the important dietary nutrients, include lycopene, beta carotene, lutein and zeaxanthin as the most effective singlet oxygen quenchers in the biological systems without producing any oxidizing products [129]. Beta carotene complements the antioxidant properties of vitamin E [130] and traps the peroxy free radicals in tissues even at low oxygen concentrations [140].

The essential micronutrient selenium acts as the defense against the ROS toxicity and also regulates the redox state of the cells [141]. The richest source of selenium is Brazil nuts which provides about 200 µg selenium per ounce; other sources are seafoods and organ meats [142]. The most vital role of selenium is in the form of antioxidant selenoproteins or selenoenzymes such as glutathione peroxidase and thioredoxin reductase [141]. Glutathione peroxidase helps to protect cells against oxidative damage from ROS and reactive nitrogen species (RNS), which are produced as byproducts of cellular metabolism and ionizing radiation from superoxide, hydrogen peroxide, hydroxyl radicals and nitric oxide and peroxynitrite [138]. Selenium functions is a chemopreventive agent which reduces oxidative stress, decreases DNA damage, and induces apoptosis and cell-cycle arrest [141]. An inverse relationship between selenium status and cancer risks in humans was reported [143,144]. When the participants of a clinical study were given 200 µg of yeast-based selenium per day for four and half years, a 50% reduction in the cancer death rate was reported as compared to the placebo group [144].

16.5.4 Fat-soluble vitamins

Vitamins D and A are effective in addressing gastrointestinal diseases. Sunlight is the richest source of vitamin D. An exposure to sunlight causes 7-dehydrocholesterol in the skin to absorb UV B rays, which is then converted into pre-vitamin D3 and further isomerizes into vitamin D3 [145]. The deficiency of vitamin D was common among patients suffering from IBD, which was correlated with the geographical disparity of IBD, justifying the higher prevalence of IBD in northern countries which are likely to get less sun exposure, as well as greater risk of IBD during winter and spring months due to the lower occurrence of UV-induced vitamin D synthesis [146].

In addition, the commonly found vitamin D deficiency in IBD patients was also correlated with tumor necrosis factor-α (TNF-α)-mediated inflammation [146]. Low levels of vitamin D have greater incidence of IBD-related surgery and hospitalization, as compared to normal vitamin D levels in patients of ulcerative colitis and Crohn's disease, who showed reduced incidences of surgery or hospitalization. Anti-TNF-α therapy is used in the treatment of IBD to treat ulcerative colitis and Crohn's disease. Considering the reported TNF-α gene suppression activity of vitamin D, the effect of vitamin D pre-treatment before the anti-TNF-α therapy was studied [147]. The results indicated that increased plasma vitamin D levels in the IBD patients could enhance the treatment efficacy as compared to the patients with lower levels of plasma vitamin D, which proved the synergistic effect of vitamin D in anti-TNF-α therapy [147]. Vitamin D supplementation was found to exhibit reduction in relapse rate with Crohn's disease. Hence, vitamin D supplementation is suggested as replacement therapy for corticosteroids and anti TNF-α therapy. Vitamin D3 was found to show synergistic effect with metformin in prevention of colon cancer as well as colitis associated colon neoplasia in animal models [148]. Vitamin A is sourced from liver, fish, meat, dairy, carrots, tomatoes and green leafy vegetables. The recent study suggested that tumor regression by HOXA5 induction could be triggered by retinoids, indicating the huge potential of vitamin A in treatment of colon cancer by eradicating cancer stem cells [149].

16.5.5 Probiotics, prebiotics and synbiotics

Probiotics are live strains of strictly selected microorganisms which bestow health benefits to the host when administered in appropriate amounts [150]. Probiotic ingestion increases host-friendly bacteria and reduces the pathogenic organisms. Clinical studies revealed the beneficial outcomes of probiotics on gastrointestinal diseases such as gastrointestinal disorders, IBD, elimination of *H. pylori* infection and diarrheas [150]. Probiotics mainly consist of various species of genus Lactobacillus or Bifidobacterium [151]. Recently, probiotics are used as the supplementation with drugs for *H. pylori* infection, due to their capability of eradicating *H. pylori* by preventing adhesion of bacteria to the gastric mucosa, causing secretion of the bacteriostatic agent reuterin which possesses anti-inflammatory properties as well as inhibitory effects due to its ability to secrete the lactic acid which is an antibacterial substance [152].

Prebiotics are a group of nondigestible dietary nutrients that positively affect the host through selective alteration of the composition or metabolism of the gut microbiota and also undergoes degradation by gut microbiota [153]. These prebiotics are composed of unique, nondigestible short-chain polysaccharide structures that are not digested by humans. The prebiotics namely fructo-oligosaccharides, galacto-oligosaccharides and trans-galacto-oligosaccharides are fermented by gut microbiota and produce short-chain fatty acids such as lactic acid, butyric acid and propionic acid, which show multiple effects on the body [153]. Fructo-oligosaccharides are naturally found in food or can also be added in the food. The consumption of prebiotic usually helps the metabolism by increasing the Lactobacillus and Bifidobacterial growth in the gut [151]. The beta-fructans oligosaccharides are the most commonly used prebiotics, which are found as natural food elements or dietary fibers present as storage carbohydrates in certain plants [154]. Fructo-oligosaccharides are abundant in chicory roots, banana, tomato and allium, whereas oligosaccharides such as raffinose and stachyose are found in beans and peas, whereas inulin is found in garlic [154]. The positive effects of prebiotics were observed in improving acute colitis in animal model in which a novel oral prebiotic fucoidan and a fucoidan polyphenol complex resulted in significant improvements in symptoms of IBD [155].

Synbiotics refers to the combination of prebiotics and probiotics promoting beneficial gut microflora. Synbiotics were created to overcome some difficulties associated with probiotics in their survival of the GIT [150]. The effects of the hexose-correlated prebiotic compound in combination with probiotic longum BB536 was examined in rats. The study results showed that the combo of both prebiotic and probiotic exerted the highest anti-inflammatory effect. Also, at certain doses, the combo exhibited a higher effect in colitis, which provides the preclinical basis for synergistic use of the synbiotics in treatment of IBD [156].

16.5.6 Polyphenols

Polyphenols are diverse antioxidant, anti-inflammatory, antimicrobial and anti-carcinogenic compounds. Dietary polyphenols are natural plant-derived compounds with a wide array of botanical sources including food and beverages namely tea, coffee, wine, olives, grapes, cereals, dark chocolate and cocoa and turmeric, with catechins, curcumnoids and anthocyanins as the key players of gastroprotective effects. Disruption of gut microbiota equilibrium (dysbiosis) plays a pivotal role in the development of several gastrointestinal disorders. Dietary polyphenols possess the ability to modulate gut microbiota composition and function and membrane permeability to impact gut metabolism and immunity [157].

The prominent green tea catechin epigallocatechin gallate (EGCG) is soluble in water and absorbable in the small intestine by de-glycosylation. EGCG inhibited cancer stem cells through targeting the Wnt/β-catenin pathway and also inhibited the expression of colorectal cancer stem cell markers. EGCG downregulates the activation of the Wnt/β-catenin pathway along with suppression of cell proliferation and induction of apoptosis, while its upregulation diminished the inhibitory effects of EGCG on colorectal cancer stem cells [158]. EGCG was effective on chemoresistant colon stem-like cancer cells in combination with the drug 5-fluorouracil than when the drug was used alone [159]. Another study showed higher therapeutic efficiency when EGCG was administered after anticancer treatment with doxorubicin on Ehrlich's ascites grafted mice carcinoma cells. Doxorubicin-loaded 6-O-(3-hexadecyloxy-2-hydroxyporply)-hyaluronic acid nanoparticles exhibited ~38-fold increase in efficiency when catechin was orally administered via gavage, as compared to the use of drug alone [160].

Curcumin is a yellow-colored hydrophobic polyphenol present in the Indian spice turmeric and derived from the rhizome of the herb Curcuma longa. Turmeric contains three natural analogues such as curcuminoids, in which curcumin is the most abundant (77%), as compared to demethoxycurcumin (17%) and bisdemethoxycurcumin (3%). Curcumin exhibited improved endoscopic healing in peptic ulcers patients, as well as alleviated the symptoms in patients with nonulcer dyspepsia. A new zinc (II)-curcumin complex demonstrated prevention of cold-restraint stress-induced gastric ulcers in mice, which showed significant gastroprotective effect associated with increased mRNA expression of HSP70 and diminution of increased inducible nitric oxide synthase (iNOS) mRNA expression in the mucosa. Curcumin prevented indomethacin-induced gastric ulcerations in rats through prevention of peroxidase inactivation as well as enhancement of ROS scavenging [161]. The curcumin polyphenols mostly undergo degradation by gut microflora. Among various subunits, tetrahydrocurcumin was found to be potentially effective in IBD and colorectal cancer due to its significant anti-inflammatory action. Tetrahydrocurcumin may also conquer the poor bioavailability of hydrophobic curcumin in the treatment of IBD [162]. In comparison to other metabolites, a 6-fold increase in antiproliferative potential was reported with dimethoxycurcumin. The anti-inflammatory and anticancer effects of curcumin occur via different mechanisms of action: (i) suppression of carcinogens in the body, (ii) changes in expression of proteins and (iii) suppression of the action of drug-degrading enzymes. The curcumin showed potential to inhibit the activation of NF-kB10, a mediator of inflammation [163]. The curcumin has been found to be a potential adjuvant for amino salicylates in the maintenance therapy for ulcerative colitis because of its broad-spectrum anti-inflammatory effects compared to amino salicylates. The patients receiving curcumin along with drugs exhibited lesser recurrence as compared to those receiving drug alone [164].

Anthocyanins are members of the flavonoid group of phytochemicals, abundantly found in red-, purple-, blue- and black-colored fruits and vegetables such as blackberries, blueberries, grapes and eggplants. The most recognized colorful anthocyanins are bioflavonoid phytochemicals, which possess the free-radical scavenging and antioxidant capacities as well as other health benefits [165]. Anthocyanins move through the small intestine into the colon, where they undergo degradation by natural microbiota as in the case of the curcumnoids. The anti-inflammatory potential of anthocyanin C3G11 was measured by the magnitude of cytokine-triggered inflammatory response using the human intestinal HT-29 cell line. When compared with a commonly used anti-inflammatory drug 5-amino salicylic acid for IBD, C3G was able to reduce cytokine-induced inflammatory response [166]. Anthocyanins such as glycosides of cyanidin and delphinidin were found to protect the GIT from fat-rich diet-induced alterations in redox signaling, barrier integrity and dysbiosis [167].

16.5.7 Polyunsaturated Fatty Acids

A fatty acid consists of an aliphatic hydrocarbon chain with methyl and carboxyl groups at opposite ends, whereas PUFAs contain more than one double bond in their structure. Biologically important long chain PUFAs can be divided into two groups: omega-3 (n-3) fatty acids and omega-6 (n-6) fatty acids. The n-3 PUFAs contain the first double bond at C3, whereas n-6 PUFA contains the first double bond at C6. The examples of n-3 PUFAs include alpha-linolenic acid (ALA, 18:3), eicosapentaenoic acid (EPA, 19:5) and docosahexaenoic acid (DHA, 22:6). The examples of n-6 PUFAs include linoleic acid (LA, 18:2) and arachidonic acid (AA, 20:4). The essential omega-3 PUFA consists of linear carbon chains with multiple double bonds, and mostly consist of ALA13 (C18:3, n3), EPA14 (C20:5, n3) and DHA15 (C22:6, n3) [168].

Since all essential fatty acids cannot be endogenously synthesized in the body, they can be supplied from an external source as either food or supplementation. For instance, ALA is derived from foods such as canola, soybeans and flaxseeds, whereas DHA and EPA are available from fish oil supplementation and marine supplementation such as salmon, trout and blue fin tuna. The use of omega-3 PUFA in IBD has confirmed that exogenous administration of active metabolites derived from PUFAs like lipoxin A4 derived from AA, resolvins derived from EPA, DHA and DPA; maresin 1 derived from DHA and protectins derived from DPA improved disease and inflammatory outcomes in ulcerative colitis patients without causing immunosuppression or other side effects [169]. In a randomized, open-label, cross-over trial, the study participants were treated with 4 g mixed eicosapentaenoic acid/docosahexaenoic acid in soft-gel capsules and Smartfish drinks for a period of 8 weeks. It was revealed that omega-3 PUFA supplementation produced a reversible increase in several short-chain fatty acid-producing bacteria irrespective of the method of administration [170].

16.5.8 Phytosterols

Phytosterols or phytostenols are plant-derived sterols which possess structural similarity to cholesterol but contain additional double bonds and methyl or ethyl group side chains. The phytosterols are mainly found in vegetables, nuts, fruits and seeds. Sitosterol, campesterol and stigmasterol are major dietary phytosterols comprising 65%, 30% and 3% of dietary phytosterol intake, respectively. These phytosterols are one of the most discussed natural components in context to health-enhancing benefits with limited evidence on their gastroprotection effects [171]. The phytosterol pre-treatment alleviated the clinical symptoms and exerted a protective effect against dextran sulphate sodium-induced colonic inflammation. The protective effect was brought by decreasing infiltration of inflammatory cells as well as an accelerating mucosal healing, which might be attributed to their antioxidant action along with regulation of the gut microbiota [172]. Phytosterols also played a role in the restoration of the intestinal motor pattern, suggesting its role in the management of IBD and other inflammatory diseases of the intestine [171].

16.5.9 Other nutraceuticals

Plants such as senna and cascara are widely employed plant laxatives rich in anthraquinone glucosides. The anthraquinone drugs show anti-constipation effect due to their ability of modifying motility patterns and increasing colonic fluid volume. Sennosides, active constituents in dried leaflets of *Cassia senna*, did not show carcinogenic effect in rats after daily dosing of up to 300 mg/kg/day for a period of two years without causing a genotoxic risk for patients taking senna extracts. Anthraquinones cause apoptosis of colonic epithelial cells, followed by their phagocytic uptake *via* macrophages, which appears as a lipofuscin-like pigment that darkens the colonic mucosa. This condition is known as pseudomelanosis coli [173]. Dried bark of *Cascara sagrada* contains anthraquinone glycosides such as cascarosides A, B, C, D and a small amount of anthraquinone glycosides. Clinical studies showed improved stool frequency and consistency with cascara [174].

Psyllium husk is derived from the seeds of *Plantago ovata*. It consists of highly branched and gel-forming polymer arabinoxylan. This polymer is rich in arabinose and xylose and possess limited digestibility in humans [175]. Psyllium is one of the most used bulk laxatives for constipation which act purely mechanically by absorbing excess water while stimulating normal bowel elimination. It demonstrated increased stool frequency and improved stool consistency by trapping the large quantities of water in the intestine, easing defecation and altering the colonic environment [175]. However, psyllium causes loss of appetite in patients due to delay in gastric emptying if taken before meals. In addition, its texture may cause negative effects on the patient's compliance with the treatment [78]. The study suggested that mixed fibers from fiber supplements were well-tolerated and more effective in reducing flatulence and bloating while being equally effective in improving constipation compared to psyllium [176].

Aloe vera gel, an extract of *Aloe barbadensis*, shows hepato-protective, anti-inflammatory and anti-ulcerative effects. In a non-placebo-controlled study, it was reported that aloe vera can alleviate abdominal pain, discomfort and flatulence in IBS patients with constipation, while it was unable to improve urgency, frequency and consistency of stool in these patients [177]. In a double-blind, randomized, controlled trial, aloe vera gel was administered to patients with active ulcerative colitis for a period of four weeks. The results showed a greater effect on alleviating symptom than placebo; however, the effect was not statistically significant [178]. Another study reported the use of aloe vera as an effective and safe treatment option for patients with IBS compared to placebo [179].

Bael (*Aegle marmelos*) trees are found in tropical and subtropical countries, and both ripe and unripe fruits can be consumed. The pretreatment of ripe fruit pulp of the aqueous extract of *Aegle marmelos* for 14 days was found to decreased mean ulcer index, increased enterochromaffin cell count, 5-hydroxytryptamine (5-HT) content as well as adherent mucosal thickness in all ulcerated gastric tissues in adult albino rats [180,181]. On the other hand, unripe bael fruit extract exhibited a dose-dependent reduction in intestinal inflammation by protecting mast cell degranulation in acetic acid and indomethacin-induced IBD in Wistar rats [182].

Garlic (*Allium sativum* L.) is a globally consumed spice which contains diverse bioactive compounds, such as allicin, alliin, diallyl sulfide, diallyl disulfide, diallyl trisulfide, ajoene and *S*-allyl-cysteine that exhibit several potential bioactivities such as antioxidant, anti-inflammatory, anticancer, hepatoprotective and digestive system protective [183,184]. Bulbs of the plant *Allium sativum* is divided into several fleshy cloves, which are edible. Garlic oil was capable of preventing ethanol-induced gastric injury in rats. This protective effect was attributed to its antioxidant activity mediated through decreased lipid peroxidation and increased antioxidant enzyme levels brought about by ethanol. Another study showed the effects of garlic preparations on the gastric mucosa. A newly developed endoscopic air-powder delivery system was used for direct administration of garlic preparations into the stomach. Among three preparations, raw garlic powder caused severe damage and erosion in the mucosa. Boiled garlic powder caused reddening of the mucosa, whereas aged garlic extract did not cause any undesirable effects [185]. Also, direct administration of powdered enteric-coated products caused reddening of the mucosa, whereas an oral enteric-coated tablet caused loss of epithelial cells in the ileum. The study suggested that safety precautions must be used in choosing a garlic preparation to avoid undesirable effects, including gastrointestinal problems [185].

Honey is mostly colored, viscous, sweet liquid that is prepared by different species of honeybees from the nectar of flowers. Natural honey and *Nigella sativa* (black seed/kalaunji) have been used as a natural remedy, usually as a topical preparation for wound healing. The beneficial effects of honey occur due to its capacity of stimulating tissue growth, enhancing re-epithelization, minimizing scar formation due to acidity, as well as hydrogen peroxide content, osmotic effect, antioxidant and immunostimulatory effects [186]. A study has shown the equal effectiveness of both natural honey and *Nigella sativa* seeds in healing acetylsalicylic acid-induced gastric ulcers in rats [187]. In addition, honey can inhibit the growth of *H. pylori*, which is the main cause of gastritis, peptic ulcer and gastric adenocarcinoma.

Amla (Indian gooseberry) is the strongest rejuvenative among Indian medicinal plants. The ethanolic extract of fruits of *Phyllanthus emblica* showed antiulcer activity through its antioxidative properties by modulation of IL-10 level in a dose-dependent manner [188]. Amla extract at oral doses 250 and 500 mg/kg significantly inhibited the development of gastric lesions in various experimental rat models including pylorus ligation Shay rats; indomethacin, hypothermic restraint stress-induced gastric ulcer and necrotizing agents [189]. It also caused significant reduction of the pyloric ligation-induced basal gastric secretion, titratable acidity and gastric mucosal injury indicating antisecretory, antiulcer and cytoprotective properties of amla extract [190].

Glycyrrhizin is derived from liquorice, the root of *Glycyrrhiza glabra*, which is a widely employed folk medicine in the treatment of gastrointestinal disorders. Its extracts showed enhanced potential for healing of ulceration in the stomach and esophagus due to its antioxidant effect [191]. The antiulcer drug carbenoxolone, is a succinate derivative of glycyrrhetinic acid which is used to promote healing of ulcers [192]. The effect of glycyrrhizin extract and knockout extract (glycyrrhizin-eliminated extract from whole crude extract) indicated the possibility of glycyrrhizin to cause synergistic suppression of iNOS expression when coexisted with the other constituents present in liquorice extract. The knock-out extract proved to be a fruitful approach in determining actual pharmacological functions of target natural compound in the phytochemical mixture [193].

16.6 Concluding remarks

Gastrointestinal diseases are prevalent in the elderly due to various reasons including declined gastrointestinal functions and malnutrition. Different nutraceuticals have demonstrated potential biological effects in treatment of various gastrointestinal diseases by acting as the substrate or inhibitors of specific enzymes or receptors during various biochemical events that occur during disease pathology and progression. The escalating usage of these nutraceuticals in management of gastrointestinal diseases is attributed to a general belief of nontoxicity and lack of side effects as compared to traditional pharmaceutical treatments, as evidenced by huge commercial market of nutraceuticals. This fact motivates the elderly patients to use nutraceuticals as safer alternative to pharmaceuticals for reducing the gastrointestinal disease symptoms. As the mechanisms of actions and toxicity issues of nutraceuticals are ill-understood in the humans, the caution must be exercised in the application of nutraceuticals for the treatment of gastrointestinal disorders.

Conflict of Interest

None.

References

1. Grassi M, Petraccia L, Mennuni G, et al. Changes, Functional Disorders, and Diseases in the Gastrointestinal Tract of Elderly. *Nutr Hosp.* 2011;26(4):659–668.
2. Kaur D, Rasane P, Singh J, et al. Nutritional Interventions for Elderly and Considerations for the Development of Geriatric Foods. *Curr Aging Sci.* 2019;12(1):15–27.
3. da Costa JP, Vitorino R, Silva GM, Vogel C, Duarte AC, Rocha-Santos T. A Synopsis on Aging-Theories, Mechanisms and Future Prospects. *Ageing Res Rev.* 2016:29:90–112.
4. Booth FW, Roberts CK, Laye MJ. Lack of Exercise is a Major Cause of Chronic Diseases. *Compr Physiol.* 2012;2(2):1143–211.
5. Goyal RK, Chaudhury A. Physiology of Normal Esophageal Motility. *J Clin Gastroenterol.* 2008;42(5):610–9.
6. Debi U, Sharma M, Singh L, Sinha A. Barium Esophagogram in Various Esophageal Diseases: A Pictorial Essay. *Indian J Radiol Imaging.* 2019;29(2):141–154.
7. Patel DA, Lappas BM, Vaezi MF. An Overview of Achalasia and its Subtypes. *Gastroenterol Hepatol.* 2017;13(7):411–421.
8. Aslam M, Vaezi MF. Dysphagia in the Elderly. *Gastroenterol Hepatol.* 2013;9(12):784–95.
9. Besanko LK, Burgstad CM, Mountifield R, et al. Lower Esophageal Sphincter Relaxation is Impaired in Older Patients with Dysphagia. *World J Gastroenterol.* 2011;17(10):1326–31.

10. Pandolfino JE, Roman S. High-Resolution Manometry: An Atlas of Esophageal Motility Disorders and Findings of GERD using Esophageal Pressure Popography. *Thorac Surg Clin*. 2011;21(4):465–75.

11. Martinucci I, de Bortoli N, Giacchino M, et al. Esophageal Motility Abnormalities in Gastroesophageal Reflux Disease. *World J Gastrointest Pharmacol Ther*. 2014;5(2):86–96.

12. Clarrett DM, Hachem C. Gastroesophageal Reflux Disease (GERD). *Mo Med*. 2018;115(3):214–218.

13. Rémond D, Shahar DR, Gille D et al. Understanding the Gastrointestinal Tract of the Elderly to Develop Dietary Solutions That Prevent Malnutrition. *Oncotarget*. 2015;6(16):13858–98.

14. O'Mahony D, O'Leary P, Quigley EM. Aging and Intestinal Motility: A Review of Factors that Affect Intestinal Motility in the Aged. *Drugs Aging*. 2002;19(7):515–27.

15. Shimamoto C, Hirata I, Hiraike Y, Takeuchi N, Nomura T, Katsu K. Evaluation of gastric motor activity in the elderly by electrogastrography and the (13)C-acetate breath test. *Gerontology*. 2002;48(6):381–6.

16. Nakae Y, Onouchi H, Kagaya M, Kondo T. Effects of Aging and Gastric Lipolysis on Gastric Emptying of Lipid in Liquid Meal. *J Gastroenterol*. 1999;34(4):445–9.

17. Saffrey MJ. Cellular Changes in the Enteric Nervous System During Ageing. *Dev Biol*. 2013;382(1):344–55.

18. Wade RP. Aging and Neural Control of the GI Tract I. Age-related Changes in the Enteric Nervous System. *Am J Physiol Gastrointest Liver Physiol*, 2002;283:G489–G495.

19. Kim SE. Colonic Slow Transit Can Cause Changes in the Gut Environment Observed in the Elderly. *J Neurogastroenterol Motil*. 2017;23(1):3–4.

20. Knowles CH, Farrugia G. Gastrointestinal Neuromuscular Pathology in Chronic Constipation. *Best Pract Res Clin Gastroenterol*. 2011;25(1):43–57.

21. Kim HJ, Kim N, Kim YS, et al. Changes in the Interstitial Cells of Cajal and Neuronal Nitric Oxide Synthase Positive Peuronal Cells with Aging in the Esophagus of F344 Rats. *PLoS One*. 2017;12(11):e0186322.

22. Zizzo MG, Frinchi M, Nuzzo D, et al. Altered Gastrointestinal Motility in an Animal Model of Lesch-Nyhan Disease. *Auton Neurosci*. 2018;210:55–64.

23. Bitar K, Greenwood-Van Meerveld B, Saad R, Wiley JW. Aging and Gastrointestinal Neuromuscular Function: Insights From Within and Outside the Gut. *Neurogastroenterol Motil*. 2011;23(6):490–501.

24. Dockray GJ. Topical Review. Gastrin and Gastric Epithelial Physiology. *J Physiol*. 1999;518(Pt 2):315–24.

25. Hildebrand P, Lehmann FS, Ketterer S, et al. Regulation of Gastric Function by Endogenous Gastrin Releasing Peptide in Humans: Studies with a Specific Gastrin Releasing Peptide Receptor Antagonist. *Gut*. 2001;49(1):23–8.

26. Turner JR, Liu L, Fligiel SE, Jaszewski R, Majumdar APN. Aging Alters Gastric Mucosal Responses to Epidermalgrowth Factor and Transforming Growth Factor-alpha. *Am J Physiol Gastrointest Liver Physiol*. 2000;278:G805–G810.

27. Ebner R, Derynck R. Epidermal Growth Factor and Transforming Growth Factor-alpha: Differential Intracellular Routing and Processing of Ligand-Receptor Complexes. *Cell Regul*. 1991;2(8):599–612.

28. Fukatsu K, Kudsk KA. Nutrition and Gut Immunity. *Surg Clin North Am*. 2011;91(4):755–70.

29. Das SK, Balasubramanian P, Weerasekara YK. Nutrition Modulation of Human Aging: The Calorie Restriction Paradigm. *Mol Cell Endocrinol*. 2017;455:148–157.

30. Majumdar AP. Regulation of Gastrointestinal Mucosal Growth During Aging. *J Physiol Pharmacol*. 2003;54 Suppl 4:143–54.

31. Sokic-Milutinovic A, Todorovic V, Milosavljevic T, Micev M, Drndarevic N, Mitrovic O. Gastrin and Antral G cells in Course of *Helicobacter pylori* Eradication: Six Months Follow Up Study. *World J Gastroenterol*. 2005;11(27):4140–7.

32. Burkitt MD, Varro A, Pritchard DM. Importance of Gastrin in the Pathogenesis and Preatment of Gastric Tumors. *World J Gastroenterol.* 2009;15(1):1–16.
33. Golemis EA, Scheet P, Beck TN, et al. Molecular Mechanisms of the Preventable Causes of Cancer in the United States. *Genes Dev.* 2018;32(13–14):868–902.
34. Armaghany T, Wilson JD, Chu Q, Mills G. Genetic Alterations in Colorectal Cancer. *Gastrointest Cancer Res.* 2012;5(1):19–27.
35. Tamura G. Alterations of Tumor Suppressor and Tumor-Related Genes in the Development and Progression of Gastric Cancer. *World J Gastroenterol.* 2006;12(2):192–8.
36. Pilotto A, Franceschi M. *Helicobacter pylori* Infection in Older People. *World J Gastroenterol.* 2014;20(21):6364–73.
37. Katelaris PH, Seow F, Lin BP, Napoli J, Ngu MC, Jones DB. Effect of Age, *Helicobacter pylori* Infection, and Gastritis with Atrophy on Serum Gastrin and Gastric Acid Secretion in Healthy Men. *Gut.* 1993;34(8):1032–7.
38. Zullo A, Hassan C, Romiti A, et al. Follow-up of Intestinal Metaplasia in the Stomach: When, How and Why. *World J Gastrointest Oncol.* 2012;4(3):30–6.
39. Dukowicz AC, Lacy BE, Levine GM. Small Intestinal Bacterial Overgrowth: A Comprehensive Review. *Gastroenterol Hepatol.* 2007;3(2):112–22.
40. Jones KD, Berkley JA. Severe Acute Malnutrition and Infection. *Paediatr Int Child Health.* 2014;34(Suppl 1):S1–S29.
41. Keller J, Layer P. The Pathophysiology of Malabsorption. *Viszeralmedizin.* 2014;30(3):150–4.
42. Cavalcoli F, Zilli A, Conte D, Massironi S. Micronutrient Deficiencies in Patients with Chronic Atrophic Autoimmune Gastritis: A Review. *World J Gastroenterol.* 2017;23(4):563–572.
43. Campbell AK, Miller JW, Green R, Haan MN, Allen LH. Plasma Vitamin B-12 Concentrations in an Elderly Latino Population Are Predicted by Serum Gastrin Concentrations and Crystalline Vitamin B-12 Intake. *J Nutr.* 2003;133(9):2770–6.
44. Stein J, Connor S, Virgin G, Ong DE, Pereyra L. Anemia and Iron Deficiency in Gastrointestinal and Liver Conditions. *World J Gastroenterol.* 2016;22(35):7908–25.
45. Wood RJ, Serfaty-Lacrosniere C. Gastric Acidity, Atrophic Gastritis, and Calcium Absorption. *Nutr Rev.* 1992;50(2):33–40.
46. Serra S, Jani PA. An Approach to Duodenal Biopsies. *J Clin Pathol.* 2006;59(11):1133–50.
47. Worwag EM, Craig RM, Jansyn EM, Kirby D, Hubler GL, Atkinson AJ Jr. D-xylose Absorption and Disposition in Patients with Moderately Impaired Renal Function. *Clin Pharmacol Ther.* 1987;41(3):351–357.
48. Arora S, Kassarjian Z, Krasinski SD, Croffey B, Kaplan MM, Russell RM. Effect of Age on Tests of Intestinal and Hepatic Function in Healthy Humans. *Gastroenterology.* 1989;98:1580–1585.
49. Evans C. Malnutrition in the Elderly: A Multifactorial Failure to Thrive. *Perm J.* 2005;9(3):38–41.
50. Wysokiński A, Sobów T, Kłoszewska I, Kostka T. Mechanisms of the Anorexia of Aging - A Review. *Age (Dordr).* 2015;37(4):9821.
51. Hickson M. Malnutrition and Ageing. *Postgrad Med J.* 2006;82(963):2–8.
52. Hoffman R. Micronutrient Deficiencies in the Elderly – Could Ready Meals be part of the solution? *J Nutr Sci.* 2017;6:e2.
53. Ling PR, Bistrian BR. Comparison of the Effects of Food versus Protein Restriction on Selected Nutritional and Inflammatory Markers in Rats. *Metabolism.* 2009;58(6):835–42.
54. Das SK, Moriguti JC, McCrory MA, et al. An Underfeeding Study in Healthy Men and Women Provides Further Evidence of Impaired Regulation of Energy Expenditure in Old Age. *J Nutr.* 2001;131(6):1833–8.

55. Austin J, Marks D. Hormonal Regulators of Appetite. *Int J Pediatr Endocrinol.* 2009;2009:141753.

56. Pilgrim AL, Robinson SM, Sayer AA, Roberts HC. An Overview of Appetite Decline in Older People. *Nurs Older People.* 2015;27(5):29–35.

57. Boyce JM, Shone GR. Effects of Ageing on Smell and Taste. *Postgrad Med J.* 2006;82(966):239–41.

58. Wang H, Zhou M, Brand J, Huang L. Inflammation and Taste Disorders: Mechanisms in Taste Buds. *Ann N Y Acad Sci.* 2009;1170:596–603.

59. Mathey MF, Siebelink E, de Graaf C, Van Staveren WA. Flavor Enhancement of Food Improves Dietary Intake and Nutritional Status of Elderly Nursing Home Residents. *J Gerontol A Biol Sci Med Sci.* 2001;56(4):M200–5.

60. Kazemi S, Savabi G, Khazaei S, et al. Association between Food Intake and Oral Health in Elderly: SEPAHAN Systematic Review no. 8. *Dent Res J (Isfahan).* 2011;8(Suppl 1):S15–20.

61. Kossioni AE. The Association of Poor Oral Health Parameters with Malnutrition in Older Adults: A Review Considering the Potential Implications for Cognitive Impairment. *Nutrients.* 2018;10(11):1709.

62. Tardy AL, Pouteau E, Marquez D, Yilmaz C, Scholey A. Vitamins and Minerals for Energy, Fatigue and Cognition: A Narrative Review of the Biochemical and Clinical Evidence. *Nutrients.* 2020;12(1):228.

63. Mundi MS, Patel J, McClave SA, Hurt RT. Current Perspective for Tube Feeding in the Elderly: From Identifying Malnutrition to Providing of Enteral Nutrition. *Clin Interv Aging.* 2018;13:1353–64.

64. Atalay BG, Yagmur C, Nursal TZ, Atalay H, Noyan T. Use of Subjective Global Assessment and Clinical Outcomes in Critically Ill Geriatric Patients Receiving Nutrition Support. *JPEN J Parenter Enteral Nutr.* 2008;32(4):454–9.

65. Alibhai SM, Greenwood C, Payette H. An Approach to the Management of Unintentional Weight Loss in Elderly People. *CMAJ.* 2005;172(6):773–80.

66. Singh M. Mood, Food, and Obesity. *Front Psychol.* 2014;5:925.

67. Yau YH, Potenza MN. Stress and Eating Behaviors. *Minerva Endocrinol.* 2013;38(3):255–67.

68. Hoogendijk EO, Flores Ruano T, Martínez-Reig M, et al. Socioeconomic Position and Malnutrition among Older Adults: Results from the FRADEA Study. *J Nutr Health Aging.* 2018;22(9):1086–91.

69. Whitelock E, Ensaff H. On Your Own: Older Adults' Food Choice and Dietary Habits. *Nutrients.* 2018;10(4):413.

70. Glisky EL. Changes in Cognitive Function in Human Aging. In: Riddle DR, ed. *Brain Aging: Models, Methods, and Mechanisms.* Boca Raton, FL: CRC Press/Taylor & Francis; 2007.

71. Vetta F, Ronzoni S, Taglieri G, Bollea MR. The Impact of Malnutrition on the Quality of Life in the Elderly. *Clin Nutr.* 1999;18(5):259–67.

72. Liao DH, Zhao JB, Gregersen H. Gastrointestinal Tract Modelling in Health and Disease. *World J Gastroenterol.* 2009;15(2):169–76.

73. Saltzman JR, Russell RM. The Aging Gut. Nutritional Issues. *Gastroenterol Clin North Am.* 1998;27(2):309–24.

74. Dumic I, Nordin T, Jecmenica M, Stojkovic Lalosevic M, Milosavljevic T, Milovanovic T. Gastrointestinal Tract Disorders in Older Age. *Can J Gastroenterol Hepatol.* 2019;2019:6757524.

75. Patricia JJ, Dhamoon AS. Physiology, Digestion. [Updated 2020 Sep 18]. In: *StatPearls* [Internet]. Treasure Island (FL): StatPearls Publishing; 2020.

76. Abell TL, Werkman RF. Gastrointestinal Motility Disorders. *Am Fam Physician.* 1996;53(3):895–902.

77. Bharucha AE, Chakraborty S, Sletten CD. Common Functional Gastroenterological Disorders Associated with Abdominal Pain. *Mayo Clin Proc.* 2016;91(8):1118–32.

78. Gao X, Liu J, Li L, Liu W, Sun M. A Brief Review of Nutraceutical Ingredients in Gastrointestinal Disorders: Evidence and Suggestions. *Int J Mol Sci.* 2020;21(5):1822.

79. Razak PA, Richard KM, Thankachan RP, Hafiz KA, Kumar KN, Sameer KM. Geriatric Oral Health: A Review Article. *J Int Oral Health.* 2014;6(6):110–6.

80. Kaye AD, Baluch A, Scott JT. Pain Management in the Elderly Population: A Review. *Ochsner J.* 2010;10(3):179–87.

81. Miranda-Rius J, Brunet-Llobet L, Lahor-Soler E, Farré M. Salivary Secretory Disorders, Inducing Drugs, and Clinical Management. *Int J Med Sci.* 2015;12(10):811–24.

82. Shaker R. Oropharyngeal Dysphagia. *Gastroenterol Hepatol (N Y).* 2006;2(9):633–4.

83. Sebastian S, Nair PG, Thomas P, Tyagi AK. Oropharyngeal Dysphagia: Neurogenic Etiology and Manifestation. *Indian J Otolaryngol Head Neck Surg.* 2015;67(Suppl 1):119–23.

84. Raber-Durlacher JE, Brennan MT, Verdonck-de Leeuw IM, et al. Swallowing Dysfunction in Cancer Patients. *Support Care Cancer.* 2012;20(3):433–43.

85. Buchholz DW. Dysphagia Associated with Neurological Disorders. *Acta Otorhinolaryngol Belg.* 1994;48(2):143–55.

86. Rao SSC, Mudipalli RS, Mujica VR, Patel RS, Zimmerman B. Effects of Gender and Age on Esophageal Biomechanical Properties and Sensation. *Am J Gastroenterol.* 2003;98(8):1688–95.

87. Wilcox CM. Overview of Infectious Esophagitis. *Gastroenterol Hepatol.* 2013;9(8):517–9.

88. Vakil N, van Zanten SV, Kahrilas P, Dent J, Jones R; Global Consensus Group. The Montreal Definition and Classification of Gastroesophageal Reflux Disease: A Global Evidence-Based Consensus. *Am J Gastroenterol.* 2006;101(8):1900–20; quiz 1943.

89. Chait MM. Gastroesophageal Reflux Disease: Important Considerations for the Older Patients. *World J Gastrointest Endosc.* 2010;2(12):388–96.

90. Ates F, Francis DO, Vaezi MF. Refractory Gastroesophageal Reflux Disease: Advances and Treatment. *Expert Rev Gastroenterol Hepatol.* 2014;8(6):657–67.

91. Badillo R, Francis D. Diagnosis and Treatment of Gastroesophageal Reflux Disease. *World J Gastrointest Pharmacol Ther.* 2014;5(3):105–12.

92. Sipponen P, Maaroos HI. Chronic Gastritis. *Scand J Gastroenterol.* 2015;50(6):657–67.

93. Dholakia KR, Dharmarajan TS, Yadav D, Oiseth S, Norkus EP, Pitchumoni CS. Vitamin B12 Deficiency and Gastric Histopathology in Older Patients. *World J Gastroenterol.* 2005;11(45):7078–83.

94. Madisch A, Andresen V, Enck P, Labenz J, Frieling T, Schemann M. The Diagnosis and Treatment of Functional Dyspepsia. *Dtsch Arztebl Int.* 2018;115(13):222–32.

95. Brun R, Kuo B. Functional Dyspepsia. *Therap Adv Gastroenterol.* 2010;3(3):145–64.

96. Walker MM, Talley NJ. Functional Dyspepsia in the Elderly. *Curr Gastroenterol Rep.* 2019;21(10):54.

97. Narayanan M, Reddy KM, Marsicano E. Peptic Ulcer Disease and *Helicobacter pylori* Infection. *Mo Med.* 2018;115(3):219–24.

98. Sheh A, Fox JG. The Role of the Gastrointestinal Microbiome in *Helicobacter pylori* Pathogenesis. *Gut Microbes.* 2013;4(6):505–31.

99. Pilotto A, Franceschi M, Maggi S, Addante F, Sancarlo D. Optimal Management of Peptic Ulcer Disease in the Elderly. *Drugs Aging.* 2010;27(7):545–58.

100. Khaghan N, Holt PR. Peptic Disease in Elderly Patients. *Can J Gastroenterol.* 2000;14(11):922–8.

101. McCrea GL, Miaskowski C, Stotts NA, Macera L, Varma MG. Pathophysiology of Constipation in the Older Adult. *World J Gastroenterol.* 2008;14(17):2631–8.

102. De Giorgio R, Ruggeri E, Stanghellini V, Eusebi LH, Bazzoli F, Chiarioni G. Chronic Constipation in the Elderly: A Primer for the Gastroenterologist. *BMC Gastroenterol.* 2015;15:130.

103. Schuster BG, Kosar L, Kamrul R. Constipation in Older Adults: Stepwise Approach to Keep Things Moving. *Can Fam Physician.* 2015;61(2):152–8.
104. Vancamelbeke M, Vermeire S. The Intestinal Barrier: A Fundamental Role in Health and Disease. *Expert Rev Gastroenterol Hepatol.* 2017;11(9):821–34.
105. Center for Disease Control and Prevention. Available from: https://www.cdc.gov/ibd/what-is-IBD.htm.
106. LeBlanc JF, Wiseman D, Lakatos PL, Bessissow T. Elderly Patients with Inflammatory Bowel Disease: Updated Review of the Therapeutic Landscape. *World J Gastroenterol.* 2019;25(30):4158–71.
107. Katz S, Feldstein R. Inflammatory Bowel Disease of the Elderly: A Wake-Up Call. *Gastroenterol Hepatol (N Y).* 2008;4(5):337–47.
108. Kilcoyne A, Kaplan JL, Gee MS. Inflammatory Bowel Disease Imaging: Current Practice and Future Directions. *World J Gastroenterol.* 2016;22(3):917–32.
109. Kurniawan I, Kolopaking MS. Management of Irritable Bowel Syndrome in the Elderly. *Acta Med Indones.* 2014;46(2):138–47.
110. Sanchez C, Chinn BT. Hemorrhoids. *Clin Colon Rectal Surg.* 2011;24(1):5–13.
111. Yamamoto M, Ikeda M, Matsumoto T, et al. Hemorrhoidectomy for Elderly Patients Aged 75 Years or More, Before and After Studies. *Ann Med Surg.* 2020;55:88–92.
112. Lohsiriwat V. Hemorrhoids: From Basic Pathophysiology to Clinical Management. *World J Gastroenterol.* 2012;18(17):2009–17.
113. Schussman LC, Lutz LJ. Outpatient Management of Hemorrhoids. *Prim Care.* 1986;13(3):527–41.
114. Matrana MR, Margolin DA. Epidemiology and Pathophysiology of Diverticular Disease. *Clin Colon Rectal Surg.* 2009;22(3):141–6.
115. Comparato G, Pilotto A, Franzè A, Franceschi M, Di Mario F. Diverticular Disease in the Elderly. *Dig Dis.* 2007;25(2):151–9.
116. Salzman H, Lillie D. Diverticular Disease: Diagnosis and Treatment. *Am Fam Physician.* 2005;72(7):1229–34.
117. Dekker E, Tanis PJ, Vleugels JLA, Kasi PM, Wallace MB. Colorectal Cancer. *Lancet.* 2019;394(10207):1467–80.
118. Millan M, Merino S, Caro A, Feliu F, Escuder J, Francesch T. Treatment of Colorectal Cancer in the Elderly. *World J Gastrointest Oncol.* 2015;7(10):204–20
119. Kuipers EJ, Grady WM, Lieberman D, et al. Colorectal Cancer. *Nat Rev Dis Primers.* 2015;1:15065.
120. Kordatou Z, Kountourakis P, Papamichael D. Treatment of Older Patients with Colorectal Cancer: A Perspective Review. *Ther Adv Med Oncol.* 2014;6(3):128–40.
121. Njeze GE. Gallstones. *Niger J Surg.* 2013;19(2):49–55.
122. Tanaja J, Lopez RA, Meer JM. Cholelithiasis. [Updated 2020 Aug 10]. In: *StatPearls* [Internet]. Treasure Island (FL): StatPearls Publishing; 2020.
123. Johnson CD. ABC of the Upper Gastrointestinal Tract. Upper Abdominal Pain: Gall Bladder. *BMJ.* 2001;323(7322):1170–3.
124. Jones MW, Weir CB, Ghassemzadeh S. Gallstones (Cholelithiasis) [Updated 2020 Oct 10]. In: *StatPearls* [Internet]. Treasure Island, FL: StatPearls Publishing; 2020.
125. Dahiya S, Dahiya R. Chapter 11. Delivery Strategies and Formulation Approaches of Anticancer Nutraceuticals. In: Gupta SV, Pathak YV. (eds.). *Advances in Nutraceutical Applications in Cancer - Recent Research Trends and Clinical Applications.* 1st edition, CRC Press, Taylor & Francis Group: Boca Raton, FL, 2019; 239–67.
126. Global Nutraceuticals Market (2018 to 2027) - Analysis and Forecasts by Type & Application. Available from: https://www.globenewswire.com/news-release/2020/04/29/2024120/0/en/Global-Nutraceuticals-Market-2018-to-2027-Analysis-and-Forecasts-By-Type-Application.html.
127. Holscher HD. Dietary Fiber and Prebiotics and the Gastrointestinal Microbiota. *Gut Microbes.* 2017;8(2):172–84.

128. Lattimer JM, Haub MD. Effects of Dietary Fiber and its Components on Metabolic Health. *Nutrients*. 2010;2(12):1266–89.
129. Dhingra D, Michael M, Rajput H, Patil RT. Dietary Fibre in Foods: A Review. *J Food Sci Technol*. 2012;49(3):255–66.
130. Das L, Bhaumik E, Raychaudhuri U, Chakraborty R. Role of Nutraceuticals in Human Health. *J Food Sci Technol*. 2012;49(2):173–83.
131. Ho KS, Tan CY, Mohd Daud MA, Seow-Choen F. Stopping or Reducing Dietary Fiber Intake Reduces Constipation and its Associated Symptoms. *World J Gastroenterol*. 2012;18(33):4593–6.
132. Anderson JW, Baird P, Davis RH Jr, et al. Health Benefits of Dietary Fiber. *Nutr Rev*. 2009;67(4):188–205.
133. Srinivasan K. Role of Spices Beyond Food Flavoring: Nutraceuticals with Multiple Health Effects. *Food Rev Int*. 2005;21:167–88.
134. Mathew B, Biju R. Neuroprotective Effects of Garlic: A Review. *Libyan J Med*. 2008;3(1):23–33.
135. Pazyar N, Feily A. Garlic in Dermatology. *Dermatol Reports*. 2011;3(1):e4.
136. Thomson M, Alnaqeeb MA, Bordia T, Al-Hassan JM, Afzal M, Ali M. Effects of Aqueous Extract of Onion on the Liver and Lung of Rats. *J Ethnopharmacol*. 1998;61(2):91–9.
137. Tan BL, Norhaizan ME, Liew WP, Sulaiman Rahman H. Antioxidant and Oxidative Stress: A Mutual Interplay in Age-Related Diseases. *Front Pharmacol*. 2018;9:1162.
138. Voll LM, Abbasi AR. Are there Specific In Vivo Roles for Alpha- and Gamma-Tocopherol in Plants? *Plant Signal Behav*. 2007;2(6):486–8.
139. Lobo V, Patil A, Phatak A, Chandra N. Free Radicals, Antioxidants and Functional Foods: Impact on Human Health. *Pharmacogn Rev*. 2010;4(8):118–26.
140. Jung S, Wu K, Giovannucci E, Spiegelman D, Willett WC, Smith-Warner SA. Carotenoid Intake and Risk of Colorectal Adenomas in a Cohort of Male Health Professionals. *Cancer Causes Control*. 2013;24(4):705–17.
141. Kurutas EB. The Importance of Antioxidants Which Play the role in Cellular Response Against Oxidative/Nitrosative Stress: Current State. *Nutr J*. 2016;15(1):71.
142. Tinggi U. Selenium: Its Role as Antioxidant in Human Health. *Environ Health Prev Med*. 2008;13(2):102–8.
143. National Institute of Health, Office of Dietary Supplements. Available from: https://ods.od.nih.gov/factsheets/Selenium-HealthProfessional.
144. Cai X, Wang C, Yu W, et al. Selenium Exposure and Cancer Risk: An Updated Meta-analysis and Meta-regression. *Sci Rep*. 2016;6:19213.
145. Kadkol S, Diamond AM. The Interaction Between Dietary Selenium Intake and Genetics in Determining Cancer Risk and Outcome. *Nutrients*. 2020;12(8):2424.
146. Wacker M, Holick MF. Sunlight and Vitamin D: A Global Perspective for Health. *Dermatoendocrinol*. 2013;5(1):51–108.
147. Fletcher J, Cooper SC, Ghosh S, Hewison M. The Role of Vitamin D in Inflammatory Bowel Disease: Mechanism to Management. *Nutrients*. 2019;11(5):1019.
148. Dadaei T, Safapoor MH, Asadzadeh Aghdaei H, et al. Effect of Vitamin D3 Supplementation on TNF-α Serum Level and Disease Activity Index in Iranian IBD patients. *Gastroenterol Hepatol Bed Bench*. 2015;8(1):49–55.
149. Li W, Wang QL, Liu X, et al. Combined Use of Vitamin D3 and Metformin Exhibits Synergistic Chemopreventive Effects on Colorectal Neoplasia in Rats and Mice. *Cancer Prev Res*. 2015;8(2):139–48.
150. Ordóñez-Morán P, Dafflon C, Imajo M, Nishida E, Huelsken J. HOXA5 Counteracts Stem Cell Traits by Inhibiting Wnt Signaling in Colorectal Cancer. *Cancer Cell*. 2015;28(6):815–29.
151. Markowiak P, Śliżewska K. Effects of Probiotics, Prebiotics, and Synbiotics on Human Health. *Nutrients*. 2017;9(9):1021.

152. Fijan S. Microorganisms with Claimed Probiotic Properties: An overview of Recent Literature. *Int J Environ Res Public Health.* 2014;11(5):4745–67.
153. Homan M, Orel R. Are Probiotics Useful in *Helicobacter pylori* Eradication? *World J Gastroenterol.* 2015;21(37):10644–53.
154. Davani-Davari D, Negahdaripour M, Karimzadeh I, et al. Prebiotics: Definition, Types, Sources, Mechanisms, and Clinical Applications. *Foods.* 2019;8(3):92.
155. Looijer-van Langen MA, Dieleman LA. Prebiotics in Chronic Intestinal Inflammation. *Inflamm Bowel Dis.* 2009;15(3):454–62.
156. Lean QY, Eri RD, Fitton JH, Patel RP, Gueven N. Fucoidan Extracts Ameliorate Acute Colitis. *PLoS One.* 2015;10(6):e0128453.
157. Ocón B, Anzola A, Ortega-González M, et al. Active Hexose-correlated Compound and Bifidobacterium Longum BB536 Exert Symbiotic Effects in Experimental Colitis. *Eur J Nutr.* 2013;52(2):457–66.
158. Kumar Singh A, Cabral C, Kumar R, et al. Beneficial Effects of Dietary Polyphenols on Gut Microbiota and Strategies to Improve Delivery Efficiency. *Nutrients.* 2019;11(9):2216.
159. Chen Y, Wang XQ, Zhang Q, et al. (-)-Epigallocatechin-3-Gallate Inhibits Colorectal Cancer Stem Cells by Suppressing Wnt/β-Catenin Pathway. *Nutrients.* 2017;9(6):572.
160. Toden S, Tran HM, Tovar-Camargo OA, Okugawa Y, Goel A. Epigallocatechin-3-gallate Targets Cancer Stem-like Cells and Enhances 5-Fluorouracil Chemosensitivity in Colorectal Cancer. *Oncotarget.* 2016;7(13):16158–71.
161. Lee WH, Loo CY, Bebawy M, Luk F, Mason RS, Rohanizadeh R. Curcumin and its Derivatives: Their Application in Neuropharmacology and Neuroscience in the 21st century. *Curr Neuropharmacol.* 2013;11(4):338–78.
162. Mei X, Xu D, Xu S, Zheng Y, Xu S. Gastroprotective and Antidepressant Effects of a New Zinc(II)-Curcumin Complex in Rodent Models of Gastric Ulcer and Depression Induced by Stresses. *Pharmacol Biochem Behav.* 2011;99(1):66–74.
163. Stearns ME, Amatangelo MD, Varma D, Sell C, Goodyear SM. Combination Therapy with Epigallocatechin-3-gallate and Doxorubicin in Human Prostate Tumor Modeling Studies: Inhibition of Metastatic Tumor Growth in Severe Combined Immunodeficiency mice. *Am J Pathol.* 2010;177(6):3169–79.
164. Dulbecco P, Savarino V. Therapeutic Potential of Curcumin in Digestive Diseases. *World J Gastroenterol.* 2013;19(48):9256–70.
165. Triantafyllidi A, Xanthos T, Papalois A, Triantafillidis JK. Herbal and Plant Therapy in Patients with Inflammatory Bowel Disease. *Ann Gastroenterol.* 2015;28(2):210–20.
166. Lila MA. Anthocyanins and Human Health: An In Vitro Investigative Approach. *J Biomed Biotechnol.* 2004;2004(5):306–13.
167. Serra D, Paixão J, Nunes C, Dinis TC, Almeida LM. Cyanidin-3-glucoside Suppresses Cytokine-induced Inflammatory Response in Human Intestinal Cells: Comparison with 5-Aminosalicylic Acid. *PLoS One.* 2013;8(9):e73001.
168. Cremonini E, Daveri E, Mastaloudis A, Adamo AM, Mills D, Kalanetra K, Hester SN, Wood SM, Fraga CG, Oteiza PI. Anthocyanins protect the gastrointestinal tract from high fat diet-induced alterations in redox signaling, barrier integrity and dysbiosis. *Redox Biol.* 2019;26:101269.
169. Ratnayake WM, Galli C. Fat and Fatty Acid Terminology, Methods of Analysis and Fat Digestion and Metabolism: A Background Review Paper. *Ann Nutr Metab.* 2009;55(1–3):8–43.
170. Kaur N, Chugh V, Gupta AK. Essential Fatty Acids as Functional Components of Foods- A Review. *J Food Sci Technol.* 2014;51(10):2289–303.
171. Watson H, Mitra S, Croden FC, et al. A Randomised Trial of the Effect of Omega-3 Polyunsaturated Fatty acid Supplements on the Human Intestinal Microbiota. *Gut.* 2018;67(11):1974–83.

172. Gupta C, Prakash D. Nutraceuticals for Geriatrics. *J Tradit Complement Med.* 2014;5(1):5–14.

173. Aldini R, Micucci M, Cevenini M, et al. Antiinflammatory Effect of Phytosterols in Experimental Murine Colitis Model: Prevention, Induction, Remission Study. *PLoS One.* 2014;9(9):e108112.

174. Morales MA, Hernández D, Bustamante S, Bachiller I, Rojas A. Is Senna Laxative Use Associated to Cathartic Colon, Genotoxicity, or Carcinogenicity? *J Toxicol.* 2009;2009:287247.

175. Cirillo, C.; Capasso, R. Constipation and Botanical Medicines: An Overview. *Phytother. Res.* 2015;29:1488–93.

176. Jalanka J, Major G, Murray K, et al. The Effect of Psyllium Husk on Intestinal Microbiota in Constipated Patients and Healthy Controls. *Int J Mol Sci.* 2019;20(2):433.

177. Erdogan A, Rao SSC, Thiruvaiyaru D, et al. Randomised Clinical Trial: Mixed Soluble/Insoluble Fibre vs. Psyllium for Chronic Constipation. *Aliment Pharm Ther.* 2016;44:35–44.

178. Khedmat H, Karbasi A, Amini M, Aghaei A, Taheri S. Aloe vera in Treatment of Refractory Irritable Bowel Syndrome: Trial on Iranian Patients. *J Res Med Sci.* 2013;18(8):732.

179. Davis K, Philpott S, Kumar D, Mendall M. Randomised Double-blind Placebo-controlled Trial of Aloe vera for Irritable Bowel Syndrome. *Int J Clin Pract.* 2006;60(9):1080–6.

180. Langmead L, Feakins RM, Goldthorpe S, et al. Randomized, Double-blind, Placebo-controlled Trial of Oral Aloe vera Gel for Active Ulcerative Colitis. *Aliment Pharmacol Ther.* 2004;19(7):739–47.

181. Singh P, Dutta SR, Guha D. Gastric Mucosal Protection by Aegle Marmelos Against Gastric Mucosal Damage: Role of Enterochromaffin Cell and Serotonin. *Saudi J Gastroenterol.* 2015;21(1):35–42.

182. Hong SW, Chun J, Park S, Lee HJ, Im JP, Kim JS. *Aloe vera* Is Effective and Safe in Short-term Treatment of Irritable Bowel Syndrome: A Systematic Review and Meta-analysis. *J Neurogastroenterol Motil.* 2018;24(4):528–35.

183. Behera JP, Mohanty B, Ramani YR, Rath B, Pradhan S. Effect of Aqueous Extract of Aegle marmelos Unripe Fruit on Inflammatory Bowel Disease. *Indian J Pharmacol.* 2012;44(5):614–8.

184. Shang A, Cao SY, Xu XY, et al. Bioactive Compounds and Biological Functions of Garlic (*Allium sativum* L.). *Foods.* 2019;8(7):246.

185. Khosla P, Karan RS, Bhargava VK. Effect of Garlic Oil on Ethanol Induced Gastric Ulcers in Rats. *Phytother Res.* 2004;18(1):87–91.

186. Hoshino T, Kashimoto N, Kasuga S. Effects of Garlic Preparations on the Gastrointestinal Mucosa. *J Nutr.* 2001;131(3s):1109S–13S.

187. Javadi SMR, Hashemi M, Mohammadi Y, MamMohammadi A, Sharifi A, Makarchian HR. Synergistic Effect of Honey and Nigella sativa on Wound Healing in Rats. *Acta Cir Bras.* 2018;33(6):518–23.

188. Hashem-Dabaghian F, Agah S, Taghavi-Shirazi M, Ghobadi A. Combination of Nigella sativa and Honey in Eradication of Gastric *Helicobacter pylori* Infection. *Iran Red Crescent Med J.* 2016;18(11):e23771.

189. Chatterjee A, Chattopadhyay S, Bandyopadhyay SK. Biphasic Effect of Phyllanthus emblica L. Extract on NSAID-Induced Ulcer: An Antioxidative Trail Weaved with Immunomodulatory Effect. *Evid Based Complement Alternat Med.* 2011;2011:146808.

190. Sairam K, Rao CV, Babu MD, Kumar KV, Agrawal VK, Goel RK. Antiulcerogenic Effect of Methanolic Extract of Emblica Officinalis: An Experimental Study. *J Ethnopharmacol.* 2002;82(1):1–9.

191. Jalilzadeh-Amin G, Najarnezhad V, Anassori E, Mostafavi M, Keshipour H. Antiulcer Properties of *Glycyrrhiza glabra* L. Extract on Experimental Models of Gastric Ulcer in Mice. *Iran J Pharm Res*. 2015;14(4):1163–70.
192. Asl MN, Hosseinzadeh H. Review of Pharmacological Effects of *Glycyrrhiza* sp. and its Bioactive Compounds. *Phytother Res*. 2008;22(6):709–24.
193. Uto T, Morinaga O, Tanaka H, Shoyama Y. Analysis of the Synergistic Effect of Glycyrrhizin and other Constituents in Licorice Extract on Lipopolysaccharide-induced Nitric Oxide Production using Knock-out Extract. *Biochem Biophys Res Commun*. 2012;417(1):473–8.

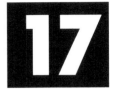

Oro-Dental Challenges during Aging and Nutraceuticals

Anita Patel
Sankalchand Patel University

Satish Patel
Prabhu Dental Clinic

Dhavalkumar Patel
Leading Pharma LLC

Jayvadan Patel
Sankalchand Patel University

Contents

DOI: 10.1201/9781003110866-17

17.1 Oral health, general health and quality of life

Oral health is very important to the general health and comfort of elder people. The mouth has been interpreted as "the window to your overall health". The oral cavity reflects a person's health and welfare throughout life. Oral diseases can have an impact on lots of aspects of overall health conditions. Oral and other diseases also contribute to common risk factors. As the possibility of chronic conditions rises with age, it is essential to inspect the interaction of these diseases with oral disease and their collective influence on overall health among elder people [1]. Over recent years, much research has confirmed the effect of oral health on the quality of life and overall health [2,3]. The linkage between oral health and overall health is mostly well-defined among the elder populace. Problems with dentures, gums as well as teeth can notably influence the overall comfort of an older individual and their aptitude to become old positively. The incident of pain, continued existence of dental eruptions, difficulty with eating and chewing, and awkwardness about the shape of teeth or else about missing, faded, or broken teeth can negatively distress people's daily life, confidence, and well-being [3,4].

Deprived oral health can restrict food selections and weaken the enjoyment of eating [5]. Some researchers described that the more the number of missing teeth, the inferior the quality of life [6]. Several investigations point out that extensive tooth loss impairs chewing effectiveness [7]. Having 20 teeth is considered essential for efficient dentition [8], and chewing with detachable dentures is at least 30%–40% less efficient as compared to chewing with ordinary teeth [9]. Elders with extensive or entire tooth loss are more prone to replace with easier-to-chew foodstuffs like those rich in saturated fats and cholesterol for foods rich in carotenes, fiber, and vitamin C [10,11]. Among elder individuals, tooth loss has been connected with both weight loss as well as overweight [12,13].

Extensive and total tooth loss might limit the societal relationships and restrain familiarity. Tooth loss can have an effect on verbal communication, which in turn restricts social relations, depreciates from the look, and reduces self-respect [14,15]. Untreated oral ailments will not work out if remain untreated and can greatly affect the quality of life. Distress from untreated oral disorders can limit regular activities of everyday life and upset sleep. In advanced conditions, dental caries entail the soft tissue of the tooth and demolish the structure of the tooth leaving just root portions that can cause ulcerations and swelling [16]. Periodontitis can tear down the underneath tissues of the teeth and lead to abscesses that give rise to swelling, blood loss, and soreness [17]. Dental caries and periodontitis, if remain untreated, eventually result in tooth loss [18].

Deprived oral health can also augment the dangers to overall health and with compromised chewing as well as eating capability have an effect on food ingestion [10,12]. Failing to avert or manage the development of oral ailment may amplify the hazard of unfavorable health effects. A current Cochrane methodical assessment establishes facts that the management of periodontal illness enhanced metabolic power in elder persons with type 2 diabetes [19]. An additional latest investigation establishes that invasive dental practices such as tooth removal and periodontal treatment likely preventable with early treatment and prevention amplified the occurrence of ischemic stroke as well as myocardial infarctions [20]. Several studies also confirmed a similar relationship between oral sanitation and optimistic health effects. Two methodical analyses found that superior oral hygiene care can avert respiratory diseases and casualty from pneumonia in elderly citizens in hospitals [21,22]. A different latest investigation establishes that regular tooth brushing was linked with lesser risks of cardiovascular disease [23].

Likewise, systemic disorders and/or the undesirable side effects of their therapies can cause a bigger risk of oral diseases, dry mouth, and distorted sense of taste along with the smell. The high incidence of multi-medication treatments at a later age may further complicate the effect on oral health and oral health care [4]. Chronic health states produce a gigantic burden on the health of elder persons as well as the whole healthcare organization. Regular dental care not only averts periodontal infection but also assists to stratify elder patients who are at considerable risk for more severe systemic conditions.

17.2 Age-related oral changes

With aging, the look and structure of teeth have a propensity to transform [24]. Yellowing or darkening of the teeth is caused by alterations in the thickness as well as the composition of the fundamental dentin and its covering, the enamel [25,26]. Abrasion and slow destruction also carve up alterations in tooth appearance [27]. Nerves, blood vessels, and lymphatic vessels entering aged pulp reveal progressive mineralization of the nerve sheath, arteriosclerotic alterations, and degenerative transforms, respectively. The death of the nerve that takes place in aged pulp clarifies why aged teeth are often painless [28].

The number of blood vessels entering a tooth and the enamel decrease with age, leading to reduced sensitivity [25]. Through lesser sensitivity to environmental stimuli, the response to trauma or caries might diminish. The cementum, a substance that covers the root surface progressively thickens, with the total width roughly tripling between 10 and 75 years of age. Because of the highly organic nature of cementum, it is less resistant to environmental agents, such as sugar, acids from soft drinks, and tobacco, which has a drying effect [29]. Age-related alterations in the oral mucosa and hormonal or nutritional deficiencies bring about diminished keratinization, dryness, and thinning of the structure of epithelial [30]. Furthermore, the width as well as fiber content of the periodontal tendon, a part of the attachment apparatus of the periodontium, diminishes with age [31]. One more common situation found in older persons is a gingival recession but is not considered a normal age-dependent oral alteration. Gingival recession exposes the cementum, possibly leading to root caries [32].

Teeth play an important role in speaking, smiling, chewing, and appearance. However, as you age, teeth and gums present with unique dilemmas. Saliva, a clear fluid present in the oral cavity, has a very important role in oral as well as dental health. It helps out in speaking, chewing, and shielding the teeth from decay, gums from infection, and the oral cavity from the progress of thrush /candidiasis and other bacterial and viral infections [33]. Alterations in the oral cavity as a result of aging are seen in the oral hard as well as soft tissues and also in bones, the temporomandibular joints, and the oral mucus membrane. While elder patients maintain their natural teeth for longer, the clinical image consists of normal physiological age changes in combination with pathological causes. The clinical consequence with an aging populace maintaining more of its natural teeth for longer, dental experts should be expecting to monitor oral age-related alterations more often [25].

With the increase in age, there are changes seen in mucous membranes of the lips, buccal and palatal tissues, and floor of the mouth. The patient's chief complaints are mainly burning sensation, pain, and dryness of the mouth or cracks in the lips. Chewing and swallowing become very difficult, and the taste is altered. The epithelial membrane is thin and easily injured. It heals slowly because of impaired circulation [34].

Probably the most common manifestation of aging of the tongue is depapillation, which usually begins at the apex and lateral borders. Tongue often appears to be smooth and glossy or red and inflamed. The size of the tongue probably does not vary with age. Glossodynia and glossopyrosis are the most common problems occurring in senescence. Lingual tissue changes are commonly associated with alteration in taste sensation. This reduced perception of taste can be because of some gradual nerve degeneration and hyperkeratinization of the epithelium which may occlude taste bud ducts and pores.

However, tooth loss can lead to a wider tongue by virtue of the overdevelopment of the tongue's intrinsic musculature [34].

Oral health and its inferences to one's general health are often unnoticed as not important by the general populace in addition to the ever-rising elderly people. The condition of the anatomical structures in the mouth (e.g., gums, palate, teeth, and tongue) can imitate the general health status of a person. Though numerous pathologies modify the ordinary flora of the mouth in all age groups, elder persons normally present with certain alterations in their mouth which are usual for their age [35]. Dental professionals must be aware of pathologic findings against normal findings in the mouth that are regular with aging. Oral alterations in elder people have common implications ranging from the physical to the mental and societal comfort of the person [36].

17.3 Oral health problems in elder populace

Oral health declines with age leading to high levels of tooth loss, dental caries, dry mouth, and the prevalence rates of periodontal disease, ill-fitting denture, mucosal lesions, oral ulceration, xerostomia, and oral cancer and has been obvious in the elder populace with deprived oral health worldwide. Attrition, abrasion, and dental carry rise with age, while periodontitis affects persons of all ages but is most frequent in the aged person. The fraction of pathological tooth wear in elder populace is three times that found in populace aged 26–30 years. Edentulism rises with age and in the 75 years and elder with 9.6% being males and 31.5% females [24,37,38]. The most common oral issues found in the elderly population are as follows.

17.3.1 Root carries

Root caries can occur at any age, but it is one of the noteworthy dental problems among the elder populace nowadays. Root caries is the main reason for tooth loss in elder people, and tooth loss is the most important oral health-related depressing variable of quality of life for old people [39]. The occurrence of root caries in patients elder than 60 years is two times that of 30-year-olds [40]; 64% of individuals elder than 80 years have root caries, and up to 96% have coronal caries (on top of the gum) [41]. Elderly individuals are more vulnerable to root caries attributable to poor oral hygiene, occasional cleaning as well as dental examinations, not enough use of fluoride-containing oral hygiene products, salivary gland dysfunction, and detachable partial dentures, which can entrap plaque around the teeth, thus favoring the development of caries [42]. Risk factors for coronal as well as root caries lead to augmented exposure to cariogenic bacteria, like *Streptococcus mutans*, *Lactobacillus*, and *Actinomyces* [40]. Data also have revealed relationships of food and oral habits and other variables on root caries (Figure 17.1) [43].

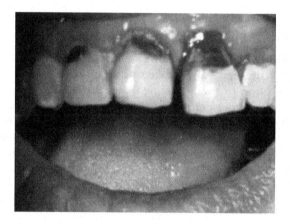

Figure 17.1 *Root caries: black discoloration on root surfaces.*

17.3.2 Tooth loss

Tooth loss or edentulism is widespread among older people all over the world [44] and is greatly associated with socio-economic conditions. Functional dentitions, as considered by the presence of no less than 20 natural teeth, are observed to be most common among old people of high socio-economic class contrary to persons of low socio-economic class [45]. Partial or total tooth loss is an age-related condition that is caused primarily by severe dental caries and periodontitis, thereafter leading to teeth extraction [46,47]. A relatively small number of epidemiological studies of tooth loss at age have been carried out in developing countries. On the other hand, in countries where access to oral health checks is inadequate and teeth are often pulled out as a result of pain, discomfort, or deficiency in materials needed dental treatment [3]. Tooth loss adversely influences eating habits and difficulty in food intake [38]. Extensive tooth loss diminishes chewing ability, and it also affects food options; for example, edentulous people tend to circumvent dietary fiber and have preference foods rich in saturated fats and cholesterols [10]. Edentulousness is made known to be an independent risk factor for weight loss [12] and, in addition to the problem with chewing, the old-age populace might have societal handicaps related to communication. Tooth loss has also been connected with a higher risk of ischemic stroke [48] and poor mental health [49].

17.3.3 Periodontal disease

Worldwide, the percentage of the subjects with Community Periodontal Index score 4 (deep pockets) ranges from approximately 5%–70% among the elder community [24]. Epidemiological investigations confirm that poor oral sanitation or elevated levels of dental plaque are linked with high occurrence rates and harshness of periodontal disorder [50]. Little education, no routine dental check-ups, a small number of teeth present, and habitual smoking have independent effects on the development of periodontal diseases in elder adults [51,52].

17.3.3.1 Gingivitis

Plaque is a biofilm that consists of gram-negative bacteria along with endotoxins that build up on the surface of the teeth at the gingival boundaries, resulting in gingival inflammation known as gingivitis [53]. Gingivitis is described by edema of the gingival tissue, which frequently bleeds easily with gentle brushing as well as periodontal probing. Additional reasons for gingivitis consist of trauma and the use of tobacco. Though gingivitis is more widespread in elder persons, age only is not a risk factor for gingivitis [40]. It can be inverted with good quality oral cleanliness; otherwise, it might step forward to periodontitis.

17.3.3.2 Periodontitis

Periodontitis represented in Figure 17.2 occurs when gingival inflammation induces the periodontal ligament to separate from the cementum as well as tooth structure, resulting in an augmented depth of the gingival pocket, loosening of the tooth, and, eventually, tooth loss [54].

Periodontitis is bound up with anaerobic bacteria, like *Aggregatibacter actinomycetemcomitans*, *Bacteroides forsythus*, and *Porphyromonas gingivalis*. Lots of elder individuals are liable to periodontal detachment and tooth loss as a result of poor oral sanitation and gingival depression [55]. Moreover, poor oral health and poor general health are interrelated, primarily because of common risk factors; for example, severe periodontal disease is associated with diabetes mellitus [56–58], ischemic heart disease [59], and chronic respiratory disease [60,61].

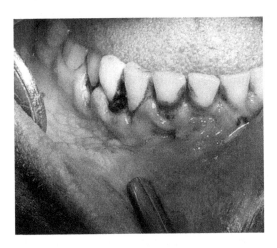

Figure 17.2 *Periodontitis: an infection of gum.*

17.3.4 Candidiasis

Though it is expected that *Candida* species are present in the normal oral flora of healthy adults [62], but certain circumstances raise the danger of overgrowth specifically in elder individuals. These circumstances consist of the pathogenicity of individual *Candida* strains; local factors like denture irritation, steroid inhaler use, tobacco use, and xerostomia; and systemic factors like antibiotic use, chemotherapy, endocrine disorders, immunodeficiency, malabsorption, malnutrition, radiation therapy, and systemic corticosteroid use [63,64].

17.3.5 Xerostomia

Xerostomia, the subjective feeling of dry mouth resulting from decreased saliva production, affects 29%–57% of elder persons [65,66], and the condition is reported in just about 30% of the people aged 65 and older [67]. Saliva lubricates the oral cavity, averts decay by promoting remineralization of teeth, and defends against bacterial and fungal infections [55]. In addition to dry mouth, clinical manifestations of xerostomia comprise a burning sensation, changes in taste, and difficulty with swallowing and speech [65]. Although salivary flow does not decline with age alone, certain medications and illnesses increase the risk of xerostomia in elder persons [65,68,69]. The medications mostly accountable for dry mouth are antihistamines, antipsychotics, atropinics, beta blockers, and tricyclic antidepressants; accordingly, the complaint of dry mouth is most frequent in patients treated for hypertension, urinary disorders, or psychiatric [67,70].

17.3.6 Denture-related conditions

Denture stomatitis is a widespread oral mucosal lesion of clinical significance in old-age populaces. The occurrence rate of stomatitis is accounted within the range of 11%–67% in whole denture wearers [71,72]. In several cases of denture stomatitis, colonization of yeast to the fitting surface of the prosthesis is experiential. Additional factors of stomatitis comprise allergic reaction to the denture base material or symptoms of the systemic disorder [73,74]. The incidences of denture stomatitis show a relationship strongly to denture sanitation or the quantity of denture plaque. The practice of denture at night [74], ignorance of denture-soaking at night and make use of faulty and inappropriate dentures [75] are as well risk factors for denture stomatitis, as is alcohol and tobacco consumption [74]. It is observed that the lower the level of education, the higher the incidence of stomatitis, and finally, the longer since the previous dental appointment, the higher the probability of denture-related lesions [3]. Other denture-related lesions consist of denture hyperplasia as well as traumatic ulcers; their occurrence rates in old-age denture wearers vary from 4% to 26% [72,76]. Denture hyperplasia is most common in persons with ill-fitting and/or unretentive dentures [77].

Both types of lesions have been experiential more often among complete denture wearers than in individuals wearing detachable partial dentures. Furthermore, low education, alcohol and tobacco use, and irregular dental visits are factors linked with an augmented prevalence rate of denture-related lesions [76].

17.3.7 Oral cancer

Oral cancer stands as the main threat to the health of the elderly in both high as well as low-income countries. It comprises an oral cavity, lip, and pharyngeal cancer and is the eighth most common cancer globally [78]. Age-specific rates for cancer of the oral cavity raise more and more with age, the majority of cases taking place in the age groups higher than 60 years. The occurrence of precancerous lesions of the oral mucous membrane (Figure 17.3) such as leukoplakia (a situation that involves white patches or spots inside the mouth) and lichen planus (an ongoing inflammatory situation that affects mucous membranes inside the mouth) in elder people ranges from 1.0% to 4.8% and 1.1% to 6.6%, correspondingly [76,79,80]. Leukoplakia is more recurrent among men, while lichen planus is linked with the female gender [76,79] Tobacco use is the most important determinant of oral cancer and premalignant lesions [81] counting leukoplakia, but too much consumption of alcohol is also a noteworthy factor with respect to these situations [80]. Socio-economic status such as low levels of education [79] as well as income [82] is a risk factor for leukoplakia. Cancer and its management can both be responsible for the most important anatomical alterations in the oral cavity and the modification of basic functions, including chewing, speaking, and/or swallowing, to a large extent impairing the quality of life of survivors [83].

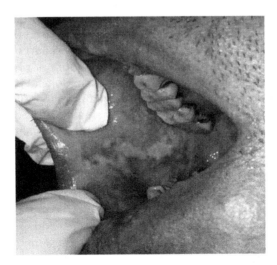

Figure 17.3 *Precancerous lesions of the oral mucous membrane.*

17.4 Need for nutraceuticals for the elder

In elder adults, there is an augmented risk of nutritional deficiencies exclusively as a result of an unbalanced diet. They have a slower metabolic rate, reduced physical activity, and altered hunger, satiety, smell, thirst, and taste sensations [84]. In addition, elder adults develop systemic problems like arthritis, cardiovascular diseases, degenerative diseases of the central nervous system, diabetes, lung diseases, and obesity as a result of increased risk of chronic low-grade inflammation and immunosenescence. These afterward result in weakened mobility, feeding problems, tooth loss from deprived oral health, changes in salivary flow as a result of medications, and swallowing complexities. In consequence, the aged develop the first choice for soft and micronutrient lacking foods. Therefore, there is an urgent requirement to identify the nutraceuticals that would make their oral as well as systemic health better by overcoming the effects of aging [84,85].

"Nutraceuticals" (a combination of the words "nutrition" and "pharmaceutical") speak about any substance considered to be a food or a food component that presents medicinal and health benefits, together with the prevention and treatment of disease [86]. Nutraceuticals do not have formal regulatory definitions, but they can be generally defined to comprise functional foods, nutritional supplements, and medicinal foods [87]. Odontonutraceuticals is a new word launch to identify those bioactive phytochemicals which can present health-promoting effects and averts oral diseases in which "odonto" arises from the Greek word odontos for "tooth", while the term nutraceuticals refers to bioactive phytochemicals [88]. It symbolizes pleiotropic phytotherapeutic agents in dentistry as they normalize different biochemical as well as molecular targets [89]. It might play a momentous role in the care of dental patients and also in managing multifaceted oral disorders. Fascinatingly, the latest findings propose that plant extracts, composed of a variety of bioactive components, are more effective than individual compounds, due to additive and/or synergistic effects [89,90]. A plethora of plants have been an excellent source of pharmaceuticals, and epidemiological investigations have recognized the role of nutraceuticals in the management of degenerative diseases, as per their neuroprotective, anti-inflammatory, and anticancer properties [91]. The active components present in nutraceuticals that are normally produced by plants as secondary compounds come out to facilitate plants overcome traumatic conditions. The valuable properties of nutraceuticals can be ascribed to the varieties of phytochemicals, such as anthocyanin glycosides, flavonoids, triterpenoids, and proanthocyanidin oligomers [92–94]. Odontonutraceuticals comprise green tea, probiotics, grapes, and cocoa seed extracts that are rich in polyphenols, flavonoids, and proanthocyanidins, vitamins A, B, C, D, and E, and minerals like magnesium, calcium, zinc, and copper [85,89,92,95].

17.5 Nutraceuticals for improving oral health of elders

Nutraceuticals, comprising nutritional supplements as well as functional foods, are a $152 billion global market. The percentage of people aged 65 years and more using nutraceuticals is greater than for any other age group and has twofold in current years. Aging is closely related to diminished immunity, increased morbidity and mortality arising from contagious agents, and deprived nutritional status. Deficiencies in vitamin E, vitamin B6, folate, zinc, and selenium are most common, and deficits in these micronutrients have been documented to affect immunity depressingly. As a result, if nutraceuticals can get better micronutrient status, the regular use of nutraceuticals by the aged people may provide an opportunity to improve invulnerability in this at-risk populace [92]. Numerous nutraceuticals are found to be advantageous in the prevention of certain age-related oral problems and so show a guarantee for improving public health. This section highlights the role of different nutraceuticals in the prevention of oral disease in elders.

17.5.1 Vitamins

Vitamin supplementations alone or in combination (multivitamins) are increasingly used of all nutraceuticals suggested to aged citizens. Vitamins play a fascinating role in the avoidance and treatment of a number of pathological oral conditions.

17.5.1.1 Vitamin A

Vitamin A helps in preserving periodontal health and averts disease progression. Furthermore, the role of vitamin A in the immune system can be as well essential for maintaining some bacteria at satisfactory levels and for preventing over-inflammation [96].

17.5.1.2 Vitamin D

An active form of vitamin D is 1, 25-dihydroxycholecalciferol, and it helps in bone remodeling. In addition, vitamin D plays an imperative role in altering the immune system of an individual, thus suppressing inflammation by inhibiting inflammatory cells. Therefore, vitamin D plays a vital role in the improvement of the health of periodontal tissues [97,98].

17.5.1.3 Vitamin C

Vitamin C alleviates the collagen structure by hydroxylation and preserves the integrity of connective tissues such as the alveolar bone, cementum, and periodontal ligament. Moreover, vitamin C improves the immune system and speeds up the wound-healing process. In the supplemented diet with vitamin C, reduced receptor activator of nuclear factor-κB ligand expression in periodontal diseases was seen, and also osteoclastogenesis stimulation was reduced [99]. Vitamin C alters the pathogenesis of periodontitis and has shown the importance of this vitamin being revealed in preserving the health of the periodontium [100–103]. Vitamin C has a defensive role in maintaining bone health in aged men in general and especially in smokers. A similar positive result was not experiential in women. Shielding effects of vitamin C on bone health can be predictable, as the vitamin can counter the effects of oxidative stress, which plays a role in the decline of bone by resorption. It is fascinating to note that nutritional vitamin C from fruits and vegetables had a superior role to play than supplemental vitamin C. This may be correlated to the variation in the cellular uptake and following processing of vitamin C in elder individuals [104].

17.5.1.4 Vitamin E

Vitamin E is recognized for its antioxidant action [105]. It impedes the production of reactive oxygen species (ROS) by terminating the free radical chain reaction. Vitamin E has been identified to defend periodontal health by increasing the nitric oxide synthases levels and avoids oxidative stress [106,107].

17.5.1.5 Vitamin B complex

Vitamin B complex has been identified to prevent gingival inflammation, restore periodontal health, and can positively influence periodontal wound healing processes [108].

17.5.2 Minerals

Vitamin D together with calcium plays an imperative role in preserving the periodontium, and it also helps in preserving the cementum and alveolar bone height [90]. However, the evidence is lacking, and magnesium has shown a positive relationship with periodontal disease suppression [90].

17.5.3 Polyphenols

Recent evidence supports the role of nutraceuticals in combating diseases, especially through the anti-inflammatory and anticarcinogenic actions of explicit antioxidants known as polyphenols [109–111]. Polyphenols are a class of plant-based chemical compounds referred to as phytochemicals. The "polyphenol" covers more than 8,000 types of phenolic structures, the most popular flavonoids, lignans, phenolic acids, and stilbenes. The antioxidant properties of these phytochemicals promote oral health by lessening the risk of inflammation and reducing the risk of tumor production as well as oxidative stress [112–114]. Plentiful investigations support the role of polyphenols in the prevention of periodontal disease. In an *in-vitro* study, Bodet et al. [115] reported strong evidence that cranberry polyphenols decreased the inflammatory actions of all three red complex species by partially deactivating their inflammatory enzymes, as a result probably averting degradation of the collagen in the periodontal sulcus. Catechins mostly found in green tea displayed a similar inhibitory effect in *Porphyromonas gingivitis* [116]. Black tea extract potentiated an extremely vulnerable antibacterial effect against *Porphyromonas gingivitis* and considerably lessen inflammatory factors, stopping gingival cellular damage [117]. Shahzad and his group investigated the antifungal potential of 14 polyphenols for inhibition and adhesion properties of *Candida albicans*. In this investigation, they used reference strains and isolates collected from the bloodstream, dentures as well as oral cavity. Out of 14, 7 polyphenols, namely, caffeic acid, curcumin, gallic acid, naringenin, pyrocatechol, pyrogallol, and quercetin, confirmed effective against growth and exhibited dose-dependent effect. Curcumin mainly found in turmeric and pyrogallol mostly present in cocoa powder, coffee, and beer were the most valuable polyphenols in decreeing biofilm. Researchers showed that both curcumin and pyrogallol appreciably suppressed genes that coded for adhesion molecules in biofilm growth by 50%–70% [118].

17.5.4 Curcumin

Curcumin is a natural nutraceutical with identified anti-neoplastic activities. A variety of systematic investigations have confirmed that curcumin having multiple and varied molecular pathways of action entailed in carcinogenesis as well as tumor formation. Investigational *in-vitro* and *in-vivo* studies have revealed the anti-tumor effects of curcumin on oral squamous cell carcinoma (OSCC) as a single agent as well as in combination with presently existing conventional therapies. It should be renowned that the *in-vitro* studies are in fact a mixture of oral and oropharyngeal cell lines, and hence, upcoming studies must take into consideration the necessary differences between squamous cell carcinomas of the oropharynx and squamous cell carcinomas of the oral cavity in terms of etiopathogenesis, morbidity, and mortality and look into each of them independently. Chakravarti and coworkers showed that curcumin is a potent inhibitor of constitutive and interleukin-6 induced signal transducer and activator of transcription 3 (STAT3) phosphorylation, and so, it has the aptitude to suppress proliferation of head and neck squamous carcinoma (HNSCC) cell lines [119]. Abuzeid and his team recently demonstrated that a novel curcumin analog (FLLL32) inhibited the active form of STAT3 in HNSCC cells and induced a potent antitumor effect [120]. Researchers reported that curcumin increased the expression and function of cytochrome P450 (CYP) 1A1 and/or CYP1B1 in OSCC of the tongue cells, indicating that it has chemopreventive properties mediated by the inhibition of carcinogen bioactivation [121]. A more current investigation also revealed that curcumin is a potent inhibitor of CYP 1B1 in OSCC [122]. Lin and coworkers demonstrated momentous inhibitory effects of curcumin on the proliferation and the growth of a human OSCC cell line (SAS) inoculated subcutaneously to mice. The cytotoxic effect of curcumin was mostly at the G2/M phase of the cell cycle [123].

17.5.5 Flavonoids

Flavonoids consist of plenty of naturally occurring organic compounds and present in a great variety of plants comprising fruits, grains, nuts, seeds, tea, vegetables, and wine. Flavonoids have many clinical effects and so extensively used in dentistry [124]. Flavonoids, like hesperidin, genipin, and proanthocyanidin have been verified beneficial in promoting oral health. Hesperidin protects dentine collagen and stimulates mineral deposition on root surface caries [125,126]. Green tea extract has been publicized to diminish abrasion as well as erosion and make easy protection of the dentine matrix, *in-vitro* and *in-situ* [127]. Cranberry extract slows down the development of dental biofilm and diminishes plaque formation [128]. Quercetin belongs to the flavonol class and mostly found in citrus fruit. It has a collagen cross-linking effect and provokes the growth of bone mass [129]. Naringin, a flavonoid glycoside, principally present in apples and onions. It displays a strong affinity toward collagen and strengthens the quality of bone [130]. Proanthocyanidin, a plant flavonoid, has been reported to have a remineralization effect on artificial root caries [126,131]. Proanthocyanidin is widespread in elm trees, grape seed, and pine bark [127]. It is also present in vegetables and fruits but in lower concentrations.

The grape seed extract is a rich source of proanthocyanidin, generally employed as natural antioxidants as well as free-radical scavengers, which has been shown to strengthen collagen-based tissues by rising collagen cross-links [132]. Researchers examined the effect of grape seed extract on the remineralization and demineralization of the collagen-rich root tissue of human teeth [131]. Proanthocyanidin from cranberries slows down the surface-adsorbed glucosyltransferases and acid production by *Streptococcus mutans* [133]. Researchers have also shown that proanthocyanidin increases collagen synthesis and speeds up the conversion of soluble collagen to insoluble collagen during growth. Proanthocyanidin-treated collagen matrices were revealed to be nontoxic and defied enzyme digestion *in-vitro* and *in-vivo* [134].

17.5.6 Tea

Tea is one of the most popular and studied beverages in the field of oral health. Different varieties of teas with diverse phenolic composition have displayed abilities to have an effect on oral pathogens. In the context of anticaries action, oolong tea extract was shown to act against *Streptococcus mutans* by reducing the production of lactic acid, lessening the feasibility of bacteria, reducing the production of glucosyltransferases, and dropping bacterial adherence to hydroxyapatite discs, an effect also depicted for green tea [135,136].

In respect to anti-periodontal action, the anti-inflammatory effect of tea and its phenolic components have been described. A variety of tea extracts from black, white, green, and oolong tea were distinguished as exerting anti-adhesive and antimicrobial activity against *Porphyromonas gingivitis*, in addition to reducing the action of virulence-related proteins, comprising collagenase, matrix metalloproteinase 9, and neutrophil elastase from this bacterium. The anti-inflammatory action was perceived as a reduction of the secretion of pro-inflammatory cytokines, counting interleukin (IL)-6, IL-8, and chemokine ligand 5, after pretreatment with tea extracts [137].

17.5.7 Carotenoids

Carotenoids, as nutraceuticals, have inhibitory effects on the development of inflammatory diseases. They neutralize the ROS activation that can provoke oxidative stress, which gives rise to excessive tissue damages. Carotenoids can defend the damages of tissue cells from some unwanted diseases induced by inflammation like periodontitis [138]. β-Carotene, a chief carotenoid, is a vitamin A precursor that has anti-cancer or antioxidant effects. It has been documented that nutritional intakes of β-carotene were related to decrease in periodontal pocket depth after periodontal therapy in nonsmokers, but not smokers, with chronic periodontitis [139]. β-Cryptoxanthin, one of the key carotenoids, is present in large quantities in fruits and vegetables like carrot, papaya, and paprika [140]. Nishigaki and team members reported that β-cryptoxanthin reduced appreciably PG-induced production of IL-6 and IL-8 in human periodontal ligament cells [141]. Lycopene, carotenoids mostly found in tomato, exhibits antioxidant property [142]. Arora and the group reported that systemic lycopene administration suppressed salivary IL-1 levels, resultant in the suppression of periodontal inflammation [143]. Belludi and the team also confirmed that lycopene is a useful carotenoid in patients with periodontitis clinically [144].

17.5.8 Probiotics

Probiotics contain beneficial bacterial strains, and they help in decreasing the pathogenic bacteria which cause periodontal disease. *Lactobacillus reuteri* showed a significant change in the plaque flora which was pathogenic [99]. Probiotics are also useful in the prevention of dental caries, gingivitis, periodontitis, halitosis, malodour, etc. [145].

Investigators examined that administration of probiotics reduced oral candida counts in aged people; this finding may offer a new approach for controlling oral yeast infections. Yet, there is a paucity of information concerning the contributions of probiotics to oral health [146]. Studies have shown that probiotics containing *Lactobacillus rhamnosus* GG and *Lactobacillus casei* or *Bifidobacterium* DN-173 010 have drastically reduced the growth of oral *streptococci* and dental caries risk [147]. Mouth washes with chosen strains of *Lactobacillus reuteri* or tablets having 6.7×108 colony-forming units of *Lactobacillus salivarius* and Xylitol (280 mg/tablet) have revealed the lessening in gingivitis and plaque buildup [148]. Studies have shown that 14-day intake of *Lactobacillus reuteri* led to the establishment of the strain in the oral cavity and significant reduction of gingivitis and plaque in patients with moderate to severe gingivitis [147]. Consumption of probiotic cheese containing *Lactobacillus rhamnosus* GG and *Propionibacterium freudenreichii* ssp. *shermanii* JS revealed a decrease in *Candida albicans* count [148]. Elder patients with gingivitis, periodontitis, and pregnancy gingivitis were locally treated by culture supernatant of a *Lactobacillus acidophilus* strain, and it was observed that momentous recovery was reported for nearly all patients. There has been considerable attention observed among elders in using probiotics in the management of periodontal disease. The probiotic strains used in these investigations comprise *Lactobacillus brevis* (CD2), *Lactobacillus reuteri*, *Lactobacillus salivarius* WB21, *and Bacillus subtilis*. *Lactobacillus reuteri* and *Lactobacillus brevis* have enhanced gingival health, as considered by reduced bleeding of gum [149,150]. When cheese containing *Lactobacillus rhamnosus* strains GG and LC705 and *Propionibacterium freudenreichii* ssp. *shermanii* JS was consumed by a test group of the aged populace for 16 weeks, the number of elevated oral yeast counts reduced, but no alters were experiential in mucosal lesions, which confirmed that there is the noteworthy effect of probiotic bacteria on oral candida infection in elders [151].

17.5.9 Coenzyme Q10

Coenzyme Q10 is the most important endogenous lipid-soluble antioxidant present in all organisms. The thrilling new discovery by scientific researchers recommends that CoQ10 is an important antioxidant readily used by the body and delaying a variety of progress of diseases [152]. Coenzyme Q10 is a nutraceutical available over the counter simply. Ubiquinol10 is a reduced form of Coenzyme Q10, used as an endogenous antioxidant which amplified the amount of coenzyme Q10 in the gingival disease and proficiently suppressed periodontal inflammation [153].

17.5.10 Resveratrol

Resveratrol isolated from grape has been employed as an antioxidant in anticancer therapy and also to lessen oral mucosal and gingival inflammation [99].

17.5.11 Cranberry

Cranberry inhibits the formation of the biofilm and prevents adherence to *Porphyromonas gingivitis*, thereby preventing periodontal disease [99].

17.5.12 Aloe vera

Aloe vera gel heals the mucosal wounds, and it can alleviate the pain of patients with oral lichen planus disease [154].

17.6 Conclusion

In conclusion, odontonutraceuticals are estimated to stand for promising agents toward multi-factorial oral disorders and to attain more and more importance within the scientific/clinical scenario. Their efficacy, in elder dental patients, needs to be supported by further evidence, and in these terms, we strongly emphasize a systematic approach to verify phytochemical efficacy, raising the pyramid of evidence-based dentistry, where the preclinical research is the essential prerequisite for clinical studies, which in turn represent the apex of evidence.

References

1. Griffin SO, Jones JA, Brunson D, Griffin PM, Bailey WD. Burden of oral disease among older adults and implications for public health priorities. *Am J Public Health.* 2012; 102(3):411–418.
2. Sischo L, Broder HL. Oral health-related quality of life. *J dent Res.* 2011; 90(11):1264–1270.
3. Petersen PE, Yamamoto T. Improving the oral health of older people: The approach of the WHO global oral health programme. *Community Dent Oral Epidemiol.* 2005; 33:81–92.
4. Inglehart MR, Bagramian RA, eds. *Oral Health Related Quality of Life.* Chicago, IL: Quintessence Publishing Co. Inc. 2002; 13–28.
5. Beaudette JR, Fritz PC, Sullivan PJ, Ward WE. Oral health, nutritional choices, and dental fear and anxiety. *Dent J (Basel).* 2017; 5(1):8.
6. Garcia RI, Henshaw MM, Krall EA. Relationship between periodontal disease and systemic health. *Periodontol 2000.* 2001; 25:21–36.
7. Sarita PT, Witter DJ, Kreulen CM, Van't Hof MA, Creugers NH. Chewing ability of subjects with shortened dental arches. *Community Dent Oral Epidemiol.* 2003; 31(5):328–334.
8. Chalub LLFH, Ferreira RC, Vargas AMD. Influence of functional dentition on satisfaction with oral health and impacts on daily performance among Brazilian adults: A population-based cross-sectional study. *BMC Oral Health.* 2017; 17(1):112.
9. Sharma AJ, Nagrath R, Lahori M. A comparative evaluation of chewing efficiency, masticatory bite force, and patient satisfaction between conventional denture and implant-supported mandibular overdenture: An *in-vivo* study. *J Indian Prosthodont Soc.* 2017; 17:361–372.
10. Walls AWG, Steele JG, Sheiham A, Marcenes W, Moynihan PJ. Oral health and nutrition in older people. *J Public Health Dent.* 2000; 60(4):304–307.
11. Ervin RB, Dye BA. The effect of functional dentition on healthy eating index scores and nutrient intakes in a nationally representative sample of older adults. *J Public Health Dent.* 2009; 69(4):207–216.

12. Ritchie CS, Joshipura K, Silliman RA, Miller B, Douglas CW. Oral health problems and significant weight loss among community-dwelling older adults. *J Gerontol A Biol Sci Med Sci.* 2000; 55(7):M366–M371.

13. Sheiham A, Steele JG, Marcenes W, Finch S, Walls AW. The relationship between oral health status and body mass index among older people: A national survey of older people in Great Britain. *Br Dent J.* 2002; 192(12):703–706.

14. Eli I, Bar-Tal Y, Kostovetzki I. At first glance: Social meanings of dental appearance. *J Public Health Dent.* 2001; 61(3):150–154.

15. Starr JM, Hall R. Predictors and correlates of edentulism in the healthy older people. *Curr Opin Clin Nutr Metab Care.* 2010; 13(1):19–23.

16. Monse B, Heinrich-Weltzien R, Benzian H, Holmgren C, van Palenstein Helderman W. PUFA - An index of clinical consequences of untreated dental caries. *Community Dent Oral Epidemiol.* 2010; 38(1):77–82.

17. Herrera D, Roldán S, González I, Sanz M. The periodontal abscess (I). Clinical and microbiological findings. *J Clin Periodontol.* 2000; 27(6):387–394.

18. Burt BA, Eklund SA. *Dentistry, Dental Practice, and the Community.* St. Louis, MO: Elsevier Saunders. 2005; 224.

19. Simpson TC, Needleman I, Wild SH, Moles DR, Mills EJ. Treatment of periodontal disease for glycaemic control in people with diabetes. *Cochrane Database Syst Rev.* 2010; 12(5):CD004714.

20. Minassian C, D'Aiuto F, Hingorani AD, Smeeth L. Invasive dental treatment and risk for vascular events a self-controlled case series. *Ann Intern Med.* 2010; 153(8):499–506.

21. Sjogren P, Nilsson E, Forsell M, Johansson O, Hoogstraate J. A systematic review of the preventive effect of oral hygiene on pneumonia and respiratory tract infection in elderly people in hospitals and nursing homes: Effect estimates and methodological quality of randomized controlled trials. *J Am Geriatr Soc.* 2008; 56(11):2124–2130.

22. Pace CC, McCullough GH. The association between oral microorganisms and aspiration pneumonia in the institutionalized elderly: Review and recommendations. *Dysphagia.* 2010; 25(4):307–322.

23. de Oliveira C, Watt R, Hamer M. Toothbrushing, inflammation, and risk of cardiovascular disease: Results from Scottish Health Survey. *BMJ.* 2010; 340:c2451.

24. Razak AP, Richard KMJ, Thankachan RP, Hafiz KA, Kumar KN, Sameer KM. Geriatric oral health: A review article. *J Int Oral Health.* 2014; 6(6):110–116.

25. Sharanya H. Age related dental problems. *J Pharm Sci & Res.* 2015; 7(6):347–349.

26. Berg R, Morgenstern NE. Physiologic changes in the elderly. *Dent Clin North Am.* 1997; 41(4):651–668.

27. Barbour ME, Rees GD. The role of erosion, abrasion and attrition in tooth wear. *J Clin Dent.* 2006; 17(4):88–93.

28. Carvalho TS, Lussi A. Age-related morphological, histological and functional changes in teeth. *J Oral Rehabil.* 2017; 44(4):291–298.

29. Yamamoto T, Hasegawa T, Yamamoto T, Hongo H, Amizuka N. Histology of human cementum: Its structure, function, and development. *Jpn Dent Sci Rev.* 2016; 52(3):63–74.

30. Andreescu CF, Mihai LL, Raescu M, Tuculina MJ, Cumpata CN, Ghergic DL. Age influence on periodontal tissues: A histological study. *Rom J Morphol Embryol.* 2013; 54(3 Suppl):811–815.

31. Ren Y, Maltha JC, Stokroos L, Liem RS, Kuijpers-Jagtman AM. Age-related changes of periodontal ligament surface areas during force application. *Angle Orthod.* 2008; 78(6):1000–1005.

32. Heasman PA, Ritchie M, Asuni A, Gavillet E, Simonsen JL, Nyvad B. Gingival recession and root caries in the ageing population: A critical evaluation of treatments. *J Clin Periodontol.* 2017; 44(Suppl. 18):S178–S193.

33. Kumar B, Kashyap N, Avinash A, Chevvuri R, Sagar MK, Shrikant K. The composition, function and role of saliva in maintaining oral health: A review. *Int J Contemp Dent Med Rev.* 2017; Article ID 011217.
34. Meenakshi A, Vadodaria J. Geriatric nutrition: A prosthodontic review. *Int J Oral Health Med Res.* 2018; 5(1):72–76.
35. Scully C, Ettinger RL. The influence of systemic diseases on oral health care in older adults. *J Am Dent Assoc.* 2007; 138:7S–4S.
36. Pugliese S, Kashi AR. Changes in the oral cavity with age. In: Rosenthal R, Zenilman M, Katlic M, eds. *Principles and Practice of Geriatric Surgery.* Springer, New York. 2011; 501–512.
37. Loe H. Oral Hygiene in the prevention of caries and periodontal disease. *Int Dent J.* 2000; 50:129–139.
38. Nagaratnam N, Nagaratnam K, Cheuk G. Oral issues in the elderly. In: *Geriatric Diseases.* Cham: Springer. 2017; 1–8.
39. Saunders Jr. RH, Meyerowitz C. Dental caries in older adults. *Dent Clin North Am.* 2005; 49(2):293–308.
40. MacDonald DE. Principles of geriatric dentistry and their application to the older adult with a physical disability. *Clin Geriatr Med.* 2006; 22(2):413–434.
41. Warren JJ, Cowen HJ, Watkins CM, Hands JS. Dental caries prevalence and dental care utilization among the very old. *J Am Dent Assoc.* 2000; 131(11):1571–1579.
42. Hahn CL, Liewehr FR. Innate immune responses of the dental pulp to caries. *J Endod.* 2007; 33:643–651.
43. Steele JG, Sheiham A, Marcenes W, Fay N, Walls AW. Clinical and behavioural risk indicators for root caries in older people. *Gerodontology.* 2001; 18(2):95–101.
44. Petersen PE. The World Oral Health Report 2003: Continuous improvement of oral health in the 21st century – The approach of the WHO Global Oral Health Programme. *Community Dent Oral Epidemiol.* 2003; 31(Suppl. 1):3–24.
45. Sande AR, Suragimath A, Bijjaragi S, Mathur A. Geriatric dentistry in India: An oral medicine perspective. *J Indian Acad Oral Med Radiol;* 2014; 26:298–301.
46. Guiglia R, Musciotto A, Compilato D, et al. Aging and oral health: Effects in hard and soft tissues. *Curr Pharm Des.* 2010; 16:619–630.
47. Shimazaki Y, Soh I, Koga T, Miyazaki H, Takehara T. Risk factors for tooth loss in the institutionalized elderly; a six-year cohort study. *Community Dent Health* 2003; 20:123–127.
48. Joshipura KJ, Hung H-C, Rimm EB, Willett WC, Ascherio A. Periodontal disease, tooth loss, and incidence of ischemic stroke. *Stroke.* 2003; 34:47–52.
49. Kisely S. No mental health without oral health. *Can J Psychiatry.* 2016; 61(5):277–282.
50. Lertpimonchai A, Rattanasiri S, Vallibhakara SA, Attia J, Thakkinstian A. The association between oral hygiene and periodontitis: A systematic review and meta-analysis. *Int Dent J.* 2017; 67(6):332–343.
51. Locker D, Leake JL. Risk indicators and risk markers for periodontal disease experience in older adults living independently in Ontario, Canada. *J Dent Res.* 1993; 72:9–17.
52. Ogawa H, Yoshihara A, Hirotomi T, Ando Y, Miyazaki H. Risk factors for periodontal disease progression among elderly people. *J Clin Periodontol.* 2002; 29:592–597.
53. Paster BJ, Olsen I, Aas JA, Dewhirst FE. The breadth of bacterial diversity in the human periodontal pocket and other oral sites. *Periodontol 2000.* 2006; 42:80–87.
54. Loesche W. Dental caries and periodontitis: Contrasting two infections that have medical implications. *Infect Dis Clin North Am.* 2007; 21(2):471–502.
55. Hazzard WR, Blass J, Halter J, Ouslander J, Tinetti M, eds. *Principles of Geriatric Medicine and Gerontology.* 5th ed. New York: McGraw-Hill Professional 2003; 1–35.
56. Preshaw PM, Alba AL, Herrera D, et al. Periodontitis and diabetes: A two-way relationship. *Diabetologia.* 2012; 55(1):21–31.

57. Taylor GW, Loesche WJ, Terpenning MS. Impact of oral diseases on systemic health in the elderly: Diabetes mellitus and aspiration pneumonia. *J Public Health Dent.* 2000; 60(4):313–320.
58. Mealey BL, Oates TW. Diabetes mellitis and periodontal diseases. *J Periodontol.* 2006; 77(8):1289–1303.
59. Dhadse P, Gattani D, Mishra R. The link between periodontal disease and cardiovascular disease: How far we have come in last two decades? *J Indian Soc Periodontol.* 2010; 14(3):148–154.
60. Gomes-Filho IS, Passos JS, da Cruz SS. Respiratory disease and the role of oral bacteria. *J Oral Microbiol.* 2010; 2:5811.
61. El-Solh AA, Pietrantoni C, Bhat A, et al. Colonization of dental plaques: A resevoir of respiratory pathogens for hospital-acquired pneumonia in institutionalized elders. *Chest.* 2004; 126(5):1575–1582.
62. Cho T, Nagao J-I, Imayoshi R, Tanaka Y. Importance of diversity in the oral microbiota including candida species revealed by high-throughput technologies. *Int J Dent.* 2014; 2014: Article ID 454391.
63. Neville BW, ed. *Oral & Maxillofacial Pathology.* 2nd ed. Philadelphia, PA: W.B. Saunders. 2002; 210–214.
64. Epstein JB, Gorsky M, Caldwell J. Fluconazole mouthrinses for oral candidiasis in postirradiation, transplant, and other patients. *Oral Surg Oral Med Oral Pathol Oral Radiol Endod.* 2002; 93(6):671–675.
65. Guggenheimer J, Moore PA. Xerostomia: Etiology, recognition and treatment. *J Am Dent Assoc.* 2003; 134(1):61–69.
66. Saunders R, Friedman B. Oral health conditions of community-dwelling cognitively intact elderly persons with disabilities. *Gerodontology.* 2007; 24(2):67–76.
67. Ship JA, Pillemer SR, Baum BJ. Xerostomia and the geriatric patient. *J Am Geriatr Soc.* 2002; 50:535–543.
68. Bergdahl M, Bergdahl J. Low unstimulated salivary flow and subjective oral dryness: Association with medication, anxiety, depression, and stress. *J Dent Res.* 2000; 79:1652–1658.
69. Shetty SR, Bhowmick S, Castelino R, Babu S. Drug induced xerostomia in elderly individuals: An institutional study. *Contemp Clin Dent.* 2012; 3(2):173–175.
70. Thomson WM, Chalmers JM, Spencer AJ, Slade GD. Medication and dry mouth: Findings from a cohort study of older people. *J Public Health Dent.* 2000; 60:12–20.
71. Al-Maweri SA, Al-Jamaei AA, Al-Sufyani GA, Tarakji B, Shugaa-Addin B. Oral mucosal lesions in elderly dental patients in Sana'a, Yemen. *J Int Soc Prev Community Dent.* 2015; 5(Suppl 1):S12–S19.
72. Dhankar K, Ingle NA, Chaudhary A, Kaur N. Geriatric dentistry: A review. *J Oral Health Comm Dent.* 2013; 7(3)170–173.
73. Naik AV, Pai RC. A study of factors contributing to denture stomatitis in a north Indian community. *Int J Dent.* 2011; 2011: Article ID 589064.
74. Pattanaik S, Vikas BVJ, Pattanaik B, Sahu S, Lodam S. Denture stomatitis: A literature review. *J Ind Acad Oral Med Radiol.* 2010; 22(3):136–140.
75. Atashrazm P, Sadri D. Prevalence of oral mucosal lesions in a group of Iranian dependent elderly complete denture wearers. *J Contemp Dent Pract.* 2013; 14(2):174–178.
76. Jainkittivong A, Aneksuk V, Langlais RP. Oral mucosal conditions in elderly dental patients. *Oral Dis.* 2002; 8:218–223.
77. Veena KM, Jagadishchandra H, Sequria J, Hameed SK, Chatra L, Shenai P. An extensive denture-induced hyperplasia of maxilla. *Ann Med Health Sci Res.* 2013; 3(Suppl1):S7–S9.
78. Petersen PE, Bourgeois D, Ogawa H, Estupinan-Day S, Ndiaye C. The global burden of oral diseases and risk to oral health. *Bull World Health Organ.* 2005; 83(9):661–669.
79. Reichart PA. Oral mucosal lesions in a representative cross-sectional study of aging Germans. *Community Dent Oral Epidemiol.* 2000; 28:390–398.

80. Garcia-Pola Vallejo MJ, Martinez Diaz-Canel AI, Garcia Martin JM, Gonzalez Garcia M. Risk factors for oral soft tissue lesions in an adult Spanish population. *Community Dent Oral Epidemiol.* 2002; 30:277–285.

81. Thomas G, Hashibe M, Jacob BJ, et al. Risk factor for multiple oral premalignant lesions. *Int J Cancer.* 2003; 107:285–291.

82. Hashibe M, Jacob BJ, Thomas G, et al. Socioeconomic status, lifestyle factors and oral premalignant lesions. *Oral Oncol.* 2003; 39:664–671.

83. Torres-Carranza E, Infante-Cossio P, Hernandez-Guisado JM, Hens-Aumente E, Gutierrez-Perez JL. Assessment of quality of life in oral cancer. *Med Oral Patol Oral Cir Bucal.* 2008; 13(11):E735–E741.

84. Spackman SS, Bauer JG. Periodontal treatment for older adults. In: Newman MG, Takei HH, Klokkevold PR, Carranza FA, eds. *Carranza's Clinical Periodontology.* 10th ed. New Delhi: Elsevier 2007; 675–692.

85. Gaur S, Agnihotri R. Green tea: A novel functional food for the oral health of older adults. *Geriatr Gerontol Int.* 2014; 14:238–250.

86. Gupta SC, Kim JH, Prasad S, Aggarwal BB. Regulation of survival, proliferation, invasion, angiogenesis, and metastasis of tumor cells through modulation of inflammatory pathways by nutraceuticals. *Cancer Metastasis Rev.* 2010; 29(3):405–434.

87. Gupta C, Prakash D. Nutraceuticals for geriatrics. *J Tradit Complement Med.* 2015; 5(1):5–14.

88. Varani EM, Iriti M. Odonto nutraceuticals: Pleioyropic photo therapeutic agents for oral health. *Pharmaceuticals.* 2016; 9(1):10–13.

89. Gonzalez-Vallinas M, Gonzalez-Castejon M, Rodriguez-Casado A, Ramirez de Molina A. Dietary phytochemicals in cancer prevention and therapy: A complementary approach with promising perspectives. *Nut Rev.* 2013; 71(9):585–599.

90. Iriti M, Vitalini S, Fico G, Faoro F. Neuroprotective herbs and foods from different traditional medicines and diets. *Molecules.* 2010; 15:3517–3555.

91. Zhao J. Nutraceuticals, nutritional therapy, phytonutrients and phytotherapy for improvement of human health: A perspective on plant biotechnology application. *Recent Pat Biotechnol.* 2007; 1:75–97.

92. Sharma G, Prakash D, Gupta C. Phytochemicals of nutraceutical importance: Do they defend against diseases? In: Prakash D, Sharma G, eds. *Phytochemicals of Nutraceutical Importance.* Wallingford: CABI International Publishers. 2014; 1–19.

93. Kennedy DO, Wightman EL. Herbal extracts and phytochemicals: Plant secondary metabolites and the enhancement of human brain function. *Adv Nutr.* 2011; 2:32–50.

94. Salminen A, Kauppinen A, Kaarniranta K. Phytochemicals suppress nuclear factor-kappaB signaling: Impact on health span and the aging process. *Curr Opin Clin Nutr Metab Care.* 2012; 15:23–28.

95. Sharma R. Nutraceuticals and nutraceutical supplementation criteria in cancer: A literature survey. *Open Nutraceut J.* 2009; 2:92–106.

96. Petti S, Cairella G, Tarsitani G. Nutritional variable related to gingival health in adolescent girls. *Community Dent Oral Epidemiol.* 2000; 28:407–413.

97. Bikle DD. Vitamin D metabolism, mechanism of action, and clinical applications. *Chem Biol.* 2014; 21:319–329.

98. Gil A, Plaza-Diaz J, Mesa MD. Vitamin novel actions. *Ann Nutr Metab.* 2018; 72:87–95.

99. Pendyala GS, Joshi SR, Mopagar V, et al. Nutraceutical basis for drug delivery in periodontal disease. *Pravara Med Rev.* 2020; 12(03):87–90.

100. Pushparani DS, Nirmala S, Theagarayan P. Low serum vitamin C and Zinc is associated with the development of oxidative stress in type 2 diabetes mellitus with periodontitis. *Int J Pharm Sci Rev Res.* 2013; 23(2):259–264.

101. Iwasaki M, Moynihan P, Manz MC et al. Dietary antioxidants and periodontal disease in community-based older Japanese: A 2-year follow-up study. *Public Health Nutr.* 2013; 16(2):330–338.

102. Iwasaki M, Manz MC, Taylor GW, Yoshihara A, Miyazaki H. Relations of serum ascorbic acid and alpha-tocopherol to periodontal disease. *J Dent Res.* 2012; 91(2):167–172.

103. Van der Putten GJ, Vanobbergen J, De Visschere L, Schols J, de Baat C. Association of some specific nutrient deficiencies with periodontal disease in elderly people: A systematic literature review. *Nutrition.* 2009; 25:717–722.

104. Sahni MT, Hannan D, Gagnon DJ, Blumberg LA, Cupples DP, Kiel KL. Tucker High vitamin C intake is associated with lower 4-year bone loss in elderly men. *J Nutr.* 2008; 138:1931–1938.

105. Traber MG, Atkinson J. Vitamin E, antioxidant and nothing more. *Free Radic Biol Med.* 2007; 43:4–15.

106. Varela-Lopez A, Battino M, Bullon P, Quiles JL. Dietary antioxidants for chronic periodontitis prevention and its treatment. A review on current evidences from animal and human studies. *Ars Pharm.* 2015; 56:131–140.

107. Wong RSY, Radhakrishnan AK. Tocotrienol research: Past into present. *Nutr Rev.* 2012; 70:483–490.

108. Kulkarni V, Bhatavadekar NB, Uttamani JR. The effect of nutrition on periodontal disease: A systematic review. *J Calif Dent Assoc.* 2014; 42:302–311.

109. Singhal K, Raj N, Gupta K, Singh S. Probable benefits of green tea with genetic implications. *J Oral Maxillofac Pathol.* 2017; 21:107–114.

110. Varela-López A, Bullón P, Giampieri F, Quiles JL. Non-Nutrient, naturally occurring phenolic compounds with antioxidant activity for the prevention and treatment of periodontal diseases. *Antioxidants (Basel).* 2015; 4:447–481.

111. Iriti M, Varoni EM. Chemopreventive potential of flavonoids in oral squamous cell carcinoma in human studies. *Nutrients.* 2013; 5:2564–2576.

112. Ding Y, Yao H, Yao Y, Fai LY, Zhang Z. Protection of dietary polyphenols against oral cancer. *Nutrients.* 2013; 5:2173–2191.

113. Liu RH. Health-promoting components of fruits and vegetables in the diet. *Adv Nutr.* 2013; 4:384S–392S.

114. Scalbert A, Johnson IT, Saltmarsh M. Polyphenols: Antioxidants and beyond. *Am J Clin Nutr.* 2005, 81(suppl 1):215S–217S.

115. Bodet C, Piche M, Chandad F, Grenier D. Inhibition of periodontopathogen-derived proteolytic enzymes by a high-molecular-weight fraction isolated from cranberry. *J Antimicrob Chemother.* 2006; 57:685–690.

116. Okamoto M, Sugimoto A, Leung KP, Nakayama K, Kamaguchi A, Maeda N. Inhibitory effect of green tea catechins on cysteine proteinases in *Porphyromonas gingivalis.* *Oral Microbiol Immunol.* 2004; 19:118–120.

117. Bedran TBL, Morin M-P, Palomari Spolidorio D, Grenier D. Black tea extract and its theaflavin derivatives inhibit the growth of periodontopathogens and modulate interleukin-8 and β-defensin secretion in oral epithelial cells. *PLoS One.* 2015; 10:e0143158.

118. Shahzad M, Sherry L, Rajendran R, Edwards CA, Combet E, Ramage G. Utilising polyphenols for the clinical management of *Candida albicans* biofilms. *Int J Antimicrob Agents.* 2014; 44:269–273.

119. Chakravarti N, Myers JN, Aggarwal BB. Targeting constitutive and interleukin-6-inducible signal transducers and activators of transcription 3 pathway in head and neck squamous cell carcinoma cells by curcumin (diferuloylmethane). *Int J Cancer.* 2006; 119(6):1268–1275.

120. Abuzeid WM, Davis S, Tang AL, et al. Sensitization of head and neck cancer to cisplatin through the use of a novel curcumin analog. *Arch Otolaryngol Head Neck Surg.* 2011; 137(5):499–507.

121. Rinaldi AL, Morse MA, Fields HW, et al. Curcumin activates the aryl hydrocarbon receptor yet significantly inhibits (-)-benzo(a)pyrene-7R-trans-7,8-dihydrodiol bioactivation in oral squamous cell carcinoma cells and oral mucosa. *Cancer Res.* 2002; 62(19):5451–5456.

122. Walle T, Walle UK. Novel methoxylated flavone inhibitors of cytochrome P450 1B1 in SCC-9 human oral cancer cells. *J Pharm Pharmacol.* 2007; 59(6):857–862.
123. Lin YC, Chen HW, Kuo YC, Chang YF, Lee YJ, Hwang JJ. Therapeutic efficacy evaluation of curcumin on human oral squamous cell carcinoma xenograft using multimodalities of molecular imaging. *Am J Chin Med.* 2010; 38(2):343–358.
124. Sankari SL, Babu NA, Rani V, Priyadharsini C, Masthan KM. Flavonoids – Clinical effects and applications in dentistry: A review. *J Pharm Bioallied Sci.* 2014; 6(Suppl 1):S26–S29.
125. Hiraishi N, Sono R, Islam MS, Otsuki M, Tagami J, Takatsuka T. Effect of hesperidin *in vitro* on root dentine collagen and demineralization. *J Dent.* 2011; 39:391–396.
126. Pavan S, Xie Q, Hara AT, Bedran-Russo AK. Biomimetic approach for root caries prevention using a proanthocyanidin-rich agent. *Caries Res.* 2011; 45:443–447.
127. Fine AM. Oligomeric proanthocyanidin complexes: History, structure, and phytopharmaceutical applications. *Altern Med Rev.* 2000; 5:144–151.
128. Habauzit V, Sacco SM, Gil-Izquierdo A, et al. Differential effects of two citrus flavanones on bone quality in senescent male rats in relation to their bioavailability and metabolism. *Bone.* 2011; 49:1108–1116.
129. Trivedi R, Kumar A, Gupta V, et al. Effects of Egb 761 on bone mineral density, bone microstructure, and osteoblast function: Possible roles of quercetin and kaempferol. *Mol Cell Endocrinol.* 2009; 302:86–91.
130. Wong RW, Rabie AB. Effect of naringin collagen graft on bone formation. Biomaterials. 2006; 27:1824–1831.
131. Xie Q, Bedran-Russo AK, Wu CD. *In vitro* remineralization effects of grape seed extract on artificial root caries. *J Dent.* 2008; 36:900–906.
132. Yamakoshi J, Saito M, Kataoka S, Kikuchi M. Safety evaluation of proanthocyanidin-rich extract from grape seeds. *Food Chem Toxicol.* 2002; 40:599–607.
133. Duarte S, Gregoire S, Singh AP, et al. Inhibitory effects of cranberry polyphenols on formation and acidogenicity of Streptococcus mutans biofilms. *FEMS Microbiol Lett.* 2006; 257:50–56.
134. Han B, Jaurequi J, Tang BW, Nimni ME. Proanthocyanidin: A natural crosslinking reagent for stabilizing collagen matrices. *J Biomed Mater Res A.* 2003; 65:118–124.
135. Matsumoto M, Hamada S, Ooshima T. Molecular analysis of the inhibitory effects of oolong tea polyphenols on glucan-binding domain of recombinant glucosyltransferases from Streptococcus mutans MT8148, FEMS. *Microbiology Letters.* 2003; 228(1):73–80.
136. Sasaki H, Matsumoto M, Tanaka T, Maeda M, Nakai M, Hamada S, Ooshima T. Antibacterial activity of polyphenol components in oolong tea extract against Streptococcus mutans. *Caries Res.* 2004; 38(1):2–8.
137. Zhao L, La VD, Grenier D. Antibacterial, antiadherence, antiprotease, and anti-inflammatory activities of various tea extracts: Potential benefits for periodontal diseases. *Journal of Medicinal Food.* 2013; 16(5):428–436.
138. Naruishi K. Carotenoids and periodontal infection. *Nutrients.* 2020; 12:269–277.
139. Dodington DW, Fritz PC, Sullivan PJ, Ward WE. Higher intakes of fruits and vegetables, β-carotene, vitamin C, α-tocopherol, EPA, and DHA are positively associated with periodontal healing after nonsurgical periodontal therapy in nonsmokers but not in smokers. *J Nutr.* 2015; 145:2512–2519.
140. Hirata N, Ichimaru R, Tominari T, et al. Beta-Cryptoxanthin inhibits lipopolysaccharide-induced osteoclast differentiation and bone resorption via the suppression of inhibitor of NF-κB kinase activity. *Nutrients.* 2019; 11:368.
141. Nishigaki M, Yamamoto T, Ichioka H, et al. β-cryptoxanthin regulates bone resorption related-cytokine production in human periodontal ligament cells. *Arch Oral Biol.* 2013; 58:880–886.
142. Salehi B, Sharifi-Rad R, Sharopov F, et al. Beneficial effects and potential risks of tomato consumption for human health: An overview. *Nutrition.* 2019; 62:201–208.

143. Arora N, Avula H, Avula JK. The adjunctive use of systemic antioxidant therapy (lycopene) in nonsurgical treatment of chronic periodontitis: A short-term evaluation. *Quintessence Int.* 2013; 44:395–405.

144. Belludi SA, Verma S, Banthia R, et al. Effect of lycopene in the treatment of periodontal disease: A clinical study. *J Contemp Dent Pract.* 2013; 14:1054–1059.

145. Janczarek M, Bachanek T, Mazur E, Chałas R. The role of probiotics in prevention of oral diseases. *Postepy Hig Med Dosw.* 2016; 70(0):850–857.

146. Burton JP, Chilcott CN, Tagg JR. The rationale and potential for the reduction of oral malodour using Streptococcus salivarius probiotics. *Oral Dis.* 2005; 11 (Suppl. 1):29–31.

147. de Vrese M, Schrezenmeir J. Probiotics, prebiotics, and synbiotics. *Adv Biochem Eng Biotechnol.* 2008; 111:1–66.

148. Reddy RS, Swapna LA, Ramesh T, Singh TR, Vijayalaxmi N, Lavanya R. Bacteria in oral health – Probiotics and prebiotics a review. *Int J Biol Med Res.* 2011; 2:1226–1233.

149. Krasse P, Carlsson B, Dahl C, Paulsson A, Nilsson A, Sinkiewicz G. Decreased gum bleeding and reduced gingivitis by the probiotic Lactobacillus reuteri. *Swed Dent J.* 2006; 30:55–60.

150. Twetman S, Derawi B, Keller M, Ekstrand K, Yucel-Lindberg T, Stecksen-Blicks C. Short-term effect of chewing gums containing probiotic Lactobacillus reuteri on the levels of inflammatory mediators in gingival crevicular fluid. *Acta Odontol Scand.* 2009; 67:19–24.

151. Hatakka K, Ahola AJ, Yli-Knuuttila H, et al. Probiotics reduce the prevalence of oral candida in the elderly-a randomized controlled trial. *J Dent Res.* 2007; 86:125–130.

152. Kadir AKMS, Rabbi AA, Rahman MM. CoEnzyme Q10: A new horizon in the treatment of periodontal diseases. *Int Dent J Stud Res.* 2017; 5(1):1–6.

153. Prakash S, Sunitha J, Hans M. Role of coenzyme Q10 as an antioxidant and bienergiger in periodontal diseases. *Ind J Pharmacol.* 2010; 42:334–337.

154. Thongprasom K, Carrozzo M, Furness S, Lodi G. Interventions for treating oral lichen planus. *Cochrane Database Syst Rev.* 2011; 6(7):CD001168.

Role of Nutraceuticals in Human Postnatal Stem Cell Aging

Shikha Sharma
Institute For Stem Cell Biology and Regenerative Medicine

Avinash Sanap
Dr. D. Y. Patil Vidyapeeth
Savitribai Phule University of Pune

Kalpana Joshi
Sinhgad College of Engineering affiliated to Savitribai Phule Pune University

Ramesh Bhonde
Regenerative Medicine Laboratory

Contents

DOI: 10.1201/9781003110866-18

18.1 Introduction

Over 60 years ago, Leonard Hayflick and Paul Moorhead described senescence for the first time [1]. Senescence exhibits diverse functions based on the age of an organism [2]. It plays a beneficial role during embryonic development in body shaping, in tissue regeneration and as a cancer barrier in young individuals. Senescent number increases during aging and leads to low chronic inflammation via senescence-associated secretory phenotype (SASP), produces reactive oxygen species (ROS) and results in an altered microenvironment which supports cancer progression and age-related diseases. Senescence is associated with cessation of proliferation, increased β-galactosidase activity, cell cycle inhibitors including p21 and p16, lysosomal enzyme activity, DNA double-stranded break, changes in chromatin structure and activation of the DNA damage repair pathway [3]. Compared to quiescent cells, senescent cells have lost the ability to re-enter the cell cycle and are unaffected by growth factors or stimuli. Moreover, senescent cells are also different from terminally differentiated cells which are derived from undifferentiated precursors through defined development programming. Both cells undergo irreversible cell cycle arrest [4]. Terminally differentiated cells including neurons, adipocytes and hepatocytes also have the propensity to undergo senescence during aging or oncogenic stimulus or genetic damage indicating that senescence can also occur independently of cell cycle arrest [4]. Several other factors that contribute to senescence include telomere erosion (replicative senescence), in response to some chemical or physical factors, stress-induced senescence due to overexpression of oncogenes, increased ROS production, ER stress, DNA damage, and chromatin structure dysfunction [5].

18.1.1 Replicative senescence

Cell normally undergoes normal mitosis for proliferation and eventually reaches a stage of cell cycle arrest when its proliferation capacity exhausts leading to replicative senescence. Replicative senescence was originally defined in fibroblast with its finite proliferative capacity around 50 passages [6]. Senescence is promoted by various intrinsic and extrinsic factors such as oxidative stress,

DNA damage, mitochondrial dysfunction, chemotherapeutic agents, and irradiation [7]. Mostly the senescence is mediated by damage in DNA repair pathway components such as ATM and ATR which modulates cell cycle checkpoint genes including CHK1, CHK2, and CDKs leading to cell cycle arrest. The main cell cycle arrest proteins include p53/p21^{CIP1} and p16^{INK4a}/Rb which are overexpressed and used as markers for senescence [8,9]. Shortening of telomeres results in the exposure of uncapped free end of double-stranded DNA which is recognized as double-stranded break by DNA damage response which promotes the replicative senescence [10,11]. A decrease in telomeric length is also regarded as the biomarker for replicative senescence [12].

18.1.2 Stress-induced premature senescence

Stress-induced premature senescence results from the DNA damage caused by various factors such as oxidative stress, oncogenes overexpression, radiation, etc. independent of telomere length [13,14]. Various oncogenes including ras, Raf, c-Myc, Akt, and E2F3 have been found to elicit senescence suggesting its role in tumor suppression [15–18]. During oncogenic induced senescence (OIS), initial hyperproliferation leads to the activation of oncogenes that induces DDR. Mitotic signals induce DNA replication origin which leads to the accumulation of DNA damage due to the stalled replication forks and activation of DDR [19–21]. Persistent DDR associated with irreparable DNA damage generally induces senescence [22]. In contrast to replicative senescence in OIS, DDR occurs independently of telomere length but is associated with telomeric dysfunction [23]. Irrespective of the mechanism that drives DNA damage, DDR is associated with increased expression of γ-H2AX, p53-binding protein 1, ATM, ATR, CHK1, CHK2, and p53/p21^{CIP1} axis [11,24].

18.1.3 Mechanism of senescence

The prominent mechanism that underlies the senescence is the induction of the p53 and p16^{INK4a}/Rb tumor suppressor networks [25]. p53 activation regulates a wide range of gene regulatory networks associated with the proliferation of cells [26]. Importantly, p53 regulate the expression of cyclin-dependent kinase inhibitor (CDKi) p21^{CIP1} in senescent cells which in turn inhibit the activity of CDK2 leading to the hypo-phosphorylation of Rb and cell cycle exit [24]. Indeed, the suppression of p53 signaling was found to be implicated with the onset of cellular senescence [27–30]. Moreover, if the stress resulting in senescence is transient, p53 induction leads to a quiescent state by activating the DNA repair process and resuming the cell cycle [31]. However, persistent stress leads to the activation of p16^{INK4a} involved in the suppression of CDK4 and CDK6 implicated in long-lasting arrest [32]. Indeed, p21^{CIP1} is associated with the onset of senescence, whereas p16^{INK4a} leads to sustainable growth arrest [32,33]. In addition, transient cell cycle arrest or DNA damage also induces p21^{CIP1} expression suggesting its use as senescent markers only with the combination of other markers [4]. p16^{INK4a} and p19^{ARF} have been implicated in senescent cell cycle arrest. p16INK4a blocks CDK4 and CDK6, whereas p19ARF prevents degradation of p53 [4]. p16INK4a has been known as the most prominent marker of senescence, and its expression increases during aging [34,35]. However, p16INK4a has been also detected in non-senescence cells including cancer cells, macrophages and lymphocytes with inactivated Rb indicating its role in senescence and differentiation [33]. Taken together, it is important to use a combination of markers for deducing senescent phenotype.

18.1.4 Senescence-associated secretory phenotype

Senescence cells secrete a wide range of soluble and insoluble factors termed SASP which have been implicated in modulating the signal of their surrounding environment [36,37]. SASP secretome includes cytokines, growth factors, chemokines, extracellular matrix proteases, and several signaling molecules. However, its composition varies and depends on the cell type and factors inducing senescence. Senescent cells influence the surrounding cells through various signaling mechanisms including NOTCH/JAG1, ROS production, exosomes, and cargo transfer via cytoplasmic bridges and exert various beneficial and detrimental effects [38–41]. Indeed, the SASP effect is pleiotropic. SASP exerts its anti-tumorigenic effect by promoting senescence to the cells exposed to stressed conditions through its paracrine factors including IL-6R, insulin-like growth factor binding protein 7 (IGFBP7) or CXCR2, IL8 and several chemokines [42–44]. Conversely, SASP can also promote tumorigenesis through its proinflammatory and inflammatory mediators [4]. In addition, SASP also regulates the recruitment of immune cells including NK cells, Th1 cells, and macrophages in inducing or preventing the formation of senescent cells [4]. SASP has also been associated with aging and age-related diseases. A low level of inflammation has been shown to exist in many age-related pathologies. Elimination of the senescent cells was shown to be related to the low level of proinflammatory cytokines such as IL-1α, IL-6, and TNF-α in the kidney, fat and skeletal muscle of aged mice [45–48]. Importantly, only a small fraction of cells are senescent in aging tissue speculating the other beneficial effects of removing these senescent cells. Finally, the injury-driven secretome of senescent cells also promotes stemness.

18.1.5 Mechanism of SASP

The SASP is controlled at various stages such as transcription, mRNA stability, translation and secretion and depends on the autocrine and paracrine feedback loop. Multiple signaling pathways are known to play a vital role in mediating SASP including DDR, cGAS/STING, and p38 MAP kinase which mostly leads to the activation of NF-kB and CCAAT/enhancer-binding protein-β (C/EBPβ) [49–54]. Activated NF-kB and C/EBPβ regulate the transcription of key components of inflammatory SASP including IL-6 and IL-8 which in turn also act in an autocrine feed-forward loop to upregulate SASP signaling [42–55]. IL-1α is also regarded as the master regulator of SASP signaling and can partially recapitulate inflammatory SASP [56]. Furthermore, blocking NLRP3 inflammasome is important for the processing and activation of IL-1β reducing the SASP [57]. Moreover, the mTOR pathway plays a vital role in SASP regulation. It has been implicated in the phosphorylation of the translation repressor protein 4EBP vital for the IL-1α and MAPKAPK2 translation important for SASP regulation [58,59]. MAPKAPK2 blocks ZFP36L1 which leads to the degradation of proinflammatory SASP components indicating the indirect role of mTOR regulation. In addition, OIS stimulates the upregulation of SASP components by linking protein synthesis and autophagy in the TOR-autophagy spatial coupling compartment (TASCC) [60]. However, blocking autophagy by GATA also controls SASP [61]. However, the mechanism described here mostly covers the pro-inflammatory SASP as this is highly conserved among the various forms of senescence.

18.2 Features of cellular senescence

18.2.1 SA β-galactosidase activity

Senescence-associated β-galactosidase (SA β-gal) activity is the most widely used senescence marker. This enzyme is present in cell lysosomes under normal physiological conditions (pH 4.0–4.5). During senescence, SA β-gal activity increases due to an increase in lysosomal content at pH 6.0 and is detected in senescent cells [62–64]. Late passage normal fibroblasts deficient in GLB1 (gene encoding lysosomal beta D galactosidase) underwent replicative senescence without expressing SA β-gal activity indicating that it is nonessential for senescence [63]. Hildebrand et al. identified α-fucosidase as an alternative senescence biomarker whose expression was induced in all types of cellular senescence and higher than SA β-gal activity [65]. Young et al. stated the activation of autophagy during senescence which is associated with the PI3K-mTOR pathway. Further, they observed that ULK3 (autophagy-related gene) promotes autophagy and senescence while blocking autophagy delays senescence phenotype and its secretome [66]. In addition, various cells stain positive for SA β-gal activity including osteoclasts, Kupffer cells, and macrophages suggesting the requirement for the additional markers for senescence [67,68]. Georgakopoulou et al. identified lipofuscin as an additional marker for senescence, and it was observed to colocalize with SA β-gal activity in senescent cells under *in vitro* and *in vivo* conditions [69].

18.2.2 Morphological changes

Senescent cells are characterized as enlarged, flat and vacuolized with multiple or enlarged nuclei. Modification in the shape is dependent on the expression of the scaffolding protein caveolin 1 and the Rho GTPases Rac1 and CDC42. ER stress has been associated with vacuolation by the unfolded protein response [70,71]. In addition, senescent cells associate with the neighbouring cells by cytoplasmic bridges that function as a signal via direct intercellular protein transfer [40]. Under *in vivo* conditions, senescent cells exhibit the morphology according to the tissue architecture. Biran et al. identified the increased size of SA β-gal cells in aged mice [72].

18.2.3 Cell cycle arrest

Cellular senescence is defined as the irreversible cell cycle arrest at the G1 phase. Cell cycle progression is mediated by CDK/cyclin complexes. Interaction between cyclins and CDKs is inhibited by CDKIs in senescent cells. Activation of cyclin D1-cdk4/6 and cyclin E1-cdk2 leads to the progression of the G1/S phase. DNA damage, telomere erosion or activated oncogenes induce the ATM/p53/p21 pathway and trigger senescence-associated G1 cell cycle arrest. p21 blocks DNA replication as well as dephosphorylation of pRb by Cdk2 and Cdk4/6 complexes which are the key hallmark of senescence. p16 is often used as a biomarker for senescence and is known to inhibit the cell cycle progression at G1 to S phase by blocking cyclin D1-associated kinases CDK4 and CDK6.

18.2.4 Nuclear shape

Senescence is associated with an increase in nuclear size and alteration in nuclear lamina which can lead to genetic instability [73]. Freund et al. have found that senescence induced in primary human and murine cells by DNA damage, oncogene expression, or replicative exhaustion leads to the loss of lamin B1 protein through p53 or pRB tumor suppressor-dependent pathway suggesting its role as a senescence biomarker [74]. Senescence is also related to the altered chromatin structure leading to heterochromatin state with senescence-associated heterochromatin foci (SAHFs) which may result in the suppression of genes associated with proliferation [75].

18.3 Mesenchymal stem cells

Stem cells are the precursor biological cells that possess the ability to self-renew and multilineage differentiation potential [76]. Mesenchymal stem cells (MSCs) are non-hematopoietic, multipotent stem cells that can differentiate into multilineage cells including chondroblasts, adipocytes and osteoblasts [77]. The International Society for Cellular Therapy (ISCT) states minimal guidelines to define MSCs as plastic adherent cells positive for CD105, CD90 and CD73 and negative for CD34, CD45, CD14 or CD11b, CD19 or CD79a and HLA-DR cell surface markers as well as capable of multilineage differentiation potential [77]. They can be isolated from multiple tissues including skin, dental pulp, adipose tissue, bone marrow, placenta, umbilical cord, amniotic membrane, and cord blood cells, etc. [78]. MSCs have been implicated in the treatment of various diseases including diabetes, limb ischemia, cardiac ischemia, ischemic stroke, multiple sclerosis, liver failure, liver cirrhosis, graft versus host disease, osteoarthritis, amyotrophic lateral sclerosis, amyloidosis, rheumatoid arthritis and respiratory distress syndrome [78].

18.3.1 Mesenchymal stem cells and senescence

MSCs proliferate by mitosis and have a finite lifespan in vitro and thereby undergo replicative senescence after undergoing several rounds of population doubling (PD) [1]. MSCs exhibit around 30–40 maximum number of PD [79,80]. MSCs exhibit heterogeneity toward proliferation rate depending on the age, tissue source, donor and culture conditions [81]. Umbilical cord-derived MSCs (UC-MSCs) exhibit shorter PD time as compared to bone-marrow-derived MSCs (BM-MSCs) and adipose-tissue-derived MSCs (AD-MSCs) [82]. In addition, BM-MSCs have more proliferation ability than muscle-derived stem cells and AD-MSCs [83]. MSC function declines with aging. MSCs isolated from the younger donor exhibit increased proliferation as compared to the MSCs derived from the old donor [78]. Younger MSCs have a better capability to inhibit the proliferation of allogeneic peripheral blood nuclear cells than aged MSCs [84]. Aged MSCs also exhibit SASP phenotype, thereby affecting the behaviour of neighbouring cells via autocrine/paracrine mechanism by accelerating senescence [84]. Indeed, the culture system also has a profound effect on the proliferation of MSCs. The three-dimensional culture shows more expansion ability than the two-dimensional culture [78].

Furthermore, cell cycle progression is faster in smaller cells as compared to larger senescent cells [85] which may be due to the prolonged G1/G0 phase and decreased S phase in senescent MSCs [86]. A decrease in the proliferation rate of MSCs is associated with increased expression of senescence-associated β-galactosidase (SA-β gal). The elevated levels of SA-β gal along with the formation of reactive oxygen species (ROS) and telomere shortening results in the morphological change in cells and senescence [87]. Increased cell size and granularity elevates the autofluorescence of MSCs which is positively correlated with the senescent cell formation [88]. Morphologically, MSCs during early passage are short and fibroblast-like spindle shape but become enlarged and irregular with more podia and actin stress fibre while undergoing senescence [84]. Oja et al. reported that MSCs between passage 1–3 have uniform morphology while they begin to enlarge from passage 5 with subsequent passaging [89]. This indicates that MSCs don't proliferate infinitely but undergo replicative senescence with growth arrest after several passages which are also referred to as developmental senescence. MSCs can undergo premature aging due oxidative stress resulting from stress-induced senescence or oncogenic induced senescence [87]. Various reports indicate that ROS plays an important role in mediating senescence in MSCs [90–92]. Altered levels of ROS and antioxidant enzymes including superoxide dismutase (SOD) promote growth arrest in senescent MSCs [92]. Moreover, senescence in MSCs is manifested by elevated p21/p53 and p16 expression levels [84].

Additionally, the senescent population in MSC culture can be isolated based on cell surface marker profile. Gnani et al. revealed that CD146 expression was downregulated in MSCs isolated from aged donors than young donors as well as in extensive cultured MSCs [93]. Moreover, Jin et al. found that low expression of CD146 in MSCs is associated with senescence [94]. Madsen et al. reported that surface marker CD264 is present on the aged MSCs [95]. In another study, the same group revealed that bone marrow mesenchymal stem cells (BM-MSCs) exhibiting CD264 expression also showed an increased level of SA-β-gal activity along with reduced colony-forming efficiency and differentiation [96]. However, further studies are needed to validate their use as senescent markers as this marker profile difference could be associated with the functional changes during aging.

18.3.2 Implications of senescence on MSC function

Senescence in MSCs is associated with reduced proliferation, differentiation and altered gene expression as well as chromosome structure (Figure 18.1). MSCs undergoing senescence shows a gradual decrease in the DNA methylation pattern with a concomitant decrease in dnmt1 and dnmt3b altering the expression of specific genes [97]. In addition, the expression of Nanog, oct4 and TERT is also altered in senescent MSCs indicating its influence on the stemness of MSCs [87]. MSCs mainly mediate their function through the paracrine mechanism by secreting various cytokines, growth factors and exosomes

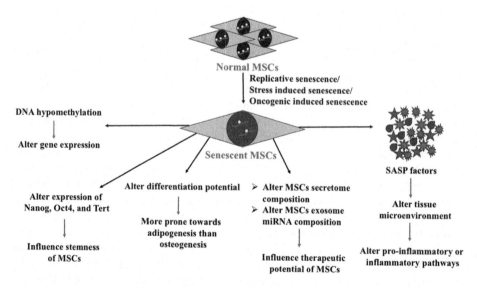

Figure 18.1 *Effect of senescence on the biological functions of MSCs.*

[98,99]. MSC-derived exosomes contain various growth factors, cytokines, miRNAs, lncRNAs and mRNAs which are implicated in regulating immune responses in the body. Senescence influences the biological function of MSCs by altering the composition of MSCs secretome. miRNAs in the exosomes of senescent MSCs are largely altered [99]. Moreover, senescent MSCs secrete SASP factors including cytokines, growth and chemotactic factors which can modulate the tissue microenvironment by altering pro-inflammatory or inflammatory pathways [87]. Moreover, senescence also alters the differentiation potential of MSCs which limits their potential application in stem cell therapy. Senescent MSCs tend to differentiate more toward adipogenesis than osteogenesis [100]. Senescent MSCs subjected to osteogenesis showed a decrease in the expression level of bone formation markers such as alkaline phosphatase and osteocalcin [101]. Hence, rejuvenating the function of MSCs for autologous transplantation is crucial for regenerative medicine therapy. Therefore, there is a dire need to maintain the characteristic of MSCs including self-renewal and differentiation before using them for therapeutic purposes. Recent work suggests that senescence is a modifiable risk factor that may help to overcome premature aging.

18.3.3 Senescence regulation by senolytics and senostatics

Senescence is controlled by two types of compounds such as senolytics and senostatics. Senolytic drugs cause apoptosis of senescent cells, while senostatics compounds reduce the cell progression toward senescence or SASP generation [102,103]. Zhu et al. reported the first time about the combination of quercetin and dasatinib in mediating apoptosis in senescent cells [103]. Combination of quercetin and dasatinib are the most well-described senolytics in controlling the senescent cell population. Other senolytic compounds include Panobinostat, BCL inhibitor ABT-737, HSP90 inhibitors or cardiac glycosides [6]. Senostatics also prevent the formation of senescent cells by inhibiting the p53 pathway. Well-known senostatics compounds include metformin and rapamycin [6].

18.4 Nutraceutical-based senolytics and senostatics

Synthetic compounds exert senolytic and senostatics effects, but they induce systematic side effects which can be deleterious to healthy cells. However, the present research is focused on the identification of nutraceuticals exhibiting anti-senescence properties. Nutraceuticals are bioactive compounds derived from natural products including plant material and have antioxidant and anti-inflammatory properties [6]. Below, we have discussed few nutraceutical compounds acting either as senolytics or senostatics in controlling proliferation and senescence. Figure 18.2 shows potential nutraceuticals as anti-senescence compounds for MSCs.

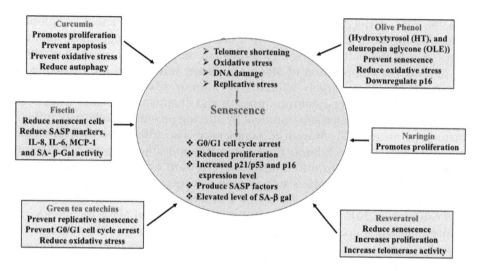

Figure 18.2 *Potential nutraceuticals compound for preventing senescence in MSCs.*

18.4.1 Omega 3 polyunsaturated fatty acids

Polyunsaturated fatty acids (PUFAs) are classified into omega-6 PUFAs, including docosahexaenoic acid (DHA) and eicosapentaenoic acid (EPA) and omega-6 PUFAs, such as arachidonic acid (AA). Omega 3 PUFAs need to be sourced from dietary components in mammals [104]. Omega 3 PUFAs have been implicated in aging, immune regulation, anti-inflammatory activity, cell differentiation and cell proliferation [105]. Peng et al. reported that both DHA and EPA decreased myoblast cell proliferation with a concomitant increase in G1 phase and decrease in S-phase through a mechanism involving MAPK-ERK [106]. In another study, it was shown that DHA and EPA suppressed myoblast differentiation with a significant decrease in the level of muscle-related genes including IGF2, myoglobin, Tnnt3, Myh3 and Mylpf linking MAPK/ERK and PI3K/Akt cascade [107]. A study showed that fad3b ESCs resulted in the accumulation of omega 3 PUFAs which inhibited the cell proliferation by increasing G1 phase by downregulating the expression of cdk4 via upregulation of p21 [108]. EPA and DHA were shown to induce neuronal differentiation by exerting cell cycle arrest in neural stem cells (NSCs) by downregulating Hes1 and upregulating p27 and p21 [109]. It was found that DHA increased the number of neurospheres from both neurogenic and gliogenic neural stem/progenitor cells (NSPCs) while specifically promoting neuronal differentiation [110]. DHA was shown to stimulate the undifferentiated human AD-MSCs to upregulate angiopoietin-1 mRNA, Il-6 and Il-8 mRNAs with the decrease in the cumulative sprout length in the in vitro angiogenesis assay [111]. Recently, another study found that EPA increased the vascular structure formation and protein expression of the endothelial-specific markers including CD31, fetal liver kinase-1, and VE- cadherin, via a mechanism involving calcium, reactive oxygen species (ROS), and nitric oxide (NO) signaling implicated in the function of AMPK and PPAR-α [112].

18.4.2 Curcumin

Curcumin is a natural hydrophobic polyphenol found in the rhizomes of the *Curcuma longa* plant. It is known to exert several pharmacological properties including anti-inflammatory, anti-fungal, antiviral, anti-microbial, antioxidant, anti-cancer, anti-atherosclerotic and anti-angiogenic [113]. Attari et al. revealed that curcumin increased the survival and proliferation of rat bone marrow stem cells (rBM-MSCs) in a dose-dependent manner in 48 hours while exerting no effect on adult rat neural stem/progenitor cells (rNS/PCs). However, after 72 hours, a low dose of curcumin promoted the survival and proliferation of rBM-MSCs and rNS/PCs [114]. A study stated that curcumin treatment protects hAD-MSCs from cell death mediated by oxidative stress generated by hydrogen peroxide (H_2O_2) [115]. In another study, Yang et al. reported that curcumin treatment increased the proliferation of BM-MSCs and altered its extracellular matrix content. A study stated that curcumin promotes cell survival by reducing the expression of autophagy markers such as Atg7 and p62 and inhibits G1 to S cell cycle progression in NSCs [116]. Ormond et al. found that curcumin stimulates the proliferation of NSCs under in vitro conditions suggesting its role in the regulation of stem cell proliferation [117].

18.4.3 Quercetin

Quercetin is a well-known flavonoid known for its pharmacological properties and beneficial health effects [118]. It is widely distributed in foods, beverages and plants and is abundant in Chinese medicine including HuangqiGuizhiWuwu tang [119]. Quercetin exhibits anti-inflammatory, neuroprotective, anticarcinogenic, chemopreventive and cardioprotective functions [120–122]. Pang et al. showed that quercetin promotes the proliferation of BMMSCs [123].

Various studies have shown that quercetin promotes osteogenic differentiation of MSCs by enhancing the activation of BMP signaling and estrogen receptor pathway and their downstream mediators such as Smad1, Smad4, Runx, OSX and OPN [118,123]. Casado-Diaz et al. stated that high concentration of quercetin (10 µm) inhibited the cell proliferation and osteoblast differentiation by downregulating the expression of osteoblastogenesis genes including ALPL, collagen type1 alpha 1 (COL1A1) and osteocalcin while promoting adipogenesis by upregulating the expression of CCAAT/enhancer-binding protein alpha (CEBPA) and peroxisome proliferator-activated receptor gamma 2 (PPARG2) [124]. Baral et al. showed that quercetin and its metabolite quercetin-3-O-glucuronide (Q3GA) regulates the proliferation of NSCs. Quercetin decreases the proliferation of NSCs along with Akt phosphorylation and increased cleavage of caspase-3 and PARP, whereas Q3GA induces proliferation as well as Akt phosphorylation [125]. Another study demonstrated that quercetin induces the proliferation of NSCs in the subventricular zone after focal cerebral ischemia in adult rats [126].

18.4.4 Olive phenols

A Mediterranean diet that constitutes fish, plant-based foods and olive oil reduce the development of age-related diseases suggesting that diet components have a crucial role in the aging process [127]. The olive oil plant exhibits an increased amount of phenolic compounds that are associated with various beneficial roles by improving cardiac health, cancer prevention and exerting antimicrobial effects [128,129]. It was found that two olive phenols including hydroxytyrosol (HT), and oleuropein aglycone (OLE) prevent senescence by downregulating p16 levels and SASP levels in two different cell lines including pre-senescent human lung fibroblasts (MRC5) and neonatal human dermal fibroblasts [130]. Another study also observed the protective role of HT using UVA-induced senescence aging model of human dermal fibroblasts (HDFs) with significant reduction of SA-β-Gal staining. Further, they observed that the anti-senescence effect of HT was associated with the downregulation of MMP-1, MMP-3 and reduced expression of IL-1β, IL-6, and IL-8 [131]. OLE has been implicated in decreasing oxidative stress and inhibiting mTOR, which play a crucial role in regulating aging [132,133]. However, there is no direct evidence stating the influence of OLE in organismal aging. It is well known that proteasome machinery is involved in degrading the damaged or misfolded proteins during aging. A study found that OLE treatment can delay the senescence in human fibroblast by improving proteosome activity [134]. Further, it was observed that OLE treatment during early passage of human embryonic fibroblast resulted in the reduction of ROS levels and control of the senescence [130–136].

18.4.5 Green tea catechins

Polyphenols, particularly flavonoids, constitute the most prominent components of green tea leaves with catechins being the most abundant such as (-)-epigallocatechin-3-gallate (EGCG-59%), (-)-epigallocatechin (EGC-19%), (-)-epicatechin-3-gallate (ECG-13.6%) and (-)- epicatechin (EC-6.4%) [137,138]. Han et al. demonstrated that EGCG can prevent the replicative senescence in three different primary cells including rat vascular smooth muscle cells, human articular chondrocytes and human dermal fibroblast by suppressing p53 acetylation and downregulating its expression [139]. They further observed that EGCG treatment was able to recover the cell cycle progression comparable to control cells by preventing G0/G1 cell cycle arrest. Kumar et al. showed that EGCG treatment was able to suppress premature senescence in preadipocytes by downregulating PI3K/Akt/mTOR and AMPK signaling as well as suppressing ROS, iNOS, SASP, NF-kB, Cox-2, and p53-mediated cell cycle arrest [140]. In addition, EGCG also suppressed the anti-apoptotic protein BCL-2 and promoted cell death. These findings suggest the senolytic properties of EGCG and can be utilized for developing anti-aging therapies. Using a mouse model of brain senescence, it was found that daily consumption of green tea catechins reduced the oxidative DNA damage and memory regression in these mice. However, catechins were unable to prolong the life of these mice but was able to delay the brain senescence suggesting its role in the healthy aging of the brain [141]. A study found that EGCG was able to increase the lifespan of rats by 8–12 weeks as compared to controls. Further EGCG treatment reduced the oxidative stress and damage to the kidney and liver by downregulating the expression of NF-kB and upregulating longevity factors FoxO3a and SIRT1 suggesting its role in increasing the life span [142]. In contrast, Strong et al. observed no significant alteration in the lifespan of genetically heterogeneous mice administered with green tea extract. Taken together, only a few reports have indicated the beneficial effect of green tea extract in combating aging and age-related disorders [143].

18.4.6 Fisetin

Fisetin is a bioactive flavonoid predominantly present in various fruits and vegetables including onion, grape, persimmon, cucumber, apple, and strawberry. It is found in the highest concentration in strawberry followed by apple [144]. Fisetin exhibits antioxidant, antiproliferative and apoptotic properties. Haddad et al. showed that fisetin inhibited the growth of various cell lines including prostate cancer (PCa) cell lines (LNCaP and PC3), breast cancer (MCF-7), and normal prostate stromal cell lines (PrSC). Further, it resulted in the G2/M cell cycle arrest in PC3 cells, while in LNCaP, it caused significant G2/M cell cycle arrest, nonsignificant G1 and reduction in the S phase suggesting its antiproliferative role [145]. Another group stated that fisetin induced G1 cell cycle arrest in LNCaP cell lines by reducing the expression of cyclins D1, D2, and E along with their activating partner cyclin-dependent kinases with concomitant induction of WAF1/p21 and KIPI/p27. In addition, fisetin also resulted in apoptosis by activating caspases 3, 8 and 9 [146,147]. Murtaza et al. demonstrated that fisetin reduced the growth and proliferation of pancreatic cancer (PaC) cells with the induction of apoptosis through the suppression of DR3-mediated NF-kappaB signaling [148]. Suh et al. showed that fisetin induced apoptosis in colon cancer cells by downregulating COX2 and Wnt/EGFR/NF-kB signaling pathways [149]. A study revealed that fisetin resulted in autophagic cell death in prostate cancer cells through the downregulation of the mTOR signaling pathway [150]. Recently, it was found that fisetin induced apoptosis in TPC1 cells by downregulating the expression of JAK1 and STAT3 and by promoting oxidative damage and increasing caspase activity implicating its role in thyroid cancer treatment [151]. Sabarwal et al. observed fisetin-mediated increase in apoptotic cells through ROS production in human gastric carcinoma cells [152]. Youns et al. revealed growth inhibitory and anti-apoptotic effect of fisetin in hepatic and pancreatic cell lines by modulating predominantly CDK5 signaling, NRF2 mediated oxidative stress pathway, ERK/MAPK and glucocorticoid signaling pathways [153]. Fisetin was shown to inhibit cell proliferation of PANC-1 cells and induces autophagy through endoplasmic reticulum stress and mitochondrial stress mechanism [154]. Li et al. showed anti-proliferative and apoptotic effect of fisetin in human oral squamous carcinoma cells by repressing the PAK4 signaling pathway [155]. Fisetin was shown to reduce oxidative stress-induced senescence in murine embryonic fibroblasts. Further, it was observed that progeroid Ercc$^{-/\Delta}$ and aged wild-type mice supplemented with fisetin for over 14 weeks resulted in the reduced expression of p16 in adipose tissue along with the decrease in SASP. On the other hand, naturally aged mice at 22–24 months when treated with fisetin for 5 days showed a decrease in the population of senescent cells in white adipose tissue. In addition, in vitro human adipose tissue explants treated with fisetin resulted in the reduction of SASP markers, IL-8, IL-6, MCP-1 and SA-β-Gal activities. Moreover, fisetin supplementation to mice at 85 weeks of age increased the life span by an additional 3 months [156].

18.4.7 Resveratol

Resveratrol is a stilbenoid and phytoalexin found in various fruits and vegetables such as berries and grapes [157,158]. Resveratrol exhibits antioxidant, antitumor, phytoestrogenic and antiviral properties [157]. It was shown that resveratrol was able to overcome the senescence phenotype of SIPS model-based cell types including WI-38 human fibroblasts and HT-1080 cells with inducible ectopic p21. They further observed that cells were able to overcome cell cycle arrest with two-fold increase in the number of cells upon resveratrol treatment [159]. Xia et al. stated that resveratrol prevented the senescence of endothelial progenitor cells (EPCs) and increased their proliferation as well as migration potential. This effect was associated with the increase in telomerase activity through the activation of the PI3K-AKT pathway in a dose-dependent manner [160]. In contrast, Miller et al. observed no significant difference between control and resveratrol treated mice in increasing aging rate while rapamycin treated mice exhibited an increase in survival in males (10%) and females (18%) mice [161]. The National Institute on Aging Interventions Testing Program (ITP) revealed that agents such as curcumin and resveratrol do not affect the life span of heterogeneous mouse model [143]. KilicEren et al. demonstrated that resveratrol induced premature senescence in human dermal fibroblast through the downregulation of SIRT1 and SIRT2 [162]. Resveratrol was shown to stimulate senescence in breast and lung cancer cell lines through Rad9-dependent pathway [163]. Matos et al. demonstrated that resveratrol reduced the copper sulphate-induced premature senescence (CuSO$_4$-SIPS) in WI-38 fibroblast by modulating protein degradation pathways [164]. It was shown that resveratrol promoted S phase cell cycle arrest and oxidative and replicative stress-induced senescence in U2OS and A549 cells through p53-CXCR2 signaling [165]. MRC5 cells treated with resveratrol exhibited an increase in replication and reduced oxidative damage and senescence. These changes were associated with the decrease in the level of H3 and H4 acetylated histones along with reduced p53 expression [166]. Another study stated that resveratrol reversed the senescence induced by high fat/sucrose (HFS) diet in rats and bovine aortic endothelial cells (BAECs) induced by high glucose through SIRT1/NADPH dependent pathway [167]. Resveratrol was shown to exert anti-proliferative effect on various cancerous and noncancerous cell lines including HeLa, MDA-MB-231, HUVEC, A431, human pancreatic cells, and prostate cancer cells by modulating various pathways such as oxidative stress, p53/ p21WAF1/CIP1 and p27KIP1 pathway [168–171].

18.4.8 Naringin

Naringin (naringenin 7-O-neohesperidose) is a flavonoid that possesses antioxidant and anticancerous properties. It is also implicated in controlling cholesterol levels and for the treatment of bone disorders such as osteoarthritis and osteoporosis [172]. Naringin promotes differentiation as well as proliferation of stem cells. It increases osteogenic differentiation by upregulating the expression of genes involved in bone formation through several pathways including notch1, BMP4, and wnt-β catenin in MSCs [173,174]. It upregulates the expression of osteogenic genes such as Runx2, OCN, OXS, and Coll [173,175]. It is shown to promote the proliferation of human BM-MSCs by inducing the ERK signaling pathway [173]. It is shown to facilitate the proliferation and differentiation of human periodontal ligament stem cells (hPDLSCs) at 1 uM concentration under *in vitro* and *in vivo* conditions [176].

18.4.9 Herbs as senostatics

Joshi et al. have suggested the intervention of the 'Rasayana therapy', one of the eight branches of Ayurveda for prevention of aging and diseases through modulation of MSC properties [177]. Naturally occurring herbs are a rich source of individual bioactive phytochemicals; moreover, their interaction with macro and micro molecules may play the role of senostatics. Dhanwantharam kashaya is an ayurvedic medicine known for its role in brain function improvement, delaying senescence and downregulating the expression of p21 and cyclin D1 in WJMSCs [178]. Our study has demonstrated that *Tinospora cordifolia* and *Withania somnifera* delay senescence in WJMSCs as evidenced by reduced SA-β-gal activity and a decrease in apoptotic cells [179]. Interestingly, these herbs downregulate the expression of senescence marker p21 without affecting the stem cell characteristics (CD 90 expression) of the WJMSCs [179].

18.5 Conclusion and future direction

Mesenchymal stem cell therapy is gaining immense popularity for the treatment of various diseases. MSCs mediate their therapeutic potential either through differentiation or paracrine mechanism. Importantly, the quality of the MSCs plays a vital role in determining the treatment efficacy. MSCs are required to propagate *in vitro* for several passages for obtaining the required number of cells for transplantation purposes. MSCs cultured *in vitro* have a fine lifespan and are more prone to undergoing replicative senescence with increased passage number. Senescence alters the biological functions of MSCs through several mechanisms and reduces their cell medicinal property. This calls for the dire need to identify the bioactive compounds which can either delay or suppress the senescence phenotype for maintaining the quality and quantity of MSCs. Till now, extensive research on nutraceuticals has been carried out on exploring their role as anti-cancer agents. In recent years, few studies have shown their role in promoting the proliferation of stem cells and exert an anti-senescence effect. Despite this, still tremendous research is required to validate their role in maintaining the biological quality of stem cells. It is yet to determine whether the same bioactive compound would be effective in a similiar manner on all MSCs isolated from different tissues? It is yet to explore which nutraceutical would have the most potent proliferative or anti-senescence effect? What would be the long-term effect of nutraceuticals on the biological characteristic of MSCs? Is it possible to increase the survival rate of MSCs upon transplantation with nutraceuticals?

Acknowledgement

RB, KJ, SS and AS contributed to the concept, data collection and analysis of the manuscript. SS wrote the manuscript.

References

1. Hayflick L, Moorhead PS. The serial cultivation of human diploid cell strains. *Exp Cell Res.* 1961;25, 585–621.
2. López-Otín C, Blasco MA, Partridge L, Serrano M, Kroemer G. The hallmarks of aging. *Cell.* 2013;153(6):1194–217.
3. Bielak-Zmijewska A, Mosieniak G, Sikora E. Is DNA damage indispensable for stress-induced senescence? *Mech Ageing Dev.* 2018;170:13–21.
4. Herranz N, Gil J. Mechanisms and functions of cellular senescence. *J Clin Invest.* 2018;128(4):1238–1246.
5. de Magalhães JP, Passos JF. Stress, cell senescence and organismal ageing. *Mech Ageing Dev.* 2018;170:2–9.
6. Kaur A, Macip S, Stover CM. An appraisal on the value of using nutraceutical based senolytics and senostatics in aging. *Front Cell Dev Biol.* 2020;8:218.
7. Kuilman T, Michaloglou C, Mooi WJ, Peeper DS. The essence of senescence. *Genes Dev.* 2010;24(22):2463–2479.
8. Fumagalli M, Rossiello F, Mondello C, d'Adda di Fagagna F. Stable cellular senescence is associated with persistent DDR activation. *PLoS One.* 2014; 9(10):e110969.
9. Jackson SP, Bartek J. The DNA-damage response in human biology and disease. *Nature.* 2009;461(7267):1071–8.
10. Muñoz-Espín D, Serrano M. Cellular senescence: From physiology to pathology. *Nat Rev Mol Cell Biol.* 2014;15(7):482–96.

11. d'Adda di Fagagna F, Reaper PM, Clay-Farrace L, et al. A DNA damage checkpoint response in telomere-initiated senescence. *Nature.* 2003;426(6963):194–198.
12. Bernadotte A, Mikhelson VM, Spivak IM. Markers of cellular senescence. Telomere shortening as a marker of cellular senescence. *Aging (Albany NY).* 2016;8(1):3–11.
13. Boothman DA, Suzuki M. Stress-induced premature senescence (SIPS) – Influence of SIPS on radiotherapy. *J Radiat Res.* 2008;49:105–112.
14. González-Hunt C, Wadhwa M, Sanders L. DNA damage by oxidative stress: Measurement strategies for two genomes. *CurrOpinToxicol.* 2018;7:87–94.
15. Serrano M, Lin AW, McCurrach ME, Beach D, Lowe SW. Oncogenic ras provokes premature cell senescence associated with accumulation of p53 and p16INK4a. *Cell.* 1997;88(5):593–602.
16. Astle MV, Hannan KM, Ng PY, et al. AKT induces senescence in human cells via mTORC1 and p53 in the absence of DNA damage: Implications for targeting mTOR during malignancy. *Oncogene.* 2012; 31(15):1949–62.
17. Qian Y, Chen X. Senescence regulation by the p53 protein family. *Methods Mol Biol.* 2013; 965:37–61.
18. Ko A, Han SY, Choi CH, et al. Oncogene-induced senescence mediated by c-Myc requires USP10 dependent deubiquitination and stabilization of p14ARF. *Cell Death Differ.* 2018;25(6):1050–1062.
19. Demaria M, Ohtani N, Youssef SA, et al. An essential role for senescent cells in optimal wound healing through secretion of PDGF-AA. *Dev Cell.* 2014;31(6):722–733.
20. Di Micco R, Fumagalli M, Cicalese A, et al. Oncogene-induced senescence is a DNA damage response triggered by DNA hyper-replication. *Nature.* 2006;444(7119):638–642.
21. Bartkova J, Rezaei N, Liontos M, et al. Oncogene-induced senescence is part of the tumorigenesis barrier imposed by DNA damage checkpoints. *Nature.* 2006;444(7119):633–637.
22. Fumagalli M, Rossiello F, Clerici M, et al. Telomeric DNA damage is irreparable and causes persistent DNA-damage-response activation. *Nat Cell Biol.* 2012;14(4):355–365.
23. Suram A, Kaplunov J, Patel PL, et al. Oncogene-induced telomere dysfunction enforces cellular senescence in human cancer precursor lesions. *EMBO J.* 2012;31(13):2839–2851.
24. d'Adda di Fagagna F. Living on a break: Cellular senescence as a DNA-damage response. *Nat Rev Cancer.* 2008;8(7):512–522.
25. Lowe SW, Cepero E, Evan G. Intrinsic tumour suppression. *Nature.* 2004;432(7015):307–315.
26. Kastenhuber ER, Lowe SW. Putting p53 in context. *Cell.* 2017;170(6):1062–1078.
27. Beauséjour CM, Krtolica A, Galimi F, et al. Reversal of human cellular senescence: Roles of the p53 and p16 pathways. *EMBO J.* 2003;22(16):4212–4222.
28. Shay JW, Pereira-Smith OM, Wright WE. A role for both RB and p53 in the regulation of human cellular senescence. *Exp Cell Res.* 1991;196(1):33–39.
29. Stewart SA, Ben-Porath I, Carey VJ, O'Connor BF, Hahn WC, Weinberg RA. Erosion of the telomeric single-strand overhang at replicative senescence. *Nat Genet.* 2003;33(4):492–496.
30. Campisi J. Senescent cells, tumor suppression, and organismal aging: Good citizens, bad neighbors. *Cell.* 2005;120(4):513–522.
31. Childs BG, Durik M, Baker DJ, van Deursen JM. Cellular senescence in aging and age-related disease: From mechanisms to therapy. *Nat Med.* 2015;21(12):1424–1435.
32. Sharpless NE, Depinho RA. The mighty mouse: Genetically engineered mouse models in cancer drug development. *Nat Rev Drug Discov.* 2006;5(9):741–754.
33. Sharpless NE, Sherr CJ. Forging a signature of in vivo senescence. *Nat Rev Cancer.* 2015;15(7):397–408.
34. Krishnamurthy J, Torrice C, Ramsey MR, et al. Ink4a/Arf expression is a biomarker of aging. *J Clin Invest.* 2004;114(9):1299–1307.

35. Burd CE, Sorrentino JA, Clark KS, et al. Monitoring tumorigenesis and senescence in vivo with a p16(INK4a)-luciferase model. *Cell*. 2013;152(1–2):340–351.
36. Kuilman T, Peeper DS. Senescence-messaging secretome: SMS-ing cellular stress. *Nat Rev Cancer*. 2009;9(2):81–94.
37. Coppé JP, Desprez PY, Krtolica A, Campisi J. The senescence-associated secretory phenotype: The dark side of tumor suppression. *Annu Rev Pathol*. 2010;5:99–118.
38. Hoare M, Ito Y, Kang TW, et al. NOTCH1 mediates a switch between two distinct secretomes during senescence. *Nat Cell Biol*. 2016;18(9):979–992.
39. Nelson G, Wordsworth J, Wang C, et al. A senescent cell bystander effect: Senescence-induced senescence. *Aging Cell*. 2012;11(2):345–349.
40. Biran A, Perelmutter M, Gal H, et al. Senescent cells communicate via intercellular protein transfer. *Genes Dev*. 2015;29(8):791–802.
41. Lehmann BD, Paine MS, Brooks AM, et al. Senescence-associated exosome release from human prostate cancer cells. *Cancer Res*. 2008;68(19):7864–7871.
42. Acosta JC, O'Loghlen A, Banito A, et al. Chemokine signaling via the CXCR2 receptor reinforces senescence. *Cell*. 2008;133(6):1006–1018.
43. Kuilman T, Michaloglou C, Vredeveld LC, et al. Oncogene-induced senescence relayed by an interleukin-dependent inflammatory network. *Cell*. 2008;133(6):1019–1031.
44. Wajapeyee N, Serra RW, Zhu X, Mahalingam M, Green MR. Oncogenic BRAF induces senescence and apoptosis through pathways mediated by the secreted protein IGFBP7. *Cell*. 2008;132(3):363–374.
45. Baar MP, Brandt RM, Putavet DA, et al. Targeted apoptosis of senescent cells restores tissue homeostasis in response to chemotoxicity and aging. *Cell*. 2017;169(1):132–147. e16.
46. Baker DJ, Wijshake T, Tchkonia T, et al. Clearance of p16Ink4a-positive senescent cells delays ageing-associated disorders. *Nature*. 2011;479(7372):232–236.
47. Baker DJ, Childs BG, Durik M, et al. Naturally occurring p16(Ink4a)-positive cells shorten healthy lifespan. *Nature*. 2016;530(7589):184–189.
48. Franceschi C, Campisi J. Chronic inflammation (inflammaging) and its potential contribution to age-associated diseases. *J Gerontol A Biol Sci Med Sci*. 2014;69(1):S4–S9.
49. Coppé JP, Patil CK, Rodier F, et al. Senescence-associated secretory phenotypes reveal cell-nonautonomous functions of oncogenic RAS and the p53 tumor suppressor. *PLoS Biol*. 2008;6(12):2853–2868.
50. Rodier F, Coppé JP, Patil CK, et al. Persistent DNA damage signalling triggers senescence-associated inflammatory cytokine secretion. *Nat Cell Biol*. 2009;11(8):973–979.
51. Glück S, Guey B, Gulen MF, et al. Innate immune sensing of cytosolic chromatin fragments through cGAS promotes senescence. *Nat Cell Biol*. 2017;19(9):1061–1070.
52. Dou Z, Ghosh K, Vizioli MG, et al. Cytoplasmic chromatin triggers inflammation in senescence and cancer. *Nature*. 2017;550(7676):402–406.
53. Yang H, Wang H, Ren J, Chen Q, Chen ZJ. cGAS is essential for cellular senescence. *Proc Natl Acad Sci U S A*. 2017;114(23):E4612–E4620.
54. Freund A, Patil CK, Campisi J. p38MAPK is a novel DNA damage response-independent regulator of the senescence-associated secretory phenotype. *EMBO J*. 2011;30(8):1536–1548.
55. Chien Y, Scuoppo C, Wang X, et al. Control of the senescence-associated secretory phenotype by NF-κB promotes senescence and enhances chemosensitivity. *Genes Dev*. 2011;25(20):2125–2136.
56. Orjalo AV, Bhaumik D, Gengler BK, Scott GK, Campisi J. Cell surface-bound IL-1α is an upstream regulator of the senescence-associated IL-6/IL-8 cytokine network. *Proc Natl Acad Sci U S A*. 2009;106(40):17031–17036.
57. Acosta JC, Banito A, Wuestefeld T, et al. A complex secretory program orchestrated by the inflammasome controls paracrine senescence. *Nat Cell Biol*. 2013;15(8):978–990.

58. Laberge RM, Sun YU, Orjalo AV, et al. MTOR regulates the pro-tumorigenic senescence-associated secretory phenotype by promoting IL1A translation. *Nat Cell Biol.* 2015;17(8):1049–1061.

59. Herranz N, Gallage S, Mellone M, et al. mTOR regulates MAPKAPK2 translation to control the senescence-associated secretory phenotype. *Nat Cell Biol.* 2015;17(9):1205–1217.

60. Narita M, Young AR, Arakawa S, et al. Spatial coupling of mTOR and autophagy augments secretory phenotypes. *Science.* 2011;332(6032):966–970.

61. Kang C, Xu Q, Martin TD, et al. The DNA damage response induces inflammation and senescence by inhibiting autophagy of GATA4. *Science.* 2015;349(6255):aaa5612.

62. Kurz DJ, Decary S, Hong Y, Erusalimsky JD. Senescence-associated β-galactosidase reflects an increase in lysosomal mass during replicative ageing of human endothelial cells. *J Cell Sci.* 2000;113(20):3613–3622.

63. Lee BY, Han JA, Im JS, et al. Senescence-associated β-galactosidase is lysosomal β-galactosidase. *Aging cell.* 2006;5(2):187–195.

64. Dimri GP, Lee X, Basile G, et al. A biomarker that identifies senescent human cells in culture and in aging skin in vivo. *Proc Natl Acad Sci U S A.* 1995;92(20):9363–9367.

65. Hildebrand DG, Lehle S, Borst A, Haferkamp S, Essmann F, Schulze-Osthoff K. α-Fucosidase as a novel convenient biomarker for cellular senescence. *Cell Cycle.* 2013;12(12):1922–1927.

66. Young AR, Narita M, Ferreira M, et al. Autophagy mediates the mitotic senescence transition. *Genes Dev.* 2009;23(7):798–803.

67. Bursuker I, Rhodes JM, Goldman R. β-Galactosidase – An indicator of the maturational stage of mouse and human mononuclear phagocytes. *J Cell Physiol.* 1982;112(3):385–390.

68. Kopp HG, Hooper AT, Shmelkov SV, Rafii S. β-Galactosidase staining on bone marrow. The osteoclast pitfall. *HistolHistopathol.* 2007;22(9):971–976.

69. Georgakopoulou EA, Tsimaratou K, Evangelou K, et al. Specific lipofuscin staining as a novel biomarker to detect replicative and stress-induced senescence. A method applicable in cryo-preserved and archival tissues. *Aging (Albany NY).* 2013;5(1):37–50.

70. Cho KA, Ryu SJ, Oh YS, et al. Morphological adjustment of senescent cells by modulating caveolin-1 status. *J Biol Chem.* 2004;279(40):42270–42278.

71. Denoyelle C, Abou-Rjaily G, Bezrookove V, et al. Anti-oncogenic role of the endoplasmic reticulum differentially activated by mutations in the MAPK pathway. *Nat Cell Biol.* 2006;8(10):1053–1063.

72. Biran A, Zada L, Abou Karam P, et al. Quantitative identification of senescent cells in aging and disease. *Aging Cell.* 2017;16(4):661–671.

73. Hernandez-Segura A, Nehme J, Demaria M. Hallmarks of cellular senescence. *Trends Cell Biol.* 2018; 28(6):436–453.

74. Freund A, Laberge RM, Demaria M, Campisi J. Lamin B1 loss is a senescence-associated biomarker. *Mol Biol Cell.* 2012;23(11):2066–75.

75. Aird KM, Zhang R. Detection of senescence-associated heterochromatin foci (SAHF). *Methods Mol Biol.* 2013; 965():185–96.

76. ChagastellesPC, Nardi NB. Biology of stem cells: An overview. *Kidn Int Supplements.* 2011;1(3):63–67.

77. Dominici M, le Blanc K, Mueller I, et al. Minimal criteria for defining multipotent mesenchymal stromal cells. The International Society for Cellular Therapy position statement. *Cytotherapy.* 2006;8(4):315–317.

78. Saud B, Malla R, Shrestha K. A review on the effect of plant extract on mesenchymal stem cell proliferation and differentiation. *Stem Cells Int.* 2019;2019:7513404.

79. Banfi A, Bianchi G, Notaro R, et al. Replicative aging and gene expression in long-term cultures of human bone marrow stromal cells. *Tissue Eng.* 2002;8:901–910.

80. Baxter MA, Wynn RF, JowittSN, et al. Study of telomere length reveals rapid aging of human marrow stromal cells following in vitro expansion. *Stem Cells.* 2004;22:675–682.

81. Phinney DG. Functional heterogeneity of mesenchymal stem cells: Implications for cell therapy. *J Cell Biochem*. 2012;113:2806–2812.
82. Jin H, Bae Y, Kim M et al. Comparative analysis of human mesenchymal stem cells from bone marrow, adipose tissue, and umbilical cord blood as sources of cell therapy. *Int J Mol Sci*. 2013;14(9):17986–1800.
83. Via AG, Frizziero A, Oliva F. Biological properties of mesenchymal stem cells from different sources. *Musc Ligam Tend J*. 2012;2(3):154–162.
84. Liu J, Ding Y, Liu Z, Liang X. Senescence in mesenchymal stem cells: Functional alterations, molecular mechanisms, and rejuvenation strategies. *Front Cell Dev Biol*. 2020;8:258.
85. Ginzberg MB, Chang N, D'Souza H, et al. Cell size sensing in animal cells coordinates anabolic growth rates and cell cycle progression to maintain cell size uniformity. *eLife*. 2018;7:e26957.
86. Gaur, M. Methods and strategies for procurement, isolation, characterization, and assessment of senescence of human mesenchymal stem cells from adipose tissue. *Methods Mol Biol*. 2019;2045:37–92.
87. Zhou X, Hong Y, Zhang H, Li X. Mesenchymal stem cell senescence and rejuvenation: Current status and challenges. *Front Cell Dev Biol*. 2020;8:364.
88. Bertolo A, Baur M, Guerrero J, et al. Autofluorescence is a reliable in vitro marker of cellular senescence in human mesenchymal stromal cells. *Sci Rep*. 2019;9:2074.
89. Oja S, Komulainen P, Penttila A, Nystedt J, Korhonen M. Automated image analysis detects aging in clinical-grade mesenchymal stromal cell cultures. *Stem Cell Res Ther*. 2018;9:6.
90. Huang XR. Adipose-derived mesenchymal stem cells isolated from patients with abdominal aortic aneurysm exhibit senescence phenomena. *Oxid Med CelLongev*. 2019;2019:1305049.
91. Li X. FGF21 mediates mesenchymal stem cell senescence via regulation of mitochondrial dynamics. *Oxid Med Cell Longev*. 2019;2019:4915149.
92. Bi S. Stem cell rejuvenation and the role of autophagy in age retardation by caloric restriction: An update. *Mech Ageing Dev*. 2018;175, 46–54.
93. Gnani D, Crippa S, Della Volpe L, et al. An early-senescence state in aged mesenchymal stromal cells contributes to hematopoietic stem and progenitor cell clonogenic impairment through the activation of a pro-inflammatory program. *AgingCell*. 2019;18:e12933.
94. Jin HJ, Kwon JH, Kim M, et al. Downregulation of melanoma cell adhesion molecule (MCAM/CD146) accelerates cellular senescence in human umbilical cord blood-derived mesenchymal stem cells. *Stem Cells Transl Med*. 2016;5:427–439.
95. Madsen SD, Russell KC, Tucker HA, Glowacki J, Bunnell BA, O'Connor, KC. Decoy TRAIL receptor CD264: A cell surface marker of cellular aging for human bone marrow-derived mesenchymal stem cells. *Stem Cell Res Ther*. 2017;8:201.
96. Madsen SD, Jones SH, Tucker HA, et al. Survival of aging CD264(+) and CD264(-) populations of human bone marrow mesenchymal stem cells is independent of colony-forming efficiency. *Biotechnol Bioeng*. 2020;117:223–237.
97. Childs BG. Senescent cells: A therapeutic target for cardiovascular disease. *J Clin Invest*. 2018;128:1217–1228.
98. Ranganath SH. Harnessing the mesenchymal stem cell secretome for the treatment of cardiovascular disease. *Cell Stem Cell*. 2012;10:244–258.
99. Özcan, S. Myeloma cells can corrupt senescent mesenchymal stromal cells and impair their anti-tumor activity. *Oncotarget*. 2015;6:39482–39492.
100. Andrzejewska A. concise review: Mesenchymal stem cells: From roots to boost. *Stem Cell*. 2019;37:855–864.
101. Abuna RP. Aging impairs osteoblast differentiation of mesenchymal stem cells grown on titanium by favoring adipogenesis. *J Appl Oral Sci*. 2016;24:376–382.

102. Short S, Fielder E, Miwa S, von Zglinicki T. Senolytics and senostatics as adjuvant tumour therapy. *EBioMedicine*. 2019; 41:683–692.
103. Zhu Y, Tchkonia T, Pirtskhalava T, Gower A, Ding H, Giorgadze N, et al. The Achilles' heel of senescent cells: From transcriptome to senolytic drugs. *Aging Cell*. 2015;14:644–658.
104. Perica MM, Delaš I. Essential fatty acids and psychiatric disorders. *Nut Clin Pract*. 2011;26(4):409–425.
105. Das UN. Essential fatty acids and their metabolites as modulators of stem cell biology with reference to inflammation, cancer, and metastasis. *Cancer Metastasis Rev*. 2011; 30(3–4):311–324.
106. Peng Y, Zheng Y, Zhang Y, et al. Different effects of omega-3 fatty acids on the cell cycle in C2C12 myoblast proliferation. *Mol Cell Biochem*. 2012;367(1–2):165–173.
107. Zhang J, Xu X, Liu Y, et al. EPA and DHA inhibit myogenesis and downregulate the expression of muscle-related genes in C2C12 myoblasts. *Genes (Basel)*. 2019;10(1):64.
108. Wei Z, Li D, Zhu L, et al. Omega 3 polyunsaturated fatty acids inhibit cell proliferation by regulating cell cycle in fad3b transgenic mouse embryonic stem cells. *Lipids Health Dis*. 2018;17(1):210.
109. Katakura M, Hashimoto M, Okui T, Shahdat HM, Matsuzaki K, Shido O. Omega-3 polyunsaturated fatty acids enhance neuronal differentiation in cultured rat neural stem cells. *Stem Cells Int*. 2013;2013:490476.
110. Sakayori N, Maekawa M, Numayama-Tsuruta K, Katura T, Moriya T, Osumi N. Distinctive effects of arachidonic acid and docosahexaenoic acid on neural stem/progenitor cells. *Genes to Cells*. 2011;16(7):778–790.
111. Parshyna I, Lehmann S, Grahl K, et al. Impact of omega-3 fatty acids on expression of angiogenic cytokines and angiogenesis by adipose-derived stem cells. *Atheroscler Suppl*. 2017;30:303–310.
112. Taha A, Sharifpanah F, Wartenberg M, Sauer H. Omega-3 and Omega-6 polyunsaturated fatty acids stimulate vascular differentiation of mouse embryonic stem cells. *J Cell Physiol*. 2020;235(10):7094–7106.
113. Gorabi AM, Kiaie N, Hajighasemi S, Jamialahmadi T, Majeed M, Sahebkar A. The effect of curcumin on the differentiation of mesenchymal stem cells into mesodermal lineage. *Molecules*. 2019;24(22):4029.
114. Attari F, Zahmatkesh M, Aligholi H, et al. Curcumin as a double-edged sword for stem cells: Dose, time and cell type-specific responses to curcumin. *Daru*. 2015;23(1):33.
115. Wang N, Wang F, Gao Y, et al. Curcumin protects human adipose-derived mesenchymal stem cells against oxidative stress-induced inhibition of osteogenesis. *J Pharmacol Sci*. 2016;132(3):192–200.
116. Yang Z, He C, He J, et al. Curcumin-mediated bone marrow mesenchymal stem cell sheets create a favorable immune microenvironment for adult full-thickness cutaneous wound healing. *Stem Cell Res Ther*. 2018;9:21.
117. Ormond DR, Shannon C, Oppenheim J, et al. Stem cell therapy and curcumin synergistically enhance recovery from spinal cord injury. *PLoS One*. 2014;9(2):e88916.
118. Zhou C, Lin Y. Osteogenic differentiation of adipose-derived stem cells promoted by quercetin. *Cell Proliferation*. 2014;47(2):124–132.
119. Pang XG, Cong Y, Bao NR, Li YG, Zhao JN. Quercetin stimulates bone marrow mesenchymal stem cell differentiation through an estrogen receptor-mediated pathway. *Biomed Res Int*. 2018;2018:4178021.
120. Skibola CF, Smith MT. Potential health impacts of excessive flavonoid intake. *Free Rad Biol Med*. 2000;29(3–4):375–383.
121. Hollman PCH, Katan MB. Dietary flavonoids: Intake, health effects and bioavailability. *Food Chem Toxicol*. 1999;37(9–10):937–942.
122. Kelly GS. Quercetin. Monograph. Alternative medicine review. *J Clin Ther*. 2011;16(2):172–194.

123. Pang B, Zhao TY, Zhao LH, et al. HuangqiGuizhiWuwu decoction for treating diabetic peripheral neuropathy: A meta-analysis of 16 randomized controlled trials. *Neural Regener Res.* 2016;11(8):1347–1358.
124. Casado-Díaz A, Anter J, Dorado G, Quesada-Gómez JM. Effects of quercetin, a natural phenolic compound, in the differentiation of human mesenchymal stem cells (MSC) into adipocytes and osteoblasts. *J NutrBiochem.* 2016;32:151–162.
125. Baral S, Pariyar R, Kim J, et al. Quercetin-3-O-glucuronide promotes the proliferation and migration of neural stem cells. *Neurobiol Aging.* 2017;52:39–52.
126. Zhang LL, Cao Q, Hu ZY, Yan XH, Wu BY. Effect of quercetin on neural stem cell proliferation in the subventricular zone of rats after focal cerebral ischemia-reperfusion injury. *J Sou Med Univ.* 2011;31(7):1200–1203.
127. Omar SH. Oleuropein in olive and its pharmacological effects. *Sci Pharm.* 2010; 78(2):133–54.
128. Tuck KL, Hayball PJ. Major phenolic compounds in olive oil: Metsabolism and health effects. *JNutrBiochem.* 2002;13(11):636–644.
129. KarkovićMarković A, Torić J, Barbarić M, JakobušićBrala C. Hydroxytyrosol, tyrosol and derivatives and their potential effects on human health. *Molecules.* 2019; 24(10):2001.
130. Menicacci B, Cipriani C, Margheri F, Mocali A, Giovannelli L. Modulation of the senescence-associated inflammatory phenotype in human fibroblasts by olive phenols. *Int J Mol Sci.* 2017;18(11):2275.
131. Jeon S, Choi M. Anti-inflammatory and anti-aging effects of hydroxytyrosol on human dermal fibroblasts (HDFs). *Biomed Dermatol.* 2018;2:21.
132. Johnson SC, Rabinovitch PS, Kaeberlein M. mTOR is a key modulator of ageing and age-related disease. *Nature.* 2013;493(7432):338–345.
133. Sun W, Frost B, Liu J. Oleuropein, unexpected benefits! *Oncotarget.* 2017;8:17409.
134. Saez I, Vilchez D. The mechanistic links between proteasome activity, aging and age-related diseases. *Curr Genomics.* 2014;15(1):38–51.
135. Katsiki M, Chondrogianni N, Chinou I, Rivett AJ, Gonos ES. The olive constituent oleuropein exhibits proteasome stimulatory properties in vitro and confers life span extension of human embryonic fibroblasts. *Rejuvenation Res.* 2007;10(2):157–172.
136. Giovannelli L. Beneficial effects of olive oil phenols on the aging process: Experimental evidence and possible mechanisms of action. *Nutr Aging.* 2012;1:207–223.
137. Cabrera C, Artacho R, Gimenez R. Beneficial effects of green tea: A review. *J Am Coll Nutr.* 2006;25:79–99.
138. McKay DL, Blumberg JB. The role of tea in human health: An update. *J Am Coll Nutr.* 2002;21:1–13.
139. Han DW, Lee MH, Kim B, Lee JJ, Hyon SH, Parl JC. Preventative effects of epigallocatechin-3-O-gallate against replicative senescence associated with p53 acetylation in human dermal fibroblasts. *Oxid Med CellLongev.* 2012;2012:850684.
140. Kumar R, Sharma A, Kumari A, Gulati A, Padwad Y, Sharma R. Epigallocatechin gallate suppresses premature senescence of preadipocytes by inhibition of PI3K/Akt/mTOR pathway and induces senescent cell death by regulation of Bax/Bcl-2 pathway. *Biogerontology.* 2019;20(2):171–189.
141. Unno K, Takabayashi F, Yoshida H, et al. Daily consumption of green tea catechin delays memory regression in aged mice. *Biogerontology.* 2007;8(2):89–95.
142. Niu Y, Na L, Feng R, Gong L, Zhao Y, Li Q, Li Y, Sun C. The phytochemical, EGCG, extends lifespan by reducing liver and kidney function damage and improving age-associated inflammation and oxidative stress in healthy rats. *Aging Cell.* 2013;12(6):1041–1049.
143. Strong R, Miller RA, Astle CM, et al. Evaluation of resveratrol, green tea extract, curcumin, oxaloacetic acid, and medium-chain triglyceride oil on life span of genetically heterogeneous mice. *J Gerontol A Biol Sci Med Sci.* 2013; 68(1):6–16.

144. Khan N, Syed DN, Ahmad N, Mukhtar H. Fisetin: A dietary antioxidant for health promotion. *Antioxid Redox Signal*. 2013;19(2):151–62.
145. Haddad A, Venkateswaran V, Viswanathan L, et al. Novel antiproliferative flavonoids induce cell cycle arrest in human prostate cancer cell lines. *Prostate Cancer Prostatic Dis*. 2006;9:68–76.
146. Khan N, Asim M, Afaq F, Abu Zaid M, Mukhtar H. A novel dietary flavonoid fisetin inhibits androgen receptor signaling and tumor growth in athymic nude mice. *Cancer Res*. 2008;68(20):8555–8563.
147. Khan N, Afaq F, Syed DN, Mukhtar H. Fisetin, a novel dietary flavonoid, causes apoptosis and cell cycle arrest in human prostate cancer LNCaP cells. *Carcinogenesis*. 2008a;29(5):1049–1056.
148. Murtaza I, Adhami VM, Hafeez BB, Saleem M, Mukhtar H. Fisetin, a natural flavonoid, targets chemoresistant human pancreatic cancer AsPC-1 cells through DR3-mediated inhibition of NF-kappaB. *Int J Cancer*. 2009;125(10):2465–2473.
149. Suh Y, Afaq F, Johnson JJ, Mukhtar H. A plant flavonoid fisetin induces apoptosis in colon cancer cells by inhibition of COX2 and Wnt/EGFR/NF-kappaB-signaling pathways. *Carcinogenesis*. 2009;30(2):300–307.
150. Suh Y, Afaq F, Khan N, Johnson JJ, Khusro FH, Mukhtar H. Fisetin induces autophagic cell death through suppression of mTOR signaling pathway in prostate cancer cells. *Carcinogenesis*. 2010;31(8):1424–1433.
151. Liang, Y, Kong, D, Zhang, Y, et al. Fisetin inhibits cell proliferation and induces apoptosis via JAK/STAT3 signaling pathways in human thyroid TPC 1 cancer cells. *BiotechnolBioproc*. 2020;25, 197–205.
152. Sabarwal A, Agarwal R, Singh RP. Fisetin inhibits cellular proliferation and induces mitochondria-dependent apoptosis in human gastric cancer cells. *Mol Carcinog*. 2017;56(2):499–514.
153. Youns M, Abdel Halim Hegazy W. The natural flavonoid fisetin inhibits cellular proliferation of hepatic, colorectal, and pancreatic cancer cells through modulation of multiple signaling pathways. *PLoS One*. 2017;12(1):e0169335.
154. Jia S, Xu X, Zhou S et al. Fisetin induces autophagy in pancreatic cancer cells via endoplasmic reticulum stress- and mitochondrial stress-dependent pathways. *Cell Death Dis*. 2019;10:142.
155. Li Y, Jia S, Dai W. Fisetin modulates human oral squamous cell carcinoma proliferation by blocking PAK4 signaling pathways. *Drug Des Devel Ther*. 2020;14:773–782.
156. Yousefzadeh MJ, Zhu Y, McGowan SJ, et al. Fisetin is a senotherapeutic that extends health and lifespan. *EBioMedicine*. 2018;36:18–28.
157. Risuleo G. Resveratrol. *Nutraceuticals*. 2016;5:453–464.
158. Salehi B, Mishra AP, Nigam M, et al. Resveratrol: A double-edged sword in health benefits. *Biomedicines*. 2018;6(3):91.
159. Demidenko ZN, Blagosklonny MV. At concentrations that inhibit mTOR, resveratrol suppresses cellular senescence. *Cell Cycle*. 2009; 8(12):1901–1904.
160. Xia L, Wang XX, Hu XS, et al. Resveratrol reduces endothelial progenitor cells senescence through augmentation of telomerase activity by Akt-dependent mechanisms. *Br J Pharmacol*. 2008;155(3):387–394.
161. Miller RA, Harrison DE, Astle CM, et al. Rapamycin, but not resveratrol or simvastatin, extends life span of genetically heterogeneous mice. *J Gerontol A Biol Sci Med Sci*. 2011; 66(2):191–201.
162. KilicEren M, Kilincli A, Eren Ö. Resveratrol induced premature senescence is associated with DNA damage mediated SIRT1 and SIRT2 down-regulation. *PLoS One*. 2015;10(4):e0124837.
163. Chen KY, Chen CC, Chang YC, Chang MC. Resveratrol induced premature senescence and inhibited epithelial-mesenchymal transition of cancer cells via induction of tumor suppressor Rad9. *PLoS One*. 2019;14(7):e0219317.

164. Matos L, Gouveia AM, Almeida H. Erratum to "Resveratrol Attenuates Copper-Induced Senescence by Improving Cellular Proteostasis". *Oxid Med Cell Longev.* 2017;2017:9172085.

165. Li B, Hou D, Guo H, et al. Resveratrol sequentially induces replication and oxidative stresses to drive p53-CXCR2 mediated cellular senescence in cancer cells. *Sci Rep.* 2017;7:208.

166. Giovannelli L, Pitozzi V, Jacomelli M, et al. Protective effects of resveratrol against senescence-associated changes in cultured human fibroblasts. *J Gerontol A Biol Sci Med Sci.* 2011;66(1):9–18.

167. Tang Y, Xu J, Qu W, et al. Resveratrol reduces vascular cell senescence through attenuation of oxidative stress by SIRT1/NADPH oxidase-dependent mechanisms. *J NutrBiochem.* 2012;23(11):1410–6.

168. Rodríguez-Enríquez S, Pacheco-Velázquez SC, Marín-Hernández Á, et al. Resveratrol inhibits cancer cell proliferation by impairing oxidative phosphorylation and inducing oxidative stress. *ToxicolApplPharmacol.* 2019;370:65–77.

169. Zhai XX, Ding JC, Tang ZM, Li JG, Li YC, Yan YH, Sun JC, Zhang CX. Effects of resveratrol on the proliferation, apoptosis and telomerase ability of human A431 epidermoid carcinoma cells. *Oncol Lett* 2016;11:3015–3018.

170. Qin Y, Ma Z, Dang X, Li W, Ma Q. Effect of resveratrol on proliferation and apoptosis of human pancreatic cancer MIA PaCa-2 cells may involve inhibition of the Hedgehog signaling pathway. *Mol Med Rep.* 2014;10:2563–2567.

171. Singh SK, Banerjee S, Acosta EP, Lillard JW, Singh R. Resveratrol induces cell cycle arrest and apoptosis with docetaxel in prostate cancer cells via a p53/ p21WAF1/CIP1 and p27KIP1 pathway. *Oncotarget.* 2017;8(10):17216–17228.

172. Lavrador P, Gaspar VM, Mano JF. Bioinspired bone therapies using naringin: Applications and advances. *Drug Discov Today.* 2018;23(6):1293–1304.

173. Liu M, Li Y, Yang ST. Effects of naringin on the proliferation and osteogenic differentiation of human amniotic fluid-derived stem cells. *J Tiss Eng Regenerat Med.* 2017;11(1):276–284.

174. Yu G, Zheng GZ, Chang B et al. Naringin stimulates osteogenic differentiation of rat bone marrow stromal cells via activation of the notch signaling pathway. *Stem Cells Int.* 2016; 2016:7130653.

175. Wang H, Li C, Li J et al. Naringin enhances osteogenic differentiation through the activation of erksignaling in human bone marrow mesenchymal stem cells. *Iran J Basic Med Sci.* 2017;20(4):408–414.

176. Yin L, Cheng W, Qin Z et al. Effects of naringin on proliferation and osteogenic differentiation of human periodontal ligament stem cells in vitro and in vivo. *Stem Cells Int.* 2015;2015:758706.

177. Joshi, K, Bhonde, R. Insights from Ayurveda for translational stem cell research. *J Ayu Integr Med.* 2014;5:4.

178. Warrier SR, Haridas N, Balasubramanian S, Jalisatgi A, Bhonde R, Dharmarajan A. A synthetic formulation, Dhanwantharamkashaya, delays senescence in stem cells. *Cell Prolif.* 2013;46:283–290. doi:10.1111/cpr.12026.

179. Sanap A, Chandravanshi B, Shah T, et al. Herbal pre-conditioning induces proliferation and delays senescence in Wharton's Jelly Mesenchymal Stem Cells. *Biomed Pharmacother* 2017;93:772–8. doi:10.1016/j.biopha.2017.06.107.

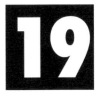

Nutraceuticals and Challenges Faced by Aging Populations in U.S. Nursing Homes

Benjamin B. Greco and Yashwant V. Pathak
University of South Florida

Contents

DOI: 10.1201/9781003110866-19

19.1 Introduction

Imagine something increasing from $2.4 to $4.5 billion per year for 19 years. That is how much the U.S. prescriptions increased between the years 1997 and 2016 (Fenton, 2019). Many believe that today's pharmaceutical industry is one of the largest markets in the entire world. A consumer in this market can find medication for just about anything they can imagine. Likewise, doctors in the medical field also have a vast quantity of medicines they are licensed to prescribe for their patients. There are also numerous alternatives to prescription medication, such as herbal therapy, which is why doctors also have to be very intelligent when it comes to medication. They are in charge of dosing the patients and need to be able to prescribe the correct amount of medication to achieve a target effect. Doctors also have to be up to date on all medications a patient is taking.

A medical professional in this field should also be able to make an educated decision on when prescription medication is prescribed. Studies have shown there are other forms of treatment than prescription drugs. This industry also plays an enormous part in the nursing homes around the United States. There is a great concern about the medications being taken and how they are being delivered to the aging patients in the nursing homes. Along with this, it is difficult for a doctor to be undeniably accurate with the number of medications there are on the market. There are prescriptions to help you use the restroom, raise, or lower your heart rate, reduce pain when you need relief, and even to strengthen your bones. Similar to prescription medication, there is "OTC", or over the counter, medicine that patients can buy at a pharmacy without a doctor's order. Some of these can include cold and flu medicine, light painkillers, and also nausea medicine. These are handy in today's society because they are relatively cheap and can provide the same results as prescription medication. This may sound great, but a downfall to OTC medicines is the lack of regulations when buying can cause misuse in the industry (Tesfamarium et al., 2019).

Nursing homes, assisted living facilities, and long-term care facilities play an extremely large role in the way people age today in the United States. Roughly, 1.4 million people in the United States live in nursing homes alone. This population is not including the people who are living in assisted living facilities or rehabilitation centers. There are many reasons people will need to live in a long-term care facility at some point in their life. Older adults move to this type of living environment because they require a certain level of assistance to accommodate their day-to-day life. They may not be as flexible or have the hand-eye coordination to get themselves ready for the day. This may seem ridiculous, but when a person gets older, their body changes along with what they can handle. Another common reason people move to long-term care facilities is that they need assistance managing their medication (Nursing Home Abuse Center, 2020).

Dementia, diabetes, eye disease, amputation, and risk of falls are all very common reasons for a person to live in a long-term care facility. These are also very common ailments in society today and as the aging population grows. For example, someone who is diagnosed with dementia has a greater risk in not remembering how to perform tasks of daily living. The person may need help showering, toileting, eating, and even dressing. Similar to dressing and eating, many people with these types of problems have a very difficult time managing their own medication. This can be dangerous because they may not be getting the correct dose of medicine, or even worse, they could even be taking the wrong medicine all together. The resident could take too much of a painkiller and could overdose before anyone has the time to save them. This is a major concern in long-term care and is a major factor in why residents need assistance every day.

19.2 Role of med-tech in nursing homes

Medication and the pharmacies providing the medication play a large role in the way nursing homes and assisted living facilities operate. In assisted living facilities, there is a position held by a person who is mainly responsible for delivering and assisting the residents with taking their scheduled medication. This is a med-tech or medication aide. Most medications are prescribed and consumed at specific times throughout the day. The role of a med-tech is to bring the medication to the resident to ensure they are able to take it within the time given by the doctor. Similar to assisted living facilities, nursing homes also have a system for administering medication to the residents. A nurse manages the medicine, on the other hand, because nursing homes are supposed to be more of a skilled facility. The role of a med-tech is very crucial to the safety of the residents because they need to ensure no one is being under- or overdosed.

19.3 Nutraceuticals, herbal medicines, and functional foods

These are the nutraceuticals, herbal medicines, and functional foods, which are now being used in nursing homes. People from all over the world have brought their knowledge of nutraceuticals to the United States, and the way they use them has spread to all parts of the country. By definition, a nutraceutical is a product derived by a food source that adds great health benefits to a person's diet. They are often combined with pharmaceutical medicines to reach a target goal for the patient in need (Journal of Nutraceuticals and Food Science, 2019). Many people believe the profits of nutraceuticals outweighs those of traditional medication. Some people even wonder if this industry could benefit those living in a long-term care facility. They feel as if the side effects of the prescription medications are detrimental and cause more harm than good.

19.4 Role of nutrition in aging populations

One question raised whether doctors and medical facilities can replace the use of prescription medication with the use of nutraceutical medicine or use them as complementary purposes. Several reports in many epidemiological studies have shown the effects of appropriate diet on better outcomes as part of the disease treatment (Everitt et al., 2006). To add to that, lifestyle strategies such as natural nutrition and nutritional supplementation have been identified as target options for those living in aging populations (Brown et al., 2010; Polidori et al., 2012; Polidori and Schulz, 2014).

Having good nutritional habits at an older age is a benefit in itself. There is evidence that shows that a diet full of specific food groups such as vegetables, fruits, and fish can reduce the prevalence of some of the main ailments in aging groups. Some of these include cancer, diabetes, and cardiovascular disease (Grant, 1999; Panza et al., 2004; Sofi et al., 2008; Frisardi et al., 2010). Studies like these have come out to show how eating healthy and eating foods with great nutraceutical value have a strong effect on the people who consume them. These have been a key role in how professionals in the medical field look at nutrition and how they will begin to understand them even more.

19.5 Challenges faced by aging populations in nursing homes

Some of the most common challenges faced by residents and patients in long-term care facilities are dementia described by cognitive impairment, financial situations, and sustainability. Cognitive impairment is an umbrella term that includes vision abnormalities, depression, poor cerebral blood flow, and memory problems. There are many researchers who are curious as to if we can substitute traditional medicine for nutraceutical treatment.

Financial issues play a role when discussing prescription medication because there are many older adults who cannot afford medicine without insurance. This may lead to other problems such as not being able to have a medication or having to use an alternative that may not have the same effects. If a healthy diet is introduced to an aging population of lower economic status, their need for prescription medication may decrease because they are receiving the adequate amount of nutrients they need. This correlates with sustainability because they will need to continue their diet. The benefits of a healthy diet present themselves after a period of consistency. This will allow the body to adapt to the change in food intake and learn where to send the nutrients absorbed after consumption. Although these problems in long-term care facilities are confined, there is a strong empirical finding that medication and healthy foods can work together to benefit older adults.

19.6 Concept of nutraceuticals, herbal medicine, and functional food in aging populations

A functional food has many different compounds inside with biochemical and physiological elements that benefit human health (Ferrari, 2004). The American Dietetic Association has created a few concepts to better understand how these substances affect a person's life, especially in an aging population (Bloch and Thomson 1995). A chemopreventive agent is a nutritive or non-nutritive component that has been investigated for its anticarcinogenic effects in people. Some foods that hold these properties are vegetables and plants (Ferrari, 2004). Being able to prevent and fight cancer in older populations is vital for survival in some cases. As you age, the immune system becomes weaker, meaning if an older person is diagnosed with cancer, they would have to be extremely worried about their compromised immune system.

Their next term is phytochemical, which is a substance found in fruits and vegetables that can be ingested daily and exhibit the ability to regulate a person's metabolism (Ferrari, 2004). Just as most bodily functions do as we age, our metabolism slows down. Having the ability to regulate or have a normal metabolism as you age will help with many issues experienced by older adults in long-term care facilities. One of these issues is digestion. If the metabolism is slow, the rate at which food is digested is also slowed down. If an older adult cannot digest food properly, they will eat less during the day. That is not ideal as an older adult should be receiving adequate nutrition throughout the day.

19.7 Increasing consumption of herbal products by aging populations

Herbal medicine usage in older populations is an important topic because the older population is growing very rapidly. Therefore, there are many older adults who take a diverse quantity of herbal medicines along with traditional medication (González-Stuart, 2011). It is important for patients and doctors to know how different herbal supplements interact with prescription medication already being taken. Since this is still a developing sector of medicine, there are many sources of misinformation, mainly on the internet, which is another reason healthcare providers should be up to date on the most advanced information if they are going to suggest herbal medicines to a patient.

19.8 Nutraceuticals/functional foods: Dementia and blood flow

About 22% of the population living in nursing homes and assisted living facilities have some form of cognitive impairment that inhibits their ability to live on their own (Nursing Home Abuse Center, 2020). There are many different aspects of nutraceuticals, which can benefit a person who is suffering from these age-related issues. Nutraceuticals can be broken down further into micronutrients and vitamins, which have different characteristics and benefits to an older adult's health.

An example of a diet, which is full of herbal origin materials, is the Mediterranean diet. This diet is characterized by a high intake of fish and plant-based foods. Olive oil is used as a source of monounsaturated fat and there is also a moderate consumption of wine. This combination is considered healthy because of the synergistic action between the components. Synergistic action is important because it is responsible for creating and releasing chemicals that protect the brain (Mecocci et al., 2014). A person suffering from cognitive impairment would benefit from this type of mechanism because their brain is the most affected by the disease.

Along with this, diseases such as diabetes mellitus and hypertension are very sensitive to changes in micronutrients. This could be extremely important for researchers because they can study how a diet like this can change risk factors and prevent vascular pathology (De la Torre, 2010; Polidori et al., 2012; Feart et al., 2013). If this method can be used in long-term care facilities around the country, we may see an increase to resilience against dementia in the aging population, along with other forms of diseases. This alone could replace different medications that are used to control the disease.

19.9 Dementia and flavonoids

A person in a long-term care facility or the family of a resident may be curious as to what makes a food capable of treating a person suffering from dementia. First, there are flavonoids, which have metabolites that interact with neuronal-glial pathways that involve neuronal survival and function (Spencer, 2010; Williams and Spencer, 2012). These metabolites ensure neural function by stimulating changes in cerebral blood flow. This is very beneficial to a person who is suffering from vascular dementia because they are not receiving enough oxygen to the brain, and flavonoids can allow for increased blood flow. There is a possibility that if used correctly, this form of flavonoid-based nutraceutical can replace similar prescription medication. There are several such products available which can be used in aging populations in nursing homes.

19.10 Challenges with cerebral functions in aging populations

Two very commonly used herbal origin products that have an effect on cerebral function and blood flow are memantine and rivaroxaban (warfarin). Although these two medications can cause actions in the body that will contribute to further blood flow, there are many other side effects and actions a person may not want. In two studies conducted on memantine, 815 subjects were studied with moderate to severe vascular dementia (Areosa and Sheriff, 2003).

From their findings, it appears that memantine, an NMDA receptor antagonist, has a positive effect on patients with vascular dementia. In another study, although an overall blood flow increase was not noticed after taking memantine, an increased blood flow was recorded around the hippocampus. This is a major region of the brain involved in learning a memory. This means that these cells are more protected now because they are getting the oxygen and nutrients they need to remain stable and keep the hippocampus safe (Kanaya and Hanyu, 2017). Along with the benefit of blood flow to the brain, there are other great uses for memantine, but there are also negative side effects that an older adult may want to avoid. In a study done on the effects of memantine, one adverse effect displayed in users of memantine is dizziness (Grossberg and Thomas, 2009). This is extremely dangerous in a long-term care facility because their stability is already compromised. They live in that setting because they are unable to move around safely and adding something that causes dizziness to the equation is irresponsible. Another negative side effect of memantine observed by Grossberg and Thomas was hallucination. About dementia, a common symptom is a person having slight to severe hallucinations. It may be counterintuitive for an older adult to be prescribed a medication that may cause hallucinations if they are already experiencing them. These hallucinations are dangerous because they can lead a person to harming themselves or others around them. Hallucinations are also negative for an older adult because they come along with paranoia, agitation, increased heart rate, and fear of being alone. The reason older adults move to long-term care facilities is to have an easier life. Drugs that induce these forms of effects are counter-productive for adaptation to a new environment and social progression.

19.11 Warfarin and nutraceuticals

The next medication that is being given to older adults that has the ability to increase cerebral function by increasing blood flow is warfarin. This medication can also act in the same way flavonoids do in the body. Warfarin is a vitamin K antagonist, which means it counters the action of vitamin K (Kaithoju, 2015). Vitamin K allows blood to coagulate, and warfarin slows down the coagulation factor in blood. It does this by eliminating the vitamin K-dependent coagulation factors (Chen et al., 2018).

This type of medication is considered to be a "blood thinner" by ending the action of vitamin K-dependent coagulation factors. The blood then acts as if it is thinner and allows for better flow around the body. Increased blood flow through the body is beneficial for someone with decreased cerebral function because the blood delivered the appropriate amount of oxygen and nutrients to the brain for proper function. This idea may seem like a solution on the surface, but this medication is not designed specifically for the brain. Warfarin affects the entire body and could cause problems after long-term usage. About brain function, warfarin displays a few negative effects on the brain.

First, the threat of micro bleeds is greatly increased in patients taking this medicine. Though it has prevention against ischemic stroke, warfarin does show in increased intracranial bleeding compared to other forms of anticoagulant drugs. This cranial bleeding, or micro bleeding, can even cause injury to the brain, and in the long term leads to dementia (Chen et al., 2018). One risk factor relating this medication's effects to long-term care facilities is hemorrhaging after a fall. If a resident has a fall and hits their head, there is no way of immediately deciding if there is a brain bleed occurring. Blood thinners and anticoagulants make it extremely difficult for the body to repair a bleed after injury. Naturally, the blood coagulates at an injury to control the bleeding, this is why scabs and bruises form. If the presence of an anticoagulant drug is in the person's system, the body will not be able to stop the bleeding naturally and the person could die as a result of internal bleeding. Both of these medications are not specifically intended to create more blood flow to the brain, but sometimes they are prescribed because their beneficial effects out way their adverse effects. This is a common issue in long-term care facilities because doctors are always trying to decide which medication is the best for their patient to take. As mentioned earlier, they also have to be able to decipher which medications can be taken together. Nutraceutical preparations may help to resolve these issues.

19.12 Flavonoid-based nutraceuticals for aging populations

This is where the beauty of nutraceuticals could be used. Many foods anyone can buy in the supermarket have great nutraceutical value that could benefit older adults the same way medications can. Let us take caffeine and cocoa for example. In relation to vascular dementia and creating better blood flow to the brain, caffeine and cocoa have been shown to be vasodilators, which means it allows better blood flow in a person's body. There are many ways an older adult can consume caffeine and cocoa such as coffee, tea, chocolate, and even some breakfast cereals. In the flavonoid group, there are two specific flavanols, catechin and epicatechin, which are found in cocoa and caffeine. There has been research over the past 10 years that shows how these two flavanols show diverse beneficial effects, particularly relating to vascular function (Francis et al., 2006). If an older adult consumes cocoa, the flavanols inside will contribute to the hemodynamics of that person, which is the system of that person's blood flow. It has been inferred that one action of cocoa flavanols on cerebral blood flow has helped in improving performance on visual and cognitive tasks (Scholey et al., 2010; Field et al., 2011). The next product with nutraceutical attributes an older adult can take to allow for better cerebral blood flow is coffee. Coffee is a great choice because it has caffeine in it. When ingested, caffeine initially has a vasoconstrictive effect, but very soon after there is a vasodilation effect (Echeverri et al., 2010). This helps to create better blood flow to the brain because vasodilation is the opening of arteries and veins. We intend for this action to occur because the increased blood flow to the brain will deliver the appropriate oxygen and nutrients to preserve brain cells.

Along with the benefits of these flavanols, there could be some negative side effects experienced. Adverse effects from these two flavonoids can vary from person to person and depend on certain factors such as method of consumption, tolerance, and pre-existing conditions. One example is an older adult should not consume high amounts of caffeine if they have pre-existing cardiovascular issues. There have been numerous studies to show that caffeine increases cardiovascular risk (LaCroix et al., 1986). This means the increased blood flow causes an increase in the older adult's heart rate, leading to the heart overworking. This in a normal, healthy patient tends to be fine, but in an older adult, the heart may not be able to handle the added stress caused by the caffeine. This could lead to a heart attack, stroke, or even an aneurism. If a doctor is going to recommend a patient to increase their caffeine intake throughout the day, he or she should be extremely conclusive about the effects the caffeine will have on the patient. Likewise with an increased intake of cocoa. They must know what medications a person is taking that may interact with the cocoa and give the best method for a person to use both simultaneously.

In the flavonoid category, there are other flavonoids that create similar effects for older adults in society today. There are also many other foods on the market that carry various nutraceutical benefits of flavonoids. Older adults are very sensitive to what they consume every day. This may be a key to eliminating harmful medications and replacing them with a healthy diet full of nutraceutical benefits.

19.13 Nutraceuticals/functional foods: memory loss

Another commonly affected function of the brain when it comes to aging and cognitive impairment is memory. As you get older, your ability to learn and remember new information begins to become more difficult. Luckily, this is normal in all aging adults and should not be confused with a form of dementia. One should be concerned when the inability to remember has a negative effect on the person's ability to care for themselves. You will see common occurrences such as forgetting where the remote is, losing reading glasses, and forgetting to start the dishwasher. If an older adult starts forgetting how to properly take their medication, does not remember how to drive, and is incapable of dressing themselves, then a stronger symptom of dementia is presenting itself. As one could imagine there are many different medications on the pharmaceutical market designed to assist older adults suffering from memory loss due to cognitive impairment.

Along with the flavonoids mentioned before, two more assist with memory loss in both normal aging populations and those who are diagnosed with dementia. The first flavanol is quercetin, one of the most studied flavanols, which is found in apples, caper, green tea, and onions (Kelsey et al., 2010). Its primary function is to prevent endothelial apoptosis caused by oxidants, by its antioxidant properties (Dong et al., 2012). The quercetin is experimented in order to increase cell survival in neurotoxic conditions (Heo and Lee, 2004). Neurotoxic conditions are disorders in the brain that have been caused by exposure to neurotoxic substances such as particles of metal, bacterial toxins, and even pesticides. In similar studies, the effects of quercetin have demonstrated the ability to improve memory and hippocampal synaptic plasticity. Along with quercetin, there is kaempferol, which is widely distributed in humans' daily diet (Aherne and O'Brien, 2002). In a study, kaempferol protects PC12 cells in the brain and improves cognitive learning ability and memory (Spencer, 2009).

19.14 Ginkgo Biloba-Based nutraceuticals and cognitive functions in aging populations

An older adult who is looking to substitute medications, which are designed to improve cognitive function and memory, have many great food options with these nutraceutical benefits. A few choices of food that have nutraceutical levels of quercetin and kaempferol are spinach, chives, and kale. All of these are natural foods that can be found in a normal grocery store and offer many more benefits such as vitamins and minerals. One plant that has been studied extensively for these nutraceuticals is Ginkgo Biloba (GB). GB is a plant whose herbal extracts are often used as a treatment to improve cognitive function. Extracts of GB contain a few components such as quercetin, kaempferol, and terpenoid lactones that appear to be responsible for its neuroprotective properties (Rendeiro et al., 2012). In general, extracts of GB are studied for its potential to treat memory and cognitive impairment. Hemodynamic, neurotransmitter, and free-radical effects have been shown by these extracts. This is important because all of these biological functions may be relevant to aging and age-related disorders (MacLennan et al., 2002; Brown et al., 2010). For this reason, several studies have been done on people and beneficial effects of Gb in prevention and treatment of older adults with neurodegenerative disorders such as Alzheimer's disease were shown. Several improvements to a person's cognitive function such as performance, memory, and attention were observed.

19.15 Herbal medicine: marijuana in older adults

One of the most highly talked about and controversial forms of herbal medicine on the market is medical marijuana (can we refer to it as nutraceuticals?) With very strict federal laws and newly rising lenient state laws, questions about the use of marijuana as a medicine become more prevalent in today's society.

Although the stereotype of a traditional marijuana user is a teenager or young adult who uses the product in a recreational way to experience its psychoactive effects, many people use it as relief for illness. In addition, there is a large population of older adults, independent and assisted living, who can use marijuana for its benefits. There have been many "qualifying conditions" a person can have that will allow them to receive a prescription for medical marijuana. Some of these conditions include Alzheimer's disease, arthritis, Parkinson's disease, PTSD, and multiple sclerosis (Karst, 2018).

19.16 CBD products and aging populations in nursing homes

Older adults mainly focus on medical marijuana and its derivatives, like CBD, to help manage pain from injuries and ailments such as arthritis, diabetic neuropathy, migraines, and cancer (Huntsberry-Lett, 2019). Older adults are generally more likely to choose this over prescription medications because their side effects may not be controlled by standard drug treatments (D'Souza et al, 2018). One of the most common adverse effects older adults experience while taking prescription painkillers is nausea. This can occur because the chemicals within the drug irritate the person's stomach lining, causing an uncomfortable feeling and induce vomiting. The use of marijuana could possibly substitute an older adult's prescription pain killer. Peripheral nerves that detect pain contain abundant receptors for cannabinoids, the active molecule in marijuana. These cannabinoids are said to block the peripheral nerve pain signals (Mack and Joy, 2000).

19.17 Herbal medicine: why marijuana?

Another factor to think about when considering why older adults may choose marijuana over prescription medication is the natural aspect of marijuana. The belief is that because marijuana is a plant, it is safer to consume than man-made prescription medicine (Minerbi, 2019). To add, there have been tested ways to extract cannabinoids from the plant to be consumed by mouth or inhaled as a vapor. Many older adults lean toward these methods because there is far less stigma related to marijuana use with these than traditional smoking. The safety of the effects of medical marijuana, in different forms, is further favored by reports of its effects on children with seizures. The perception of marijuana as a "nondrug" is attractive to the older community when it is available in forms contrary to traditional medications (Minerbi, 2019).

The last reason an older adult may use medical marijuana rather than traditional medication is because of close family suggestions. An older adult may be more open to ideas from close relatives that mean well. They understand the family has empathy for what the older adult is going through and may suggest other forms of medicine to relieve symptoms of ailment. The older adult knows the family is trying to improve his or her quality of life, so they may consider different ideas presented from the ones they love. They may also trust the family when it comes to this topic because there could be someone who also uses marijuana and can give personal feedback about the way it makes them feel. The older adult potentially will experiment with marijuana in the presence of that family member as a form of security.

19.18 Cost effectiveness: Pharmaceuticals

Global healthcare spending has been rising sharply over the past decade, and prescription drug costs are a major factor. Recent public discussion about extremely high prescription prices have made this topic very popular in the media and during political meetings (Grong et al., 2017). The cost of prescription medication even found its way into the most two recent presidential debates (Ward, 2015). Many examples of high-price prescription medication are all over social media. One of the mentioned examples is a medication called imatinib, brand name Gleevec. This medication is used for myeloid leukemia, and the price has tripled since the FDA has allowed for a new indication (Grong et al., 2017). The cost of this medication was $31,930 in 2005 and has been raised to $118,000 per year. This is a massive increase and was immediately a huge problem for patients who could not afford treatment. Another example is a medication called sofosbuvir. This medicine costs $84,000 for only a 12-week dose, or $1,000 per pill. This has actually caused many insurance companies to refuse coverage for this routine hepatitis c medication (Grong et al., 2017).

This increase in prescription medication leads to the next issue, which is that governments and insurance agencies are struggling to keep up with the increasing cost of all medications (Radhakrishnan, 2015). In December 2015, the U.S. government issued a warning about the increasing price of sofosbuvir and how it can affect the country's healthcare system. The report stated the company who created the drug and set a "benchmark price" to later allow the price to be raised. They did this knowingly it would decrease the number of eligible patients who had previously qualified for the treatment. This could have a huge negative impact on the older adults of America. Most older adults in the United States are using their social security benefits and discounted healthcare to be able to acquire necessary medication. If the governments and insurance companies are having trouble funding the needs of the older community, it would hinder the ability of the older adults to receive these medicines.

19.19 Cost effectiveness: Nutraceuticals

As stated before, many healthy nutraceuticals and functional foods can be found directly in a grocery store or supplement supply shop. Along with this, nutraceuticals have gained substantial attention because of their nutritional and safety profiles. Along with this, Indian economists and market research agencies have championed the Indian nutraceutical market as a "potential engine of growth" (Street, 2014). This sketches out the politics of the expansion of affordable, fast moving, nutraceutical products and functional foods. These ideas also illustrate the impact of fast-moving nutraceuticals on Indian communities. It showed how the transition into using functional foods can be achieved and how low-income families can feed their families while also providing nutraceutical benefits (Street, 2014).

We can relate this to what is happening in the United States because of our level of Americans living in poverty and our number of older adults. Many of these families are living from paycheck to paycheck and, unfortunately, cannot afford medical insurance or treatment. Similar to the older adult community, who are relying on social security and Medicare to cover the costs of their medicine. Some of these older adults may be able to cut down on how much they need to spend each year if their cost of medications decreases. Although they would have to spend their money out of pocket to receive nutraceutical foods, the cost should still be significantly lower than having to spend out of pocket on prescription medication. Even though the cost of this market is relatively low compared to the pharmaceutical market, it does have room to grow. The gaining popularity of this industry will increase the cost of certain products and will eventually compete with traditional prescriptions. The cost of herbal and functional foods is increasing with other commodities (Dahiya, 2013). This goes to show how one day older adults will have to be aware of functional food prices if they will continue to supplement for prescription medicine.

19.20 Conclusion

The pharmaceutical industry is a major moneymaker in the United States. Almost every single person at one point in his or her life has been prescribed a medication to treat an ailment. This shows how the industry will always be used and needed as patients continue to use their products. Although prescription medications are designed to treat specific illness or injury, many people believe they can supplement healthy eating habits for prescription medication. Older adults might be at the top of this list because they are the leaders in buying prescription medication in the United States. There are many instances where doctors or pharmacists believe the supplementation of foods that have nutraceutical values can benefit older adults in the same way prescription medication can. The reason for this is that, generally, healthy foods do not have negative effects associated with them. On the other hand, many medications older adults take have adverse effects. People who use natural substances often say they do so because they are generally safer and do not cause any problems as prescription medicine does.

Nutraceuticals and functional food offer health benefits associated with them. Many older adults living in long-term care facilities often face issues such as memory loss, vascular distress, and dementia. Certain flavanols, a nutraceutical, are found in foods such as vegetables and plants and are studied because of their effects on memory and cerebral function.

Herbal medicine is also important to understand because although similar, it is different from nutraceuticals. Herbal medication has also been used for an extremely long time, and uses of different herbs and plants can benefit people in medicinal ways. Medical marijuana is a very large discussion in society today regarding herbal treatments. Its strict federal laws and lenient state laws cause this type of treatment to be very controversial. Users of this herbal treatment are very impressed with the effects, and many believe it alleviates pain, nausea, and other symptoms of serious illness. Although numerous studies have been done, some people believe the media and politics have a great part in why it is not available throughout the country.

References

Aherne, S. A., and O'Brien, N. M. (2002). Dietary flavonols: Chemistry, food content, and metabolism. *Nutrition* 18, 75–81. doi:10.1016/S0899-9007(01)00695-5.

Areosa, S. A., and Sherriff, F. (2003). Memantine for dementia. *Coch Database Syst Rev.* (3):CD003154. doi:10.1002/14651858.cd003154.

Baskys, A., and Hou, A. (2007). Vascular dementia: Pharmacological treatment approaches and perspectives. Retrieved December 21, 2020, from https://www.ncbi.nlm.nih.gov/pmc/articles/PMC2685259/.

Bloch, A., and Thomson C. (1995). Position of the American dietetic association: Phytochemicals and functional foods. *J Am Diet Assoc.* 95: 493–496.

Brown, L. A., Riby, L. M., and Reay, J. L. (2010). Supplementing cognitive aging: a selective review of the effects of ginkgo biloba and a number of everyday nutritional substances. *Exp Aging Res.* 36, 105–122. doi:10.1080/03610730903417960.

Chen, N., Lutsey, P. L., Maclehose, R. F., Claxton, J. S., Norby, F. L., Chamberlain, A. M., and Alonso, A. (2018). Association of oral anticoagulant type with risk of dementia among patients with nonvalvular atrial fibrillation. *J Am Heart Assoc,* 7(21). doi:10.1161/jaha.118.009561.

Dahiya, K. (2013). Nutraceuticals and their impact on human health. *J Plant Biochem Physiol.* 1(4). doi:10.4172/2329–9029.1000e111.

De la Torre, J. C. (2010). Vascular risk factor detection and control may prevent Alzheimer's disease. *Ageing Res Rev.* 9, 218–25. doi:10.1016/j.arr.2010.04.002.

Dong, Z. H., Zhang, C. Y., and Pu, B. H. (2012). Effects of ginkgo biloba tablet in treating mild cognitive impairment. *Zhongguo Zhong Xi Yi Jie He Za Zhi* 32, 1208–1211.

D'Souza, D. C., Hauser, W., Schauer, G. L., Han, B. H., Devinsky, O., Leal-Galicia, P., et al. (2018). Medical cannabis for older patients. Retrieved January 25, 2021, from https://link.springer.com/article/10.1007/s40266-018-0616-5#citeas.

Echeverri, D., Montes, F. R., Cabrera, M., Galán, A., and Prieto, A. (2010). Caffeine's vascular mechanisms of action. *Int J Vasc Med.* 2010, 1–10. doi:10.1155/2010/834060.

Everitt, A. V., Hilmer, S. N., Brand-Miller, J. C., Jamieson, H. A., Truswell, A. S., Sharma, A. P., et al. (2006). Dietary approaches that delay age-related diseases. *Clin Interv Aging.* 1, 11–31. doi:10.2147/ciia.2006.1.1.11.

Féart, C., Samieri, C., Allès, B., and Barberger-Gateau, P. (2013). Potential benefits of adherence to the Mediterranean diet on cognitive health. *Proc Nutr Soc.* 72, 140–152. doi:10.1017/S0029665112002959.

Field, D. T., Williams, C. M., and Butler, L. T. (2011). Consumption of cocoa flavanols results in an acute improvement in visual and cognitive functions. *Physiol Behav.* 103, 255–260. doi:10.1016/j.physbeh.2011.02.013.

Frisardi, V., Panza, F., Solfrizzi, V., Seripa, D., and Pilotto, A. (2010). Plasma lipid disturbances and cognitive decline. *J Am Geriatr Soc.* 58, 2429–2430. doi:10.1111/j.1532-5415.2010.03164.x.

Ferrari, C.K.B. (2004). Functional foods, herbs and nutraceuticals: towards biochemical mechanisms of healthy aging. *Biogerontology* 5, 275–289 (2004). doi:10.1007/s10522-004-2566-z.

Fenton, T. (2019, March 11). How many pills do Americans consume? Retrieved December 06, 2020, from https://www.tctimes.com/news/how-many-pills-do-americans-consume/article_7f2144c4-41cf-11e9-b2dc-67a9260a317a.html.

Facts and Statistics about U.S. Nursing Homes. (2020, June 26). Retrieved December 11, 2020, from https://www.nursinghomeabusecenter.org/informative/facts-statistics-nursing-homes/.

Francis, S. T., Head, K., Morris, P. G., and Macdonald, I. A. (2006). The effect of flavanol-rich cocoa on the fMRI response to a cognitive task in healthy young people. *J Cardiovasc Pharmacol* 47(Suppl. 2), S215–S220. doi:10.1097/00005344-200606001-00018.

González-Stuart, A. (2011). Herbal product use by older adults. *Maturitas*, 68(1), 52–55. doi:10.1016/j.maturitas.2010.09.006.

Grant, W. B. (1999). Dietary links to Alzheimer's disease: 1999 update. *J Alzheimers Dis* 1, 197–201.

Gronde, T. V., Uyl-de Groot, C. A., & amp; Pieters, T. (2017). Addressing the challenge of high-priced prescription drugs in the era of precision medicine: A systematic review of drug life cycles, therapeutic drug markets and regulatory frameworks. *PLoS One.* 12(8). doi:10.1371/journal.pone.0182613.

Grossberg, G., and Thomas, S. (2009). Memantine: A review of studies into its safety and efficacy in treating Alzheimer's disease and other dementias. *Clin Inter Aging* 367. doi:10.2147/cia.s6666.

Heo, H. J., and Lee, C. Y. (2004). Protective effects of quercetin and vitamin C against oxidative stress-induced neurodegeneration. *J Agric Food Chem.* 52, 7514–7517. doi:10.1021/jf049243r.

Huntsberry-Lett, A. (2019). Medical marijuana for seniors: Weighing the risks, benefits and out-of-pocket costs. Retrieved from https://www.agingcare.com/articles/medical-marijuana-for-seniors-weighing-the-risks-benefits-and-out-of-pocket-costs-443881.htm.

Journal of Nutraceuticals and Food Science. (2019). Retrieved December 13, 2020, from https://www.imedpub.com/scholarly/nutraceuticals-journals-articles-ppts-list.php.

Kaithoju, S. (2015). Ischemic stroke: Risk stratification, warfarin treatment and outcome measure. *J Atrial Fibrillat.* 8(4), 1144. doi:10.4022/jafib.1144.

Kanaya, K., Hanyu, H. (2017, June 27). The effectiveness and difference of memantine and donepezil – Relating to changes in cerebral blood flow and clinical efficacy. Retrieved December 21, 2020, from https://www.imedpub.com/articles/the-effectiveness-and-difference-of-memantine-and-donepezil--relating-tochanges-in-cerebral-blood-flow-and-clinical-efficacy.php?aid=19607.

Kanowski, S., and Hoerr, R. (2003). Ginkgo biloba extract EGb 761 in dementia: Intent-to-treat analyses of a 24-week, multi-center, double-blind, placebo-controlled, randomized trial. *Pharmacopsychiatry* 36, 297–303. doi:10.1055/s-2003-45117.

Karst A. (2018). Weighing the benefits and risks of medical marijuana use: A brief review. *Pharmacy* 2018; 6(4):128. https://doi.org/10.3390/pharmacy6040128.

Kelsey, N. A., Wilkins, H. M., and Linseman, D. A. (2010). Nutraceutical antioxidants as novel neuroprotective agents. *Molecules* 15, 7792–7814. doi:10.3390/molecules15117792.

LaCroix, Z., Mead, A., and Liang, K. (1986). Coffee consumption and the incidence of coronary heart disease. *N Engl J Med.* 315(16), 977–982.

Mack A, Joy J. *Marijuana as Medicine? The Science Beyond the Controversy*. Washington, DC: National Academies Press (US); 2000. 4, MARIJUANA AND PAIN. Available from: https://www.ncbi.nlm.nih.gov/books/NBK224384/.

Maclennan, K. M., Darlington, C. L., and Smith, P. E. (2002). The CNS effects of ginkgo biloba extracts and ginkgolide *B Progr Neurobiol*. 67, 235–257. doi:10.1016/S0301-0082(02)00015-1.

Mecocci, P., and Polidori, M. C. (2012). Antioxidant clinical trials in mild cognitive impairment and Alzheimer's disease. *Biochim Biophys Acta* 1822, 631–638. doi:10.1016/j.bbadis.2011.10.006.

Mecocci, P., Tinarelli, C., Schulz, R., and Polidori, M. (2014, June 03). Nutraceuticals in cognitive impairment and Alzheimer's disease. Retrieved December 17, 2020, from https://www.frontiersin.org/articles/10.3389/fphar.2014.00147/full.

Minerbi, A., Häuser, W., and Fitzcharles, MA. Medical cannabis for older patients. *Drugs Aging* 36, 39–51 (2019). doi:10.1007/s40266-018-0616-5.

Panza, F., Solfrizzi, V., Colacicco, A. M., D'Introno, A., Capurso, C., Torres, F., et al. (2004). Mediterranean diet and cognitive decline. *Public Health Nutr*. 7, 959–963. doi:10.1079/PHN2004561.

Polidori, M. C., and Schulz, R. J. (2014). Nutritional contributions to dementia prevention: main issues on antioxidant micronutrients. *Genes Nutr*. 9, 382. doi:10.1007/s12263-013-0382-2.

Radhakrishnan, P. (2015). Commentary: Making middle income countries pay full price for drugs is a big mistake. *BMJ*. doi:10.1136/bmj.h3757.

Rendeiro, C., Guerreiro, J. D., Williams, C. M., and Spencer, J. P. (2012). Flavonoids as modulators of memory and learning: molecular interactions resulting in behavioural effects. *Proc Nutr Soc*. 71, 246–262. doi:10.1017/S0029665112000146.

Scholey, A. B., French, S. J., Morris, P. J., Kennedy, D. O., Milne, A. L., and Haskell, C. F. (2010). Consumption of cocoa flavanols results in acute improvements in mood and cognitive performance during sustained mental effort. *J Psychopharmacol*. 24, 1505–1514. doi:10.1177/0269881109106923.

Sofi, F., Cesari, F., Abbate, R., Gensini, G. F., and Casini, A. (2008). Adherence to Mediterranean diet and health status: meta-analysis. *Br Med J*. 337, a1344aq. doi:10.1136/bmj.a1344.

Spencer, J. P. (2009). The impact of flavonoids on memory: physiological and molecular considerations. *Chem Soc Rev*. 38, 1152–1161. doi:10.1039/b800422f.

Spencer, J. P. (2010). Beyond antioxidants: The cellular and molecular interactions of flavonoids and how these underpin their actions on the brain. *Proc Nutr Soc*. 69, 244–260. doi:10.1017/S0029665110000054.

Street, A. (2014). Food as pharma: Marketing nutraceuticals to India's rural poor. *Crit Publ Health* 25(3), 361–372. doi:10.1080/09581596.2014.966652.

Ward, A. (2015). Pharmaceuticals: Value over volume. *Financial Times*. Sept, 24.

Williams, R. J., and Spencer, J. P. (2012). Flavonoids, cognition, and dementia: Actions, mechanisms, and potential therapeutic utility for Alzheimer disease. *Free Radic Biol Med*. 52, 35–45. doi:10.1016/j.freeradbiomed.2011.09.010.

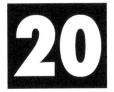

Neurodegenerative Mechanistic Pathways with Focus on Ayurveda Point of View and Applications of Nutraceuticals

Ghuncha Ambrin
University of Massachusetts Dartmouth

Lei Wang
Prime Bio, Inc.
Institute of Advanced Sciences

Raj Kumar
Institute of Advanced Sciences

Bal Ram Singh
Prime Bio, Inc.
Institute of Advanced Sciences

Contents

DOI: 10.1201/9781003110866-20

Nutraceuticals can be defined as a food, its product, herbs and a combination of such possessing health-benefitting properties. Nutraceuticals range from dietary nutrient supplements to genetically designed foods, herbal products, beverages, soups, vegetables, fruits and processed foods, like cereals, etc., and also food items prepared in specific way with combination and cooking (Prakash, Prakash et al. 2010). Although nutraceuticals are mainly represented by vitamins, minerals and amino acids, and over 1,000 other probiotic compounds have been identified till date (Makkar 2018), most traditions throughout the world have certain understanding of using, and also not using, certain food items under certain health-related conditions. Traditionally, people have consumed local plants and animals as food, which meant to eat food seasonably and, in most cases, locally. With the advent of technology for transportation and communication, nonlocal foods have become common, and thus a better understanding of the nutritional values of such food in relevant situations is important. Modern scientific examination of nutraceuticals will be helpful to integrate traditional practices, or even develop new ones, with modern healthcare standards.

Eastern healthcare systems, such as traditional Chinese medicine, or Ayurveda, the traditional Indian medicine, naturally incorporate nutraceuticals as part of addressing diseases and adverse health conditions, most of which is geared toward preventing diseases rather than treating them. However, treatment regimes are also comprehensive to include lifestyle, diet and herbs.

20.1 Neurodegeneration

Neurodegeneration basically refers to losing the cellular function and structure of nerve cells. The term neurodegeneration is usually understood to be a term used for neuron-related pathological conditions, primarily affecting the neurons in the brain. Diseases like tumors, edema, hemorrhage, etc. are not considered as neurodegenerative disease as these are not neuron-based disease. Similarly, any deformity or complications to the supporting cells or neuronal attributes are not considered as neurodegenerative diseases. When neurons die of known causes like poisoning, hypoxia or infection also does not fall under the term neurodegeneration.

According to the National Institute of neurological Disorders and Stroke, there are 600 neurological disorders (Brown 2005), which are mostly dominated by Alzheimer's disease (AD) and Parkinson's disease (PD). About 50 million people are diagnosed with neurological disorders every year in the United States. What causes neurodegeneration is still not known, though the etiology may consist of one or several factors that could be the cause of neurodegeneration, including environmental agents, chemical agents, lifestyle habits, genetic mutations, age, etc.

It is a fairly accepted fact that in several cases, the accumulation of misfolded proteins leads to neurodegeneration as seen in AD, of PD, but there is supportive evidence of the protective role of such protein aggregation as we see in Huntington's disease (HD) (Holmberg, Staniszewski et al. 2004, Okazaki, Fu et al. 2010, Atkin, Farg et al. 2014). What triggers neurodegeneration with subsequent loss of cells is still unknown. Do all the neurodegenerative diseases follow the same pathway? Not all neuropathological diseases have the same causative agent and have one or multiple different pathways. Activation of one pathway can exacerbate the other in many cases, and the reason for the initiation of the disease is still unknown, but once it is triggered, it builds up over time leading to synaptic impairment and neurodegeneration (Przedborski, Vila et al. 2003). In this section, we examine some common factors and mechanism that are seen in neuropathology, which mostly comprises the accumulation of toxic substances, mitochondrial dysfunction and pTau aggregation leading to apoptosis of the neuronal cells. Four different types of physiological cell deaths have been defined in the pathological conditions: necrosis, apoptosis, autophagy and cytoplasmic (Clarke 1990) which are controlled by specific mechanisms (Uchiyama 2001). In this section, we discuss in detail the mechanisms and pathways that are commonly involved in inflammation and neurodegeneration leading to cell death.

20.1.1 Dysfunction of the macroautophagy pathway

The onset of many neurodegenerative diseases occurs due to the accumulation of toxic proteins in different cellular organelles like the endoplasmic reticulum, mitochondria and others in both soluble and nonsoluble forms, and the inability of the regulation of these toxic proteins ultimately by the dysfunction of the ubiquitin-proteasome or macroautophagy pathway.

There are usually three pathways for the clearance of the proteins that are no longer needed by the physiological systems: (i) ubiquitin-proteasome pathway, (ii) autophagy-lysosome pathway and (iii) chaperone-mediated autophagy (Rubinsztein 2006). It has been suggested that the ubiquitin-proteasome pathway forms the dominant pathway in the clearance of the protein aggregates. The autophagy-lysosome and chaperone-mediated pathways are employed when the substance is not cleared by the proteasome. Proteasome and ubiquitin are the cytosolic-based protein complexes which are involved in the regulation of other proteins in the biological system. There are several aspects of this process which need to be considered. What are the functions of the ubiquitin-proteasome pathway? How does the ubiquitin-proteasome complex work in the removal of the unneeded proteins? And how does its inability to clean up lead to neurodegeneration?

The main function of the ubiquitin-proteasome pathway is the removal of the misfolded and unwanted proteins. This pathway has recently been identified as a mechanism that control the synaptic components, including postsynaptic receptors and the scaffolding protein that holds them in place. For achieving its various functions, the components of the ubiquitin-proteasome pathway are recruited to dendritic spines in response to the synaptic activity (Atkin and Paulson 2014). It contributes to maintaining synaptic plasticity and regulates cytoskeleton reorganization. Apart from these functions, the pathway plays a major role in response to DNA damage, oxidative stress and progression of cell cycle. In normal healthy cells, the misfolded endoplasmic reticulum proteins are translocated back into the cytosol where they are degraded by the proteasome after being covalently modified by ubiquitin, conjugated through its carboxy terminus. E1 (ubiquitin-activating enzyme), E2 (ubiquitin-conjugating enzyme) and E3 (ubiquitin ligase) are the three enzymes that have been implicated in this type of conjugation. E1 hydrolyzes the ATP and forms thioester-linked conjugate between itself and ubiquitin. E2 receives ubiquitin from E1 and forms a similar thioester intermediate with ubiquitin, and E3 binds both E2 and the substrate and transfers ubiquitin to the target protein resulting in the formation of polyubiquitin chain. Chains of four or more ubiquitin molecules form a recognition signal and are shuttled to the proteasome by chaperones. At the proteasome, the protein needs to be unfolded to pass through the narrow passage of the proteasome barrel (Rubinsztein 2006). In most cases, a decreased proteasome pathway activity leads to the intracellular aggregation, and a substantial loss of synaptic connections is observed. What causes this failure? It is still not clear if the aggregation itself is the sole cause of the accumulation of toxic proteins, but a failure of the quality control pathway for the elimination of these unwanted proteins or how the ubiquitin pathway becomes impaired in disease states and at what stage of the disease does the dysregulation of the pathway occurs. Failure of ubiquitination, proteasomal degradation, imbalance in ubiquitination/de-ubiquitination and genetic mutation may characterize the failure of the pathway. Different pathways are taken pertaining to different diseases but resulting in the same outcome, i.e., the dysfunction of the ubiquitin-proteasome pathway. Improper processing of the protein at the endoplasmic reticulum, cleavage of the proteins in Golgi bodies and mitochondrial dysfunction. In general, we can say that the protein accumulation (Lewy bodies or Aβ fibrils and Aβ plaques) can influence the cell surface receptor activation, resulting in the inhibition of E3 and thereby blocking the degradation of cyclin B1 (regulatory protein in mitosis) and preventing ubiquitination. This pathway can cumulatively partake in the dysfunction of the ubiquitin-proteasome pathway and degradation of the proteasome or each one of the steps can individually affect the disruption of the proteasomal activity, resulting in the aggregation of protein and neurodegeneration.

The proteins have access to both the pathways, ubiquitin-proteasome being the most dominant. When the proteasome is not able to assist in clearance of a protein, the autophagy-lysosome pathway assumes a dominant role. In a typical cell, the aggregated proteins and damaged organelles are degraded by macroautophagy utilizing autophagosome (Figure 20.1b). The fusion between autophagosome and lysosome results in the formation of autolysosome, which is the final critical step for autophagy. It targets aggregated proteins and damaged organelles such as mitochondria (mitophagy), endoplasmic reticulum (ERphagy), peroxisomes (pexophagy), etc. (Iwata, Edashige et al. 1990, Lamb, Dooley et al. 2013). Once all the protein is degraded in the autolysosomes, they are assumed to become lysosome that can undergo another fusion with the autophagosome. Increased accumulation of autophagic compartments, impairment of the lysosome-autophagy system, and retarded maturation to autolysosomes lead to accumulation of the aggregated proteins and dysfunctional organelles. This develops into excessive oxidative stress promoting cell death leading to neurodegeneration.

Chaperone-mediated autophagy contributes to the recycling of the excess protein subunits during oxidative stress, by degradation of the oxidized proteins. It does not target organelles. Proteins that are degraded under these conditions are the ones that are no longer needed and are broken down for the recycling of the amino acid. All the chaperone-mediated autophagy substrate proteins are tagged with at least one amino acid motif biochemically related to pentapeptide (KFERQ) (Dice and Terlecky 1990). The tagged proteins are recognized by the chaperones, which are then transferred to the lysosomal membrane and translocated into its lumen and degraded (Figure 20.1c). Abnormal binding of chaperone-mediated pathway motifs and inefficient translocation of accumulated proteins into the lysosomal lumen lead to lysosomal leakage and destabilization of the lysosomal membrane, which further results in the accumulation of oxidative damage and reduced cellular viability (Cuervo and Wong 2014). Additionally, the toxic effects of the accumulated aberrant proteins lead to neuronal demise. Chaperone-mediated autophagy does not function in isolation but is actively coordinated with both ubiquitin proteasome pathway and autophagy-lysosome pathway.

The downregulation of the different pathways utilized for the clearing up of the aggregated protein in neuronal cells is not the only reason for neurodegeneration. The accumulation of the toxic complexes along with the aggregated proteins leads to the dysregulation of lipids and carbohydrate metabolism. All the neurodegenerative diseases progress very slowly, taking over several years to reach the end stage.

20.1.2 Oxidative stress in neurodegeneration

Mitochondria are the powerhouse of the cell. It is responsible for the generation of adenosine triphosphate (ATP) and for maintaining calcium homeostasis. They are also responsible for apoptosis and metabolic activity through fission (process of creating new mitochondria)/fusion (helps mitigate stress by mixing the contents of partially damaged mitochondria). They contain many redox enzymes and generate reactive oxygen species (ROS). Mitochondrial dysfunction has been implicated in several neurodegenerative diseases, regulating oxidative phosphorylation, which is essential for regulating the mitochondrial structure (Federico, Cardaioli et al. 2012). Evidence of direct involvement of

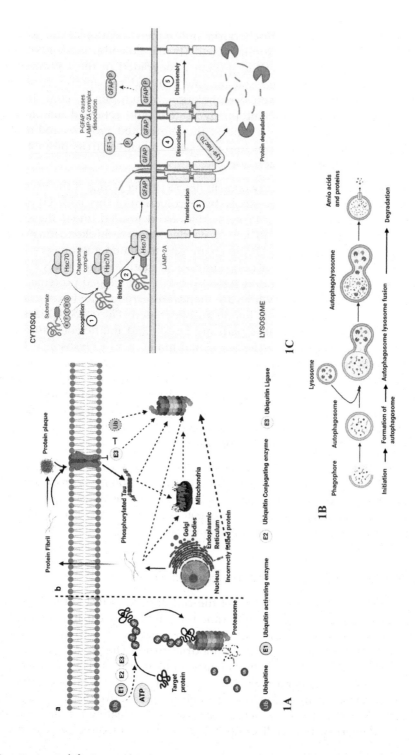

Figure 20.1 Autophagy is a strictly regulated lysosomal pathway that removes cellular debris and misfolded proteins. There are three different autophagic routes: 1. macrophage, 2. microautophagy and 3. chaperone-mediated autophagy. **(1A) a. Schematics for Macroautophagy: The ubiquitin-proteasome pathway in healthy cells.** Ubiquitin (Ub) is bound to E1, ubiquitin activating enzyme by the thioester bond requiring ATP. The molecule is then passed to E2, ubiquitin-conjugated enzyme through trans esterification. Ubiquitin ligase, E3 brings the compound closer to the substrate to facilitate the transfer of ubiquitin to the target residue. E3's can exist as multi subunit complex. Chains of four or more ubiquitin molecule can form recognition signal, allowing the substrate to be shuttled to the proteasome by set of proteins called chaperones. Target proteins are unfolded before passing through the narrow pore of the proteasome. It removes the ubiquitin and catalyzes the unfolded protein strips into peptides and releases them back into the cytosol. This mechanism facilitates the removal on unwanted and misfolded proteins, making way for the newly formed proteins required by the system. **(1A) b. Schematics of the pathway for the dysregulation of the ubiquitin-proteasome resulting in protein aggregation.** Mutation of the precursor proteins in the endoplasmic reticulum results in cleavage of misfolded proteins in the Golgi bodies which are transcytosed into the cell. The accumulation of the fibrils outside the cells results in the accumulation of these fibrils forming aggregates (e.g. plaques in Alzheimer's disease and Lewy bodies in Parkinson's disease). These protein aggregates not only activate the cell surface receptors which proceed to inhibit the E3, ubiquitin ligase resulting in the dysregulation of the ubiquitin complex formation with the target proteins, but also increase the aggregation of phosphorylated tau (ptau) in the cell. Additionally, the fibrils and protein aggregation disrupt the mitochondrial membrane. All these pathways can work together or separately, facilitating the degradation of the proteasome. **(1B) Schematics for lysosome-mediated autophagy (macroautophagy):** Cytoplasmic material is removed by the expanding membrane sac, phagophore resulting in the formation of autophagosome, a double membrane vesicle. The outer membrane of the autophagosome fuses with the lysosome exposing the single autosome membrane to the lysosomal hydrolases. The cargo contained in the membrane compartment of the autosome is subsequently lysed. The inner membrane of the autophagosome is degraded along with the enclosed cargo. The amino acid and the proteins are released into the cytosol by the lysosomal membrane permease. **(1C) Schematics for chaperone-mediated autophagy (CMA).** Recognition is initiated by the KEFRQ motif bearing substrate protein by hsc70 co chaperones in the cytosol. The substrate-chaperone complex is bound to the LAMP 2A on the lysosomal membrane. Translocation leads to the unfolding of the bound protein leading to subsequent protein degradation. Once the protein is degraded, the LAMP-2A complex is disassembled.

mitochondrial genetic defect has been implicated in various neurodegenerative diseases, such as in Fredrich's ataxia (Beal 2005), a disease that is also known as spinocerebellar degeneration. The disease damages parts of the brain, spinal cord and heart. In several other neurodegenerative diseases, there is indirect involvement of aggregated proteins with mitochondrial proteins as in the case of AD and HD. Increased production of free radicals and reduced amount of ATP production can lead to several neurodegenerative diseases, like AD, PD, ALS and HD (Avila, Perry et al. 2010). Electron transport chain (ETC) is a collection of inner membrane proteins forming large complexes essential for the synthesis of ATP (Figure 20.2). The absence or dysfunction of any of these complexes leads to protein aggregation in the mitochondria. This hindrance leads to the ROS imbalance (i.e., production and removal) resulting in the oxidative stress (Trushina and McMurray 2007, Morais and De Strooper 2010). In this section, we elaborate on the role of complexes (I–IV) in ETC and their impact on neurodegeneration. In ETC, the electrons are transferred from one complex to the other in a series of redox reactions. Energy released is used by several complexes to pump proton in the intermembrane space from the mitochondrial matrix. This creates a proton gradient. NADH is at the highest energy level, transferring its e- directly to Complex I, pumping the proton directly from the matrix to the intermembrane space. Complex I catalyzes the transfer of electron to the ubiquinone pool. This is one of the main sites of e- release. Most of the neurodegenerative diseases are known to be caused by the inhibition, mutation, or dysfunction of the Complex I (Andreazza, Shao et al. 2010). Aggregation of misfolded proteins like Aβ plaques, phosphorylated Tau (pTau), αSynuclein, Lewy bodies and copper-zinc superoxide dismutase type 1 (SOD1) impairs Complex I (Coussee, De Smet et al. 2011), facilitating the reaction of the e- with the oxygen species, resulting in ROS production leading to oxidative stress. Complex II is one of the main sites for both the Krebs cycle and mitochondrial respiratory chain. Additional e- from $FADH_2$ is fed from Complex II but does not have sufficient energy to release the proton into the intermembrane space and hence transfers its e- to the ubiquinone (Q). ROS generated at this site can have both beneficiary as well as pathological role. Complex III transfers the electron from Q to cytochrome c (cyt c), thereby pumping proton into the intermembrane matrix, hence playing a role in forming the potential gradient. Deficiency of Complex III (Haut, Brivet et al. 2003, Kilbride, Gluchowska et al. 2011) results in decreased oxidative phosphorylation, impairing energy generation. Complex IV or cytochrome c oxidase (COX) catalyzes the e- from cyt c to reduce molecular O_2, forming two water molecules coupling with the proton release into the intermembrane space. This is the terminal stage of the electron transport chain. ATP synthase catalyzes formation of ATP from ADP using the energy from the proton motive force (proton electro gradient). Loss of the ATP generation due to mitochondrial electron transporter dysfunction leads to severe neuronal damage (Golpich, Amini et al. 2017). Various proteins have been identified that maintain the mitochondrial ETC, like PTEN-induced putative kinase 1 (PINK1- protective role against cell death) (Lin, Liou et al. 2009), protein deglycase DJ-1 (Parkinson disease protein 7- potential ROS sensor) (Irrcher, Aleyasin

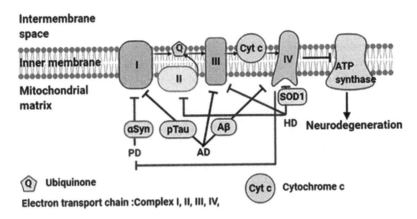

Intermembrane space

Inner membrane

Mitochondrial matrix

Cyt c

ATP synthase

HD Neurodegeneration

αSyn pTau Aβ

PD AD

SOD1

Q Ubiquinone

Cyt c Cytochrome c

Electron transport chain :Complex I, II, III, IV,

Figure 20.2 Schematics of the electron transport chain (ETC) in mitochondria displaying neurodegeneration. Several proteins in the inner membrane form large complexes I through IV which participate in the ETC. Impairment of the ETC results in several neurological disorders like AD, PD, HD and ALS. Deficiency of mitochondrial complexes I, III and IV results in AD pathology, mitochondrial complex I and IV deficiency in PD, and mitochondrial complex II, III and IV deficiency in HD. The combined mitochondrial complex deficiencies caused by increase in the expression of hyperphosphorylated tau and Ab plaques, alpha synuclein, and mSOD1 result in promoting the accumulation of aggregated/misfolded of these protein in AD, PD and HD, respectively.

et al. 2010), and leucine-rich repeat kinase 2 (LRRK2 or dardarin-mediating mitochondrial function) (Lin and Beal 2006). These have also been associated with quality control and regulating mitochondrial dynamics. Their dysfunction reduces mtDNA level which leads to disruption of the ETC, inducing apoptosis. Furthermore, transcription factors such as peroxisome proliferator-activated receptors PPAR-γ receptors have been identified in neuroinflammation. PPAR-γ is known as the main regulatory factor in the target gene modulation with PPAR response element (PPRE) in their promoters, such as those encoding for oxidative stress, inflammation (COX-2), inducible nitric oxide synthase (iNOS), nuclear factor-kappaB (NF-κB) and apoptosis (Kiaei 2008).

Mitochondria are a very dynamic organelle of the cell and regulate cell survival as well as cell death. Altered mitochondrial dynamics and mutations lead to its dysfunction (Baker and Haynes 2011). Mitochondrial dysfunctions reflect damage and decrease in its function resulting in neuroinflammation and neurodegeneration.

20.2 Calcium dysregulation in the mechanism of neurodegenerative disease

Every aspect of the cellular functionality is regulated by calcium ions (Ca^{2+}). These include signal transduction, motility, exocytosis, excitability and transcription. The alterations in the Ca^{2+} ions across the plasma membrane and intracellular organelles integrate the diverse functions of the cell. Several checkpoints in the cells measure and control the Ca^{2+} influx. These checkpoints are present in the plasma membrane and the membranes of mitochondria and endoplasmic reticulum, like G protein coupled receptors (GPCRs), ion channels, Ca^{2+} binding proteins and transcriptional networks, etc. Higher Ca^{2+} ion gradient is maintained by the Ca^{2+} buffering proteins and the membrane intrinsic Ca^{2+} transport proteins for pumping Ca^{2+} into the extracellular matrix (ECM). An array of proteins binds to the Ca^{2+} to trigger the cellular processes. Dysregulation of cellular Ca^{2+} ions results in degeneration and cell death.

The interaction of the aggregated misfolded protein with the plasma membrane leads to the formation of pores, transferring Ca^{2+} into the cytosol. This influx of Ca^{2+} leads to the depolarization resulting in an increase in intracellular Ca^{2+} concentration coupled to receptor stimulation N-methyl-D-aspartate receptor (NMDAR), α-amino-3-hydroxy-5-methyl-4-isoxazolepropionic acid receptor (AMPAR), etc. Once the intracellular homeostatic Ca^{2+} gradient is compromised, it enters excitotoxicity state. Because of the excitotoxic state, the cell inhibits the capability of Ca^{2+} removal. Together with misfolded protein aggregation and hyperphosphorylation, the cell enters a pathological state. The two main organelle that partake in neurodegeneration due to dysregulation of calcium, primarily are mitochondria and endoplasmic reticulum.

Calcium in mitochondria regulates the ATP synthase (Complex V) and can store large amounts of Ca^{2+} in matrix. Calcium in the mitochondria diffuses across the outer membrane through the large pores and is transported across the inner membrane through the ion channels. The resting electric potential between cytoplasm and the inner mitochondria is -150 to $-200\,mV$ and is created by the active transportation of protons. In stressful conditions, mitochondria accumulate large amounts of Ca^{2+} ions from the cytosol, triggering a vicious cycle exacerbating Ca^{2+} overload. Increase in Ca^{2+}overload and misfolded protein aggregation blocks Complexes III, IV and V, thereby decreasing ATP production and increases reactive oxygen species (ROS) production and depolarization (Canevari, Abramov et al. 2004, Marambaud, Dreses-Werringloer et al. 2009). The crosstalk between Ca^{2+} ions and ROS plays a key role in exacerbating neurodegenerative process in the brain (Figure 20.3).

Regulated (fast and specific) calcium release from endoplasmic reticulum controls many neuronal functions including synaptic plasticity and electric (action potential) or chemical (action potential) cell stimulation. It forms a calcium tunnel, facilitating the movement of calcium, bypassing the cytoplasmic routes. Additionally, the endoplasmic reticulum provides passage for the transportation of various molecules and signals toward their destination, which are controlled by the free Ca^{2+} release and uptake in the endoplasmic reticulum. Disruption of calcium signaling in endoplasmic reticulum in the brain leads to gradual and progressive selective loss in neuronal functions

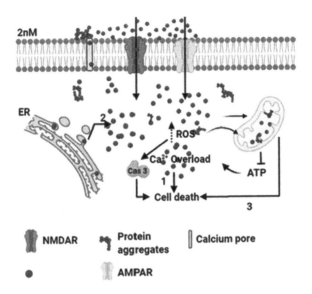

Figure 20.3 *Schematics for calcium regulated neurodegeneration. The extracellular concentration of calcium ion is maintained as 2mM. Protein aggregates in the interacts with the plasma membrane forming pores allowing for the Ca^{2+} ions to penetrate inside the cells. The aggregate interaction with the plasma membrane also depolarizes the membrane resulting in the transport of Ca^{2+} ions across the NMDAR and AMPAR. There are three direct pathways of calcium dysregulation leading to heterogenous group of neurological disorders. 1. Influx of Ca^{2+} in the cell cytosol can lead to cell death. 2. Depletion of Ca^{2+} by endoplasmic reticulum results in Ca^{2+} overload in the cytosol. This leads to increased production of ROS, activating Caspase 3 (Cas3), triggering cell death. 3. Protein aggregates in the mitochondria causes Ca^{2+} overload in the organelle, leading to inhibition of ATP synthesis resulting in ROS overload. This is a cyclic process exacerbating ROS production and Ca^{2+} overload, prompting cell death.*

leading to neurodegeneration. Several studies indicate the contribution of ER stress leading to neurodegeneration (Xiang, Wang et al. 2017, Ghemrawi and Khair 2020). In the neuronal cells, the endoplasmic reticulum extends from soma to the dendritic spines and plays a vital role in regulation of calcium levels by releasing Ca^{2+} ions to and from the cytosol through Ca^{2+} channels located on its membrane. The crosstalk between the aggregated proteins and Ca^{2+} leads to release and depletion of aggregated Ca^{2+} stores from the endoplasmic reticulum, increasing ROS production. This results in activation of caspase 3 with its end in cell death (Hashimoto, Ishii et al. 2018). The progression of neurological diseases is affected by the glial cells which are also controlled by calcium signaling. Ca^{2+} released from the endoplasmic reticulum triggers the Ca^{2+}-driven receptors on the glial cells leading to the glial activation.

20.3 Secondary effects of Ca²⁺ in neurodegeneration

Several inputs for the nucleus aimed at the long-lasting cellular response is directly controlled by the intra-endoplasmic reticulum free Ca^{2+}. Ca^{2+} alters the Ca^{2+}-dependent gene transcription. Increased Ca^{2+} induces neuronal NO synthesis leading to production of ROS resulting in neurodegeneration and ultimately cell death (Yamamoto, Wajima et al. 2007).

In aging brain, calpain is activated due to the increased level of Ca^{2+} in the cytosol. The activated calpains (Gafni, Hermel et al. 2004) cleave several proteins which are required for normal functioning of the neurons, thereby resulting in neuronal degeneration and apoptosis.

Neurodegenerative disease results in massive death of neurons everyday (100,000), leading to cognitive decline and decrease in brain weight. Only a few specific neurodegenerative diseases result in death, while others facilitate the onset of secondary health issues.

Ayurveda diagnoses neurological problems to arise from the imbalance of the vata dosha, which can be connected to the availability and movement of oxygen (Joy, Kumar et al. 2015). Additionally, Ayurveda considers neurological issues to be connected to consciousness, which is exactly located inside the brain, rather it is located outside in the universe, which can be quantum mechanically described to be linked to operate through cytoskeleton. And such operation is mediated by oxygen through the electron transport chain. Oxygen is thus the operational link the universe uses to monitor, record, maintain internal stability, for coordination and management of the ecology of life (Joy, Kumar et al. 2015). The connection between consciousness and microtubules has been addressed in clinical studies by establishing involvement aberrant microtubules with pathology of consciousness (Matell and Meck 2004, Hameroff 2012, Joy, Kumar et al. 2015, Venkatasubramanian 2015). As oxidation and oxygenation is important for the production of reactive oxygen species that are addressed by several nutraceuticals as antioxidants in preventing diseases, these concepts comply with the modern scientific standards of nutraceuticals and the concept of traditional medical system like Ayurveda for the etiology of neurodegeneration. According to Joy (Joy, Kumar et al. 2015), the primary target and aim of every disease and disorder in the ecology of life is to impair oxygenation the outcome of which is the disruption of homeostatic regulation, a concept that might also link the body physiology and natural conditions like seasonal changes.

20.4 Neuronal Regeneration

Neuronal regeneration is a concept in which neuronal tissues can regrow or repair to generate new neurons, axons, synapses and other supportive cells. Although neuronal regeneration is a relatively recent concept, researchers thought, for centuries, that the adult CNS (central nervous system) neurons are not capable to regenerate. This created a "central dogma of neuroscience". This long-held dogma of neuroscience is based on the following observations: (i) structure of the brain remains fixed after birth, (ii) new neurons are not being added to the adult mammalian brain, and (iii) neither mitotic figures nor various development stages had been seen in the adult brain. Further, this dogma assumed that neurogenesis or production of new neuron occurs during development and stops before puberty.

However, this long-held dogma was challenged by Joseph Altman during the 1960s, as he demonstrated neurogenesis in adult rat and cats (Altman 1962, Altman 1963) especially in neocortex, dentate gyrus and olfactory bulb. Later, Michael Kaplan and others demonstrated mitosis in the subventricular zone utilizing the ultrastructural characteristics of neuron (Kaplan and Bell 1984, Kaplan 1985). The discovery of glial precursor cells in the adult brain and their ability to regenerate further substantiated this concept (Gallo and Deneen 2014). It is now established that neural stem cells (NSCs) reside in the human mammalian brain and contribute to brain plasticity throughout life. There are two major regions where endogenous neural stem cells reside, the subventricular zone (SVZ) and the subgranular zone (SGZ) within the dentate gyrus of the hippocampus. Adult NSCs can transition between quiescent and active state, and can generate progenitor cells, neurons and other supportive cells, such as astrocytes and glial cells.

An important aspect in the neuronal regeneration concept is the fact that CNS neurons are relatively (in comparison to PNS) very difficult to regenerate (Figure 20.4), why? How to stimulate CNS regeneration program has been very difficult. The following are the major reasons:

A. **The inhospitable neuritogenesis environment of CNS**:
   Basis of this hypothesis is based on the fact that regeneration is possible in the peripheral nervous system (PNS) but not in the CNS. In PNS, after injury, denervated Schwann cells proliferate along with extending cytoplasmic processes which promote regeneration. These processes initiate the lining of endoneurial tubes as a Band of Bungner to support the axonal growth. Additionally, the distal potion of the axon undergoes a degeneration program known as Wallerian degeneration, and debris are cleared by glial cells, predominantly macrophages.
   In contrast, the degeneration process is not robust and regeneration processes are inhibited by inhibitory molecules in the CNS, some of them upregulated or release after the neuronal injury. In response to injury, the CNS undergoes a reactive gliosis or glial scarring (Fawcett and Asher 1999, Fournier and Strittmatter 2001), which contributes to the hostile environment for neurite outgrowth. However, the formation of glial scar is not the real cause of lack of re-growth of damaged

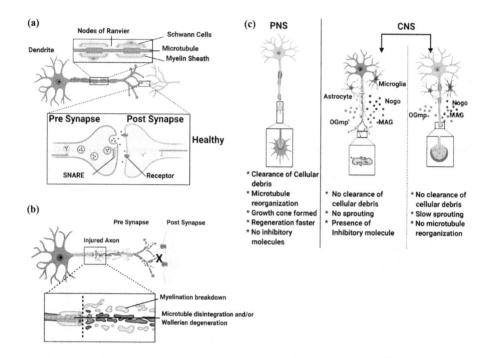

Figure 20.4 *(a) A healthy neuron. All the elements of healthy communication between neurons are shown (myelination, microtubules organization, exocytosis/endocytosis processes, neurotransmitter release, etc.). (b) An injured neuron. After injury, breakdown of myelination, microtubules disintegration, and Wallerian disintegration are the general characteristics of injury-induced disintegration. (c) Regeneration in the PNS and CNS. Regeneration in CNS neurons is a complex and difficult process compared to PNS neurons, and the major reasons are listed.*

neurons. Along with these processes, there are several molecules which contribute toward poor clearance of myelin debris. The main inhibitory molecules are NogoA and oligodendrocyte myelin-associated glycoprotein (OMgp) produced by oligodendrocytes, chondroitin sulphate proteoglycan (CSPGs) produced mainly by glia (astrocyte and oligodendrocyte precursors), myelin-associated glycoprotein (MAG) produced by myelinating glia, semaphoring 3A by perivascular and meningeal cells, and tenascin-C from astrocytes (Fawcett, Schwab et al. 2012).

B. **Age of neurons**:

As the neurons mature, they start expressing adult neuronal markers. In the developmental window, intrinsic ability is lost with neuronal maturity. Cell-autonomous factors also affect the expression of growth associated genes leading to the failure (or limit) of regeneration in CNS.

C. **Inhibitory signaling pathways**:

The process of CNS axonal regeneration appears to be quite different from the development process. During development process, there is a changing pattern of growth permitting and inhibiting molecules in the vicinity of the growth cone. In contrast, there is a sustained and injury-induced re-expression of the inhibitory molecules into the adulthood of neurons, which primarily depends on the internal state of the growth cone. Examples of these internal inhibitory molecules are semaphorins, ephrins, netrins and slits. These molecules are involved in the activation of Rho-family GTPases and in the growth cone collapse as well. Rho-family (RhoA, Rac1, Cdc42, etc.) is an important regulator of actin cytoskeleton organization. RhoA regulates cell contractility and the assembly of actin fibers, Rac1 stimulates the formation of lamellipodia (in which the actin filament that are nucleated into branched structures), and Cdc42 regulates filopodia (contains unbranched actin fibers). Inhibition of RhoA promotes axonal sprouting (Fu, Hue et al. 2007). ROCK2 pathways associated with RhoA also regulate axonal regeneration. Epidermal growth factor receptor (EGFR), protein kinase C, LIM kinase, Slingshot phosphatase and cofilin are other molecules involved in the axonal regeneration inhibition signaling (Huebner and Strittmatter 2009).

20.5 Experimental approaches to stimulate neuronal/axonal regeneration in CNS

As mentioned above, neuronal degeneration is a complex process. Therefore, the strategies for neuronal regeneration would not be a single targeted approach. It would be a combinatorial strategy that includes stimulation/inhibition of intrinsic and extrinsic pathways.

A. **Intrinsic mechanisms**:

One of the major reasons for PNS regeneration is the activation of intrinsic signaling network through regeneration promoting gene expression. Although this program is not activated after CNS axotomy, promoting regeneration promoting gene expression and manipulation of transcription factors along with coordinated effort of regulators of intraneuronal growth programs could start intrinsic pathways for neuronal regeneration, for example, activation of transcription factors such as CREB, RARβ2, STAT3, Smad1 and SnoN in regeneration and sprouting in dorsal root ganglion (DRG) (Gao, Deng et al. 2004, Wong, Yip et al. 2006, Bareyre, Garzorz et al. 2011, Parikh, Hao et al. 2011). Other potential genes of interest would be KLF7, p53, STAT3, SOX11 and SOCS3.

B. **External modification of the injured environment**:

The extracellular milieu of the inured CNS neurons is significantly different from that of the developing CNS neuron. One of the approaches involved in promoting CNS regeneration is by grafted peripheral nerves (David and Aguayo 1981). Other approaches could be deletion of myelin-associated inhibitory molecules, degrading or neutralizing the regeneration inhibiting molecules, and transplantation of neural stem cells.

C. **Promote growth enhancing environment**:

Introduction of trophic support (such as neurotrophins) and cell adhesion molecules (like integrin family) facilitates enhanced axonal growth and communication with extracellular matrices (ECM).

D. **Epigenetic mechanisms**:

Recent experiments on chromatin dynamics explain the epigenetics mechanisms which could be useful in axonal regeneration. Inhibition of HDAC (histone deacetylases) promotes neurite outgrowth *in vitro* (Gaub, Tedeschi et al. 2010). Inhibition of HDAC not only increases acetylation but also results in the increased expression of transcription p53. This, in turn, results in increased expression of the p53 targeting genes which include regeneration associated genes, GAP-43 and SCG10 (Finelli, Wong et al. 2013).

An effective regeneration of neurons includes activation of axonal growth molecules, removal or inactivation of inhibitory molecules, and by the introduction of cells that provide a more supportive growth environments (such as Schwann cell implants). However, axonal regeneration is one of the major goals of any regeneration therapy. However, only axonal regeneration is not enough to restore normal neuronal function. Therefore, general requirements for an effective regeneration strategy include both descriptive and functional tests (depicted in Figure 20.5).

20.6 Insight into neuronal regeneration from traditional medicinal system

Ayurveda, the traditional Indian medicine (TIM), and traditional Chinese medicine (TCM) are the most ancient medical traditions. Several herbs are mentioned in TIM and TCM which could be useful in tissue regeneration. There are eight branches of Ayurveda: Kayachikitsa (internal medicine), Baala chikitsa (pediatrics), Graha chikitsa (demonology), Urdhvanga Chikitsa (disease of head and neck), Shalya chikitsa (surgery), Visha chikitsa (toxicology), Jara chikitsa (rejuvenation) and Vrsha chikitsa (aphrodisiac therapy). Jara chikitsa is also known as rasayana therapy which refers to rejuvenative therapy and immunomodulation. Rasayana possesses an important quality of enhancement of Rasa (essence) to promote health and vigor of the tissues. They have three basic mechanisms – Rasa (nutrient effect), Agni (digestion and metabolism) and Srotas (microcirculation and tissue perfusion). As the

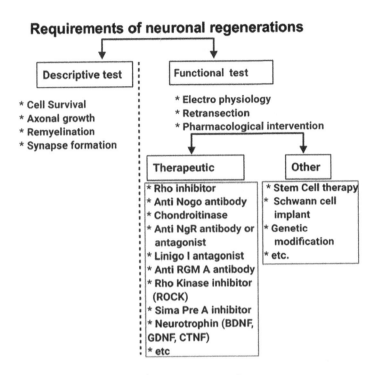

Figure 20.5 *Major requirements for any regeneration program.*

Rasa reaches the Dhatu (Tissue), they can start the rejuvenative functions. Rasayana therapy along with panchakarma and swasthavritta (daily routine as suggested by Ayurveda) improves metabolism, eliminates wastes from the Dhatu and improves Dosha's imbalance. Additionally, this leads to the reduction of catabolism processes in Dhatus that results in strengthening effects on body.

Rasayana drugs are effective in aging, degenerative, autoimmune and metabolic diseases. The activity of rasayana depends upon the method of extraction, formulation, dosage, metabolic state/age of the patient and type of tissues. For example, Medhya rasayana is for the brain and Hridya rasayana is for the heart. However, scientific studies on rasayanas are only preliminary and mainly concentrate on the pharmacological activities. Their potential in rejuvenating tissue through improving the quality of plasma, normalization of digestion and metabolism, and improving perfusion of nutrients should be tested.

In addition to be known for memory enhancement and rejuvenation of cognitive functions, Ayurvedic medicinal herbs are known to modulate the neuroendocrine-immune systems (Murphy and Frigo 1993, Rege, Thatte et al. 1999, Mishra, Singh et al. 2000, Schlebusch, Bosch et al. 2000, Govindarajan,

Vijayakumar et al. 2005). For the treatment and management of acute and chronic neurological diseases, several herbs and supplements are recommended, including Ashwagandha, Brahmi, turmeric and Shankhpushpi that are very popular to improve brain functions (Farooqui and Manly 2018).

20.7 Nutraceuticals in the traditional eastern plants and practices

Nutraceuticals are food substances that fall into the categories between food and pharmaceuticals. They are food or part of the food that provides medical or health benefits. Certain types of diet, functional components from food, herbal products, or dietary supplements can all be considered as nutraceuticals.

In Eastern cultures, such as Chinese and Indian cultures, food is an essential part of daily life not only because we need to eat to survive, but food is also believed to bring harmony to the body and generate closeness to families and relationships. Significant proportions of food are prepared in specific ways and consumed at specific times/seasons to optimize the benefits that nutraceuticals can offer. Freshness is one of the most critical aspects of all Chinese cooking. Unlike the fast-food society of the United States, Chinese tradition, for example, is to shop daily from the local market to ensure freshness (Roberts 1999). They also pay much attention to the food's texture, flavor, color and aroma. With the development of the modern nutritional sciences, it has been proved that pigments and aroma substances from food offer health benefits after consumption. The extractions from these food components are considered functional molecules and made into dietary supplements.

High importance is placed on freshness and flavor of produce or food. All the vegetables, poultry and ingredients have to be fresh. The timing on the cooking is very crucial. Dishes must not be overcooked, and the texture of the food has to be just right with the freshness and tenderness remaining. Soup is also essential in Cantonese cuisine. It consists of different ingredients and herbs and is boiled to a rich and tasty soup before it is served. There are many kinds of soups, and each soup has its own function or purpose.

Chinese artichoke (*S. affinis* tubers), a widely consumed root vegetable that can be eaten raw, pickled, dried or cooked, has been shown to efficiently protect human cells (Caco-2, SHSY-5Y and K562) against t-BHP-induced oxidative damage (Venditti, Frezza et al. 2017). The marker compounds identified were oligosaccharide stachyose and the organic acid, succinic acid, as well as phenylethanoid and iridoid glycosides. The macronutrient profile was dominated by carbohydrates (36.9% dw), whereas potassium (2.36%) was the most abundant micro-nutrient.

Butylphthalide (3-n-butylphthalide or NBP) is one of the chemical constituents in celery oil, along with sedanolide, which is primarily responsible for the aroma and taste of celery. Studies in animal models suggest that butylphthalide has neuroprotective effects (Xiong, Huang et al. 2012). In 2002, NBP was approved in China for the treatment of cerebral ischemia (Abdoulaye and Guo 2016). In rats, after exposure to CO, the upregulation of both calpain 1 and CaMK II proteins is the mechanism of cognitive dysfunction. The administration of NBP could balance the expressions of calpain 1 and CaMK II proteins and improve cognitive function through maintaining ultrastructural integrity of hippocampus, and thus may play a neuroprotective role in brain tissue in rats with CO poisoning (Bi, Sun et al. 2017).

Sometimes when the Chinese feel a deficiency in their health or strength, they usually seek a traditional method first, which is to use herbs and special ingredient soups to replenish the energy level and to stay healthy.

Chinese herbs can enhance brain and neuronal system health including but not limited to Longan Arillus, Viticis Fructus, Icariin, Jujuboside, Stachys sieboldii and ginseng. Among them, Stachys sieboldii and ginseng have been the most studied that have demonstrated significant modification roles in multi-pathways involved in neurodegeneration and healthy functions of brain.

Stachys sieboldii (SS) is a popular Chinese herbal medicine. SS extract reduces the acetylcholinesterase activity and significantly increases acetylcholine and choline acetyltransferase activity in the brain. In a subsequent mechanism study, SS is shown to regulate mRNA expression levels of neuronal plasticity molecules such as (nerve growth factor) NGF, brain-derived neurotrophic factor (BDNF)-cAMP response element binding (CREB) protein signaling pathways, and their downstream molecules such as Bcl-2 and Egr-1 by downregulating the neuronal apoptosis targets in both hippocampus and frontal cortex. SS has a similar function to nootropic drugs by inhibiting cholinergic abnormalities, and neuronal apoptosis targets, and ultimately increasing the expression of BDNF-CREB (Ravichandran, Kim et al. 2018).

Ginseng, derived from the roots of Panax ginseng Meyer (Araliaceae), is a traditional Chinese herbal medicine, and has been used as a medication for thousands of years in East Asian countries, such as Japan, China and Korea (Attele, Wu et al. 1999). Drinking ginseng tea or putting thin slices of ginseng under the tongue as dietary supplements are also traditional ways for Chinese to enjoy the beneficial effects of ginseng.

The active ingredients in ginseng include ginsenosides, ginseng polysaccharides, volatile oils (terpenoids, alcohols, fatty acids, etc.), peptides and amino acids (Christensen 2009). Ginseng has been proven to have significant roles in the treatment of neurodegenerative and neurological disorders. The beneficial effects of ginseng include modifying neurogenesis, anti-apoptotic and antioxidant properties, inhibition of mitochondrial dysfunction, receptor-operated Ca^{2+} channels, amyloid beta aggregation, and microglial activation as well as modulation of neurotransmitters (Christensen 2009, Shin, Kwon et al. 2015, Choi, Lee et al. 2021).

Ginsenosides, also known as ginseng saponins, are the first active ingredients isolated from ginseng. A variety of pharmacologically beneficial effects of ginsenosides have been identified in vitro and in vivo in animal models related to neurodegenerative diseases, such as AD (Cho 2012). It is well known that amyloid β-protein (Aβ) induces oxidative stress in neuronal cells, resulting in cell death (Uttara, Singh et al. 2009). Pretreatment of PC12 cells with ginsenosides inhibits Aβ-induced ROS overproduction and lipid peroxidation and decreases lactate dehydrogenase release, MDA production, and SOD activity, thereby improving the rate of cell survival. Ginseng also contains gintonin which is a novel ginseng-derived G protein-coupled lysophosphatidic acid (LPA, 1-acyl-2-hydroxy-sn-glycero-3-phosphate) receptor ligand (Kim, Lee et al. 2018). Administration of fermented ginseng extract in a mouse model of AD improved memory function and reduced Aβ formation in the brain (Kim, Kim et al. 2013). Oral administration of white ginseng extract to Aβ oligomer-injected mice restored the reduced synaptophysin and choline acetyltransferase activity (Choi, Kim et al. 2017). This evidence demonstrates the neuroprotective effects of ginseng as demonstrated in Figure 20.6.

Ashwagandha (*Withania somnifera*, fam. Solanaceae), or Indian ginseng, is a common herb used in Ayurvedic medicine as an adaptogen or antistress agent (Farooqui, Farooqui et al. 2018). Apparently, the only reason it is called Indian ginseng is that it has similar influence on the human body. Ashwagandha root contains a large variety of compounds including 12 alkaloids, 40 withanolides, and several sitoindosides and flavonoids (Farooqui, Farooqui et al. 2018). Withaferin A (WL-A) and withanolide A, components which produce antistress, antioxidant, and immunomodulatory effects in acute models of experimental stress, are among the constituents showing similar pharmacokinetic profiles, except for the oral bioavailability (Patil, Gautam et al. 2013). According to Ayurvedic Evidence-Based Complementary and Alternative Medicine, Ashwagandha constituents provide a number of healthful effects such as youthful state of physical and mental health and increase in happiness (Farooqui, Farooqui et al. 2018). Ashwagandha has beneficial effects for children, middle-aged and elderly by improving body's defenses against chronic diseases through cell-mediated immunity, through producing potent antioxidant and anti-inflammatory effects that protect against cellular damage caused by free radicals, and through inflammatory mediators (Farooqui, Farooqui et al. 2018). As shown in Figure 20.7, Ashwagandha root is proposed to produce beneficial effects in AD by inhibiting the activation of NF-κB, blocking β-amyloid (Aβ) production, reducing apoptotic cell death, restoring synaptic function, and enhancing antioxidant effects through the migration of Nrf2 to the nucleus, where it increases the expression of antioxidant enzymes (Farooqui, Farooqui et al. 2018). Proteomics experimental results have revealed that WL-A activates the translocation of Nrf2 to the nucleus, where the transcription factor upregulates the expression of neuroprotective proteins, such as heme oxygenase-1 (Narayan, Seeley et al. 2015, Sun, Li et al. 2016).

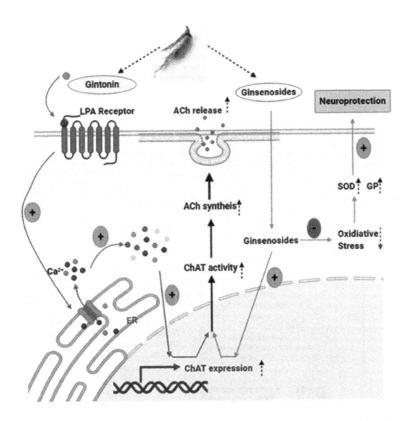

Figure 20.6 *Gintonin and ginsenosides are the two functional molecules from ginseng. (a) Gintonin induces signal transduction on the mammalian cell plasma membrane via LPA receptors. This leads to intracellular responses through the regulation of ion channels. (b) Ginsenosides induce an increase in acetylcholine synthesis and upregulate the expression of ChAT, resulting in an increase in the levels of acetylcholine and vesicular acetylcholine transporter, both of which are required for cholinergic neurotransmission. In addition, these ginsenosides decreased oxidative stress and have neuroprotective function.*

Experiments with the ethanolic extracts of Ashwagandha root on human neuroblastoma SK-N-SH cells have suggested that in dendrite extension, neurite outgrowth and synapse formation (Tohda, Kuboyama et al. 2000, Kuboyama, Tohda et al. 2005). In cultured rat cortical neurons with axonal and dendritic atrophy and pre- and postsynaptic loss upon treatment with Aβ, it was demonstrated that these neurodegenerative conditions were abrogated by treatment with WL-A (Kuboyama, Tohda et al. 2005). WL-A that also attenuates the gene expression of semaphorin 3A that promotes neural regeneration is also downregulated by WL-A (Farooqui, Farooqui et al. 2018). It is believed that Ashwagandha root constituents have a beneficial effect on neurodegenerative

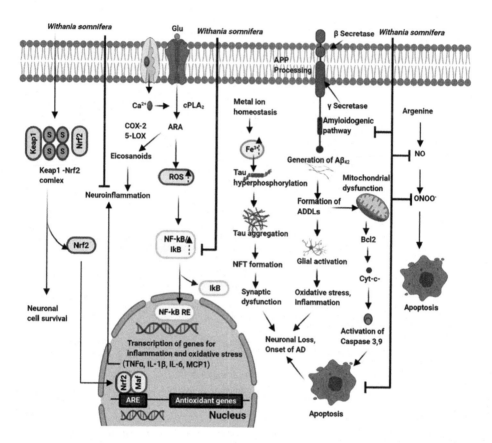

Figure 20.7 *A diagram showing proposed target sites for the action of Ashwagandha (Withania somnifera). Glutamate (Glu); NMDA receptor (NMDA-R); phosphatidyl-choline (PtdCho); cytosolic phospholipase A2 (cPLA2); cyclooxygenase-2 (COX-2); 5-lipoxygenase (5- LOX); arachidonic acid (ARA); reactive oxygen species (ROS); nuclear factor-κB (NF-κB); nuclear factor-κB-response element (NF-κB-RE); inhibitory subunit of NF-κB (I-κB); tumor necrosis factor-α (TNF-α); interleukin-1β (IL-1β); interleukin-6 (IL-6); monocyte chemoattractant protein-1 (MCP-1); nuclear factor E2-related factor 2 (Nrf2); kelch-like ECH-associated protein 1 (Keap1); anti-oxidant response element (ARE); small leucine zipper proteins (Maf); heme oxy-genase (HO-1); NADPH quinine oxidoreductase (NQO-1); γ-glutamate cystein ligase (γ-GCL); B-cell lymphoma 2 (Bcl-2); cytochrome (cyto-c); amyloid precursor protein (APP); β-amyloid (Aβ); Aβ-derived diffusible ligand (ADDL); and Alzheimer's disease (AD). (Adopted from Farooqui et al. (2018).)*

diseases, which may be mediated by their neurite promoting, antioxidant, anti-inflammatory, antiapoptotic and anxiolytic activities, in addition to their ability to improve mitochondrial dysfunction and restore energy levels and increased antioxidant defenses such as reduced glutathione (Singh, Bhalla et al. 2011) (Figure 20.7).

Although pharmacological characteristics of Ashwagandha is examined in detail, a preliminary study suggested improvement in auditory verbal working memory, reaction time and social cognition in patients with bipolar disorders with the addition of Withania somnifera (500 mg/day) adjunctively to medications (Chengappa, Bowie et al. 2013). In animal studies, WL-A has shown restoration of Aβ (25–35)-induced memory deficit in mice and recovers the decline of axons, dendrites and synapses in the cerebral cortex and hippocampus. Ashwagandha is a safe herb (Choudhary, Bhattacharyya et al. 2017), although a few people experience diarrhea or nausea after consuming the root. It should not be taken with barbiturate-type sedatives, since the herb can increase the effectiveness of these drugs. Ashwagandha can cross the blood-brain barrier and lower inflammation in the brain. Thus, WL-A can be an important candidate for the treatment of dementia and neurodegenerative diseases, as it is able to repair damaged neuronal networks (Singh, Bhalla et al. 2011).

Other Ayurvedic plants used to treat neurological disorders include Brahmi (*Bacopa monnieri*), which belongs to the family Scrophulariaceae and is found throughout the Indian subcontinent in wet, damp and marshy areas and is not only used for the treatment of a number of nervous system disorders such as insomnia, anxiety and epilepsy but also used for enhancing memory and the intellect (Roodenrys, Booth et al. 2002). Additionally, rhizome of Curcuma longa, which belongs to the family *Zingiberaceae*, has antioxidant, anti-inflammatory and cancer chemo-preventive properties; reduces oxidative damage; improves cognitive functions related to the aging process; and alleviates AD conditions (Farooqui, Farooqui et al. 2018).

20.8 How nutraceuticals help achieve balance for the body

In Eastern culture, illness is considered to be related to an imbalance that can be influenced with dietary intake. For the food intake, Chinese, for example, are not too concerned about eating within the five food group guidelines as suggested by the agencies in the Western world, although some of those can be perhaps adopted according to the Eastern cultures as well. There is more emphasis on how to eat to balance Yin (negative) and Yang (positive), which are the opposing and complementary energy forces that are believed to determine the natural order of the universe. The importance of balancing Yin and Yang forces has been a part of Chinese thought for thousands of years that applies to the social, political, medical and dietary usage. Yin and Yang have to be balanced to achieve the harmonious and healthy state for the body; otherwise, conflict and disease will occur. Different foods can be grouped into Yin or Yang categories. Figure 20.8 demonstrates the theory of achieving optimal health by consuming Yin Yang-balanced food and herbs.

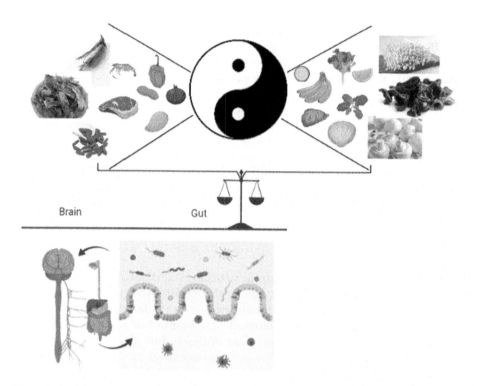

Figure 20.8 *Yin-Yang balance of food and body. The food items on the white side are Yang (positive) and on the black side are Yin (negative). In the Chinese dualism concept, food from both Yin and Yang groups can complement each other, and the balanced food consumption will help achieve optimum health and benefit the intestinal physiology. Some examples of the food and herbs belonging to the Yin and Yang groups are listed. The Yang group includes ginseng, Icariin, wolfberry, shrimp, beef, red pepper, peanuts, mango and onion. The Yin group includes cucumbers, bananas, oysters, Chinese green, oranges, mustard green, clams and mushrooms. As shown in the lower section, there are bidirectional links between the central and enteric nervous systems, known as the gut-brain-axis (GBA), the brain and gut constantly interact and communicate through this complex connection.*

In India, Ayurveda, a system of healthcare encompassing lifestyle, food and herbs, classifies three types of body constitution (*dosha*) – *prakriti* (nature) – *vata* (air), *pitta* (fire) and *kapha* (water), and an individual is born with a unique combination of these three constitutions (*tridosha*). To maintain health, one needs to maintain a balance of those natural constitution combinations under the varying conditions of daily, fortnightly, monthly and yearly cycles, seasonal foods, herbs and lifestyles (sleeping, yoga-meditation, manner of speaking, thoughts, etc.), and their combinations based on age, gender, geographical locations, social situations, etc. Ayurveda derives its fundamental principles of classification and association with nature from the five fundamental elements of matter – ether, air, fire, water and earth, signifying to their functional attributes of vibrations, flow, heat, fluidity and grossness. Ayurveda framework is quite comprehensive encompassing, the five elements which form the basis of power of the senses (hearing, touching, seeing, tasting and smelling), five organs of senses (ear, skin, eye, tongue and nose) and five organs of action (mouth and tongue, hand, legs, reproductive and excretory). These features together with mind and intellect influence and get influenced by the body's *dosha* constitution, providing the basis for diseases when there is imbalance, or to balance the body *dosha* constitution with behavioral and dietary alterations. Ayurveda considers the gastric system as the main source of impact on the *dosha* constitution, as it reflects the imbalance and can also be used to balance the *tridosha* (Lad 1984). This provides the traditional, cultural and philosophical basis of nutraceuticals to be integral part of Ayurveda.

Depending on the geographical and climate differences in China, there are many different cuisines in different areas. Each province has its own unique style of cooking; the locally available food items and seasonings are also unique. In the cold and damp areas of Northern China, people are promoting hot and spicy foods such as chilies, onions and garlic. They believe these foods will increase blood circulation and help get rid of the coldness and dampness. Generally, people from Southern China like to eat more mild and cooling foods because of the warmer climate. These foods reduce the hotness and dryness.

The Western concept of the chemistry of acid and alkali to explain food is a materialistic and current scientific approach to balance. The Western approach is also focused on how the food eaten creates the metabolic energy. But both the Eastern and Western theories agree that live biological system is not static, everything is constantly moving, changing and shifting, just as the acid and alkali ratio, tridosha balance, or the Yin Yang balance shift in our bodies. Our life force can be improved and maintained by changing what we eat. The closer food is to its natural state, and the less sophisticated, processed, or refined it is, the more nutritional value is shared with our bodies.

The first modern mention of the phrase 'you are what you eat' came from the 1826 work Physiologie du Gout, ou Medetations de Gastronomie Transcendante, in which French author Anthelme Brillat-Savarin wrote: "Tell me what you eat and I will tell you what you are", although Indian poet, Kabir, had said the same thing in 14th century – "the type of food you eat determines the type of mind you have". Food does have profound effects on the wholesome and well-being of one's body. Upon food consumption, the body's first direct contact with food and nutrients happens in the mouth with taste buds on the tongue. Ayurveda system puts a heavy emphasis on the tastes, classifying food tastes as sweet, sour, salty, bitter, pungent and astringent. These tastes can modulate the body tridosha. For example, sweet taste decreases vata and pitta, but increases kapha. Sour taste decreases vata but increases pitta and kapha. Chemical and biochemical mechanism of such effect is not known. However, given that the taste bud cells act as chemosensory processors, and involve several transmitters such as acetylcholine, serotonin, norepinephrine, GABA and ATP (Roper 2013), these are clearly impactful to the brain. In fact, taste impairment leads to major neurological disorders such as head trauma, multiple sclerosis and seizure disorders. Also, such impairment is also known to cause neurodegenerative diseases such as idiopathic Parkinson's disease and dementia, mild cognitive impairment and Alzheimer's disease (DeVere 2017).

When the food further moves down the digestive system, its contact in the gastro-intestinal (GI) tract is not only important for the nutrient absorption, but also for important neurological roles. Recent studies have demonstrated that the gut-brain axis is a coordinated communication system that not only maintains homeostasis, but also significantly influences higher cognitive functions and emotions as well as neurological and behavioral disorders (Abdullah, Defaye et al. 2020). In the meantime, the gut microbiota plays a crucial role in the bidirectional gut-brain axis that integrates the gut and central nervous system (CNS) activities (Wang, Zhang et al. 2020). There has been some great progress in characterizing the bidirectional interactions between the central nervous system, the enteric nervous system, and the gastrointestinal tract. Preclinical studies have suggested a prominent role for the gut microbiota in these gut-brain interactions (Mayer, Tillisch et al. 2015, Foster, Lyte et al. 2016). Dietary nutrients and functional molecules from Chinese herb or traditional medicine have profound effects in gut microbiota and can modify the gut-brain axis. Similarly, a positive association between Ayurvedic body constitution and skin, oral and gut microbiome has been established (Chaudhari, Dhotre et al. 2019, Jnana, Murali et al. 2020). This may also explain why dietary or natural products have beneficial effects on multiple pathways involved in neuro-degeneration diseases. Compared to the therapeutic interventions which focus on specific pathways, nutraceuticals have multifaceted effects, and the food-based approaches are believed to target multiple pathways in a slow but more physiological manner without causing severe adverse effects.

During neurodegeneration, the innate immune system is activated (Heneka, McManus et al. 2018), and the inflammatory signaling is an important type of interaction in the gut-brain axis (Rea, Dinan et al. 2016). Supplementation with SS increases beneficial intestinal microflora (Ruminococcaceae and Akkermansia muciniphila) and decreases the community of harmful microflora (Enterobacteriaceae including *Escherichia coli* and Bacteroides sp.). In the mice model, SS shows a significantly lower mRNA expression of cytokines IL-6 and IL-10 in mesenteric lymph node compared with that in the control (Na, Moon et al. 2020).

Ursolic acid (UA) is a main ingredient of several traditional Chinese herbal medicines used in the treatment of intestinal damage and bacterial dysbiosis liver diseases (Wan, Liu et al. 2019). The most well-known function of this plant-derived triterpene compound is its strong antioxidant effects (Jabeen, Ahmad et al. 2018). In PC12 cells, UA could assert its neuroprotective effects by inhibiting ROS production induced by amyloid beta peptide (Yoon, Youn et al. 2014).

In another study, UA has been shown to capture oxygen free radicals in the P450 monoamine oxidase system and liver microsome, thus exerting a strong inhibitory effect on lipid peroxidation (Misra, Sharma et al. 2017). A recent study has shown that UA could protect against CDDP-induced ototoxicity by inhibiting oxidative stress and TRPV1-mediated Ca^{2+}-signaling in the cochlear cells (Di, Xu et al. 2020).

In Ayurvedic system also, an herbal product known as triphala has phytochemicals such as quercetin and gallic acid promote the growth of Bifidobacteria and Lactobacillus species while inhibiting the growth of undesirable gut residents such as E. coli (Peterson, Denniston et al. 2017).

Gut microbiota is also influenced by different seasons (Shor, Brown et al. 2020). This may help to explain the importance of eating seasonal local food. The compositions of the gut microbiota are influenced by both the internal factors and environmental factors. In the traditional eastern culture like China and India, change of the seasons is a very important time and involves the preparation of specific types of food. This may be the wisdom passed on for several 1,000 years to achieve the harmony of seasonal shifts and physiological adjustments and enhance the gut microbiota composition.

Season is considered a major factor in disturbing the body dosha balance in the Ayurvedic system; diet, seasonal change and lifestyle interactively affect the tridosha either directly or with interactions through mind (Figure 20.9).

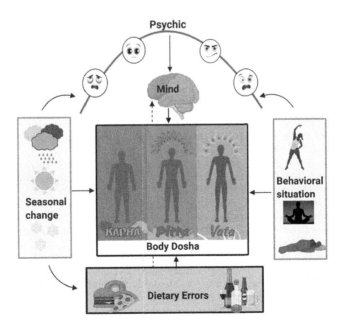

Figure 20.9 *Interconnection of body dosha with mind, diet, behavior and seasons to maintain a balance.*

Besides achieving the systematic balance in the human body, looking into the cells in multicellular organisms, they also have their own mechanisms to achieve balance to perform normal function or encounter challenges. The major basic functions of neuronal cells are to grow, migrate, respond and adapt to external stimuli and to survive or die. In addition, neurons had to evolve adaptations to survive despite multiple insults and the deleterious effects of the aging process as neuronal cells do not reproduce under normal conditions. A study on the two major calpain isoforms in the brain, calpain-1 and calpain-2, has revealed that calpain-1 and calpain-2 exhibit opposite functions in both synaptic plasticity and neurodegeneration. Calpain-1 activation is required for the induction of long-term potentiation (LTP) and is generally neuroprotective, while calpain-2 activation limits the extent of potentiation and is neurodegenerative (Baudry and Bi 2016). This fits right into the Yin and Yang theories for the optimal health.

Acknowledgement

This work was in part supported by a grant from the Maryada Family Foundation.

References

Abdoulaye, I. A. and Y. J. Guo (2016). "A review of recent advances in neuroprotective potential of 3-N-butylphthalide and its derivatives." *Biomed Res Int* **2016**: 5012341.

Altman, J. (1962). "Are new neurons formed in the brains of adult mammals?" *Science* **135**(3509): 1127–1128.

Altman, J. (1963). "Autoradiographic investigation of cell proliferation in the brains of rats and cats." *Anat Rec* **145**: 573–591.

Andreazza, A. C., L. Shao, J. F. Wang and L. T. Young (2010). "Mitochondrial complex I activity and oxidative damage to mitochondrial proteins in the prefrontal cortex of patients with bipolar disorder." *Arch Gen Psychiatry* **67**(4): 360–368.

Atkin, G. and H. Paulson (2014). "Ubiquitin pathways in neurodegenerative disease." *Front Mol Neurosci* **7**: 63.

Atkin, J. D., M. A. Farg, K. Y. Soo, A. K. Walker, M. Halloran, B. J. Turner, P. Nagley and M. K. Horne (2014). "Mutant SOD1 inhibits ER-Golgi transport in amyotrophic lateral sclerosis." *J Neurochem* **129**(1): 190–204.

Attele, A. S., J. A. Wu and C. S. Yuan (1999). "Ginseng pharmacology: multiple constituents and multiple actions." *Biochem Pharmacol* **58**(11): 1685–1693.

Avila, J., G. Perry and P. Martinez-Martin (2010). "Prospects on the origin of Alzheimer's disease." *J Alzheimers Dis* **20**(2): 669–672.

Baker, B. M. and C. M. Haynes (2011). "Mitochondrial protein quality control during biogenesis and aging." *Trends Biochem Sci* **36**(5): 254–261.

Bareyre, F. M., N. Garzorz, C. Lang, T. Misgeld, H. Buning and M. Kerschensteiner (2011). "In vivo imaging reveals a phase-specific role of STAT3 during central and peripheral nervous system axon regeneration." *Proc Natl Acad Sci U S A* **108**(15): 6282–6287.

Baudry, M. and X. Bi (2016). "Calpain-1 and Calpain-2: The Yin and Yang of synaptic plasticity and neurodegeneration." *Trends Neurosci* **39**(4): 235–245.

Beal, M. F. (2005). "Mitochondria take center stage in aging and neurodegeneration." *Ann Neurol* **58**(4): 495–505.

Bi, M. J., X. N. Sun, Y. Zou, X. Y. Ding, B. Liu, Y. H. Zhang, D. D. Guo and Q. Li (2017). "N-Butylphthalide Improves Cognitive Function in Rats after Carbon Monoxide Poisoning." *Front Pharmacol* **8**: 64.

Brown, J. A. (2005). "What's new in neurological surgery." *J Am Coll Surg* **200**(6): 932–936.

Canevari, L., A. Y. Abramov and M. R. Duchen (2004). "Toxicity of amyloid beta peptide: tales of calcium, mitochondria, and oxidative stress." *Neurochem Res* **29**(3): 637–650.

Chaudhari, D., D. Dhotre, D. Agarwal, A. Gondhali, A. Nagarkar, V. Lad, U. Patil, S. Juvekar, V. Sinkar and Y. Shouche (2019). "Understanding the association between the human gut, oral and skin microbiome and the Ayurvedic concept of prakriti." *J Biosci* **44**(5).

Chengappa, K. N., C. R. Bowie, P. J. Schlicht, D. Fleet, J. S. Brar and R. Jindal (2013). "Randomized placebo-controlled adjunctive study of an extract of withania somnifera for cognitive dysfunction in bipolar disorder." *J Clin Psychiatry* **74**(11): 1076–1083.

Cho, I. H. (2012). "Effects of panax ginseng in neurodegenerative diseases." *J Ginseng Res* **36**(4): 342–353.

Choi, J. G., N. Kim, E. Huh, H. Lee, M. H. Oh, J. D. Park, M. K. Pyo and M. S. Oh (2017). "White ginseng protects mouse hippocampal cells against amyloid-beta oligomer toxicity." *Phytother Res* **31**(3): 497–506.

Choi, S. H., R. Lee, S. M. Nam, D. G. Kim, I. H. Cho, H. C. Kim, Y. Cho, H. Rhim and S. Y. Nah (2021). "Ginseng gintonin, aging societies, and geriatric brain diseases." *Integr Med Res* **10**(1): 100450.

Choudhary, D., S. Bhattacharyya and S. Bose (2017). "Efficacy and safety of ashwagandha (Withania somnifera (L.) Dunal) root extract in improving memory and cognitive functions." *J Diet Suppl* **14**(6): 599–612.

Christensen, L. P. (2009). "Ginsenosides chemistry, biosynthesis, analysis, and potential health effects." *Adv Food Nutr Res* **55**: 1–99.

Clarke, P. G. (1990). "Developmental cell death: morphological diversity and multiple mechanisms." *Anat Embryol (Berl)* **181**(3): 195–213.

Coussee, E., P. De Smet, E. Bogaert, I. Elens, P. Van Damme, P. Willems, W. Koopman, L. Van Den Bosch and G. Callewaert (2011). "G37R SOD1 mutant alters mitochondrial complex I activity, Ca(2+) uptake and ATP production." *Cell Calcium* **49**(4): 217–225.

Cuervo, A. M. and E. Wong (2014). "Chaperone-mediated autophagy: roles in disease and aging." *Cell Res* **24**(1): 92–104.

David, S. and A. J. Aguayo (1981). "Axonal elongation into peripheral nervous system "bridges" after central nervous system injury in adult rats." *Science* **214**(4523): 931–933.

DeVere, R. (2017). "Disorders of Taste and Smell." *Continuum (Minneap Minn)* **23**(2, Selected Topics in Outpatient Neurology): 421–446.

Dice, J. F. and S. R. Terlecky (1990). "Targeting of cytosolic proteins to lysosomes for degradation." *Crit Rev Ther Drug Carrier Syst* **7**(3): 211–233.

Farooqui, A. A., T. Farooqui, A. Madan, J. H. Ong and W. Y. Ong (2018). "Ayurvedic medicine for the treatment of dementia: mechanistic aspects." *Evid Based Complement Alternat Med* **2018**: 2481076.

Farooqui, A. A. and T. Manly (2018). "When attended and conscious perception deactivates fronto-parietal regions." *Cortex* **107**: 166–179.

Fawcett, J. W., M. E. Schwab, L. Montani, N. Brazda and H. W. Muller (2012). "Defeating inhibition of regeneration by scar and myelin components." *Handb Clin Neurol* **109**: 503–522.

Fawcett, J. W. and R. A. Asher (1999). "The glial scar and central nervous system repair." *Brain Res Bull* **49**(6): 377–391.

Federico, A., E. Cardaioli, P. Da Pozzo, P. Formichi, G. N. Gallus and E. Radi (2012). "Mitochondria, oxidative stress and neurodegeneration." *J Neurol Sci* **322**(1–2): 254–262.

Finelli, M. J., J. K. Wong and H. Zou (2013). "Epigenetic regulation of sensory axon regeneration after spinal cord injury." *J Neurosci* **33**(50): 19664–19676.

Foster, J. A., M. Lyte, E. Meyer and J. F. Cryan (2016). "Gut microbiota and brain function: An evolving field in neuroscience." *Int J Neuropsychopharmacol* **19**(5).

Fournier, A. E. and S. M. Strittmatter (2001). "Repulsive factors and axon regeneration in the CNS." *Curr Opin Neurobiol* **11**(1): 89–94.

Fu, Q., J. Hue and S. Li (2007). "Nonsteroidal anti-inflammatory drugs promote axon regeneration via RhoA inhibition." *J Neurosci* **27**(15): 4154–4164.

Gafni, J., E. Hermel, J. E. Young, C. L. Wellington, M. R. Hayden and L. M. Ellerby (2004). "Inhibition of calpain cleavage of huntingtin reduces toxicity: Accumulation of calpain/caspase fragments in the nucleus." *J Biol Chem* **279**(19): 20211–20220.

Gallo, V. and B. Deneen (2014). "Glial development: the crossroads of regeneration and repair in the CNS." *Neuron* **83**(2): 283–308.

Gao, Y., K. Deng, J. Hou, J. B. Bryson, A. Barco, E. Nikulina, T. Spencer, W. Mellado, E. R. Kandel and M. T. Filbin (2004). "Activated CREB is sufficient to overcome inhibitors in myelin and promote spinal axon regeneration in vivo." *Neuron* **44**(4): 609–621.

Gaub, P., A. Tedeschi, R. Puttagunta, T. Nguyen, A. Schmandke and S. Di Giovanni (2010). "HDAC inhibition promotes neuronal outgrowth and counteracts growth cone collapse through CBP/p300 and P/CAF-dependent p53 acetylation." *Cell Death Differ* **17**(9): 1392–1408.

Ghemrawi, R. and M. Khair (2020). "Endoplasmic reticulum stress and unfolded protein response in neurodegenerative diseases." *Int J Mol Sci* **21**(17).

Golpich, M., E. Amini, Z. Mohamed, R. Azman Ali, N. Mohamed Ibrahim and A. Ahmadiani (2017). "Mitochondrial dysfunction and biogenesis in neurodegenerative diseases: Pathogenesis and treatment." *CNS Neurosci Ther* **23**(1): 5–22.

Govindarajan, R., M. Vijayakumar and P. Pushpangadan (2005). "Antioxidant approach to disease management and the role of 'Rasayana' herbs of Ayurveda." *J Ethnopharmacol* **99**(2): 165–178.

Hameroff, S. (2012). "How quantum brain biology can rescue conscious free will." *Front Integr Neurosci* **6**: 93.

Hashimoto, S., A. Ishii, N. Kamano, N. Watamura, T. Saito, T. Ohshima, M. Yokosuka and T. C. Saido (2018). "Endoplasmic reticulum stress responses in mouse models of Alzheimer's disease: Overexpression paradigm versus knockin paradigm." *J Biol Chem* **293**(9): 3118–3125.

Haut, S., M. Brivet, G. Touati, P. Rustin, S. Lebon, A. Garcia-Cazorla, J. M. Saudubray, A. Boutron, A. Legrand and A. Slama (2003). "A deletion in the human QP-C gene causes a complex III deficiency resulting in hypoglycaemia and lactic acidosis." *Hum Genet* **113**(2): 118–122.

Heneka, M. T., R. M. McManus and E. Latz (2018). "Inflammasome signalling in brain function and neurodegenerative disease." *Nat Rev Neurosci* **19**(10): 610–621.

Holmberg, C. I., K. E. Staniszewski, K. N. Mensah, A. Matouschek and R. I. Morimoto (2004). "Inefficient degradation of truncated polyglutamine proteins by the proteasome." *EMBO J* **23**(21): 4307–4318.

Huebner, E. A. and S. M. Strittmatter (2009). "Axon regeneration in the peripheral and central nervous systems." *Results Probl Cell Differ* **48**: 339–351.

Irrcher, I., H. Aleyasin, E. L. Seifert, S. J. Hewitt, S. Chhabra, M. Phillips, A. K. Lutz, M. W. Rousseaux, L. Bevilacqua, A. Jahani-Asl, S. Callaghan, J. G. MacLaurin, K. F. Winklhofer, P. Rizzu, P. Rippstein, R. H. Kim, C. X. Chen, E. A. Fon, R. S. Slack, M. E. Harper, H. M. McBride, T. W. Mak and D. S. Park (2010). "Loss of the Parkinson's disease-linked gene DJ-1 perturbs mitochondrial dynamics." *Hum Mol Genet* **19**(19): 3734–3746.

Iwata, M., K. Edashige and K. Saeki (1990). "Activation of protein kinase C by myristate and its requirements of Ca2+ and phospholipid." *Physiol Chem Phys Med NMR* **22**(4): 211–218.

Jnana, A., T. S. Murali, K. P. Guruprasad and K. Satyamoorthy (2020). "Prakriti pheno-types as a stratifier of gut microbiome: A new frontier in personalized medicine?" *J Ayurveda Integr Med* **11**(3): 360–365.

Joy, B., S. N. Kumar, A. R. Radhika and A. Abraham (2015). "Embelin (2,5-Dihydroxy-3-undecyl-p-benzoquinone) for photodynamic therapy: study of their cytotoxicity in cancer cells." *Appl Biochem Biotechnol* **175**(2): 1069–1079.

Kaplan, M. S. (1985). "Formation and turnover of neurons in young and senescent animals: An electronmicroscopic and morphometric analysis." *Ann N Y Acad Sci* **457**: 173–192.

Kaplan, M. S. and D. H. Bell (1984). "Mitotic neuroblasts in the 9-day-old and 11-month-old rodent hippocampus." *J Neurosci* **4**(6): 1429–1441.

Kiaei, M. (2008). "Peroxisome proliferator-activated receptor-gamma in amyotrophic lateral sclerosis and huntington's disease." *PPAR Res* **2008**: 418765.

Kilbride, S. M., S. A. Gluchowska, J. E. Telford, C. O'Sullivan and G. P. Davey (2011). "High-level inhibition of mitochondrial complexes III and IV is required to increase gluta-mate release from the nerve terminal." *Mol Neurodegener* **6**(1): 53.

Kim, J., S. H. Kim, D. S. Lee, D. J. Lee, S. H. Kim, S. Chung and H. O. Yang (2013). "Effects of fermented ginseng on memory impairment and beta-amyloid reduction in Alzheimer's disease experimental models." *J Ginseng Res* **37**(1): 100–107.

Kim, K. H., D. Lee, H. L. Lee, C. E. Kim, K. Jung and K. S. Kang (2018). "Beneficial effects of Panax ginseng for the treatment and prevention of neurodegenerative diseases: Past findings and future directions." *J Ginseng Res* **42**(3): 239–247.

Kuboyama, T., C. Tohda and K. Komatsu (2005). "Neuritic regeneration and synaptic recon-struction induced by withanolide A." *Br J Pharmacol* **144**(7): 961–971.

Lad, V. (1984). "Ayurveda, the science of self healing – A practical Guide." *Motilal Banarasi Das Delhi(India)*.

Lamb, C. A., H. C. Dooley and S. A. Tooze (2013). "Endocytosis and autophagy: Shared machinery for degradation." *Bioessays* **35**(1): 34–45.

Lin, M. T. and M. F. Beal (2006). "Mitochondrial dysfunction and oxidative stress in neuro-degenerative diseases." *Nature* **443**(7113): 787–795.

Lin, T. K., C. W. Liou, S. D. Chen, Y. C. Chuang, M. M. Tiao, P. W. Wang, J. B. Chen and J. H. Chuang (2009). "Mitochondrial dysfunction and biogenesis in the pathogenesis of Parkinson's disease." *Chang Gung Med J* **32**(6): 589–599.

Makkar, H. P. S. (2018). "Review: Feed demand landscape and implications of food-not feed strategy for food security and climate change." *Animal* **12**(8): 1744–1754.

Marambaud, P., U. Dreses-Werringloer and V. Vingtdeux (2009). "Calcium signaling in neu-rodegeneration." *Mol Neurodegener* **4**: 20.

Matell, M. S. and W. H. Meck (2004). "Cortico-striatal circuits and interval timing: Coincidence detection of oscillatory processes." *Brain Res Cogn Brain Res* **21**(2): 139–170.

Mayer, E. A., K. Tillisch and A. Gupta (2015). "Gut/brain axis and the microbiota." *J Clin Invest* **125**(3): 926–938.

Mishra, L. C., B. B. Singh and S. Dagenais (2000). "Scientific basis for the therapeutic use of Withania somnifera (ashwagandha): a review." *Altern Med Rev* **5**(4): 334–346.

Misra, R. C., S. Sharma, Sandeep, A. Garg, C. S. Chanotiya and S. Ghosh (2017). "Two CYP716A subfamily cytochrome P450 monooxygenases of sweet basil play similar but nonredundant roles in ursane- and oleanane-type pentacyclic triterpene biosyn-thesis." *New Phytol* **214**(2): 706–720.

Morais, V. A. and B. De Strooper (2010). "Mitochondria dysfunction and neurodegenerative disorders: cause or consequence." *J Alzheimers Dis* **20**(Suppl 2): S255–263.

Murphy, B. M. and L. C. Frigo (1993). "Development, implementation, and results of a suc-cessful multidisciplinary adverse drug reaction reporting program in a university teaching hospital." *Hosp Pharm* **28**(12): 1199–1204, 1240.

Na, E., K. H. Moon and S. Y. Lim (2020). "Effect of Stachy sieboldii MIQ. supplementation on modulating gut microflora and cytokine expression in mice." *Comb Chem High Throughput Screen*.

Narayan, M., K. W. Seeley and U. K. Jinwal (2015). "Identification and quantitative analysis of cellular proteins affected by treatment with withaferin a using a SILAC-based proteomics approach." *J Ethnopharmacol* **175**: 86–92.

Okazaki, K., Y. J. Fu, Y. Nishihira, M. Endo, T. Fukushima, T. Ikeuchi, K. Okamoto, O. Onodera, M. Nishizawa and H. Takahashi (2010). "Alzheimer's disease: report of two autopsy cases with a clinical diagnosis of corticobasal degeneration." *Neuropathology* **30**(2): 140–148.

Parikh, P., Y. Hao, M. Hosseinkhani, S. B. Patil, G. W. Huntley, M. Tessier-Lavigne and H. Zou (2011). "Regeneration of axons in injured spinal cord by activation of bone morphogenetic protein/Smad1 signaling pathway in adult neurons." *Proc Natl Acad Sci U S A* **108**(19): E99–107.

Patil, D., M. Gautam, S. Mishra, S. Karupothula, S. Gairola, S. Jadhav, S. Pawar and B. Patwardhan (2013). "Determination of withaferin A and withanolide A in mice plasma using high-performance liquid chromatography-tandem mass spectrometry: application to pharmacokinetics after oral administration of Withania somnifera aqueous extract." *J Pharm Biomed Anal* **80**: 203–212.

Peterson, C. T., K. Denniston and D. Chopra (2017). "Therapeutic uses of triphala in ayurvedic medicine." *J Altern Complement Med* **23**(8): 607–614.

Prakash, V. B., S. Prakash, R. Sharma and S. K. Pal (2010). "Sustainable effect of Ayurvedic formulations in the treatment of nutritional anemia in adolescent students." *J Altern Complement Med* **16**(2): 205–211.

Przedborski, S., M. Vila and V. Jackson-Lewis (2003). "Neurodegeneration: what is it and where are we?" *J Clin Invest* **111**(1): 3–10.

Ravichandran, V. A., M. Kim, S. K. Han and Y. S. Cha (2018). "Stachys sieboldii Extract Supplementation Attenuates Memory Deficits by Modulating BDNF-CREB and Its Downstream Molecules, in Animal Models of Memory Impairment." *Nutrients* **10**(7).

Rea, K., T. G. Dinan and J. F. Cryan (2016). "The microbiome: A key regulator of stress and neuroinflammation." *Neurobiol Stress* **4**: 23–33.

Rege, N. N., U. M. Thatte and S. A. Dahanukar (1999). "Adaptogenic properties of six rasayana herbs used in Ayurvedic medicine." *Phytother Res* **13**(4): 275–291.

Roberts, J. A. G. (1999). *A Concise History of China.* Cambridge: Harvard University Press.

Roodenrys, S., D. Booth, S. Bulzomi, A. Phipps, C. Micallef and J. Smoker (2002). "Chronic effects of Brahmi (Bacopa monnieri) on human memory." *Neuropsychopharmacology* **27**(2): 279–281.

Roper, S. D. (2013). "Taste buds as peripheral chemosensory processors." *Semin Cell Dev Biol* **24**(1): 71–79.

Rubinsztein, D. C. (2006). "The roles of intracellular protein-degradation pathways in neurodegeneration." *Nature* **443**(7113): 780–786.

Schlebusch, L., B. A. Bosch, G. Polglase, I. Kleinschmidt, B. J. Pillay and M. H. Cassimjee (2000). "A double-blind, placebo-controlled, double-centre study of the effects of an oral multivitamin-mineral combination on stress." *S Afr Med J* **90**(12): 1216–1223.

Shin, B. K., S. W. Kwon and J. H. Park (2015). "Chemical diversity of ginseng saponins from Panax ginseng." *J Ginseng Res* **39**(4): 287–298.

Shor, E. K., S. P. Brown and D. A. Freeman (2020). "A novel role for the pineal gland: Regulating seasonal shifts in the gut microbiota of Siberian hamsters." *J Pineal Res*: e12696.

Singh, N., M. Bhalla, P. de Jager and M. Gilca (2011). "An overview on ashwagandha: A Rasayana (rejuvenator) of Ayurveda." *Afr J Tradit Complement Altern Med* **8**(5 Suppl): 208–213.

Sun, G. Y., R. Li, J. Cui, M. Hannink, Z. Gu, K. L. Fritsche, D. B. Lubahn and A. Simonyi (2016). "Withania somnifera and Its Withanolides Attenuate Oxidative and Inflammatory Responses and Up-Regulate Antioxidant Responses in BV-2 Microglial Cells." *Neuromolecular Med* **18**(3): 241–252.

Tohda, C., T. Kuboyama and K. Komatsu (2000). "Dendrite extension by methanol extract of Ashwagandha (roots of Withania somnifera) in SK-N-SH cells." *Neuroreport* **11**(9): 1981–1985.

Trushina, E. and C. T. McMurray (2007). "Oxidative stress and mitochondrial dysfunction in neurodegenerative diseases." *Neuroscience* **145**(4): 1233–1248.

Uchiyama, Y. (2001). "Autophagic cell death and its execution by lysosomal cathepsins." *Arch Histol Cytol* **64**(3): 233–246.

Uttara, B., A. V. Singh, P. Zamboni and R. T. Mahajan (2009). "Oxidative stress and neurodegenerative diseases: a review of upstream and downstream antioxidant therapeutic options." *Curr Neuropharmacol* **7**(1): 65–74.

Venditti, A., C. Frezza, D. Celona, A. Bianco, M. Serafini, K. Cianfaglione, D. Fiorini, S. Ferraro, F. Maggi, A. R. Lizzi and G. Celenza (2017). "Polar constituents, protection against reactive oxygen species, and nutritional value of Chinese artichoke (Stachys affinis Bunge)." *Food Chem* **221**: 473–481.

Venkatasubramanian, G. (2015). "Understanding schizophrenia as a disorder of consciousness: Biological correlates and translational implications from quantum theory perspectives." *Clin Psychopharmacol Neurosci* **13**(1): 36–47.

Wang, H., S. Zhang, F. Yang, R. Xin, S. Wang, D. Cui and Y. Sun (2020). "The gut microbiota confers protection in the CNS against neurodegeneration induced by manganism." *Biomed Pharmacother* **127**: 110150.

Wong, L. F., P. K. Yip, A. Battaglia, J. Grist, J. Corcoran, M. Maden, M. Azzouz, S. M. Kingsman, A. J. Kingsman, N. D. Mazarakis and S. B. McMahon (2006). "Retinoic acid receptor beta2 promotes functional regeneration of sensory axons in the spinal cord." *Nat Neurosci* **9**(2): 243–250.

Xiang, C., Y. Wang, H. Zhang and F. Han (2017). "The role of endoplasmic reticulum stress in neurodegenerative disease." *Apoptosis* **22**(1): 1–26.

Xiong, N., J. Huang, C. Chen, Y. Zhao, Z. Zhang, M. Jia, Z. Zhang, L. Hou, H. Yang, X. Cao, Z. Liang, Y. Zhang, S. Sun, Z. Lin and T. Wang (2012). "Dl-3-n-butylphthalide, a natural antioxidant, protects dopamine neurons in rotenone models for Parkinson's disease." *Neurobiol Aging* **33**(8): 1777–1791.

Yamamoto, S., T. Wajima, Y. Hara, M. Nishida and Y. Mori (2007). "Transient receptor potential channels in Alzheimer's disease." *Biochim Biophys Acta* **1772**(8): 958–967.

Yoon, J. H., K. Youn, C. T. Ho, M. V. Karwe, W. S. Jeong and M. Jun (2014). "p-Coumaric acid and ursolic acid from Corni fructus attenuated beta-amyloid(25–35)-induced toxicity through regulation of the NF-kappaB signaling pathway in PC12 cells." *J Agric Food Chem* **62**(21): 4911–4916.

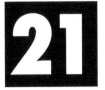

Regulations and Intellectual Property Rights in Anti-aging Nutraceuticals

Vishal Katariya, Shruti Ashok Sawant Desai, and Sajal Yenkar
Katariya and Associates

Contents

21.1 Introduction

Modern medicinal methodologies to treat or cure an ailment are an attractive new way to help cure sufferings of many, which were untreatable by the

DOI: 10.1201/9781003110866-21

age-old traditional medicinal methods due to various reasons like financial hurdles, nonaccess to high-tech medicinal facilities, unavailability of high-precision medicine for the ailment, etc.

"Nutraceuticals" in recent years have emerged as a solution to all these problems and have helped people to get a healthy route to attain good health. This modern revolutionized method of treatment has seen a different approach from experts and officials around the world in terms of their classification, utility, rights, gains, advantages, etc. While some are "for" to such modern methods, some also criticize it to be vague and less studied to be authenticated as an effective medicine for treating diseases or curing ailments.

"Nutraceutical" is a very broad term and encompasses foods or part of foods, any naturally occurring substances that when consumed give physiological benefits. The food and drug regulatory associations world-wide classify nutraceuticals as "unregulated", this classification has led to many controversies in the use and effectiveness or standardization of nutraceuticals for treating a particular disease.

However, such nutrient-packed, energy-filled nutritious pharmaceutics were a quick bloomer especially in industry related to "anti-aging" or "age-related defect" curing or reversing products or medicines. Pharmaceutical industries have realized the growing potential of nutraceuticals in the ever-growing industry of anti-aging medicines/products due to their advantages over pharmaceutics.

Nutraceuticals can be dietary food supplements or medicines that act as natural remedies over various types of ailments or diseases. Nutraceuticals is a broad term that includes food items with health benefits for various disorders, diseases and ailments.

Aging can be defined as a phenomena or process where an individual's body internally as well as externally undergoes maturation and wearing such that the outer effect is what we call as old-age and related health issues. Aging in scientific terms is the onset of "senescence" of cells. According to Britannica, "Aging is progressive physiological changes in an organism that lead to senescence, or a decline of biological functions and of the organism's ability to adapt to metabolic stress." Most of the outcomes of aging on the human body are due to the result of activity of free radicals in the body that continuously work to eliminate dead, aging degenerative cells in the body and skin. Naturally in our body vitamins, antioxidants, carotenoids, flavonoids, etc. help to reverse or slow down the harmful effect of these free radicals. It is thus clearly seen that the anti-aging factors or substances are most of the nutrients that are present in our day-to-day life foods. These foods packed with vitamins, antioxidants, catenoids, flavonoids etc. are nothing but the nutraceuticals that help in reversing age-related effects on the body and are termed as "anti-aging nutraceuticals". These nutraceuticals prove a noninvasive way for patients with skin-related disorders as a cure and also aid in reversing age-related diseases/

ailments. Thus, nutraceuticals is a broader term that encompasses all types of nutraceuticals, one of them being the "anti-aging nutraceuticals".

21.2 IPR and nutraceuticals industry

IPRs are a bundle of legal rights which are granted by the government of a country to an inventor or a creator for protecting the inventions or creations of the intellect. The basic principle of IP Rights is to provide an applicant with a set of exclusive legal rights that helps the inventor or creator to benefit and protect their work. Broadly, IP can be divided into two kinds – Industrial Property which includes patents for inventions, trademarks, industrial designs and geographical indications; and Copyright which covers literary works (such as novels, poems and plays), films, music, artistic works (e.g., drawings, paintings, photographs and sculptures) and architectural design [1]. Intellectual property enables inventors and creators to not only protect their respective works but also gain monetary benefits from their products as well as earn recognition for them.

IP can be protected via any of the mentioned rights; however, the best mode for protecting "nutraceuticals" would be to obtain a patent. As mentioned, "nutraceuticals" is a broad term in itself and encompasses all and every food item that imparts health benefit to the user when consumed in the right form and appropriate quantity. Thus, nutraceuticals are nothing but the medicinal and nutritional "functional foods".

In Canada, a functional food has been defined as being "similar in appearance to conventional foods", "....consumed as part of a usual diet", whereas a nutraceutical is "a product produced from foods but sold in pills, powders, (potions), and other medicinal forms not generally associated with food".

In Britain, the Ministry of Agriculture, Fisheries and Food has developed a definition of a functional food as "a food that has a component incorporated into it to give it a specific medical or physiological benefit, other than purely nutritional benefit".

Hence, both in Canada and in Britain, a functional food is essentially a food, but a nutraceutical is an isolated or concentrated form. In America, "medical foods" and "dietary supplements" are regulatory terms (see below); however, "nutraceuticals", "functional foods", and other such terms are determined by consultants and marketers, based on consumer trends.

Food labeling regulations do not allow food labels to carry health claims in many countries. This makes it hard for companies marketing nutraceuticals to advertise the benefits of their products without a medicine license, so they may decide either not to do any research, or they may research a new product thoroughly and possibly obtain a patent [2].

A patent is an exclusive legal right granted for an invention (either a product or a process) that is novel in its conception and offers a new technical solution to any existing or pre-existing problem. Patents are most sought after because they provide an incentive to creators/inventors by recognizing their creativity in the form of a patent grant. Once a patent is granted, the invention cannot be utilized, produced, distributed, or sold without the consent of the patent owner. A patent is a valuable form of legal protection for intangibles where protection is granted for a limited amount of time – in a majority of countries for a period of 20 years. Patents not only prove to be an incentive for creators or inventors, by providing the possibility of monetary benefits for their marketable inventions, but also tend to encourage innovation and help improve the quality of life of individuals.

In order to obtain a patent for an invention, one must begin by filing an application for a patent. The application is written in a clear and precise manner with enough detail to enable a person with average intelligence and a basic understanding of the field, to use or reproduce the said invention. A patent application generally contains the title of the invention followed by a short description of the field of invention. Most countries have varying structures for their patent applications, but all of them commonly contain a description of the background and of the invention. Such descriptions can include drawings, plans or diagrams to illustrate the content in greater detail. An important section of the application is the "claims" where the inventor or creator claims certain specific features of their invention, which details the extent of protection to be granted by the patent.

Patent owners have the advantage of deciding who can or cannot use their patented inventions; however, this is only during the term of the patent duration. Patent owners can also grant licenses to other parties for using, manufacturing and distributing their inventions or sell their rights to the inventions to another party. During the patent term, the patent is made available to the public as a publication in the Official Gazette of a country; however, once it expires, the patent is no longer protected, and the invention enters the public domain where the owner has no exclusive rights to the invention anymore.

Ideally, an invention must, in general, fulfil the following conditions in order to be protected by a patent: it must have practical use; it must be novel, i.e., it should contain some new element or characteristic which does not form a part of the existing knowledge (called prior art) in its particular technical field; it must consist of an inventive step that cannot be presumed by a person with average knowledge of the technical field; and lastly the subject matter must be accepted as "patentable" under law [1]. Patenting comes with many limitations and the concept "everything under the sun can be patented" does not hold true. There are many countries that have an expansive list of what cannot be patented which differ from each country. Some of the things that are restricted from qualifying as patentable subject matter are – a scientific theory, any mathematical methods, various natural plant or animal varieties, discovering a natural substance, any method for commercial business or medical treatment. In India, there are many different ways to cover a nutraceutical product with patent protection. Patents may be obtained for a new chemical compound or a new use of a known compound or a new combination of known compounds provided there is proved enhancement in efficacy of the compound. Process or method of manufacturing such nutraceuticals may also be patented, provided that it qualifies all other requirements of being novel, inventive while also overcoming prior arts deficiency and not falling under any clauses of Sec 3.

There are various routes to obtain a patent, namely – a national application, a regional application and via the Patent Cooperation Treaty (PCT) regime. Ideally, the concept of an international patent does not exist. One could obtain a patent at any one or more national office by applying to each country they would want to obtain a patent, or one could choose to send in an application to a regional office such as the European Patent Office (EPO) or the African Regional Intellectual Property Organization (ARIPO) which eliminates the need to go to each country individually and file a patent. Once a creator/inventor decides to patent an invention and prepares a patent application, he/she can file the application at any national patent office or a regional patent office. Regional patent office services provide the advantage of requesting for a patent protection in one or more countries (that are a member of the regional office) and each country has the discretion to grant or reject a patent within its borders. The drawback however is that regional offices provide protection only in countries that fall within their regional offices. On the other hand, the WIPO-administered Patent Cooperation Treaty (PCT) allows the applicant to file a single patent application that has the same effect as national applications filed in the designated member countries. The advantage of filing a PCT application is that an applicant seeking protection may file one application and request protection in as many signatory states as required.

Another effective strategy to protect a botanical product from competition involves a type of IPR called trade secret. A trade secret essentially consists of vital information related to the product (or process) which is not disclosed to the public and is maintained as a secret for as long as possible and desired. Technically any kind of confidential information that provides a company with a competitive edge is considered a trade secret and they can consist of manufacturing or industrial secrets as well as commercial secrets [3]. The legal protection of trade secrets usually falls under the general concept of protection against unfair competition or the protection of confidential information. The subject matter of trade secrets is usually very vast and can include methods for sales and distribution, consumer profiles, advertising strategies, lists of suppliers and clients, and manufacturing processes. It is not always easy to distinguish what specifically falls under the scope of trade secrets, but the content is always circumstantial and judged individually. Unlike other IPRs, trade secrets have limited protection because a trade secret holder is only protected from unauthorized disclosure or use, often referred to as misappropriation.

Any unfair practice with respect to trade secrets usually includes industrial or commercial espionage, breach of contract and/or breach of confidence. However, if maintained, trade secrets do not expire unlike patents which have a set term of protection (usually 20 years) and can remain indefinitely until discovered or lost. There is no legal framework in most countries for trade secrets; however, in the US, every state has the liberty to form its own set of rules [4], and currently, several US states have adopted the Uniform Trade Secret Acts (UTSA). According to the World Intellectual Property Organisation (WIPO), one of the 17 specialized agencies of the United Nations responsible for promoting the protection of intellectual property throughout the world through cooperation among member countries of the organization, the unauthorized use of such information by persons other than the holder is regarded as an unfair practice and a violation of the trade secret.

In the case of "nutraceuticals", there are certain guidelines and regulations laid out by each country for granting a patent as well as for other IP rights. The following is the country-wise scenario for nutraceuticals and specifically "anti-aging"-related nutraceuticals.

21.3 Market exclusivity

For nutraceuticals, the laws of market exclusivity would be applicable only in case it can be classified as a pharmaceutical. Pharmaceutical development is an expensive, time-consuming and uncertain process that takes years to complete. A pharmaceutical drug will usually have two kinds of legal protections, namely exclusivity and patent protection. Exclusivity is a creation of law and enables the drug product to have exclusive or monopoly status in the market for a certain number of years. Patent is a government authority or license conferring a right or title for a set period, especially the sole right to exclude others from making, using, or selling an invention.

Often, patent protection expires before a new drug is approved for marketing. As a result, most pharmaceutical companies depend on the exclusivity rights granted by the appropriate authorities to recoup their considerable investment in the drug development and approval process in order to succeed in the global marketplace. Pharmaceutical companies generally obtain patents on their products or processes long before their product candidates are ready to go to market as it can take up to 12 years for a company to obtain market approval and there is often little, if any, patent protection left on the product at the time of marketing. To provide pharmaceutical companies with an opportunity to recoup their investment in drug research and development and to incentivize continuing innovation, many countries have implemented numerous provisions to extend the period during which companies can market their drugs free of generic competition. These nonpatent exclusivity provisions allow pharmaceutical companies to market products without competition from incoming generics, resulting in significant financial benefits for the original drug manufacturer. It is essential that a pharmaceutical company evaluate its exclusivity options and develop its competitive strategy early in the drug development process. The period of exclusivity differs from country to country.

In the USA, the Act governing exclusivity laws is the US Federal Food, Drug and Cosmetic Act (FDCA) and provides that the FDA cannot legally approve an application of a generic drug for that product until the exclusivity period expires. Drugs in general, can be marketed in the USA in the following forms: New Drug Application (NDA) and an Abbreviated New Drug Application (ANDA). An NDA application contains "full reports" relating to safety and efficacy investigations, whereas an ANDA is submitted to acquire marketing rights for a duplicate, or generic, version of an already-approved drug where no safety and efficacy data needs to be submitted for approval, but data pertaining to bioequivalence is a must. NDA also contains information regarding any drug products as well as their methods of use. These patents are further enlisted in the approved drug products with Therapeutic Equivalence Evaluations also known as the "Orange Book". This period of market exclusivity is independent of any patent protection that might be available upon grant of a patent and is granted to an NDA applicant as follows:

Orphan Drug Entity (ODE) a product for treating fewer than 200,000 patients in the US per year – 7 years

New Chemical Entity (NCE) – 5 years

"Other" Exclusivity – 3 years for a product other than a NCE (dependent on certain conditions and criteria)

Pediatric Exclusivity (PED) – 6 months added to existing Patents/Exclusivity

Patent Challenge – (PC) – 180 days (this exclusivity is for ANDAs only).

In Europe, the European Medicines Agency (EMEA) oversees the regulations pertaining to botanical drug products marketed as pharmaceuticals. In the past few years, the EU has expanded significantly the opportunities for drug manufacturers to obtain market exclusivity for their products, and since 1993, European drug companies have been able to obtain a supplementary protection certificate (SPC) to extend the patent for up to 5 years for certain medicinal products marketed in the EU in order to compensate them for the lengthy time period required to obtain regulatory approval of these products.

An SPC will be granted only if, at the date of application, the product

1. Is protected by patent;
2. Is the subject of the first valid marketing authorization granted to market the product for a medicinal use; and
3. Has not already been the subject of an SPC.

The SPC comes into force only after the corresponding general patent expires for a period equal to the period which elapsed between the date on which the patent application was filed and the date of the first marketing authorization, minus 5 years. The SPC term may not exceed 5 years from the date on which it takes effect. In 2005, the EU Data Exclusivity Directive 31 was brought into force under which sponsors may receive up to 11 years of exclusivity for new drugs. The exclusivity available under the Directive may include 8 years of data exclusivity, 2 years of marketing exclusivity, and a potential 1-year extension. In addition, under the EU Orphan drug regulations, which became effective in 2000, the Community and the member states may not accept or grant for 10 years, a new marketing authorization, or an application to extend an existing marketing authorization, for the same therapeutic indication as an orphan drug. Finally, Paediatric Regulation, which became effective in 2007, provides sponsors with the right to apply for a 6-month extension to the product's SPC in return for conducting pediatric studies on the product.

In Australia, market exclusivity laws are governed by the Australian orphan drugs policy which was set up in 1997. The main characteristic of the Australian Orphan Drugs Program is that it is based upon a close collaboration of the TGA with the US FDA and takes into account the FDA's orphan drug evaluations and aims at providing a 5-year exclusivity period to orphan drugs, but this is still under consideration by the Australian jurisdiction. However, the concept of market exclusivity is relatively new for the Australian markets and is still under development as substantial laws governing this concept are still not available.

In India, the concept of data exclusivity prevails and not market exclusivity. Data exclusivity is a form of exclusivity which prevents regulators from using the clinical trial test data that had been used to approve the originator's product, to also approve the chemically (or otherwise) equivalent generic product. This means that if the generic company wants to get regulatory approval during the period of data exclusivity (generally 5–10 years), it needs to duplicate the expenses and time taken to take its product through clinical trials. If the period of data exclusivity completely overlaps with the patent duration, there is usually no substantial effect as the patent would anyway prevent generics from releasing the product. However, off-patent or nonpatented products can also be granted data exclusivity – in which case they would enjoy 5–10 years of exclusivity. Data-exclusivity rights are also not necessarily "bound" by the same exceptions and flexibilities that patent rights are.

21.4 Country-specific regulations for nutraceuticals

21.4.1 United States of America (USA)

In the United States of America, the Food & Drug Administration (FDA) is a federal agency responsible for the regulations of food, drugs, additives and cosmetics. However, unlike pharmaceutical drugs, the FDA regulates nutraceuticals under a separate set of regulations than those for regulating conventional food and drug products. According to the Dietary Supplement Health and Education (DSHEA) Act of 1994, nutraceuticals are regulated as "Dietary Supplements" [5].

DSHEA defines a dietary supplement as "a product (other than tobacco) intended to supplement the diet that bears or contains one or more of the following dietary ingredients: vitamins, minerals, amino acids, herbs or other botanicals; a concentrate, metabolite, constituent, extract or combination of the ingredients listed above". On the other hand, FDA defines a drug as an article intended to diagnose, cure, mitigate, treat, or prevent disease. In case of a conventional drug or a food additive, it is mandatory for the manufacturer of drug or food additive to conduct safety studies and duly submit results of the same to the FDA. Post submission of the safety data by the manufacturer, the FDA reviews it and grants a premarket approval, if the drug or food additive is proven to be safe.

However, since dietary supplements have a separate definition and set of regulations, they need not comply with the FDA norms in order to be marketed, i.e., essentially dietary supplements can bypass the premarket testing and/or approval done by FDA. According to DSHEA, "safe" refers to no significant risk of illness. Further, according to DSHEA, the responsibility to ensure the safety of nutraceutical prior to its marketing, is of the manufacturer of the product. In addition to this, the manufacturer also has to take care of truthful and nonmisleading labeling of their products. Nevertheless, FDA is authorized to take action against any unsafe product, post its market launch. To put it simply – while it is the responsibility of the product (nutraceutical) manufacturer to ensure safety of the product before its market launch, it is not mandatory for him to get it registered with and/or approved by FDA at that stage. On parallel lines, while FDA may not play a role in safety assurance of a nutraceutical product at the premarketing stage, it still can exercise its power to enforce strict measures against the unsafe nutraceutical products already there in the market. Hence, the overall safety of the nutraceuticals marketed in the USA depends on the individual role play of the manufacturer and the FDA.

The DSHEA Act also lays down an additional criterion to be confirmed to, for dietary supplements, which is as follows:

- Be intended for ingestion in pill, capsule, tablet, powder, or liquid form
- Not be represented for use as a conventional food or as sole item of a meal/diet
- Be labeled as a "dietary supplement"

As far as labeling of the dietary supplements is concerned, DSHEA states that the label of a dietary supplement must include the following:

- Name of each ingredient
- Quantity of each ingredient

- Total weight of all ingredients, if a blend
- Identity of the plant part used
- The term "Dietary Supplement"
- Nutritional labeling information (calories, fat, sodium)

It is to be noted that a dietary supplement can be registered in the USA, only if it fits into the definition and meets all the requirements laid down by DSHEA.

21.4.2 European Union (EU)

European Food Safety Authority (EFSA) is an independent European agency set up in 2002, which provides scientific advice and communication on risks associated with the food chain. EFSA was established under the General Food Law by the EU, which deals with the risk assessment of food products. The food laws in the EU generally come under the legislation of EFSA.

In the EU, Nutraceuticals is a broad term which includes a wide range of substances which can be used as medicinal products, feed materials or feed additives. Since the EU involves multiple countries, the regulatory aspects of nutraceuticals become a little complex in this jurisdiction as compared to other major jurisdictions like USA, India, China, etc. Furthermore, since different procedures are to be followed for obtaining appropriate market authorization, the inclusion of a variety of substances under the scope of the term "nutraceuticals" in the EU, as stated above, makes a sizable difference in the regulatory aspects of market authorization in this jurisdiction.

In the EU, more or less, nutraceuticals are regulated based on their intended use. For instance, if nutraceuticals are administered with medical claims or if they exert a pharmacological effect, their use must comply with Directive 2001/82/EC of the EU legislation. Similarly, if nutraceuticals are used as feed additives for animal nutrition, they have to comply with Regulation No. 1831/2003. Furthermore, if nutraceuticals are administered as feed ingredients, they must comply with Commission Regulation (EU) No. 68/2013. The definitions of feed materials, feed additives and veterinary medicinal products are provided in food law legislation reported in Regulation (EC) No. 178/2002 [6].

The responsibility of providing opinions which are used by the European Commission to adopt legislation related to animal nutrition is on the scientific committees and panels of the EFSA. In case of veterinary medicinal products, the responsibility for marketing authorization is both granted by competent national authorities of the member states of the EU or by the European Medical Agency (EMA) [6].

It is noteworthy that when it comes to nutraceutical regulation in the EU, only "health claims" and not "medicinal claims" are allowed regarding the beneficial effects of nutraceuticals. For instance, a nutraceutical product can only claim to improve health or possibly assist in the avoidance of onset of illness, and not to cure and/or prevent the disease.

While the FDA in USA is authorized to act against any unsafe product on the market, the EFSA in EU does not have the same mandate. EFSA must authorize/approve in detail any health claim before it is considered at a national or European level prior to being put on the market following a specific request from member states, European Parliament, or stakeholders. Following the EFSA opinion, each state can decide independently to set specific approval regulations and/or authorization.

21.4.3 India

Nutraceuticals are known as "foods for special dietary uses" in India. In India, the regulatory body that legalizes nutraceutical products is the Food Safety and Standards Authority of India, commonly referred to as FSSAI, which was established under the Food Safety and Standards Act, 2006 [7]. FSSAI has been created for laying down science-based standards for articles of food and to regulate their manufacture, storage, distribution, sale and import to ensure availability of safe and wholesome food for human consumption. FSSAI acts as a single point of reference for all matters related to food safety and standards.

The Food Safety and Standards Act (FSSA), 2006 provides multiple benefits such as consolidation of eight laws governing the food sector (harmonization), alignment of international regulations, providing science-based standards, and providing clarity and uniformity in novel food areas and helping to curb corruption. According to the FSSA, "foods for special dietary use" are specially processed or formulated to satisfy particular dietary requirements, which exist because of a particular physical or physiological condition or specific diseases and disorders. These foodstuffs are presented such that their composition must differ significantly from the Indian Standard (IS) composition of ordinary foods of comparable nature, and may contain one or more of the following ingredients:

- plants or botanicals or their parts in the form of powder, concentrate or extract in water, ethyl alcohol or hydroalcoholic extract, single or combination
- minerals or vitamins or proteins or metals or their compounds or amino acids in amounts not exceeding the Recommended Daily Allowance for Indians or enzymes (within permissible limits)
- substances from animal origin
- dietary substances for use by humans that supplement the diet by increasing total dietary intake.

In the context of nutraceutical regulations, a health claim refers to a statement that suggests the relationship between food (e.g. nutraceutical) and health.

According to the nutraceutical regulations in India, "health claims" can be classified into three categories:

1. **Nutrient content claim**: This kind of claim suggests that a food has beneficial nutritional properties.
2. **Reduction of disease claim**: This kind of claim states or implies that the consumption of dietary supplements or one of its constituents significantly reduces the risk factor in development of disease. However, these kinds of claims are not allowed in India.
3. **Structure/function claim**: This kind of claim is a statement on the label of a food or dietary supplement about how the product affects the human body structure.

In order to enter and get a product registered in the Indian nutraceutical market, following are the most important requirements [7]:

- Product evaluation
- Actual product analysis
- Procuring licenses
- Developing India specific health and label claims.

Unlike the USA, wherein the approval from FDA is not mandatory prior to the nutraceutical product's entry into the market, in India, an approval from FSSAI is required for registration and entry into the market. Functional foods and beverages account for 60% of the Indian nutraceutical market share, while dietary supplements account for 40% [2]. Even after implementation of Food Safety and Standards Act 2006 and Food Safety Standard and Regulations in 2011, there is still much scope to harmonize the regulations across the country, to remove regulatory defects and ensure product quality.

21.4.4 Canada

In Canada, "Health Canada" is the agency that regulates both food and drug products. The Canadian regulatory system categorizes nutraceuticals either as a food, or as a drug, or as a Natural Health Product (NHP). The category into which a nutraceutical would fall depends on its ingredients, history of use, associated risks and presentation.

The primary classification of nutraceuticals is based on whether a therapeutic claim has been made or not. If a nutraceutical product makes a therapeutic claim, it is considered as a drug and regulated according to the drug laws. Such products are subject to drug laws of Canada, and their safety, efficacy and quality are assessed prior to being given market authorization. On the other hand, if a nutraceutical product makes a therapeutic claim, it is considered as a food and regulated according to the food laws, according to the Food and Drugs Act and Regulations.

The responsibility of regulating food within Canada is shared jointly by Health Canada and Canadian Food Inspection Agency (CFIA). Generally, a premarket approval is not required for food products in Canada. However, certain food products defined as "novel foods" according to the Food and Drug Regulations have to undergo a safety assessment by the Food Directorate before they can be marketed.

As stated before, the nutraceuticals with a therapeutic claim are subject to the requirements for drugs under the Food and Drugs Act. These products have to undergo a rigorous premarket approval process through evaluation of a drug submission replete with the requisite pre-clinical and clinical trial information to support the product's safety and efficacy. However, certain foods may be exempted from these requirements, based on the review of Health Canada. The health claims made in such cases need to be supported mainly by human studies and/or animal studies, in certain cases. Food products making function claims may enter the market without a pre-market approval. General health claims can also be made in case of nutraceuticals in Canada which do not refer to a specific or general health effect, disease, or health condition but are broad claims which promote health through healthy eating habits.

Apart from the food and drug categories described above, nutraceuticals in Canada are regulated under a third category known as Natural Health Products (NHP). NHPs include vitamins and minerals, herbal remedies, homeopathic medicines, traditional medicines, probiotics and other products like amino acids and essential fatty acids. Their route of administration is restricted to oral, topical and sublingual routes. Although NHPs are considered as a subset of drugs, they are exempted from many of the requirements of the Food and Drugs Regulations, unless specifically referenced in the National Health Products Regulations. NHPs are under the authority of the Natural and Nonprescription Health Products Directorate (NNHPD).

NHPs are required to undergo a premarket approval process and obtain a license prior to entering the market. The claims made under NHPs can be classified as traditional use claims and modern health claims [8].

21.4.5 Japan

In 1991, Japan introduced the concept of "Foods for Specified Health Use" (FOSHU) to regulate functional foods. In fact, Japan is a pioneer country to have regulations on nutraceuticals or functional foods. Thereafter in Japan, the foods classified under FOSHU need approval from the government in order to be sold for consumption as a daily diet. The Government of Japan based on comprehensive science-based evidence to support such claims of claimants approves these functional foods for use. Japan has three categories defined for such functional foods, namely, nutrition parting, sensory satisfaction purpose foods, and foods that would improve physiological functions [5].

21.4.6 Australia

In Australia, foods with medicinal benefits are termed as "complementary medicines", and "The Therapeutics Goods Act, 1989" regulates these products. The regulations are under the "Department of Health and Aging". Some of the products that are classified under this category in Australia are herbal medicines, homoeopathic medicines, traditional medicines, vitamins and minerals, nutritional supplements and aromatherapy products [5].

21.4.7 Russia

In Russia, functional foods/nutraceuticals are regulated under the category termed as "Biologically Active Dietary Supplements" (BADS). The government of Russia under its Ministry of Healthcare and Social Development has classified the following as BADS – nutraceuticals (amino acids, dietary fibers, vitamins, minerals) and para-pharmaceuticals (bioflavonoid, alkaloids, essential oils, polysaccharides). According to Russian government norms, "foodstuffs with clinically proven effectiveness" can fall under this category. These BADS are recommended as a prophylactic and as a prevention against the side effects of routine pharmaceuticals route of curing diseases to achieve complete remission for the prevention of pharmaceutical therapy induced side-effects and for the achievement of complete remission. The functional foods/BADS are given importance in Russia since the government focuses on preventive measures to cure chronic diseases rather than just forming them a part of daily diet [5].

21.4.8 China

The People's Republic of China (PRC) has defined laws and regulation for nutraceuticals, which are classified either as functional health food or nutritional supplement. The Food Safety Law of the People's Republic of China regulates the use of functional foods in their province, whether available inland or whether imported. In PRC, "functional food" means the food declared and legally approved to provide particular health-care functions.

Health foods in the following categories are allowed in the PRC, provided that they fulfil all the statutory and legal requirements, obligations as stated by the Food Safety Law, namely, immune function enhancers, foods aiding in blood lipid reduction, blood sugar reduction, weight loss, blood pressure, liver injury, protection against radioactivity, etc.; foods improving memory, nutritional anemia, skin, growth and development, constipation, endurance, etc.; foods that relieve body fatigue, foods that remove acne, chloasma, etc.; foods that increase antioxidants, bone density, etc.; and foods that improve digestion, etc. [9].

21.5 Country-specific IP norms for nutraceuticals

In the biotech, pharmaceutical and nutraceutical industries, it may often be the case that the patented claims are directed to a method of administering an old substance (probably modified) to treat a new condition (in a new way) proving enhanced efficacy over the old method. In that case, the patentee cannot go against the manufacturer of the old product directly but safeguard his own rights over the new use of the substance or the new method to obtain, isolate or manufacture it.

Thus, the IP in case of food or food-related substances, especially those that are direct products of plants, or their parts and produce as it is, were a subject matter of concern and discussion since various countries protect their biological conserves as per their own laws. A common platform, however, was sought internationally due to the World Convention on Biological Diversity which provided defined guidelines and norms for regulation over use of such biological material of any country especially when it was to be claimed as Intellectual Property Right of someone. Article 15 of the Convention addresses the terms and conditions for access to genetic resources and traditional knowledge, informed consent and benefit-sharing. It recognizes the sovereignty of states over their natural resources and provides that access to these resources shall be subject to the prior informed consent of the contracting party (signatory country) providing such resources. It also provides that access shall be based on mutually agreed terms in order to ensure the sharing of benefits arising from the commercial or other utilization of these genetic resources with the contracting party providing such resources.

In 1999, work was begun to operationalize the mandates of the CBD which resulted in the issuance in April 2002 by the CBD Secretariat of the "Bonn Guidelines on Access to Genetic Resources and Benefit Sharing," which were adopted unanimously by CBD treaty members (BGAGRBS, 2002). The Bonn Guidelines were adopted to assist contracting parties, governments, providers, users and other stakeholders in developing overall access and benefit-sharing strategies and in identifying the steps involved in the process of obtaining access to genetic resources and benefit-sharing. More specifically, the guidelines are intended to help them when establishing legislative, administrative, or policy measures on access and benefit-sharing and/or when negotiating contractual arrangements for access and benefit-sharing [10].

Further, it is pertinent to note that though uniformity to a greater extent has been achieved with respect to protection and grant of IP rights under agreements like Paris Convention and TRIPS (Trade Related Intellectual Property Rights), countries have liberty to a certain extent to exercise their own rules and regulation in granting IP, e.g., the Sec. 101 of US patent laws or Sec. 3 of Indian Patents Act. In summary, these sections of patent laws have acted to restrict inventions for the good or bad of it in granting patent right when the invention is of plant/animal origin as exists in nature, if use known, if substance known etc. One of the major reasons for the nutraceutical industry to not bloom up to its fullest extent for the past few years were these laws that treat plant products/food products differently and restrict them from being patent eligible. This scenario is slowly improving now, and therefore, the nutraceutical industry has a huge opportunity to research and develop new products in the field of nutraceuticals. The coming years will prove that these nutraceuticals have the capacity to benefit mankind in ways that will amaze the medical and scientific community worldwide.

In an interesting US Federal Circuit decision 2019, for an infringement case related to human dietary supplement the US Court of Appeals for the Federal Circuit reversed a finding by a District Court that human dietary supplements could not be patented because they were products of nature or followed natural laws. The appellate court instead found that "[w]e live in the natural world, and all inventions are constrained by the laws of nature", but courts "must be careful not to overly abstract claims" in deciding whether supplement inventions are eligible to be patented. This ruling has paved the way for industries and inventors in fields like Nutraceuticals where there is a very thin line when a product can fit the patentability criteria or be stuck under the norms of "just" being a daily diet food stuff.

In this particular case, "Natural Alternatives International, Inc." filed suit against "Creative Compounds LLC" for infringement of its patents related to CarnoSyn® beta-alanine which was a dietary supplement as sport nutrition. US Court of Appeals for the Federal Circuit inferred that the District Court erred in considering the product as natural, even though it provided added benefits to its customers which were otherwise untapped.

The Court also ruled that "using a natural product in unnatural quantities to alter a patient's natural state, to treat a patient with specific dosages outlined in the patents" is eligible for patent protections.

The Federal Circuit also found that the District Court erred in finding 'Natural Alternatives' product claims as patent ineligible. Judge Moore wrote that the "Product Claims are directed to specific treatment formulations that incorporate natural products, but they have different characteristics and can be used in a manner that beta-alanine as it appears in nature cannot. In the Product Claims, beta-alanine and glycine are incorporated into particular dosage forms." For example, claim 6 of US Patent No. 7,504,376 is directed to a "dietary supplement or sports drink" that uses a combination of glycine and one of the specified forms of beta-alanine in an amount effective to increase athletic performance. In addition, Creative Compounds' counsel admitted at oral argument that the combination of glycine and beta-alanine could have synergistic effects allowing for outcomes that the individual components did not have. As such, the appellate court reversed the decision below on the product claims at issue.

Finally, the Federal Circuit reversed on Natural Alternatives' method of manufacture claims because they "....are not directed to the natural law or product of nature, but instead are an application of the law and new use of that product...". It is directed to the manufacture of a human dietary supplement with certain characteristics. The supplement is not a product of nature, and the use of the supplement to achieve a given result is not directed to a law of nature. We do not see, therefore, how a claim to the manufacture of a non-natural supplement would be directed to the law of nature or natural product."

The Federal Circuit sent the case back to the District Court for further proceedings on Natural Alternatives' claims against Creative Compounds [11].

21.6 International treaties and convention

Nonetheless, nutraceuticals are treated differently according to the local laws of every country, and there is much of standardization when it comes to IP worldwide. Intellectual Property laws have evolved to a great extent over the years; however, owing to the international treaties and pacts, the IP laws vary to a lesser extent country-to-country. In fact, international treaties and conventions signed and ratified by member nations make it easier to follow similar guidelines for IP-related activities and norms in different countries. As mentioned earlier, nutraceuticals can be any food or related supplement from animal or plant origin that imparts health benefits; thus, treaties that enumerate guidelines and regulations for use of such biological materials in relation to IP become of prime importance while considering the nutraceuticals too.

21.6.1 The Nagoya Protocol

The Nagoya Protocol on Access to Genetic Resources and the Fair and Equitable Sharing of Benefits Arising from their Utilization to the Convention on Biological Diversity [12] is an international agreement which aims at sharing the benefits arising from the utilization of genetic resources in a fair and equitable way. The Nagoya Protocol on Access to Genetic Resources and the Fair and Equitable Sharing of Benefits Arising from their Utilization was adopted by the Conference of the Parties to the Convention on Biological Diversity at its tenth meeting on 29 October 2010 in Nagoya, Japan. In accordance with its Article 32, the protocol was opened for signature from 2 February 2011 to 1 February 2012 at the United Nations Headquarters in New York by Parties to the Convention. So far, there are 68 countries' party to the protocol with 70 ratifications and over 92 signatures. The most prominent parties to the protocol are India, European Union, South Africa and UAE.

The protocol came into force on 12 October 2014 as a supplement to the Convention for Biological Diversity (CBD), and its main objective is to equitably share the benefits gained from using genetic resources as well as provide the associated rights of indigenous communities. This protocol is an international attempt to ensure that anyone under the jurisdiction who benefits from traditional knowledge has obtained prior informed consent from the respective countries and have negotiated a fair as well as equitable deal to share those benefits.

One of the most prominent protocols is Article 10 which focuses on benefit sharing. Article 10 of the Protocol states that:

> Parties shall consider the need for and modalities of a global multilateral benefit-sharing mechanism to address the fair and equitable sharing of benefits derived from the utilization of genetic resources and traditional knowledge associated with genetic resources that occur in transboundary situations or for which it is not possible to grant or obtain prior informed consent. The benefits shared by users of genetic resources and traditional knowledge associated with genetic resources through this mechanism shall be used to support the conservation of biological diversity and the sustainable use of its components globally. [13]

A simple example is the Kani tribe of Southern India where an agreement following the protocol's guidelines ensures that the tribe receives a just share of income arising from research by the Tropical Botanical Garden and Research Institute (TBGRI) on the Arogyapacha plant (Trichopus zeylanicus travancoricus) which is traditionally used to revitalize and is now licensed and sold as "Jeevani".

21.6.2 WIPO: The Intergovernmental Committee on Intellectual Property and Genetic Resources, Traditional Knowledge and Folklore

In the fall of 2000, the WIPO established the WIPO Intergovernmental Committee on Intellectual Property and Genetic Resources, Traditional Knowledge and Folklore (hereinafter "Intergovernmental Committee" or IGC) [14]. Essentially, the mandate of the IGC is to facilitate the discussion of intellectual property issues that arise in the context of

1. access to genetic resources and benefit sharing;
2. protection of traditional knowledge, innovations and creativity; and
3. protection of expressions of folklore, including handicrafts [15].

The IGC was established in September 2000 and serves as an international forum where WIPO member states can discuss the intellectual property issues that arise in the context of access to genetic resources and benefit sharing as well as the protection of traditional knowledge and traditional cultural expressions. In 2009, the WIPO members decided that the IGC should establish an agreement, by starting formal negotiations, on one or more international legal instruments that would ensure the effective protection of genetic resources, traditional knowledge and traditional cultural expressions. Such an agreement could either be established as a recommendation for all the WIPO members or become a formal treaty that would bind the member countries which would choose to ratify it.

Since its inception, the IGC has stimulated an increased recognition of traditional knowledge (TK) within the patent system and in 2002 certain TK journals were included in the minimum documentation for applications under WIPO's PCT. Also, TK classification tools were integrated within the International Patent Classification in the year 2003. Further progress was made in 2002 when the IGC accepted technical standards for the documentation of TK which was developed at a WIPO meeting in Cochin, India.

In order to provide guidance on the IP aspects of mutually agreed terms for fair and equitable benefit-sharing related to Genetic Resources (GR), WIPO has developed, and regularly updates, an online database of relevant contractual practices. A rough draft consisting of guidelines on IP clauses relating to access and benefit-sharing agreements have been developed. Under the IGC, WIPO has also carried out numerous studies and developed many other resources (such as glossaries, surveys of national experiences, a laws database and training programs), which have proved useful for member states and others. Negotiations on TK have continued to this date and the WIPO member states may in due course decide to convene a diplomatic conference for the final adoption of one or more international instruments.

21.6.3 International Union for the Protection of New Varieties of Plants

Botanical products in general do not follow a strict regulatory procedure, but one of the factors that affect IPRs relating to botanical products are plant variety regulations. Nutraceuticals or functional foods from plant origin are such botanical products with defined, nutrition and physiological effect [16].

Internationally, approximately 72 countries, including the USA, EU, China and Central Africa, are party to the International Union for the Protection of New Varieties of Plants (UPOV) which is an intergovernmental organization with its headquarters in Geneva, Switzerland. India has the Protection of Plant Varieties and Farmers' Rights (PPVFR) Authority which was established as an effective system for protecting plant varieties, the rights of farmers as well as plant breeders.

UPOV was established by the International Convention for the Protection of New Varieties of Plants and was adopted in Paris in the year 1961. UPOV's mission is to provide and encourage an efficient system of protection for plant varieties. The aim of the UPOV is to encourage the development of new varieties of plants and provide the basis for member countries to encourage plant breeding by granting breeders of new plant varieties an intellectual property right called the "breeder's right".

Breeder's right is important because it means that the authorization of the breeder is required to propagate the variety for commercial purposes. The UPOV Convention describes and defines the acts that require the breeder's authorization when propagating material of a protected variety and, under certain conditions, for the harvested material. UPOV members may also decide to extend the protection to products which are made directly from the harvested material under certain conditions. In order to obtain this protection, the breeder must file an individual application with the authorities of the respective UPOV members entrusted with the task of granting the breeders' rights. Under the UPOV Convention, the breeder's right is granted only when the variety is new, distinct, uniform and stable and has a suitable denomination.

In India, the PPVFR encourages the development of new varieties of plants which may be considered as essential to recognize and protect the rights of the farmers with respect to their contribution made at any time in conserving, improving and making available plant genetic resources for the development of the new plant varieties [17].

The PPVFR Authority is of the view that in order to accelerate agricultural development, it is necessary to protect the plants breeder's rights as well as to encourage investment for research and development purposes of new plant varieties. India, having ratified the Agreement on Trade Related Aspects of the Intellectual Property Rights (TRIPS), had to make a provision for giving effect to the Agreement. To give effect to the aforesaid objectives, the Protection of Plant Varieties and Farmers' Rights (PPVFR) Act 2001 was enacted in India.

21.7 Conclusion

The regulatory bodies in every country across the globe monitor and regulate nutraceuticals or "anti-aging nutraceuticals" on the basis of their local laws and regulations, and further, their marketing strategies and end use get defined accordingly.

These country-wise regulations restrict globalization of nutraceuticals in many ways. The regulatory variation between countries hinders global trade and marketing. For instance, most of the countries discussed take a relaxed approach to regulation, yet China's process for dietary supplement approval involves a strict testing protocol, in line with the US process for pharmaceutical approval. Unlike DSHEA, the regulations in some countries do not provide adequate distinction between food, drug and nutraceuticals as such.

Anti-aging nutraceuticals may be criticized by some, but the underlying fact is that they are here as the need of the hour and are proving to be a game changer in the anti-aging industry. The pros and cons both work in favor of the nutraceuticals industry in the sense that due to less regulatory formalities and hurdles for nutraceutical products, companies are eager to capitalize this market and earn high returns. The present consumer market provides a time of great opportunity and urges companies to innovate this space. These companies in turn can benefit from the product by protecting it with the right IP.

Cons to be stated if any, are the restrictions caused by some countries for globalization of anti-aging nutraceuticals, due to no regulation over use of nutraceuticals in their country, causing issues of consumer safety at large.

There is a vivid need to study nutraceutical dose-related issues carefully since nutraceuticals often find themselves being categorized in the same regulatory category as common foods. Standardization of dose and method of delivery of nutraceuticals to improve efficacy and health benefits could overcome these issues. It is essential to test and regulate the use of nutraceuticals in a cost-effective and efficient manner which can address the safety issues for humans who are to consume such nutraceuticals.

In spite of all the differences in regulatory and nonregulatory rules of various countries for nutraceutical products, nothing prevents nutraceuticals from being marketed as pharmaceutical products and thus provide them the necessary protection under pharmaceutical laws when compared to the loosely wound rules and regulations for nutraceuticals.

To conclude, the manufacturers of nutraceuticals and "anti-aging nutraceuticals" in specific have a plethora of opportunities to explore various markets, with adequate protection being provided by the emerging laws across most of the developed and developing countries today.

References

1. http://www.wipo.int/edocs/pubdocs/en/intproperty/.
2. Esther Bull, Lisa Rapport, Brian Lockwood. What is a nutraceutical? *The Pharmaceutical Journal* 2000; Vol. 265 No. 7104 pp. 57–58.
3. http://www.wipo.int/sme/en/ip_business/trade_secrets/trade_secrets.htm.
4. Kewanee Oil Co. v. Bicron Corp., 416 U.S. 470, 94 S.Ct. 1879, 40 L.Ed.2d 315 (1974).
5. https://www.nutraceuticalbusinessreview.com/news/article_page/Scrutinising_the_term_nutraceutical__a_global_regulatory_perspective/100047.
6. D.E.A. Tedesco, P. Cagnardi. Regulatory guidelines for nutraceuticals in the European Union. In: Gupta R., Srivastava A., Lall R. (eds) *Nutraceuticals in Veterinary Medicine*. Springer, Cham 2019, pp 793–805. doi:10.1007/978-3-030-04624-8_58.
7. Raj K. Keservani, Anil K. Sharma, F. Ahmad, Mirza E. Baig. Chapter 19 – Nutraceutical and functional food regulations in India, Editor(s): Debasis Bagchi, In *Food Science and Technology, Nutraceutical and Functional Food Regulations in the United States and Around the World* (Second Edition), Academic Press, 2014, Pages 327-342, ISBN 9780124058705. doi:10.1016/B978-0-12-405870-5.00019-0.

8. Paula N. Brown, Michael Chan, Joseph M. Betz et. al., Chapter 2 – Regulation of Neutraceuticals in Canada and the United States, Editor: Paul A Spagnuolo, In Nutraceuticals and Human Health: The Food-to-supplement Paradigm, Royal Society of Chemistry, 2020, Pages 7-26, ISBN 978-1-78801-416-8.

9. https://food.chemlinked.com/foodpedia/china-health-food-regulation.

10. Leighton K. Chong, Lawrence J. Udell, Bernard W. Downs, Chapter 40 – Intellectual property, branding, trademark, and regulatory approvals in nutraceuticals and functional foods, Editor(s): Debasis Bagchi, *Nutraceutical and Functional Food Regulations in the United States and around the World* (3rd Edition), Academic Press, 2019, Pages 627-636, ISBN 9780128164679. doi:10.1016/B978-0-12-816467-9.00040-X.

11. https://pbnlaw.com/media-and-events/article/ 2019/03/federal-circuit-finds-dietary-supplements-patent-eligible-legal-analysis/?page=1292.

12. https://www.cbd.int/abs/about/default.shtml.

13. https://www.cbd.int/abs/bfmechanism.shtml.

14. http://www.wipo.int/tk/en/igc/.

15. http://www.wipo.int/export/sites/www/tk/en/resources/pdf/tk_brief2.pdf.

16. Om P. Gulati, Peter Berry Ottaway, Patrick Coppens, Chapter 14 – Botanical nutraceuticals, (food supplements, fortified and functional foods) in the European Union with main focus on nutrition and health claims regulation, Editor(s): Debasis Bagchi, In *Food Science and Technology, Nutraceutical and Functional Food Regulations in the United States and Around the World* (Second Edition), Academic Press, 2014, Pages 221-256, ISBN 9780124058705. doi:10.1016/B978-0-12-405870-5.00014-1.

17. http://plantauthority.gov.in/.

Dietary Supplements and Nutraceuticals in the Management of Endocrine Disorders

Aaishwarya Deshmukh
Smt. Kashibai Navale College of Pharmacy

Jayvadan Patel
Sankalchand Patel University

Contents

DOI: 10.1201/9781003110866-22

22.1 Introduction

The endocrine system is a magnificently multifaceted and exclusive system of glands secreting crucial hormones which regulate all the biochemical functions of the body as well as optimize the act of whole human body. All the organs, organ system, tissue and cells are influenced by the endocrine system in a very peculiar way. However, the disorders and disease related to the endocrine system may also range from a minor trouble to a major life threat. There may be various grounds and etiologies for endocrine disorders like biological, ecological, behavioral, nutritional or idiopathic in nature. Out of these, since nutritional patterns may aggravate or attenuate the pathogenesis and critical effect of endocrine disorders, it is indispensable to investigate not only the profile of nutrition, dietary supplements and nutraceuticals but also their perspectives in the prevention, treatment and management of diseases related to endocrine system. For example, profiling of Western diet suggests enhanced consumption of foods which are high in possible atherogenic, carcinogenic, toxigenic and may act in synergistically to induce chronic inflammation and disease. On the other hand, dietary patterns like Mediterranean Diet or, DASH Diet, are rich in whole grains, fruits, vegetables, omega-3 fatty acids and antioxidants, and may reduce risks and disorders associated with endocrine system due to their anti-inflammatory, antiatherogenic, anti-carcinogenic and anti-obesogenic effects [1].

Contamination of the environment is the result of constant global industrial development and has led to glut of chemical substances, which gets into the human body through many and one or the other way and routes. This systematic exposure of the people to industrial xenobiotics has adverse effects on the health indicators and well-being of individuals. Conversely, diet affluent in definite substances, micromolecules and macromolecules (micronutrients and macronutrients) is one of the main means for maintaining health and disease prevention, and to fulfil this purpose of supplementation with such substances, plentiful alleged nutraceutical preparations are available and promoted to and used by a large number of general populations, with or without evidence of their effects [2].

22.2 Dietary supplements and nutraceuticals

Dr. Stephen L. De Felice, founder and chairman of the Foundation of Innovation Medicine (FIM), Crawford, New Jersey, coined the term nutraceutical from "nutrition" and "pharmaceutical" in 1989 and its meaning was modified by Health Canada which defines nutraceutical as "a product isolated or purified from foods and generally sold in medicinal forms not usually associated with food and demonstrated to have a physiological benefit or provide protection against chronic disease" [3]. The effects and widespread use of nutraceuticals perfectly emphasizes and justifies 2,000-year-old Hippocrates's quote "let food be your medicine and medicine be your food". An impulsive growth has been recorded since last decade in the nutraceutical –a multi-billion dollar industry. The prime reason for this upsurge in interest is their presumed safety and potential nutritional and pharmaceutical value, even though they are not traditionally recognized nutrients but have been claimed to have positive physiological effects and multiple therapeutic benefits on the human body [4]. There is another area known as 'nutrigenomics' which encompasses essentially the interface between the nutritional environment and cellular/ genetic processes which offers a molecular explanation of phytochemicals benefitting health and wellbeing by alteration of gene expression or gene constitution and in turn leads to amendment in initiation, development and progression of different diseases. Nutrigenomics, by proving genetic information, has, therefore, an essential role in effects of nutraceuticals against aging and different diseases [5]. Foods and nutrients, also known as dietary supplements, are required for normal functioning of the body and are useful in maintaining the health of the individual and reducing the risk of various diseases not only in adults but more importantly in geriatric, pediatric and special population as well. Likewise, nutraceuticals are "medicinal foods" that have a major role in preserving well-being and health, transforming immunity and preventing/treating specific diseases. Thus, the field of nutraceutical and dietary supplements can be foreseen as one of the missing blocks in the health of an individual. Moreover, it has also been scientifically confirmed and sustained by a range of research work that establishes nutraceuticals/dietary supplements efficacious to treat and prevent various disease conditions including endocrine system [6].

In the last few years, research has established on the occurrence of a lower incidence of some diseases along with breast and prostate cancers [7,8] in the population who include phytochemicals like soy isoflavones or tea polyphenols containing food [9,10]; or have improved general health attained through specific dietary habits like that of Mediterranean diet [11]. There are number of studies showing bioactive substances having chemo-preventive activity caused by their antioxidant, antiproliferative and anti-inflammatory effects and endocrinal activities [12,13]. In addition, the use of dietary supplements/nutraceuticals is prevalent, with data indicating more or less of 75% individuals in developed countries using one or more dietary supplements or nutraceuticals [14].

22.2.1 Nutraceuticals in endocrine disease

There has been an exponential boost in the number of studies focusing on various physiological roles of nutraceuticals and their use as a therapeutic agent for management of various diseases [15–17], among which disorders related to the endocrine system are of a major apprehension. Since endocrine disorders have been seen as a major burden for the health-care system all over the world, and that the prevalence and occurrence of metabolically faulty pathologies like obesity, diabetes, polycystic ovarian syndrome and other endocrine disorders is still going to increase in both developed and developing countries in the forthcoming decade, dietary interventions by means of natural bioactive food compounds have surfaced as potential therapeutic tools for endocrine and metabolic disorders; which also exerts limited deleterious side effects [18]. Further, the currently used conventional drugs and invasive inventions like surgeries are also quite insufficient in controlling efficiently the uninhibited spread of endocrine disorders. Furthermore, the drugs pose severe adverse effects on long term usage thus making dietary interventions an apt choice as a therapeutic strategy. Many studies documented plant origin phenolic compounds, flavonoids, phytosterols, fatty acids and carotenoids to demonstrate defensive effects against not only prevention, but treatment of coronary heart disease obesity, dyslipidemia, polycystic ovarian syndrome [19–21] and many other endocrine disorders.

Apart from the contributions of nutraceuticals in prevention and treatment of disease, biological endpoints and molecular mechanisms of nutraceuticals have also been well-studied and well-documented and its quite evident that the actions depend on individual substances and comprises an exceptionally broad array of signaling molecules, receptors transduction pathways, biochemical reactions, target processes and molecules to be generalized. In reproductive pharmacology, many studies have advocated positive effects of vitamins C, E and β-carotene on female [22] and male fertility depending on age [23], as well as improvement in women with PCOS once after they reached increased levels of vitamin D [24]. In cancer chemoprevention, wide-ranging research has revealed multiple mechanisms behind antitumor actions of certain natural substances. Studies have shown polyphenol compounds of green tea altering intracellular signaling pathways, and exerting antiangiogenic and proapoptotic effects, which in turn is responsible for reduced incidences of breast and other types of cancer [25]. Few plant-derived nutraceuticals like polyphenols/flavonoids, resveratrol, curcumin quercetin, genistein and apigenin have also shown to regulate the proteins of cell cycle control, thus decreasing cancer cell proliferation [26]. Likewise, phytochemicals from cruciferous vegetables, e.g. indole-3-carbinol, restrained receptiveness to estrogen and diminished the expression of ERα in hormone-dependent cells, together with mammary and prostate cancer cells [27]. On the contrary, some studies have shown that unwarranted ingestion of micronutrients from supplements did not exert significant beneficial effects, or may even cause a health risk, e.g. use of antioxidants (vitamin C, E, or D) as dietary supplementation did not recover parameters of reproduction of sub fertile women [28]. A randomized trial "Selenium and Vitamin E Cancer Prevention Trial" (SELECT) verified an augmented occurrence of prostate cancer in male consuming vitamin E supplements in synthetic α-tocopherol forms [29]. Crucially, few phytochemicals have reported negative effects which necessitate the need to investigate the mechanism of action at the molecular level. In addition, Iso-flavones like genistein and daidzein ingested through soy-rich diet are phytoestrogens and can act as endocrine disruptors which are used in menopause symptoms-relieving preparations [30]. Flavonoids like quercetin and luteolin can cause endocrine disrupting effects in breast and endometrial cancer models [31]. Moreover, extreme concentrations of green tea epigallocatechin-3-O-gallate have shown to decrease the in vitro maturation and fertilization of oocytes and induced toxicity embryo in mouse model [32]. Some phytochemicals, at high concentrations, may also be implicated in sustaining the tumor progression [33]. In brief, a biphasic activity of phytoestrogens has been reported in cancer development in estrogen-sensitive tissues as well as the effects of phytoestrogens depended on the exposure time. At the outset, phytoestrogens did slug down cell growth and exerted antiproliferative expression signature by activating estrogen receptorβ (ERβ). However, because of genetic instability of malignant cells, the expression of ERβ may be evaded by gene deletion or promoter methylation, and in this type of late-stage cancer cells, phytoestrogens can induce a transcriptional profile promoting the proliferation of clones that exhibits high amounts of ERα but little ERβ, thus making it necessary to re-evaluate the potential benefits of phytoestrogens [34].

Further, nutraceuticals are drifting from the sphere of pseudoscience into the realm of true science with constantly rising numbers of ongoing clinical trials. Even evidence has proved about the benefits of some agents. High standards of clinical research should be applied to all potential therapeutic agents. In few under-treated conditions, where conventional pharmaceutical alternatives are not available, undesirable, or insufficient, nutraceuticals might demonstrate as an effective therapeutic choice, and a consideration should be given for incorporating these agents into guidelines and treatment recommendations. Since nutraceutical agents have different properties, mechanisms of action and anticipated effects, the substantiation must be evaluated properly for each individual agent before recommending for use in definite clinical situations. Important to note, nutraceuticals comprise a broad range of pharmaceutical-grade products which are under regulation as dietary supplements or food additives which are professed to offer multiple health benefits, and companies can sell them directly to the people without regulatory approvals that otherwise pharmaceuticals have to go through. Additionally, nutraceuticals (often derived from food sources), are marketed with the universal foundation that they would provide benefits ahead of their basic nutritional value. Historically, the authenticity has also been conciliated due to lack of high-quality scientific studies to support this, habitually overstated health-benefit claims, associated with commercialization and marketing of nutraceutical products. Slack regulatory standards are also applied to nutraceuticals compared with pharmaceutical agents, in many countries, eventually leads to unscrupulous manufacturers exploiting this. Unfortunately, some nutraceutical manufacturers have exploited in a way, which has led to stigmatization of the field, and has outshined the prospective true benefit from a selected subgroup of these products. Whereas large nutraceuticals have an uncorroborated function in evidence-based medical care, some are progressively being subjected to rigorous scientific evaluation, and some of these even appear to show benefits for the treatment or prevention of disease [35].

22.2.2 Linking endocrine disease and nutraceuticals and nutrition

Nutrition and endocrinology are linked since a long time with the notion that for stature growth, adequate nutrition is a prerequisite. The range is lengthened with appreciation of thyroid disorders which results from iodine deficiency in certain geographic areas [36]. Additionally, the relation between rickets and calcium and vitamin D deficiency was recognized leading food substances fortified with vitamin D [37]. The relationship between childhood obesity and the metabolic consequences observed thereafter in adult life is again of great concern during the last couple of decades. Moreover, the last decade is bustling with endocrine disruptors affecting various hormonal axes affecting not only the puberty but other functions in the latest generation [38]. It is quite obvious from these study data that the functional aspects of endocrine gland are affected by nutritional alterations. Thus, nutritional endocrine disorders are categorized by modification in the physiology or anatomy of the endocrine glands with resultant clinical consequences in the wake of deficiency or excess of a dietary compound. The nutrients present in the food are subdivided into major and minor nutrients, where carbohydrates, proteins and fats constitute the major nutrients, whereas vitamins and minerals constitute the minor nutrients. There has been evolution from the nutrient deficiency disorders like short stature and rickets to endocrine disorders like obesity and diabetes which accounts for nutrient excess to many disorders like thyroid dysfunction and reproductive disease related to nutrient deficiency. The range of nutritional endocrine disorders is summarized in Table 22.1.

Table 22.1 Nutritional Endocrine Disorders

Endocrine System	Alteration Pattern	Disorder
Metabolic	Carbohydrate metabolism dysfunction, insulin resistance, underutilization of glucose, malnutrition	Diabetes mellitus, metabolic syndrome, obesity, malnutrition
Thyroid	Iodine deficiency, selenium deficiency, iodine excess	Goiter/hypothyroidism, hyperthyroidism, autoimmune thyroid disease
Bone	Calcium/vitamin D deficiency, fluoride excess	Rickets/osteomalacia, osteoporosis, fluorosis
Gonads	Endocrine disruptors, dysregulation of sex hormones	Gonadal disorders
Growth	Malnutrition, growth hormone dysregulation	Growth disorders

22.3 Nutraceutical/dietary supplements in endocrine disorder

22.3.1 Diabetes

Clinical studies have verified that food rich in α-lipoic acid and omega-3 poly-unsaturated fatty acids (PUFA) displayed improvement in the body mass index (BMI), fasting plasma glucose (FBG), post-prandial glucose (PPBG), glycated hemoglobin (HbA1c) and fasting plasma insulin in type 2 diabetes patients. Not only that HOMA-IR, lipid profile, high-sensitivity C-reactive protein (HS-CRP) and oxidative stress markers such as superoxide dismutase (SOD), glutathi-one peroxidase (GSH-Px) and malondialdehyde (MDA) were also found to be improved [39]. In addition, omega-3 fatty acid supplementation at the daily dose of 4 g sustained renal functions in diabetic nephropathy and hypertri-glyceridemia. Furthermore, daily use of long-chain omega-3 polyunsaturated fatty acids at the dose of 500 mg/day decreased the occurrence of severe diabetic retinopathy in geriatric patients [40]. Flaxseeds on consumption also showed downregulation of insulin signaling target pathway- Insulin recep-tor substrate *1* (IRS-1), insulin-like growth factor binding protein (IGFBP4), IGFBP5, AKT and *nuclear factor kappa B* (NF-kB) signaling [41], which sug-gests that α-linolenic acid can boost numerous metabolic targets. Not only that, omega-3 PUFAs as a nutritional supplementation in early life can avert the onset of type 1 diabetes; and long-standing ingestion of these phyto-chemicals can repress inflammation, revive and regenerate pancreatic islets, and diminish autoimmunity markers, thereby aiding amelioration of type 1 diabetes. These study reports advocate the essential role of fatty acid in the management of diabetes.

Treatment with green tea (500 mg/kg body weight) for a period of 12 weeks in high-fat-diet-fed mice decreased the body weight, increased the energy expenditure, decreased inflammation and improved insulin sensitivity by downregulation of expression of miR-335, as a result, improved adipose tis-sue metabolism [42]. Resveratrol is the prime polyphenolic component found in grapes. Studies have been carried out to check and evaluate the effect of resveratrol. It was found to improve glucose homeostasis, reduce insulin resistance, guard pancreatic β-cells and improve insulin secretion by augment-ing the expression and/or actions of AMPK and SIRT1 in type 1 diabetic tis-sues [43,44]. In addition, resveratrol amplified the mitochondrial biogenesis, fatty acid metabolism, GLUT4 expression along with decreasing expression of NF-kB, IL-1β and IL-6 in muscle cells which possibly reinstated the skeletal muscle dysfunction [45]. These beneficial effects could be ascribed to the anti-oxidative and anti-inflammatory mechanisms of resveratrol. Data from animal studies has shown that an efficient improvement in the glucose homeostasis in the hepatic cells of type 1 diabetic animals by diminishing the activity of phosphoenolpyruvate carboxykinase [46], lactate dehydrogenase and escalat-ing hexokinase and pyruvate kinase activities in revesterol-treated animals. As far as clinical studies are concerned, data has revealed that 10–250 mg/day of revesterol for 1–3 months, respectively, is satisfactory to improve insulin sensitivity and glucose homeostasis. Abundant data have confirmed dose- and time-dependent actions of resveratrol in type 2 diabetes patients in addition to experimentally induced type 2 diabetes animal models [47,48].

22.3.1.1 Nutraceutical antidiabetic herbs

a. **Eugenia Jambolana (Jamun):**

Eugenia Jambolana has shown to exert antidiabetic effect by insulin release mechanism [49] or modification in hepatic and skeletal muscle glycogen content and changes in the levels of enzymes like hepatic glucokinase, hexokinase, glucose-6-phosphate and phosphofructokinase in diabetic mice. In a country like India, decoction of kernels of *Eugenia jambolana* has been used as household remedy for diabetes since a very long time. In recent times, studies with different extracts like aqueous, alcoholic as well as lyophilized powder at the dose of 200 mg/kg per day has shown a hypoglycemic effect. Moreover, in a study, aqueous extract of seed (2.5 and 5.0 g/kg body weight) p.o. for 6 weeks showed a hypoglycemic effect, along with a raise in total hemoglobin and antioxidant activity in diabetic rats [50].

b. **Allium sativum (Garlic):**

Allium sativum has been a proven a potent oxidative stress scavenger. Together with a strong antioxidant activity, it has also got rapid reactivity with thiol-containing proteins which are **deemed** responsible for the antihyperglycemic property [51]. Allicin, an active constituent of garlic, has shown to have major hypoglycemic activity. Different extracts like that of ethanol, petroleum ether and ethyl acetate have shown antihyperglycemic activity in alloxan-induced diabetes in rabbit.

c. **Trigonella foenum-graecum (fenugreek):**

Trigonella foenum-graecum has shown to induce glucose-induced insulin release through a direct effect on the isolated islets of Langerhans. A variety of extracts of different parts of this plant as well as components like fibers, proteins and saponins isolated from the **seeds** have been explored and found to have significant antihyperglycemic activity [52]. Trigonella seeds contain Trigonelline, and the major alkaloid component is responsible for mild hypoglycemic effect.

d. **Acacia arabica (Babhul):**

Acacia arabica releases insulin from pancreatic beta cells, which is said to be responsible for the hypoglycemic activity. Hypoglycemic effect was observed in a study when powdered seeds **of** Acacia arabica were administered orally (2–4 g/kg body weight) to normal rabbits, and the mechanism for this hypoglycemic effect was found to be the release of insulin from pancreatic beta cells [53].

e. **Aeglemarmelos (Holy Fruit Tree):**

Aegle marmelos has shown to augment utilization of glucose, either by direct stimulation of glucose uptake or via the mediation of enhanced insulin secretion. Hypoglycemic **activity** of the leaves is by its blood glucose lowering effect due to utilization of glucose and potent antioxidant activity [54].

f. *Azadirachta indica* (Neem):

Azadirachta indica has shown to inhibit action of adrenaline on glucose metabolism and leads to increase in utilization of peripheral glucose. Hydroalcoholic plant extract has shown blood glucose lowering effect in normal rats and in glucose-fed and streptozotocin-induced diabetic rats [55].

g. *Coccinia indica* (Kundru):

Coccinia indica has demonstrated to inhibit important gluconeogenic enzymes glucose-6-phosphatase and fructose-1, 6-bisphosphatase and suppress glucose synthesis, along with increase in glucose oxidation by shunt pathway through activation of its chief enzyme glucose-6-phosphate dehydrogenase [56]. Dried extract (500 mg/kg p.o.) treatment for 6 weeks in diabetic patients showed hypoglycemic activity [57].

h. *Gymnema sylvestre* (Gurmar):

Gymnema sylvestre has been traditionally used to treat diabetes in both Type I and II diabetics. It has shown to augment secretion of insulin, uphold regeneration of islet cells, and increase consumption of glucose and activities of enzymes accountable for utilization of glucose by insulin-dependent pathways. Further data suggested amplification of phosphorylase activity, reduction in gluconeogenic enzymes and sorbitol dehydrogenase, and also inhibition of glucose absorption from intestine [58].

i. *Momordica charantia* (Bitter Gourd):

Momordica charantia, which belongs to Cucurbitaceae family, has shown to increase hepatic glycogen. P-insulin, a polypeptide present in fruits and seeds, is considered similar to bovine insulin. Besides, Vicine is the hypoglycemic constituent in the seed. A study has shown reduction in blood glucose level by fruit powder in fasted alloxan-induced diabetic rats after treatment for 15 days [59].

j. *Ocimum sanctum* (Tulsi):

The aqueous extract of leaves of *Ocimum sanctum* has demonstrated significant drop in blood glucose level in normal as well as alloxan induced diabetic rats. The putative mechanism was cortisol inhibiting potency of tulsi leaves. In addition, supplementation of leaf powder for 1 month, given along with food, decreased fasting blood glucose level in normal as well as diabetic rats [60].

k. *Pterocarpus marsupium* (Vijaysar):

Diverse parts of the plant are used traditionally like bark, latex, etc. and have been investigated and reported to have anti-hyperglycemic activity [61]. Epicatechin, Marsupsin, **Pterosupin** and Pterostilbene were the active constituents isolated from the bark and heartwood of the plant which were found to possess blood sugar-lowering activity.

1. *Tinospora cordifolia* (Guduchi):

   Tinospora cordifolia belongs to Menispermaceae family, and the leaves of this plant have been studied for the anti-hyperglycemic actions in normal and alloxan-induced diabetes in rabbits in graded doses and the results have confirmed its blood glucose-lowering effects [62].

m. **Chromium intake and diabetes**:

   Chromium is a general constituent in the earth's crust and seawater and a critical cofactor in the insulin action, the deficiency of which might lead to diabetes or primary hyperglycemia. An ample range of foods like egg yolks, whole-grain products, cereals, coffee, nuts, green beans, broccoli, meat and some brands of wine and beer have trivalent chromium as their component. A small number of studies have accounted beneficial effects of chromium supplementation on the diabetes and glycemic control. However, extensive research is still awaited to come to a definite conclusion regarding the physiological role of chromium in metabolic homeostasis [63].

22.3.2 Metabolic syndrome (MetS)

22.3.2.1 Functional foods: Plant proteins

Functional foods are categorized by the components having action on metabolite levels which may be linked to particular clinical syndromes. As far as MetS is concerned, plant proteins also warrant a unique deliberation. Certainly, diets rich in protein have become a well-accepted approach to improve weight management and weight loss [64]. Not only this, increasing intake of protein rich food or protein supplements may also have a potential for the prevention of type II diabetes mellitus. Though optimum quantity and quality of proteins for these disorders are still contentious, there are, however, significant indications that, e.g. lofty intake of red meat is linked with an increased risk of type II diabetes (T2D) [65], while plant proteins are linked with some improvement in diabetes risk and management of hyperlipidemia. In recent times, Virtanen et al. [66] in a study which was a follow-up of the Kuopio Ischemic Heart Disease Risk Factor Study, undoubtedly showed that plant proteins are linked with a decline in the risk of T2D. Although, data on MetS are not so wide-ranging, but lupin and soy are the two types of proteins that have been studied extensively and in details in patients with MetS, thus providing clinical substantiation of prospective benefits [67]. Besides, some other plant proteins have also been studied and shown benefits, e.g. pea and wheat protein. Thus, functional food may also be explored for their potential in metabolic syndrome treatment and management.

22.3.2.2 Lupin

Lupin is a protein-rich grain legume which usually embodies four domestic species, i.e. Lupinusalbus (white lupin), L. luteus (yellow lupin), L. mutabilis (pearl lupin) and L. angustifolius (sweet leaf lupin). In European countries, L. Angustifolius and L. Albus both are widely available as a protein concentrate. Amazingly, lupin seeds have a feature of a restricted, close to nil, content of anti-nutritional factors for instance phytate, tannins, lectins, protease inhibitors and oligosaccharides [68]. Lupin seeds include two classes of proteins, i.e. the 7S and 11S globulins, (also conglutins α and β) besides two minor distinct proteins known as conglutin γ and δ. These proteins have been investigated for their actions on plasma cholesterol reduction (the mechanism involved is attributable majorly to an LDL-receptor (LDL-R) activating mechanism since a long time. Few studies have also shown conglutin γ to reduce glycemia in animal models as well as, moderately, in human volunteers, principally in the postprandial condition [69]. In preclinical studies, lupin proteins have exhibited hypolipidemic and a significant antiatherosclerotic effect which is quite similar to similar to soy proteins. In a recent study, the mechanism of possible action on blood glucose levels was investigated, where different soy and lupin proteins were hydrolyzed by enzymatic reactions with pepsin and trypsin, and the resultant peptides were separated and screened for their ability to inhibit an important enzyme involved in glucose metabolism that is dipeptidyl peptidase IV (DPP-IV). The result of this study justified this molecular target and its involvement in the development of T2D; since a number of drugs which are pharmacological inhibitors of this enzyme have been developed and are presently being used [70]. In the posthydrolysis study [71], Soy 1 and Lup 1, two small peptides, were isolated and both showed efficient inhibitory capability on DPP-IV (IC50s equal to 106 and 228 lm, respectively), hence demonstrating these proteins to be the sources of DPP-IV inhibitory peptides. In clinical settings, lupin proteins have been experimented in diverse conditions, primarily in hypercholesterolemia condition, and a positive effect on LDL-C and on the LDL:HDL cholesterol ratio was found, perhaps due to the mechanism exerted on the LDL-R, in two studies; that is, one in the form of supplementation and another with a mixed diet enriched with lupin. Another study showed that lupin protein in combination with a cellulose resulted in a notable hypocholesterolemic effect; a comparable range of hypocholesterolemia effect was noted after a pea protein/fiber combination as well [72]. A decrement in the levels of TG was observed in rodent studies, which seemed to be related with decreased fatty acid synthesis and amplified TG hydrolysis. However, this was not observed in studies in hypercholesterolemic individuals. Still, in a randomized study by Pavanello et al. in patients suffering from MetS [73], it was demonstrated that a lupin protein concentrate resulted in a reduction, besides LDL cholesterol (8.0%), also of non-HDL cholesterol (7.5%) as compared with a lactose-free milk powder diet. This study also showed that lupin proteins led to a 12.7% reduction of Proprotein convertase subtilisin/kexin type 9 (PCSK9), a key regulator of LDL-receptor in male patients, and thus, these data established a direct modulation of proprotein con-vertasesubtilisin/kexin type 9 and LDL-receptor via protein–protein interactions [74]. Auxiliary to the data generated in context to MetS and hypercholeterolemia, lupin proteins can also offer a prospective therapeutic strategy in T2D, perhaps also because of the lately described modulatory effect of conglutin β on the insulin signaling pathways [75]. Thus, lupin protein as a supplementation or an ingenious whole diet with lupin proteins can supply an efficient dietary tool for the management of different biochemical alterations which is the main characteristic of MetS.

22.3.2.3 Soy proteins

One of the most extensively evaluated dietary proteins for metabolic control is soy proteins. Proteins derived from glycine max are the archetype plant proteins and, per se, have gained notice, as per the report in the recent systematic review on the effects of plant versus animal protein sources on features of MetS. Apart from proteins, glycine max also contains components such as isoflavones or phytoestrogens, which has a potential estrogenic activity and possibly antiatherosclerotic effects. Isoflavones might pose potential risk for, chiefly growing children, although, there has not been any clear evidence of a considerable activity on the major components of MetS [76]. In fact, cautious extraction of isoflavones from soy has not found to change their lipid lowering and LDL-R stimulating activity in an experimental animal model. Despite the fact that there is apparent data to show that soy proteins by itself can raise the activity of LDL-R in different animal models and in familial hypercholesterolemic patients [77], declined triglyceridemia and alterations in other MetS-associated variables have been reported in a few studies. Few studies have revealed an improvement in the glucose homeostasis after consumption of soy proteins. Moreover, in a study, soy proteins and soy nuts were compared (soy nuts have higher phytoestrogen content and less protein) in post-menopausal women with MetS, the result of which showed that the soy nut regimen decreased fasting blood glucose level more significantly as compared to soy protein, along with an improvement in LDL- cholesterol reduction [78]. The HOMA index was found to be attenuated. In addition, triglyceridemia changes were also reported in a number of studies. 15%–20% reduction was observed in patients with mildly elevated plasma TG levels independent of the isoflavone content. Additionally, a comparison study was conducted in patients with moderate hypercholesterolemia who were treated with the bile acid binding resin colesevelam and who consumed 25 g/day of an insoluble fraction of partially hydrolyzed soy proteins with those who consumed similar intake of milk proteins [79]. This study demonstrated lucid benefits of soy proteins on LDL-cholesterol and a fairly higher ascend of HDL-cholesterol. Besides, the TG levels difference was modest, but non-HDL-cholesterol reduction was significant with soy proteins; along with a high significant difference in apo B levels, while fecal sterol excretion was decreased by milk proteins and considerably lifted by soy proteins. In yet another comparative study, acute intake of soy versus lupin protein was evaluated in context to glycaemia [80] in T2D patients. A soy or lupin-based beverage having 50 g glucose significantly attenuated glycaemia post- beverage for four hours, but with no significant difference between lupin and soy. But, in case of insulin response, it was rather elevated for lupin and soy, compared with the controls. Plant protein sources as compared with animal proteins led to change in the blood pressure but were mainly inconsistent; however, body changes were usually characterized by some weight reduction. Plant proteins were found to be inversely linked with body mass index (BMI) only in males and with WC in both genders; while animal protein intake was positively linked with BMI and waist circumference (WC). Current longitudinal EPIC-PANACE study showed that [81], in an isoenergetic diet, rising dietary plant source proteins by a mere 5% at the outlay of animal-source proteins decreased weight gain by nearly one kg per year in men over a 5-year period, but not in women. In a different study, consumption of animal proteins in children, especially dairy products (for periods of up to 7 years), led to an increase in weight and BMI as compared to vegetable proteins [82]. Furthermore, a study by Sirtori C.R. et al. particularly explored the effect of 30 g/day soy proteins in parallel group against animal food in patients with clinical features of MetS. The result of study showed a significant decline in body weight (1.5%) and BMI (1.5%), and usual drop in total and LDL-cholesterol as well as of non-HDL-C (7.14%) versus milk proteins were also found. Out of total 26 participating subjects, 13 showed decrement in MetS indexes nearing to normal range. Moreover, other plant protein sources (without isoflavones) have also been tested in individuals with MetS among which pea, fava bean proteins and wheat gluten didn't show any additional favorable outcome on fasting lipemia in comparison with animal source proteins [83].

22.3.2.4 Prebiotics, symbiotic and the major traits of metabolic syndrome

Very few studies have evaluated the effect of prebiotics on the metabolic traits of MetS and thus small sample sizes, heterogeneity among trial subjects, disease conditions, prebiotic supplements, intervention duration and outcomes need to be carefully considered. The result of few trials investigating the outcome of prebiotic supplementation on metabolic traits, i.e., body weight, glucose homeostasis and TG have revealed that dietary supplementation impacts only on post-prandial glucose and insulin levels without affecting other parameters. Fascinatingly, satiety was also found to be improved, even though it was self-reported, upon prebiotic intake. Needless to say, prebiotics have been associated with attenuation in Ghrelin levels and to an augmentation in peptide YY and GLP-1 secretion, all of which are involved in appetite regulation [84,85]. Individuals having BMI -25 kg/m^2 and who are carriers of diabetes, demonstrated an improvement in TG and HDL-C levels post prebiotic treatment in comparison to placebo. The same study also reported a decrement in plasma fasting insulin and TG levels post synbiotic supplementation. However, there was no change in FPG [86], alike what has been reported in a very current meta-analysis [87].

22.3.2.5 Vitamin D

Vitamin D is normally believed to exert a slight role in the control of MetS. But recent studies and the data have signified levels of vitamin D as an essential variable in MetS, besides being a significant determinant of cardiovascular risk. Vitamin D has a prime physiological role in regulating calcium homeostasis and thus bone metabolism. However, there is a rising data regarding the involvement of vitamin D on glucose metabolism, blood pressure and other metabolic traits related to MetS [88]. Vitamin D is synthesized in the skin upon ultraviolet-B radiation and metabolized by the hepatic 25-hydroxylase enzyme to 25-hydroxyvitamin D [25(OH)D] and by a renal 1a-hydroxylase to the vitamin D hormone calcitriol, also called 1,25-(OH)2 vitamin D; the active form of vitamin D. 25(OH)D levels are the marker for evaluation of vitamin D status because of the fact that 1,25- (OH)2 vitamin D is active for a maximum of 27 hours. A dose–response meta-analysis of 16 cross-sectional studies was conducted to review the relationship between 25(OH)D levels and risk of MetS which demonstrated a linear and inverse association between the two variables and the similar outcome was preserved upon modification in certain parameters like for age (middle versus elderly), sex (male versus female), assay detection method, latitude (low versus high), however, somewhat attenuated [89]. In addition, when the relative threat for MetS was measured comparing individuals in the top versus bottom tertiles of baseline 25(OH)D levels, the same results were obtained. An attenuation in the circulating 25(OH)D, i.e., of 0.27 ng/mL in vitamin D3 for each 1 kg/m² increment in BMI was observed in obese individuals [90]. Thus, in the midst of the diverse suggested hypotheses, the notion of reverse causality should be taken into deliberation. Certainly, vitamin D may be confiscated or accumulated in the adipose tissue leading to lower 25(OH)D serum levels, if there is a confirmatory notion to the inverse correlation between obesity and vitamin D levels and hence, obesity may be etiology and not a consequence of vitamin D deficiency [91].

22.3.2.6 Curcumin

Dried rhizomes of *Curcuma longa L.* (turmeric) contain polyphenolic compounds known as curcuminoids and are accountable for the orange-yellow color. Curcumin is the chief constituent comprising of about 5% of turmeric, with the structural analogues like demethoxycurcumin and bisdemethoxycurcumin. It is unstable at physiological pH and gets rapidly oxidized, which intercede topoisomerase poisoning as well as other antioxidant, anti-inflammatory and lipid-lowering effects. There are multiple properties of curcumin which act on a wide range of diseases, including MetS. The prime metabolic effect of curcumin appears to be its activity as insulin sensitizer, which is well demonstrated and documented in animal models of diabetes [92], and is also established in human studies. A study in the form of double-blind randomized trial demonstrated improvement of biomarkers of insulin sensitivity like C-peptide, HOMA-IR and HOMA for b cells in pre-diabetic patients after 9 months of treatment with 1,500 mg of curcumin in comparison to placebo group [93] and also shown to prevent T2D development (0% of curcumin-treated developed DM versus 16.4% of placebo-treated patients). Since Adiponectin and Leptin are associated with cardiovascular diseases; Aþ22.5% increase in adiponectin levels was identified, later on confirmed in a supplementary meta-analysis which reported a 77% rise together with a 26% decrease in leptin [94]. But a short treatment period offered no analogous benefit on glucose homeostasis, with, yet, a significant improvement in HDL-cholesterol (þ6.8%) and a decrement in TG (28.8) and non-HDL-C (13.6%). In yet another larger study where 117 subjects with MetS were enrolled provided assenting results, demonstrating, a prominent antioxidant and anti-inflammatory activity with a marked decrease of CRP concentrations [95]. The mechanism of curcuminoids in lipid-lowering is due to their ability to increase cholesterol efflux via ABCA1 and APOA-I expression and downregulation of gene for Niemann–Pick C1-Like 1 (NPC1L1) through the transcription factor, sterol regulatory element-binding protein 2 (SREBP2) [96]. Curcumin has also shown to downregulate PCSK9 mRNA levels through inhibition of the HNF-1a transcription factor; by up to 31%–48% in various cell lines, as a result augmenting LDL-R expression on the cell surface and LDL-C uptake [97]. And this in turn may be responsible for an additional anti-inflammatory activity.Furthermore, Curcumin exerted defense against atherosclerosis in LDLR/ mice by affecting synthesis and catabolism of fatty acids via modification of peroxisome proliferator-activated receptors (PPAR)-α and γ, cholesteryl ester transfer protein (CETP) and lipoprotein lipase (LPL) expression [98]. Unfortunately, a big limitation for extensive use of curcumin is the poor oral bioavailability which represents a major obstacle to clinical development.

22.3.2.7 Red yeast rice (RYR)

RYR is obtained from fermentation of the *Monascus purpureus* yeast in rice (Oryza sativa) and is a common ingredient of oriental cuisine. The fermentation process improves rice in bioactive components, including poly-ketides such as monacolins (compactin, monacolin K, M, L, J, X) which has a proven lipid-lowering effect as inhibitors of the 3-hydroxy-3-methyl-glutaryl-CoA (HMG-CoA) reductase. The prime monacolin in RYR is monacolin K, which shares a structural similarity with lovastatin and, for the same grounds, is classified as a drug by the US Food and Drug Administration (FDA) [99]. The European Food Safety Authority (EFSA), however, upholds the use of monacolin K from RYR preparations as a nutraceutical that has the capacity to decrease elevated LDL-C concentrations [100]. RYR is presently used in combination with other nutraceuticals which in turn can reduce daily doses and exert effects further than cholesterol reduction. Association of RYR with berberine has been found to be highly efficient in dropping TC by 0.68 mmol/L and LDL-C by 0.61 mmol/L, while raising HDL-C by 0.07 mmol/L, reducing TG and glucose by 0.16 and 0.14 mmol/L, respectively. Captivatingly, contrasting statins, this nutraceutical combination has also been found to improve the leptin-to-adiponectin ratio (17.8%), without changing adiponectin levels [101] and the same relationship resulted in an improved endothelial function and pulse wave velocity (PWV). Additionally, RYR (200 mg), in combination with berberine at the dosage of 500 mg and policosanols (10 mg), has also demonstrated improved insulin sensitivity in patients with IR, reducing the HOMA-IR by 24% [102].

22.3.3 Obesity

The management of obesity is a major challenge in this Medicare system, leading to recognition of substitute or alternative therapeutic options. Clinical trials have revealed that daily intake of fish or omega-3 supplementation augmented adiponectin levels in the blood by 14%–60%. Short-chain fatty acids have also shown to repress food intake by vagal afferent neurons activation. Moreover, eicosapentaenoic and docosahexaenoic acids have shown to improve chronic inflammation, insulin resistance and dyslipidemia associated with obesity [103]. A study has demonstrated that dietary intakes of fish oil (400 mg/kg/day) for 4 weeks could reinstate brain alterations in high-fat-diet-induced obesity model partly by restoring the inflammatory and oxidative damage parameters.

Polyphenols present in bilberry [104], grapes [105] and soybeans [106] have also shown to possess anti-obesity and anti-inflammatory properties and has been found to modulate the body weight, BMI, adiposity, fat pad, adipocyte differentiation and downregulate expression of NF-κB, TNF-α, IL-6, PPAR, SREBP-1C, ACC and CRP. These bioactive phytoconstituents alter cell signaling pathways through AMPK, MAPK and G-protein coupled receptor 120 and recover the balance of pro- and anti-inflammatory mediators secreted by adipose tissue and consequently decreases systemic inflammation and risk for metabolic diseases. The key pungent component of ginger, Gingerols exhibit exceptional anti-inflammatory properties by hindering prostaglandin synthetase and Arachidonate 5-lipoxygenase activity in RBL-1 cells and LPS induced COX-2 expression in U937 cells. A study by Saravanan et al. [107] demonstrated anti-obesity properties of gingerol by the inhibition of absorption of dietary fat in the gastrointestinal tract, and its hypophagic and hypolipidemic activities in male rats in the high-fat-diet-induced model of dietary obesity. In yet another few "in-vitro" studies on mouse 3T3-L1, pre-adipocytes displayed improvement in adipocyte differentiation and insulin-dependent glucose uptake [108].

Phytosterols stimulates nuclear hormone receptors LXRα and LXRβ which are recognized as regulators of cholesterol, lipid and glucose metabolism boost cholesterol excretion to the intestinal lumen and thus reduce the serum cholesterol; another mechanism being inhibition of the cholesterol absorption in the intestine. The dual mechanism of LXRα and LXRβ has made them an attractive drug targets for the treatment of diabetes and cardiovascular diseases [109]. Extensive data from literature clearly suggests the phytosterols such as stigmasterol and ergosterol, and their modified derivatives have a potential role in the modulation of lipid metabolism and glucose homeostasis by modulating LXR-alpha and beta expression through overexpression of ABCA1 and inadequately/not activating the lipogenic genes SREBP1C and SCD1 or FASN, respectively [110]. Since obesity is closely linked with inflammation, a possible therapeutic agent should have the capacity to fight against the consequences associated with inflammatory responses, and phytosterols, being known for anti-inflammatory properties, either by upregulating genes encoding anti-inflammatory proteins or by downregulating the genes encoding pro-inflammatory transcription factors is an exhilarating target in the treatment of obesity.

22.3.4 Thyroid disorders

Thyroid hormone synthesis and function requires micronutrients, mostly iodine and selenium. Iodine being avital constituent of thyroid hormones, its deficit can cause thyroid dysfunction and is considered as the main widespread reason for the preventable brain damage in the world. There are many disorders related to iodine deficiency which includes goiter, hypothyroidism and mental retardation. And consumption of iodized salt; an iodine supplementation results in decrease of these disorders. Moreover, high carbohydrate diet results in a higher T3 production which in turn leads to amplified iodine requirement. This elevated iodine requirement surpasses the iodine availability from environmental sources, consequential in the development of iodine deficiency disorders. Not only this, but iodine overload has also been associated with tendency for autoimmune thyroid disease and rarely hyperthyroidism, known as the Jod–Basedow phenomenon [111].

Apart from this, three diverse selenium-dependent iodothyronine deiodinases (types I, II and III) are critical in functioning of thyroid hormones and this makes selenium an essential micronutrient for optimal and favorable thyroid function. Besides, selenium also protects the thyroid from oxidative radical damage, because of its presence in the catalytic center of enzymes as selenocysteine. Few substances like thiocyanate and isoflavones introduced with food, also have been shown to interfere with micronutrients and influence thyroid function. Few other micronutrients such as iron, perchlorate, zinc and vitamin A too have an essential role in thyroid function [112]. Thus, deficiency of one or more of these micronutrients alone or together can affect iodine nutrition and thyroid physiology, stressing the significance of a balanced nutritious diet, dietary supplements or micronutrient supplementation to control and cure the disorders related to thyroid dysfunctioning [63].

22.3.4.1 Carnitine

Carnitine is a naturally occurring quaternary amine; ubiquitous in mammalian tissues; and as per the study data, as old as 40 years ago, was considered a peripheral antagonist of thyroid hormone (TH) action. Few older studies showed that carnitine contrasted the TH-induced changes related with the nitrogen balance in rats and metamorphosis of tadpoles. In more recent studies, carnitine showed inhibition of the thyroxine (T4)-induced liver and circulating concentration of both alanine aminotransferase (ALT) and aspartate aminotransferase (AST) [113]. L-carnitine has also revealed inhibition of cell entry and on the whole nuclear entry, of triiodothyronine (T3) and T4, in tissue culture experiments on human skin fibroblasts, human hepatoma cells HepG2 and mouse neuroblastoma cells NB 41A3, without inhibiting TH efflux from cells, and TH binding to isolated nuclei. These results establish that carnitine is a peripheral antagonist of TH action, and that one level of inhibition occurring at the nuclear envelope or before it [114].

Few studies have sought the effect of L-carnitine in the neoplastic setting of the thyroid and have found that L-carnitine generates metabolic energy in living cells by transporting long-chain acyl groups from fatty acids into the mitochondrial matrix. While treatment with L-carnitine has revealed to induce ATP generation in normal cells, it has shown to selectively attenuate cancer cell growth both in *in-vitro* and *in-vivo* models [115]. However, it is contradictory that the expression of carnitine palmitoyl transferase 1C (Cpt1c) (enzyme involved in this transport), has been detected at elevated levels in papillary thyroid tissues in comparison to normal ones; and Cpt1c up-regulation has been stipulated to promote cancer cell growth and metastasis in human papillary thyroid carcinomas cell lines [116]. Lately, carnitine has been established as a prospective biomarker candidate with ability differentiate between normal and thyroid cancer cells, nonetheless, additional studies are required to confirm carnitine as the diagnostic oncometabolite in thyroid cancer. Interestingly, a recent Turkish study [117] demonstrated the protective effects of amifostine (200 mg/kg ip), L-carnitine (200 mg/kg ip), or vitamin E (40 mg/kg im) in high dose radioactive iodine (131I) treatment-induced salivary gland damage in guinea pig animal model, the result of which showed that the three molecules exhibited different levels of protection against radioactive iodine treatment injury in salivary glands; yet, none of the agents could provide absolute protection.

22.3.4.2 Resveratrol

Resveratrol (3,5,40-trihydroxy-trans-stilbene) is a stilbenoid polyphenol found in a variety of vegetables and fruit, e.g. peanuts, peanut sprouts and grapes, and it appears to have a significant role as a chemo-preventive and therapeutic agent to treat different diseases [118] and thus has gained more attention among health professionals and other nutrition experts in current time.

Resveratrol has antioxidant, anti-inflammatory and antidiabetic effects, and its cardioprotective protective actions, predominantly, are related with various molecular targets, including apoptosis, inflammation, oxidative stress, angiogenesis, mitochondrial dysfunction and platelet aggregation [119]. A study conducted in a rat model of hemi-thyroid electrocauterization induced subclinical hypothyroidism (SCH), elucidated the effect and potential mechanism of resveratrol on memory and spatial learning. Resveratrol (15 mg/kg) and levothyroxine treatment in SCH rats demonstrated an inversion of learning and memory impairment in behavioral test. Resveratrol treatment of SCH rats caused attenuation in the expression of hypothalamic thyrotropin releasing hormone (TRH) mRNA and decreased plasma TSH which indicated that resveratrol treatment would reverse the hypothalamic–pituitary–thyroid (HPT) axis imbalance in SCH rats. In addition, up-regulation of syt-1 and brain-derived neurotrophic factor (BDNF) levels in the hippocampus was also revealed in the same study; to sum up, resveratrol treatment has found to improve spatial learning and memory of SHC rats [120].

Furthermore, the antiproliferative effect of resveratrol is dependent on the induction of ERK1/2-and p53-dependent antiproliferation in tumoral cells, binding to a specific receptor on plasma membrane integrin $\alpha v\beta 3$, and the accumulation of resveratrol-induced nuclear COX-2; consecutively, transcriptionally active complex is generated by COX-2 combining with ERK1/2, and eventually with p53 [121]. Physiological concentrations of thyroid hormone (TH), especially T4, hamper the antiproliferative and anticancer action of resveratrol which advocates that the *in-vivo* block of the surface receptor for TH on cancer cells, in addition to the decline in circulating levels of T4 and the substitution of T3 (to maintain a condition of euthyroidism), may possibly be used as approaches to recuperate or potentiate the clinical effectiveness of resveratrol in cancer treatment. Resveratrol has demonstrated to inhibit gene expression of sodium/iodide symporter (NIS) and function in FRTL-5 cells, declining cellular iodide uptake after 48 h treatment and the same effect was confirmed in *in-vivo* Sprague–Dawley rats [122]. In recent times, resveratrol has been explored for its antithyroid effects *in-vitro* and *in-vivo* models. Precisely, in FRTL-5 cells, resveratrol has shown to attenuate the expression of thyroid-specific genes, such as Tg, TPO, TSHR, NKX2-1, Foxe1 and PAX8, whereas in rats treated with resveratrol 25 mg/kg i.p. for 60 days, a significant elevation in serum TSH levels together with enlargement in thyroid size was observed as compared with control rats [123]. As far as the role of resveratrol as antineoplastic agent is concerned, it has been lately established that it restrains cell proliferation through STAT3 signaling involvement and reverses retinoic acid resistance of anaplastic thyroid cancer cells [124]. Moreover, since resveratrol also has a role in iodine trapping, it seems to be a promising anti-thyroid drug. On the whole, the *in-vitro* and *in-vivo* records designate resveratrol as a thyroid disruptor and a goitrogen, and a consideration should be given for potential therapeutic use of resveratrol or as a supplement.

22.3.4.3 Selenium

Selenium is a nonmetal element and an important micronutrient required for cellular function found in dietary items like meat and meat products (31%), fish and shellfish (20%), pasta and rice (12%), and bread and breakfast cereals (11%), though the highest selenium concentrations (1 mg/kg) is found in Brazil nuts and offal. Selenium exercises its nutritional physiology in the form of the amino acid seleno cysteine (SeCys) which is inserted into a group of proteins called "selenoproteins", some examples of which are antioxidant enzymes, glutathione peroxidase (GSH-Px) and thioredoxin reductase, and the three deiodinases of thyroid hormones [125].

A study has assessed the effect of selenium on CD4(+)CD25(+)Foxp3(+) regulatory T cells (Treg) employing an iodine-induced AIT model [126]; the objective of which was to elucidate clinical observations concerning decreased serum levels of thyroid autoantibodies in patients with autoimmune thyroiditis (AIT). NOD.H-2(h4) mice received 0.005% sodium iodine (NaI) water for 8 weeks for induction of AIT; while the group of selenium-treated mice received 0.3 mg/L sodium selenite in drinking water. The results of this study showed that selenium-treated mice have a higher number of Treg cells and higher Foxp3 mRNA expression in splenocytes compared to AIT mice. Additionally, lower serum Tg antibody (TgAb) titers and reduced lymphocytic infiltration were observed in selenium-treated AIT mice thyroid than untreated AIT mice. These data demonstrated that selenium supplementation can restore normal levels of CD4(+)CD25(+) T cells in mice with AIT, through the up-regulation of the Foxp3 mRNA expression [126]. Likewise, data are also available for human cell lines of thyroid malignancy ARO (anaplastic), NPA (BRAF positive papillary), WRO (BRAF negative papillary) and FRO (follicular) cells treated with 150 μM seleno-l-methionine (SM), in the thyroid oncology setting, which were assessed for viability at 24, 48 and 72 h. Seleno-methionine treatment inhibited thyroid cancer cell proliferation through the over-expression of GADD (growth arrest and DNA damage inducible) family genes and cell cycle arrest in S and G2/M phases [127]. Although these data are captivating, the offered substantiation on the association of selenium and thyroid cancer is yet unconvincing and require further studies.

22.3.5 Bone disorders

Nutrition has foremost role in the prevention and treatment of bone disorders, such as rickets, osteomalacia and osteoporosis; For bone metabolism, dietary protein is the macronutrient as well as calcium and vitamin D are the micronutrients of major importance [128].

22.3.5.1 Rickets/osteomalacia

One of the most critical factors to attain optimal peak bone mass is the adequate intake of calcium; second factor is vitamin D which is essential for intestinal calcium absorption. Low calcium due to vitamin D deficiency leads to overactivation of parathyroid gland, which in turn releases calcium and phosphorus from the bone [129], the snowballing effects is decreased bone mineralization and disorganized growth leading to characteristic deformities. Milk, dairy products, dark green vegetables and nuts are the finest sources of calcium and sunlight, fish-liver oils like cod liver oil, fatty fish, and liver of vitamin D. Nutritional rickets is defined as disorder of growing bones caused by calcium and vitamin D deficiency individually or both in combination and is characterized by late fontanelle closure, craniotabes, distended wrists and skeletal malformations. Thus, a daily intake of 400–800 IU of vitamin D together with 1,000 mg of calcium is recommended dose to prevent the nutritional bone disorders.

22.3.5.2 Osteoporosis

Osteoporosis, a disease characterized by low bone mass and microarchitectural deterioration responsible for amplified fracture risk of the bones, is yet another disorder having its association with dietary composition. Excess dietary protein is unfavorable to bone health because of risk of hypercalciuria and acidosis; Hypercalciuria is caused due to increase in glomerular filtration rate and decrease in tubular calcium reabsorption, which further results in negative calcium balance [130].

22.3.5.3 Fluorosis

Fluorosis is a skeletal disease caused by the consumption of excess fluoride [131], which forms an insoluble salt-like calcium fluoride which eventually leads to increase in bone density but decrease in bone strength. The disease characterized by pain and stiffness of joints, arthritis, enamel abnormalities, skeletal deformities and other systemic effects is best prevented by defluoridation of water prior to consumption.

22.3.6 Gonadal disorders

Nutritional excess and nutritional deficits both are responsible for a wide array of endocrine disorders including reproductive system-related dysfunctions. For example, nutritional excess state in the last century has led to a trend of increased height and early puberty in children which might be partly explained by the effects of various endocrine disruptors. Industrialization in recent years has also increased pollutants and contaminants in the nature, which are ingested knowingly or unknowingly into the human body through dietary constituents. Numerous endocrine disruptors, such as phytoestrogens, topical, and natural estrogens, pesticides, industrial chemicals and phthalates, have been recognized as agents affecting pubertal development; The putative mechanism of these endocrine disruptors have been found to be estrogenic/androgenic/antiestrogenic as well as antiandrogenic in nature [132] and might lead to precocious puberty, delayed puberty, or sexual differentiation disorders.

Furthermore, omega-3 polyunsaturated fatty acids present in fish oil ameliorated high-fat-diet-induced reproductive dysfunction in male C57BL/6 mouse by amendment in the rhythmic expression of testosterone synthesis-related genes [133]. Preclinical studies conducted in mice have revealed positive association of dietary intake of omega-3 and omega-6 polyunsaturated fatty acids with the implantation rate by modulating the uterine phospholipid fatty acid composition and arachidonic acid levels. A study by Dikshit et al. [134] demonstrated that α-linolenic acid, a major component of flaxseeds exerted anti-inflammatory and anti-pro-carcinogenic environment in the ovaries of normal hens by significantly attenuating inflammatory prostaglandin E2, ER-α, cytochrome (CYP) P450, CYP3A4, CYP1B1 and 16α-hydroxyestrone (16-OHE1), along with increased levels of CYP1A1 and 2-OHE1. These data evidently propose fatty acids can modulate the streoidogenic targets.

At present, perspectives of plant-derived compounds in improvement of fertility in humans and animals have become a blazing area of research. Polyphenols play a significant role in the continuance of healthy pregnancy through regulation of targets associated with inflammation and oxidative stress. Studies have also shown that hydroxytyrosol supplementation in the maternal diet (1.5 mg/kg of food) during the early pregnancy can help off springs gaining mean birth weight, which is suggestive of beneficial effects of polyphenols in both the pre- and post-natal developments of the offsprings [135]. These effects can be attributed to the antioxidant, anti-inflammatory and immune-modulatory properties of polyphenols. Of late, dietary polyphenols like epigallocatechin-3-gallate (EGCG) supplementation have demonstrated improvement in the quality of male and female gametes, predominantly owing to their ability to quench reactive oxygen species. Additionally, high doses (50 μM) of quercetin, catechin and resveratrol have also shown to boost antioxidant activity in human and animal semen; in that way polyphenols can be deemed as useful tools for semen cryopreservation, where they have shown to improve the sperm motility, survival and integrity of the DNA in cryopreserved samples [136]. Quite the opposite, green tea-derived polyphenols reduced the testosterone levels in the animals by declining the activities of steroidogenic enzymes [137] or by direct or indirect attenuation of P450scc and 17β-HSD in a dose-dependent manner. All these data suggest that the property of polyphenols can be successfully employed to design herbal drugs for reproductive endocrine disorders like polycystic ovarian syndrome (PCOS) wherein the hyperandrogenism lies in the core of pathology.

Research has shown that β-sitosterol has estrogen-like effects and transforms the steroidogenic pathway by altering the P450scc activity, thus impairing the conversion of cholesterol to pregnenolone. A study showed altered sexual development, changes in hormone production, decreased egg production and decreased spawning rate in fish exposed to phytosterols [138]. A reduction of reproductive steroid levels and changes in gonadal steroidogenesis was also observed in goldfish exposed to 75 μg/L 13 phytosterols [139]. In sub-chronic rodent studies, it has been found that merely at small doses (0.5–50 mg/kg/day) phytosterols caused changes in the weights of reproductive organs; e.g. when β-sitosterol was administered subcutaneously, it led to decrease in testicular weight and sperm density in male rats [140] and increase in uterine weights in female rats [141] and immature sheep (Ovisaries) [142]. Moreover, treatment of streptozotocin-induced diabetic male rats with 28-homobrassinolide (333 mg/ kg body weight) for 15 consecutive days to diminished LPO, amplified antioxidant enzyme, 3β-HSD and 17β-HSD activities, and elevated Steroidogenic Acute Regulatory Protein (StAR) and Androgen Binding Protein (ABP) expression and testosterone level in rat testis. Additionally, long-term effects of a dietary phytosterols mixture (5 mg/kg/ day), containing mainly beta sitosterol, revealed increased plasma levels of testosterone and decreased relative uterine weights in the pups of F [2] and F [4] generations in mouse model. Besides, phytosterol exposure augmented the concentrations of plasma estradiol in the female pups of F [3] generation and testicular levels of testosterone in the male pups of F [2] generations [143]. However, some degree of evidence from animal studies proposes that very high phytosterol intakes can modify testosterone metabolism by inhibiting a membrane-bound enzyme, 5α-reductase that converts testosterone to dihydrotestosterone, a more potent metabolite. A study has also demonstrated that dietary intake of coumestrol decreases the amplitude of LH pulses in ewes [144], thus signifying that phytosterols and its metabolites may act as GnRH modulators. Furthermore, in treatment of polycystic ovarian syndrome (PCOS) [female endocrine disorder, which is characterized by hyperandrogenism, insulin resistance and presence of multiple peripheral cysts in the ovaries], lower doses of phytosterol have found to be effective. A study by Maharjan and Nampoothiri [145] confirmed that phytosterols-containing nonpolar extract of Aloe vera gel at the dose of 25 μg/kg body weight for 60 days could efficiently manage the reproductive as well as metabolic complication associated with PCOS in Letrozole induced PCOS in rats. PCOS rats showed a reduction in serum testosterone and insulin level with improved estradiol and progesterone levels after treatment with nonpolar extract of Aloe vera gel, along with a decrement in transcripts level of StAR, Luteinizing Hormone Receptor, Androgen Receptor, Aromatase and IR as well as relative protein expression of StAR, 3β-HSD and aromatase expression. Moreover, consumption of phytosterols is getting recognition among menopausal women as well with escalating substantiation that they are favorable in relieving symptoms as well as in protection of certain cancers. Extensive promising evidence supports the inhibitory actions of phytosterols on various cancer like breast, ovarian and lung cancers. As a whole, however, phytosterols appear to act through multiple mechanisms, including inhibition of angiogenesis, invasion and metastasis, cell growth, carcinogen production, and through augmenting apoptotic death of cancer cells as well as [146] increase in the activity of antioxidant enzymes and thereby reduced oxidative stress.

22.3.7 Growth disorders

Malnutrition is one of the widespread causes of short stature in many countries, still prevalent in some developing countries. Marasmus is a disorder of deficiency of calories including proteins, whereas kwashiorkor is characterized by protein deficiency alone. Statural growth of a child is dependent on not only the genetic potential but also environmental influences, and underlying disease condition as well as food habits and nutrition levels. In nutritional short stature, the decline in weight precedes the linear growth failure; the impaired growth is because of the state of GH resistance with normal GH and reduced insulin-like growth factor-1 (IGF-1) levels, and the inability of growth hormones to stimulate the transcription of growth factors with inadequate nutritional support and sporadically the levels of GH are lower in states of chronic malnourishment [147].

22.4 The future of nutraceuticals

The ever-escalating nutraceutical market in recent times signifies that end users are seeking modestly processed food with extra nutritional benefits and organoleptic value. This change in the mindset of public, consecutively, is driving the expansion of nutraceutical markets globally, and it seems that this surge is destined to inhabit the landscape in the new millennium. This growth and development have propositions for the food, pharmaceutical, healthcare and agricultural industries. Many researchers believe that enzymes embody another exciting frontier in nutraceuticals. Thus, global trends to healthy products cannot be reversed at this point of time [148]. Recent advances in nutraceuticals supplied through oral or transdermal delivery system would offer well targeted health benefits with optimal bioavailability. Moreover, with the evolution of "Smart Nutraceuticals", a Futuristic "Physician's Desk Reference" would enclose information on individual genetic profiles, which could be matched with specific nutritional interventions as well; and this would be an immense enhancement over current nutritional recommendations, which being too generalized benefit only 60% of population [149].

22.5 Conclusion

Nutrients in the form of dietary intake, supplements and nutraceuticals are accountable for many well-recognized health benefits and improving the morbidity in patients having chronic diseases. Different mechanisms are stipulated, not limited to reduction of oxidative stress, changes in the signal transduction pathways, modulation of cell survival-cell death pathways, proliferation, differentiation and development of cellular and mitochondrial integrity, along with an array of biological and biochemical progressions. The existing acquaintance in the field of nutrition and disease emphasizes the necessity to evaluate the concurrent and synchronized use of nutraceuticals and pharmaceuticals that affects the cellular and molecular levels, which approaches the real practical situations. Moreover, in view of increased prevalence of endocrine disorders in recent time release, presence of dietary items in the usual doses, and the availability of nutraceuticals as supplements or add-ons for therapeutics and chemoprevention, it is has become of utmost importance to study in-depth role and contributions of dietary supplements/nutraceuticals and outline the mutual inflections of the actions of these substances in the endocrinological disorders. Since this comprehensive assessment and evaluation of interfaces of endocrine disorders and nutraceuticals, elucidation of the molecular mechanisms, and determination of intervention with endogenous hormones if any, will establish nutraceuticals/dietary supplements as adjuvant therapies or a major revolution in pharmacotherapy.

References

1. Johnson M. Dietary interventions for the potential prevention, treatment and management of endocrine disorders. *Endocrinol Metab Syndr.* 2017;6:5.
2. Mlynarcikova AB and Scsukova S. Endocrine disruptors, nutraceuticals and their simultaneous effects in hormone-sensitive tissues: A review. *RRJPPS* 2016;5(2): 12–20.
3. Gupta SK, Yadav SK, Patil SM. Nutraceutical – A bright scope and oppourtunity of indian healthcare market. *Intern J Res Develop Pharm Life Sci.* 2013;2(4):478–481.
4. Singh R, Geetanjali. Nutraceuticals: Promising health product. *Intern Res J Med Sci.* 2013;1(1):14–17.
5. Dahiya K. Nutraceuticals and their impact on human health. *J Plant Biochem Physiol.* 2013;1(4):1–3.
6. Rama CS, Shirode AR, Mundada AS, Kadam VJ. Nutraceuticals – an emerging era in the treatment and prevention of cardiovascular diseases. *Curr Pharm Biotechnol.* 2006;7(10):15–23.
7. Butler LM, Wu AH, Wang R, Koh W-P, Yuan J-M, Yu MC. A vegetable-fruit-soy dietary pattern protects against breast cancer among postmenopausal Singapore Chinese women. *Am J Clin Nutr.* 2010;91:1013–1019.
8. Nagata Y,Sonoda T, Mori M et al. Dietary isoflavones may protect against prostate cancer in Japanese men. *J Nutr.* 2007;137:1974–1979.
9. Haddad AQ, Venkateswaran V, Viswanathan L, Teahan SJ, Fleshner NE, Klotz LH. Novel antiproliferative flavonoids induce cell cycle arrest in human prostate cancer cell lines. *Prostate Cancer Prostatic Dis.* 2006;9:68–76.
10. Shrubsole MJ, Lu W, Chen Z et al. Drinking green tea modestly reduces breast cancer risk. *J Nutr.* 2009;139:310–316.
11. Mocanu MM, Nagy P, Szöllősi J. Chemoprevention of breast cancer by dietary polyphenols. *Molecules* 2015;20:22578–22620.
12. Baliga MS, Haniadka R, Pereira MM et al. Update on the chemo preventive effects of ginger and its phytochemicals. *Crit Rev Food Sci Nutr.* 2011;51:499–523.
13. Licznerska BE,Szaefer H, Murias M, Bartoszek A, Baer-Dubowska W. Modulation of CYP19 expression by cabbage juices and their active components: Indole-3-carbinol and 3, 3'-diindolylmethene in human breast epithelial cell lines. *Eur J Nutr.* 2013;52:1483–1492.
14. Barnes K, Lauren Ball L, Ben Desbrow B, Naser Alsharairi N, Faruk Ahmed F. Consumption and reasons for use of dietary supplements in an Australian university population. *Nutrition* 2016;32:524–530.

15. Singh AM, Dubey R, Paliwal RT, Saraogi GK, Singhai AK. Nutraceuticals-an emerging era in the treatment and prevention of diseases. *Int J Pharm Pharmac Sci.* 2012;4(4):39–43.

16. Sosnowska B., Penson P, Banach M. The role of nutraceuticals in the prevention of cardiovascular disease. *Cardiovasc Diagnosis Ther.* 2017;7:S21.

17. Chintale AG, Kadam VS, Sakhare RS, Birajdar GO, Nalwad DN. Role of nutraceuticals in various diseases: A comprehensive review. *Int J Pharm Pharmac Sci.* 2013;3:290–299.

18. Tremmel M., Gerdtham U.-G, Nilsson P, Saha S. Economic burden of obesity: A systematic literature review. *Int J Environ Res Public Health.* 2017;14.4:435.

19. Meriga B., GanjayiMS, Parim BN. Phytocompounds as potential agents to treat obesity-cardiovascular ailments. *Cardiovasc Hematol Agents Med Chem.* 2017;15(2):104–120.

20. Desai BN, Maharjan RH, Nampoothiri LP. Aloe barbadensis Mill. formulation restores lipid profile to normal in a letrozole-induced polycystic ovarian syndrome rat model. *Pharmacog Res.* 2012;4(2):109.

21. Reddy PS, Begum N, Mutha S, Bakshi V. Beneficial effect of Curcumin in Letrozole induced polycystic ovary syndrome. *Asian Pac J Reprod.* 2016;5(2):116–22.

22. Mora-Esteves C and Shin D. Nutrient supplementation: Improving male fertility fourfold. *Semin Reprod Med.* 2013;31:293–300.

23. Ruder EH, Hartman TJ, Reindollar RH, Goldman MB. Female dietary antioxidant intake and time to pregnancy among couples treated for unexplained infertility. *Fertil Steril.* 2014;101:759–766.

24. Anagnostis P, Karras S, Goulis DG. Vitamin D in human reproduction: A narrative review. *Int J Clin Pract.* 2013;67:225–235.

25. Li MJ, Yin Y-C, Wang J, Jiang YF. Green tea compounds in breast cancer prevention and treatment. *World J Clin Oncol.* 2014;5:520–528.

26. Shrubsole MJ, Lu W, Chen Z. Drinking green tea modestly reduces breast cancer risk. *J Nutr.* 2009;139(2):310–316.

27. Brandt JZ,Silveira LTR, Grassi TF et al. Indole-3-carbinol attenuates the deleterious gestational effects of bisphenol A exposure on the prostate gland of male F1 rats. *Reprod Toxicol.* 2014;43:56–66.

28. Showell MG, Mackenzie-Proctor R, Jordan V, Hart RJ. Antioxidants for female subfertility. *Cochrane Database Syst Rev.* 2013;8:CD007807.

29. Klein EA, Thompson Jr IM, Tangen CM et al. Vitamin E and the risk of prostate cancer: The Selenium and Vitamin E Cancer Prevention Trial (SELECT). *JAMA* 2011;306:1549–1556.

30. Katchy A, Pinto C, Jonsson P et al. Coexposure to phytoestrogens and bisphenol a mimics estrogenic effects in an additive manner. *Toxicol Sci.* 2014;138:21–35.

31. Nordeen SK, Bona BJ, Jones DN, Lambert JR, Jackson TA. Endocrine disrupting activities of the flavonoid nutraceuticals luteolin and quercetin. *Horm Cancer* 2013;4:293–300.

32. Fan YC and Chan WH. Epigallocatechin gallate induces embryonic toxicity in mouse blastocysts through apoptosis. *Drug Chem Toxicol.* 2014;37:247–254.

33. Russo M, Russo GL, Daglia M et al. Understanding genistein in cancer: The "good" and the "bad" effects: A review. *Food Chem.* 2016;196:589–600.

34. Sinha D, Sarkar N, Biswas J, Bishayee A. Resveratrol for breast cancer prevention and therapy: Preclinical evidence and molecular mechanisms. *Semin Cancer Biol.* 2016;40–41:209–232.

35. Berberich AJ, Hegele RA. Nutraceuticals in 2017: Nutraceuticals in endocrine disorders. *Nat Rev Endocrinol.* 2018;14(2):68.

36. Kopp W. Nutrition, evolution and thyroid hormone levels – A link to iodine deficiency disorders? *Med Hypotheses* 2004;62:871–875.

37. Ozkan B. Nutritional rickets. *J Clin Res Pediatr Endocrinol.* 2010;2:137–143.

38. Diamanti-Kandarakis E, Palioura E, Kandarakis SA, Koutsilieris M. The impact of endocrine disruptors on endocrine targets. *Horm Metab Res*. 2010;42:543–552.
39. Derosa G., D'Angelo A, Romano D, Maffioli P. A clinical trial about a food supplement containing α-lipoic acid on oxidative stress markers in type 2 diabetic patients. *Int J Mol Sci*. 2016;17(11):1802.
40. Rosenberg K. "Omega-3 fatty acid intake lowers risk of diabetic retinopathy". *AJN Am J Nur*. 2017;117(1):60–61.
41. Dikshit A., Gao C, Small C, Hale K, Hales DB. Flaxseed and its components differentially affect estrogen targets in pre-neoplastic hen ovaries. *J Steroid Biochem Mol Biol*. 2016;159:73–85.
42. Otton R., Bolin AP, Ferreira LT, Marinovic MP, Rocha ALS, Mori MA. Polyphenol-rich green tea extract improves adipose tissue metabolism by down-regulating miR-335 expression and mitigating insulin resistance and inflammation. *J Nutr Biochem*. 2018;57:170–179.
43. Burgess TA., Robich MP, Chu LM, Bianchi C, Sellke FW. Improving glucose metabolism with resveratrol in a swine model of metabolic syndrome through alteration of signaling pathways in the liver and skeletal muscle. *Arch Surg*. 2011;146:556–564.
44. Um JH., Park SJ, Kang H et al. AMP-activated protein kinase–deficient mice are resistant to the metabolic effects of resveratrol. *Diabetes* 2010;59(3):554–563.
45. Chen KH., Cheng M-L, Jing Y-H, Chiu DT-Y, Shiao M-S, Chenet J-K. Resveratrol ameliorates metabolic disorders and muscle wasting in streptozotocin-induced diabetic rats. *Am J Physiol-Endocrinol Metabol*. 2011;301:E853–E863.
46. Do GM, Jung UJ, Hae-Jin Park H-J et.al. Resveratrol ameliorates diabetes-related metabolic changes via activation of AMP-activated protein kinase and its downstream targets in db/b mice. *Mol Nutr Food Res*. 2012;56:1282–1291.
47. Yang SJ and Lim Y. Resveratrol ameliorates hepatic metaflammation and inhibits NLRP3 inflammasome activation. *Metabol Clin Exp*. 2014;63:693–701.
48. Kang W., Honh HJ, Guan J et al. Resveratrol improves insulin signaling in a tissue-specific manner under insulin-resistant conditions only: In vitro and in vivo experiments in rodents. *Metabol-Clin Exp*. 2012;61:424–433.
49. Achrekar S, Kaklij GS, Pote MS, Kelkar SM. Hypoglycemic activity of Eugenia jambolana and Ficus bengalenesis: Mechanism of action. *In Vivo* 1991;5(2):143–147.
50. Prince PS, Menon VP, Pari L. Hypoglycaemic activity of Syzigium cumini seeds: Effect on lipid peroxidation in alloxan diabetic rats. *J Ethnopharmacol*. 1998;61(1):1–7.
51. Rabinkov A, Miron T, Konstantinovski L, Wilchek M, Mirelman D, Weiner L. The mode of action of allicin: Trapping of radicals and interaction with thiol containing proteins. *Biochim Biophys Acta*. 1998;1379(2):233–244.
52. Anuradha CV, Ravikumar P. Restoration on tissue antioxidants by fenugreek seeds (Trigonella foenum graecum) in alloxan-diabetic rats. *Indian J Physiol Pharmacol*. 2001;45(4):408–420.
53. Wadood A, Wadood N, Shah SA. Effects of Acacia arabica and Caralluma edulis on blood glucose levels of normal and alloxan diabetic rabbits. *J Pak Med Assoc*. 1989;39(8):208–212.
54. Sachdewa A, Raina D, Srivastava AK, Khemani LD. Effect of Aegle marmelos and Hibiscus rosa sinensis leaf extract on glucose tolerance in glucose induced hyperglycemic rats (Charles foster). *J Environ Biol*. 2001;22:53–57.
55. Sharma SR, Dwivedi SK, Swarup D. Hypoglycemic, antihyperglycemic and hypolipidemic activities of Caesalpinia bonducella seeds in rats. *J Ethnopharmacol*. 1997;58:39–44.
56. Shibib BA, Khan LA, Rahman R. Hypoglycemic activity of Coccinia indica and Momordica charantia in diabetic rats: Depression of the hepatic gluconeogenic enzymes glucose-6-phosphatase and fructose-1, 6- bisphosphatase and elevation of both liver and red-cell shunt enzyme glucose-6-phosphate dehydrogenase. *Biochem J*. 1993;292(Pt 1):267–270.

57. Kamble SM, Kamlakar PL, Vaidya S, Bambole VD. Influence of Coccinia indica on certain enzymes in glycolytic and lipolytic pathway in human diabetes. *Indian J Med Sci.* 1998;52(4):143–146.

58. Asare Anane H, Huang GC, Amiel SA, Jones PM, Persaud SJ. Poster Presentations-Stimulation of insulin secretion by an aqueous extract of Gymnema sylvestre: Role of intracellular calcium. *Endocrine Abstracts.* 2005;10:1.

59. Handa SS, Chawla AS, Maninder NA. Hypoglycemic plants-a review. *Fitoterapia.* 2004;15(3):195–224.

60. Gholap S, Kar A. Hypoglycaemic effects of some plant extracts are possibly mediated through inhibition in corticosteroid concentration. *Pharmazie.* 2004;59(11):876–878.

61. Vats V, Yadav SP, Biswas NR, Grover JK. Anti-cataract activity of Pterocarpus marsupium bark and Trigonella foenum-graecum seeds extract in alloxan diabetic rats. *J Ethnopharmacol.* 2004;93(2–3):289–294.

62. Shani J, Goldsehmied A, Joseph B, Ahronson Z, Sulman FG. Hypoglycemic effect of Trigonella foenum graecum and Lupinus termis (Leguiminosae) seeds and their major alkaloids in alloxan-diabetic and normal rats. *Arch Int Pharmacodyn Ther.* 1974;210(1):27–37.

63. Hari Kumar KVS, Baruah MM. Nutritional endocrine disorders. *J Med Nut Nutraceutic.* 2012;1(1):5–8.

64. Westerterp-Plantenga MS, Nieuwenhuizen A, Tome D, Soenen S, Westerterp KR. Dietary protein, weight loss, and weight maintenance. *Annu Rev Nutr.* 2009;29:21–41.

65. Pan A, Sun Q, Bernstein AM, Manson JE, Willett WC, Hu FB. Changes in red meat consumption and subsequent risk of type 2 diabetes mellitus: Three cohorts of US men and women. *JAMA Intern Med.* 2013;173:1328–1335.

66. Virtanen HEK, Koskinen TT, Voutilainen S, Mursu J, Tuomainen TP, Kokko P, Virtanen JK. Intake of different dietary proteins and risk of type 2 diabetes in men: The Kuopio Ischaemic Heart Disease Risk Factor Study. *Br J Nutr.* 2017;117:882–893.

67. Chalvon-Demersay T, Azzout-Marniche D, Arfsten J, et al. A systematic review of the effects of plant compared with animal protein sources on features of metabolic syndrome. *J Nutr.* 2017;147:281–292.

68. Arnoldi A, Boschin G, Zanoni C, Lammi C. The health benefits of sweet lupin seed flours and isolated proteins. *J Funct Foods.* 2015;18:550–563.

69. Bertoglio JC, Calvo MA, Hancke JL, et al. Hypoglycemic effect of lupin seed c-conglutin in experimental animals and healthy human subjects. *Fitoterapia* 2011;82:933–938.

70. Scirica BM, Bhatt DL, Braunwald E, et al. Saxagliptin and cardiovascular outcomes in patients with type 2 diabetes mellitus. *N Engl J Med.* 2013;369:1317–1326.

71. Lammi C, Zanoni C, Arnoldi A, Vistoli G. Peptides derived from soy and lupin protein as dipeptidyl-peptidase IV inhibitors: In vitro biochemical screening and in silico molecular modeling study. *J Agric Food Chem.* 2016;64:9601–9606.

72. Sirtori CR, Triolo M, Bosisio R, et al. Hypocholesterolaemic effects of lupin protein and pea protein/fibre combinations in moderately hypercholesterolaemic individuals. *Br J Nutr.* 2012;107:1176–1183.

73. Pavanello C, Lammi C, Ruscica M, et al. Effects of a lupin protein concentrate on lipids, blood pressure and insulin resistance in moderately dyslipidaemic patients: A randomised controlled trial. *J Funct Foods.* 2017;37:8–15.

74. Lammi C, Zanoni C, Aiello G, Arnoldi A and Grazioso G. Lupin peptides modulate the protein-protein interaction of PCSK9 with the low density lipoprotein receptor in HepG2 cells. *Sci Rep.* 2016;6:29931.

75. Lima-Cabello E, Alche V, Foley RC, et al. Narrowleafed lupin (Lupinus angustifolius L.) beta-conglutin proteins modulate the insulin signaling pathway as potential type 2 diabetes treatment and inflammatory- related disease amelioration. *Mol Nutr Food Res.* 2017;61. doi:10.1002/mnfr.201600819.

76. Sirtori CR, Arnoldi A, Johnson SK. Phytoestrogens: End of a tale? *Ann Med.* 2005;37:423–438.

77. Lovati MR, Manzoni C, Canavesi A, et al. Soybean protein diet increases low density lipoprotein receptor activity in mononuclear cells from hypercholesterolemic patients. *J Clin Invest.* 1987;80:1498–1502.
78. Azadbakht L, Kimiagar M, Mehrabi Y, et al. Soy inclusion in the diet improves features of the metabolic syndrome: A randomized crossover study in postmenopausal women. *Am J Clin Nutr.* 2007;85:735–741.
79. Maki KC, Butteiger DN, Rains TM, et al. Effects of soy protein on lipoprotein lipids and fecal bile acid excretion in men and women with moderate hypercholesterolemia. *J Clin Lipidol.* 2010;4:531–542.
80. Dove ER, Mori TA, Chew GT, et al. Lupin and soya reduce glycaemia acutely in type 2 diabetes. *Br J Nutr.* 2011;106:1045–1051.
81. Vergnaud AC, Norat T, Mouw T, et al. Macronutrient composition of the diet and prospective weight change in participants of the EPIC-PANACEA study. *PLoS One.* 2013;8:e57300.
82. Gunther AL, Remer T, Kroke A, Buyken AE. Early protein intake and later obesity risk: Which protein sources at which time points throughout infancy and childhood are important for body mass index and body fat percentage at 7 y of age? *Am J Clin Nutr.* 2007;86 (6):1765–1772.
83. Mortensen LS, Hartvigsen ML, Brader LJ, et al. Differential effects of protein quality on postprandial lipemia in response to a fat-rich meal in type 2 diabetes: Comparison of whey, casein, gluten, and cod protein. *Am J Clin Nutr.* 2009;90:41–48.
84. Kellow NJ, Coughlan MT, Reid CM. Metabolic benefits of dietary prebiotics in human subjects: A systematic review of randomised controlled trials. *Br J Nutr.* 2014;111(7):1147–1161.
85. Cani PD, Lecourt E, Dewulf EM, et al. Gut microbiota fermentation of prebiotics increases satietogenic and incretin gut peptide production with consequences for appetite sensation and glucose response after a meal. *Am J Clin Nutr.* 2009;90(5):1236–1243.
86. Beserra BT, Fernandes R, do Rosario VA, Mocellin MC, Kuntz MG, Trindade EB. A systematic review and meta-analysis of the prebiotics and synbiotics effects on glycaemia, insulin concentrations and lipid parameters in adult patients with overweight or obesity. *Clin Nutr.* 2015;34(5):845–858.
87. Nikbakht E, Khalesi S, Singh I, Williams LT, West NP, Colson N. Effect of probiotics and synbiotics on blood glucose: A systematic review and meta-analysis of controlled trials. *Eur J Nutr.* 2016;7(1):95–106. doi:10.1007/s00394-016-1300-3.
88. Khan H, Kunutsor S, Franco OH, Chowdhury R. Vitamin D, type 2 diabetes and other metabolic outcomes: A systematic review and meta-analysis of prospective studies. *Proc Nutr Soc.* 2013;72(1):89–97.
89. Ju SY, Jeong HS, Kim DH. Blood vitamin D status and metabolic syndrome in the general adult population: A dose–response meta-analysis. *J Clin Endocrinol Metab.* 2014;99:1053–1063.
90. Pereira-Santos M, Costa PR, Assis AM, Santos CA, Santos DB. Obesity and vitamin D deficiency: A systematic review and meta-analysis. *Obes Rev.* 2015;16(4):341–349.
91. Jorde R. RCTS are the only appropriate way to demonstrate the role of vitamin D in health. *J Steroid Biochem Mol Biol.* 2017;177:10–14 doi:10.1016/ j.jsbmb.2017.05.004.
92. Seo KI, Choi MS, Jung UJ, et al. Effect of curcumin supplementation on blood glucose, plasma insulin, and glucose homeostasis related enzyme activities in diabetic db/db mice. *Mol Nutr Food Res.* 2008;52(9):995–1004.
93. Chuengsamarn S, Rattanamongkolgul S, Luechapudiporn R, Phisalaphong C, Jirawatnotai S. Curcumin extract for prevention of type 2 diabetes. *Diabetes Care* 2012;35(11):2121–2127.
94. Panahi Y, Hosseini MS, Khalili N, et al. Effects of supplementation with curcumin on serum adipokine concentrations: A randomized controlled trial. *Nutrition* 2016;32(10):1116–1122.

95. Panahi Y, Hosseini MS, Khalili N, Naimi E, Majeed M, Sahebkar A. Antioxidant and anti-inflammatory effects of curcuminoid-piperine combination in subjects with metabolic syndrome: A randomized controlled trial and an updated meta-analysis. *Clin Nutr.* 2015;34(4):1101–1108.

96. Kumar P, Malhotra P, Ma K, et al. SREBP2 mediates the modulation of intestinal NPC1L1 expression by curcumin. *Am J Physiol Gastrointest Liver Physiol.* 2011;301(1):G148–G155.

97. Tai MH, Chen PK, Chen PY, Wu MJ, Ho CT, Yen JH. Curcumin enhances cell-surface LDLR level and promotes LDL uptake through downregulation of PCSK9 gene expression in HepG2 cells. *Mol Nutr Food Res.* 2014;58(11):2133–2145.

98. Sahebkar A. Curcuminoids for the management of hypertriglyceridaemia. *Nat Rev Cardiol.* 2014;11:123.

99. Childress L, Gay A, Zargar A, to MK. Review of red yeast rice content and current Food and Drug Administration oversight. *J Clin Lipidol.* 2013;7(2):117–122.

100. Agostoni C, Bresson J-L, Susan Fairweather-Tait S et.al. Scientific opinion on the substantiation of health claims related to monacolin K from red yeast rice and maintenance of normal blood LDL cholesterol concentrations (ID 1648, 1700) pursuant to Article 13(1) of Regulation (EC) No. 1924/2006. 2011. *EFSA Journal* 2011;9(7):2304.

101. Ruscica M, Gomaraschi M, Mombelli G, et al. Nutraceutical approach to moderate cardiometabolic risk: Results of a randomized, double-blind and crossover study with Armolipid plus. *J Clin Lipidol.* 2014;8(1):61–68.

102. Affuso F, Ruvolo A, Micillo F, Saccà L, Fazio S. Effects of a nutraceutical combination (berberine, red yeast rice and policosanols) on lipid levels and endothelial function randomized, double-blind, placebo-controlled study. *Nutr Metab Cardiovasc Dis.* 2010;20(9):656–661.

103. Martínez-Fernández L, Laiglesia LM, Huerta AE, Martínez JA, Moreno-Aliaga MJ. Omega-3 fatty acids and adipose tissue function in obesity and metabolic syndrome. *Prostaglandins Other Lipid Mediat.* 2015;121 (Pt A):24–41.

104. Suzuki R.,Tanaka T, Takanashi M et al. Anthocyanidins-enriched bilberry extracts inhibit 3T3-L1 adipocyte differentiation via the insulin pathway. *Nutr Metab.* 2011;8:14.

105. Karlsen A., Paur I, Bøhnet SK et al. Bilberry juice modulates plasma concentration of NF-κB related inflammatory markers in subjects at increased risk of CVD. *Eur J Nutr.* 2010;49:345–355.

106. Kwon SH., Ahn IS, Kim SO et al. Anti-obesity and hypolipidemic effects of black soybean anthocyanins. *J Med Food.* 2007;10(3):552–556.

107. Saravanan G., Ponmurugan P, Deepa MA, Senthilkumar B. Anti-obesity action of gingerol: Effect on lipid profile, insulin, leptin, amylase and lipase in male obese rats induced by a high-fat diet. *J Sci Food Agr.* 2014;94(14):2972–2977.

108. Sekiya N, Shibahara N, Sakakibara I, Hattori N, Goto H, Terasawa K. Inhibitory effects of Oren-Gedoku-To (Huanglian- Jie-Du-Tang) on free radical-induced lysis of human red blood cells. *Phytother Res.* 2003;17:147–151.

109. Zhang Y, Chan JF, Cummins CL. Liver X receptors as therapeutic targets for managing cholesterol: Implications for inflammatory conditions. *Clin Lipidol.* 2009;4(1):29–40.

110. Marinozzi M, Castro Navas FF, Maggioni D et al. Side-chain modified ergosterol and stigmasterol derivatives as liver X receptor agonists. *J Med Chem.* 2017;60(15):6548–6562.

111. Bürgi H. Iodine excess. *Best Pract Res Clin Endocrinol Metab* 2010;24:107–15.

112. Triggiani V, Tafaro E, Giagulli VA, Sabbà C, Resta F, Licchelli B, et al. Role of iodine, selenium and other micronutrients in thyroid function and disorders. *Endocr Metab Immune Disord Drug Targets* 2009;9(3):277–94.

113. Hellthaler G, Wenzel KW, Rotzsch W. Aminotransferasen unter thyroxin und Karnitin. *Acta Biol German.* 1967;19, 641–652.

114. Benvenga S, Lakshmanan M, Trimarchi F. Carnitine is a naturally occurring inhibitor of thyroid hormone nuclear uptake. *Thyroid.* 2000;10(12):1043–1050.

115. Huang H, Liu N, Guo H, et.al. L-Carnitine Is an Endogenous hdac inhibitor selectively inhibiting cancer cell growth in vivo and in vitro. *PLoS One.* 2012;7(11):e49062.
116. Wang R, Cheng Y, Su D et.al. Cpt1c regulated by AMPK promotes papillary thyroid carcinomas cells survival under metabolic stress conditions. *J Cancer.* 2017;8:3675–3681.
117. Khatami F, Payab M, Sarvari M et.al. Oncometabolites as biomarkers in thyroid cancer: A systematic review. *Cancer Manag Res.* 2019;11:1829–1841.
118. Rauf A, Imran M, Suleria H.A.R et.al. A comprehensive review of the health perspectives of resveratrol. *Food Funct.* 2017;8:4284–4305.
119. Limmongkon A, Janhom P, Amthong A et al. Antioxidant activity, total phenolic, and resveratrol content in five cultivars of peanut sprouts. *Asian Pac J Trop Biomed.* 2017;7:332–338.
120. Ge JF, Xu YY, Li N, et al. Resveratrol improved the spatial learning and memory in subclinical hypothyroidism rat induced by hemi-thyroid electrocauterization. *Endocr J.* 2015;62:927–938.
121. Ho Y, Lin YS, Liu HL et al. Biological Mechanisms by Which Antiproliferative Actions of Resveratrol Are Minimized. *Nutrients.* 2017;9(10):1046.
122. Giuliani C, Bucci I, Di Santo S et al. Resveratrol inhibits sodium/iodide symporter gene expression and function in rat thyroid cells. *PLoS One* 2014;9(9):e107936.
123. Giuliani C, Iezzi M, Ciolli L et al. Resveratrol has anti-thyroid effects both in vitro and in vivo. *Food Chem Toxicol.* 2017;107 (Pt A):237–247.
124. Liu X, Li H, Wu ML et al. Resveratrol reverses retinoic acid resistance of anaplastic thyroid cancer cells via demethylating CRABP2 gene. *Front Endocrinol.* 2019;10:734.
125. Duntas LH and Benvenga S. Selenium: An element for life. *Endocrine.* 2015;48:756–775.
126. Xue H, Wang W, Li Y et al. Selenium upregulates CD4(+)CD25(+) regulatory T cells in iodine-induced autoimmune thyroiditis model of NOD.H-2(h4) mice. *Endocr. J.* 2010;57:595–601.
127. Kato MA, Finley DJ, Lubitz CC et al. Selenium decreases thyroid cancer cell growth by increasing expression of GADD153 and GADD34. *Nutr Cancer.* 2010;62:66–73.
128. Taylor SN, Wagner CL, Hollis BW. Vitamin D: Benefits for bone, and beyond. *Contemp Pediatr.* 2006;1:1–8.
129. Ozkan B. Nutritional rickets. *J Clin Res Pediatr Endocrinol.* 2010;2:137–43.
130. Heaney RP. Calcium, dairy products and osteoporosis. *J Am Coll Nutr.* 2000;19(2):83S–99.
131. Cauley JA, Murphy PA, Riley TJ, Buhari AM. Effects of fluoridated drinking water on bone mass and fractures: The study of osteoporotic fractures. *J Bone Miner Res* 1995;10:1076–1086.
132. Özen S, Darcan Ş. Effects of environmental endocrine disruptors on pubertal development. *J Clin Res Pediatr Endocrinol.* 2011;3:1–6.
133. Wang H, Cai Y, Shao Y et al. Fish oil ameliorates high-fat diet induced male mouse reproductive dysfunction via modifying the rhythmic expression of testosterone synthesis related genes. *Int J Mol Sci.* 2018;19:1325–1339.
134. Dikshit A, Gomes Filho MA, Eilati E et al. Flaxseed reduces the pro-carcinogenic microenvironment in the ovaries of normal hens by altering the PG and oestrogen pathways in a dose-dependent manner. *Br J Nut.* 2015;113:1384–1395.
135. Vazquez-Gomez M, Garcia-Contreras C, Torres-Rovira L et al. Polyphenols and IUGR pregnancies: Maternal hydroxytyrosol supplementation improves prenatal and early-postnatal growth and metabolism of the offspring. *PloS One.* 2017;12:e0177593.
136. Seddiki Y, da Silva FM, da Silva HM. Antioxidant properties of polyphenols and their potential use in improvement of male fertility: A review. *Biomed J Sci Tech Res.* 2017;1(3):612–616.
137. Das SK, Karmakar SN. Effect of green tea (camellia sinensis l.) leaf extract on reproductive system of adult male albino rats. *Int J Physiol Pathophysiol Pharmacol.* 2015;7:178.

138. Mahmood-Khan Z, Hall ER. Quantification of plant sterols in pulp and paper mill effluents. *Water Qual Res J Can.* 2008;43(2/3):93–102.
139. MacLatchy D, Peters L, Nickle J, Van Der Kraak G. Exposure to β-sitosterol alters the endocrine status of goldfish differently than 17β-estradiol. *Environ Toxicol Chem.* 1997;16:1895–1904.
140. Malini T, Vanithakumari G. Antifertility effects of β-sitosterol in male albino rats. *J Ethnopharmacol.* 1995;35:149–153.
141. Malini T, Vanithakumari G. Effect of beta-sitosterol on uterine biochemistry: A comparative study with estradiol and progesterone. *Biochem Mol Biol Int.* 1993;31:659–668.
142. Reed KF. Fertility of herbivores consuming phytoestrogen containing medicago and trifolium species. *Agriculture.* 2016;6(3):35.
143. Ryökkynen A, Käyhkö U-R, Mustonen A-M, Kukkonen JVK, Nieminen P. Multigenerational exposure to phytosterols in the mouse. *Reprod Toxicol.* 2005;19:535–540.
144. Montgomery G, Martin GB, Bars L, Pelletier J. Gonadotrophin release in ovariectomized ewes fed different amounts of coumestrol. *J Reprod Fert.* 1985;73:457–463.
145. Radha M and Laxmipriya N. Efficacy of Non polar extract (NPE) of Aloe barbadensis Mill. in Polycystic Ovarian Syndrome (PCOS) rodent model-an " in vivo" study". *Int J Pharmaceut Sci Res.* 2016;7:4933.
146. Woyengo TA., Ramprasath VR, Jones PJH. Anticancer effects of phytosterols. *Eur J Clin Nutr.* 2009;63(7):813–820.
147. Solomons NW, Rosenfield RL, Jacob RA, Sandstead HH. Growth retardation and zinc nutrition. *Pediatr Res.* 1976;10:923–927.
148. Pandey M, Verma RK, Saraf SA. Nutraceuticals: New era of medicine and health. *Asian J Pharmaceut Clinic Res.* 2010;3(1):11–15.
149. Ball D. Foods of the future may be tailored to fit. *Wall Street J.* Jan 23, 2003;1:116–121.

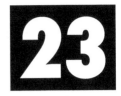

Disorders of the Urogenital System in Aging and Nutraceuticals

Aaishwarya Deshmukh
Smt. Kashibai Navale College of Pharmacy

Jayvadan Patel
Sankalchand Patel University

Contents

DOI: 10.1201/9781003110866-23

23.1 Introduction

Aging is a multivariate course of development described by numerous physical, physiological, cognitive and social modifications happening in humans; as per the gerontologist, it is defined as biological occurrences marked by heterogeneity at different levels like on cellular, somatic and molecular level, temporal continuity and the capability of being modulated. According to the "National Policy on Older Persons", elderly people are those aged 60 years or above, but then again, this senior citizen age varies globally. A country will be considered as aging, if the percentage of people aged above 65 years reaches 7% [1]. There has been a rise in percentage of elder adults in almost all the countries of the world, consistent with the data from World Population Prospects: the 2015 Revision [2], which confirms a considerable upsurge in elderly people population in recent years and this advance is going to quicken in the coming decade. Elder adults will rise by 56%, from 901 to 1.4 billion between 2015 and 2030, and by 2050, the global aged population is expected to reach nearly 2.1 billion. The existing global state ventures that adults aged above 80 years will increase from 137 million in 2017 to 425 million in 2050. Various theories explicate the progression of aging at molecular, biological, system and cellular levels, and that they are considered as programmed and damage or error theories, which suggests alterations in gene expression and cumulative damage to cells at various levels to precede aging [3]. Aging is marked by various physical, physiological and cognitive changes in the human body. Being a physiological change, a major factor in successful aging requires appropriate nutrition. Inappropriate eating habits results in the development of chronic diseases like type II diabetes mellitus, coronary heart disease, atherosclerosis, malnutrition as well as urogenital disorders, which blights the life quality and deteriorated physical and cognitive function. The decline in food intake is related with nutrient deficiencies and diseases as well.

23.1.1 Multifaceted mechanisms of the aging process

Aging is a complicated and unavoidable biological progression, connected with various chronic incapacitating health effects. The foremost reasons of mortality globally are ischemic heart disease (6.3 million), cerebrovascular accidents (4.4million), lower respiratory infections (4.3 million), diarrheal disease (2.9 million), perinatal disorders (2.4 million), chronic obstructive pulmonary disease (2.2 million), tuberculosis (2.0 million), measles (1.1 million) and lung cancer (0.9million) and is quite apparent that nutrition-modifiable disorder is accountable for a considerable proportion of deaths worldwide, may it be developing or developed countries. As far as aging is concerned, disease and debility in the geriatric population where nutrition may play a role are dyslipidemia, cardiac diseases, hypertension, cancer and stroke along with an amplified risk of developing type 2 diabetes; Alzheimer's disease, depression; physical worsening of bones and joints, osteoporosis and arthritis; cataracts and macular degeneration, pulmonary problems and infectious diseases and urogenital diseases. Maintenance of a healthy lifecycle is foremost task for health care systems day by day. Numerous genetic factors have been identified by various groups of scientists known as "longevity-related genes" which can control not only health-span but lifespan too in animal models like yeast, worms, flies and rodents. These longevity related genes are classified mainly into three conserved nutrient-sensing pathways: insulin/insulin-like growth factor-1-like signaling, target-of-rapamycin and sirtuin pathways which predominantly sense glucose, amino acid and nicotinamide adenine dinucleotide (NAD) or NAD/NADH levels in cells, respectively. Additionally, out of many aging hypotheses that have been proposed, the best projecting is the free radical hypothesis, which establishes that oxygen free radicals like reactive oxygen species are formed due to metabolism perpetrate oxidative damage to macromolecules, viz. DNA, protein and lipid, which in turn leads to biological aging and eventually death. However, free radical hypothesis of aging is not adequate enough to elaborate the core mechanisms of the aging process. Another hypothesis known as hormesis hypothesis of aging has been used often to understand the prolongevity effects prompted by the use of nutraceuticals. Hormesis theory explains the phenomenon of stimulation of immune responses in the conditions of mild stress at the organism level, the consequence of which is biologically beneficial effects and prolongation of life- and health-span. Due to multifaceted mechanisms and influences involved in the aging process, substantial exertions are being made to develop dietary interventions, which can effectively modulate mechanisms and promote healthy aging [4].

23.2 Dietary supplements and nutraceuticals

23.2.1 Dietary supplements

Nutraceuticals' use is wide ranging and strikingly escalating in countries like the United States. People have started consuming food supplements and nutraceuticals in their routine diets for numerous reasons, like vagueness about the nutrient adequacy or a yearning for an additional affirmative health standard than they recognize to be reachable from medical session, and resolution to treat from an ailment. The use of dietary supplements and nutraceuticals, for the matter of fact, is perhaps nurtured because of their extensive availability, aggressive marketing and media reports on studies signifying that nutraceuticals may benefit in not only prevention but treatment of health problems of geriatric population [5].

23.2.2 The geriatric population

The geriatric population might be anticipated to consume nutraceuticals in an endeavor to avert or treat chronic disease, to experience symptomatic relief, or to improve the morbidity and decrease the mortality. There are few studies, as old as some 50 years ago which in fact are studies specifying that almost one-fourth to one-half of the aged people consumed supplements. In a health screening program some 20 years back it was reported that Hale et al. more than 46% of the women and 34% of the men, among 3,192 ambulatory aged participants above the age of 65 years, used supplements. These participants normally used multivitamins or minerals, vitamins E and C; the reasons for consuming vitamin C as per participant's review were to prevent cold and cough, treat deficiency, for ophthalmic problems and UTIs, and vitamin E was consumed to prevent and treat deficiency disorder, and as a vasodilator in hypertensive patients. Another study in 11,888 elderly residents of a southern California retirement community stated that 62% of the male and 69% of the female consumed vitamins and minerals as supplements [6]. In yet another study, 236 elderly people from a retirement community in rural Maryland [7] were surveyed and found that 58% used supplements typically on a daily basis. Moreover, not only single multivitamin pill but products with combinations of vitamin C, potassium, calcium, B complex, vitamin E and iron were frequently consumed by geriatric population. Physicians were said to be most influential in the subjects' decision to consume these products. The study also reported that duration and the frequency of use of supplement were not related to demographics like sex, age, health status, education level or regularity of distressing about health.

23.2.3 Nutrient adequacy and supplement use

Studies specify that dietary supplementation is generally connected to subjective health acuity, well-being and balanced food and to viewpoint regarding food, vitamins and minerals [8].

A number of studies in aged population designated that dietary supplementations led to consumption of more nutrients from food than nonusers. Numerous studies show, nevertheless, that the food of several geriatric people did not meet the RDAs for quite a lot of nutrients—like folate, calcium, vitamins B6, B12, D, E and zinc [9] and that the majority of elderly people, used food which were short in iron, calcium, thiamin, vitamin A and even didn't take food supplements for these nutrients. A study by [10–11] stipulated that old people were at the increased risk of nutrient deficiency for several reasons not limited to inadequate food intake, physiological decline, disease processes, poor economic status and medical treatments.

23.3 Geriatric urology

Genitourinary system disorders are predominantly common in geriatric adults. Though there has been an overabundance of explorations related to the disorders linked with aging and the genitourinary system disorders in geriatric patients, inadequate work has focused on the pathophysiology, clinical outcomes, or natural history in aged adults; clinical studies are nonrandomized, and the majority require long-term follow-up. Moreover, the clinical studies also do not segregate result obtained from older adults from their younger counterparts, and there is a common lack of standardized operational terminology, validation and reproducible outcome measures.

23.3.1 Urinary incontinence

Urinary incontinence is a very frequent disorder observed among geriatric patients; expected ratio is between 15% and 35% of community-dwelling 60 or over old-aged people in the United States is ill with from urinary incontinence [12] and that the occurrence enhances with age in both male and female patients [13]. On the whole, the frequency of urinary incontinence was found to be 6.1% at the age of 65 years, 9.6% at the age of 75 years, 21.8% at the age between 85 and 89, and 28.2% for people aged 90 years and over. A cohort study of 7,949 elder women (mean age: 76.9±5.0 years) discovered that 41% of them reported urinary incontinence, among 14% having daily incontinent episodes [14] and stated that the urinary incontinence incidences were significantly linked with age. Few co-morbid conditions like obesity, history of stroke, chronic obstructive pulmonary disease, prior hysterectomy, reduced walk speed and deprived overall health were related strongly with augmented incontinence [15]. Urinary incontinence can have considerable negative impact on self-worth, is connected with greater rates of depression apart from impact on social facets of quality of life and daily living activities [16]. Data from a study imply that approximately 50% of housebound aged people suffer from urinary incontinence [17]. In a study from the Longitudinal Study on Aging, Coward et al. established that people staying in more populous areas are at less risk than incontinent people staying in less urbanized or populous areas [18], the reason might be comparative deficient community support services. There are additional geriatric syndromes (isolated urinary incontinence and combined urinary and fecal incontinence) that are connected with urinary incontinence like cognitive impairment and gait abnormalities, which can considerably add to the risk of functional dependence [19,20]. A study by Seidel et al.

examined the relationship between the status of cognition and continence to envisage the release placement post rehabilitation in inpatients and established that prediction of continence status at discharge could be possible if the analysis of continence and cognitive status was performed at the time of admission to rehabilitation services which in turn impacts placement decisions. Moreover, it was observed that patients who were continent at the time of admission to a nursing home were at an expressively augmented hazard for the progression to urinary incontinence and the projected occurrence of new-onset urinary incontinence was about 27% per year. Nevertheless, not only age but many risk factors have been identified for chronic incontinence like gender difference (male are more prone), dementia, or diminished mobility within 2 months in nursing-home residents [21]. Even though older-age adults are more prone for urinary incontinence, it should not be regarded as normal or foreseeable part of aging.

23.3.2 Urinary tract infections (UTIs)

In the settings of long-term care, UTIs and asymptomatic bacteriuria are prevalent in geriatric adults. Symptomatic infections are treated with antibiotics; however, the consequences of asymptomatic and recurring infections on long-term morbidity and mortality are more debatable. A prospective cohort study [22] found that UTI was not a risk factor for mortality; on the contrary, age and poor self-reported health status were noteworthy prognosticators of mortality. Though preceding longitudinal cohort study by Nordenstam et al. [23] demonstrated a substantial upsurge in 5-year mortality with bacteriuria in men, comparable finding vanished in female when those with indwelling catheters were left out from the analysis. In contrast, Nicolle et al. reported no significant survival difference between men with and without asymptomatic bacteriuria [24]. A prospective observational study by Monane et al. [25] on women both community-dwelling persons and long-term-care residents demonstrated that asymptomatic bacteriuria were present in 20% of all urine samples and in one-third of all participants over 6 months of follow-up and that disparity was observed on a month-by-month basis, along with recurrent spontaneous modifications in positive and negative specimens. These figures supports the agreement that asymptomatic bacteriuria in the aged adult does not typically warrant commencement of antibiotic therapy. In yet another randomized trial of antibiotic treatment in institutionalized geriatric female (mean age 83.4 ± 8.8 years) with asymptomatic bacteriuria, Nicolle et al. [26] instituted that short-term benefits were not associated with therapy but increased long-term risks, like reinfection with resistant organisms were observed. Likewise, Ouslander et al. [27] showed that no improvement in rates of chronic urinary incontinence was observed by treating asymptomatic bacteriuria in institutionalized elderly women. Bacteriuria is usually linked with chronic indwelling catheter use and stereotypically does not require treatment; yet UTIs related with short-term catheterization (less than 2 weeks) in geriatric adults should be taken care of. In a prospective randomized controlled trial, Harding et al. studied the effect on antibiotic therapy in 119 women with catheter-acquired UTIs and observed that infections resolved naturally in younger female than in those aged 65 years or older (89% versus 62%; P < 0.001); single-dose antibiotic therapy was usually effective in them. In another case-control study of 149 postmenopausal women, Raz et al. [28] examined the risk factors linked with recurrent UTI who were referred for evaluation and treatment of UTIs. In the same study, 53 age-matched control subjects were compared, and it was found that the case subjects tended to have at least one of the three common urologic conditions supposed to dispose them to infection: cystocele (19% versus 0%, P < 0.001), urinary incontinence (41% versus 9%, P < .001) and elevated postvoid residual urine volume (28% versus 2%, P < 0.001).

In postmenopausal women, vaginal estrogen replacement has been main of therapy for the prevention of recurrent UTIs since a long time [29]. Many patients consider cream-based preparations muddled and uncomfortable, but a randomized open parallel study by Eriksen showed good response to an estrogen-impregnated vaginal device (Estring). But the use of these devices has not been studied in a geriatric population; nonetheless, better contentment may lead to improved adherence by geriatric patients. As far as recurrent UTIs are concerned, cranberry juice and other cranberry preparations have been used as prophylactic treatments since a long time. Cranberries contain compounds which prevent bacterial adhesion to the urothelium, and there are studies which recommend the prophylactic use of cranberry products, predominantly in institutionalized older adults. Avorn et al. [30] studied the effect of cranberry juice in a randomized, double-blind, placebo-controlled trial with 153 older women (mean age 78.5 years) and found that [31] ingestion of 300 mL of cranberry juice everyday decreased the probabilities of clinically significant bacteriuria ($\geq$105 organisms) and associated pyuria to 42% as compared to control subjects (P = 0.004). In another study, Kontiokari et al. [32] compared intake of cranberrylingon berry juice, *Lactobacillus GG* and placebo in 150 women who were diagnosed with acute *Escherichia coli* UTIs and found that 20% reduction was observed in the outright recurrent UTI risk (urine culture with $\geq$105 colony-forming units of bacteria) for the female who used the juice in contrast with the control group. Furthermore, there was no difference in the relapse rate between female who consumed *Lactobacillus* and the control group. Furthermore, most of the UTIs research in elderly adults has detected patient risk factors and the bacteriology linked with infection, however, further studies must evidently state the criteria for inclusion and exclusion for subject selection.

23.3.3 Prostate diseases

Although prostate disorders like benign prostatic hyperplasia (BPH), prostatitis and chronic pelvic pain, and prostate cancer are common in male patients of all ages, the prevalence and frequency upsurge with age. There are a variety of treatment options available presently, but stress is placed on surgical therapy in the geriatric adult. BPH is one of the common prostatic disorder of old age and is caused by a stromal component proliferation of the prostate, stereotypically commencing after age of 40 years and leads to obstructive changes in the physiology and the development of lower urinary tract voiding symptoms seems to be related to this hyperplastic aging process. In a cross-sectional analysis study which was conducted on 1,557 men (mean age 51.3 years, range 40–96), Haidinger et al. [33] established that increasing age is an independent risk factor for onset of symptoms; few other studies have also supported this notion but also propose that age does not impact the consequence of successive surgery for BPH [34]. Remarkably, urinary urgency and frequency have also been correlated with increasing age in women, but outlet obstruction is uncommon. In yet another study, which was a prospective cohort analysis done on 2,280 men followed for almost 25 years, it was observed that the development of obstructive voiding symptoms for example hesitancy, urgency, decreased force, frequency, decreased caliber of urinary stream, and nocturia were exceedingly prognostic of the need for prostate surgery, and that the risk differed considerably by age [35]. The study also observed that male aged between 62 and 68 years were more likely in the need of surgery as compared to their younger counterparts. Furthermore, since last 15 years or so, there has been an overall transferal from surgery to medical therapy as the ideal initial treatment for almost all patients with BPH; this has also got tremendous boost due to development of clinically effective and safe pharmacologic agents, such as α1-adrenoceptor antagonists such as doxazosin, terazosin and tamsulosin, and 5-α-reductase inhibitors such as finasteride which ultimately has dropped the rates of surgery for BPH treatment [36–38]. In a study, Breslin et al. [39] reviewed 1,822 BPH patients in a single private practice for a period of 3 years (between July 1, 1987 and June 30, 1991) to determine that the rate of surgery drop and found that surgery dropped from 28% in the first year of the study to 8% in the last year which is similar to the timing of the improved acceptance and practice of pharmacotherapy for the treatment of BPH. In addition, review of the Medicare database by Holtgrewe recognized a 30% decline in surgery for BPH in spite of a surge in the number of elder men enrolled in the program [40]. Stirringly, phytotherapy has also gained acceptance as a treatment option for BPH lately; numerous compounds have been utilized, comprising of Serenoa repens, Pygeum africanum and Hypoxis rooperi, wherein some randomized controlled trials of these compounds have been conducted, however, exploration is considered intricate due to lack of standardization in the preparation of most of these agents. Conversely, a meta-analysis study by Wilt et al. scrutinized the data from 18 trials (2,939 men participants) and [41] found that many diverse phytotherapy preparations could improve the obstructive urinary symptoms. Still, most of these studies have constraints like limited follow-up (less than 1 year) and geriatric patients not being the prime targets [42].

Prostatitis is one of the major clinical problem prevalent in 5%–14% of men and accounts for 3%–12% of the urologist's male outpatient practice. Prostatitis affects adversely on the quality of life, with its impact scores being comparable to those of myocardial infarction, angina, or Crohn's disease [43]. Prostatitis urinary symptoms are common like LUTS symptoms (both storage or obstructive and voiding or irritative), erectile dysfunction, low libido, insufficient rigidity and premature ejaculation [44].

The National Institute of Diabetes and Digestive and Kidney Diseases has developed a new classification system for prostatitis [45] (Table 23.1). Based on the different categories of prostatitis, different phytotherapies might be sorted. For *Category I*, alternative nutraceuticals or phytotherapies should not be utilized, since cure rates are 100% with available antibiotics and appropriate supportive care. In *Category II*, patients have frequent episodes of bacterial urinary tract infection (UTI) by the same organism; treatment typically involves long-term therapeutic or suppressive doses of antibiotics. However, in this category, complementary therapy can have a supportive role. Since, extended antibiotic utilization can disrupt the normal gastrointestinal flora, along with evidence suggesting probiotics being effective in protecting the gut flora, probiotic formulations and lactobacilli culture active yogurt can be employed to prevent or lessen gastrointestinal symptoms associated with antibiotic therapy [46]. A few studies also suggest that some probiotic treatments may reduce recurring UTIs, at least in women [47–49]. Zinc is known to be a constituent of antibacterial factor in seminal fluid, and studies of chronic prostatitis have shown attenuated levels in semen, [50] though an additional recent study did find no difference [51]. Additionally, supplementation did not augment the prostatic fluid levels, thus there is no compelling substantiation about zinc assisting in treatment of infection/ symptoms or prevent recurrence in category II prostatitis. Cranberry juice, although used extensively in the treatment of UTIs particularly in women, have not showed any protective effect in UTIs of men with category II prostatitis. Additionally, unsafe interactions with warfarin have also been reported [52]. Moreover, men with prostatitis are sensitive to acid loads in their diet, and cranberry juice being highly acidic may make symptoms worse. For *Category III* prostatitis patients, phytotherapies have revealed highest potential, which is the mainly the commonest of the clinical prostatitis syndromes. The symptoms are quite similar

Table 23.1 Prostatitis Syndrome Classification by the National Institute of Diabetes and Digestive and Kidney Diseases

Class	Name
I	Acute bacterial prostatitis
II	Chronic bacterial prostatitis
III	Chronic prostatitis/chronic pelvic pain syndrome
	A. Inflammatory
	B. Noninflammatory
IV	Asymptomatic inflammatory prostatitis

to those observed in chronic bacterial prostatitis (category II) but are devoid of infection and perhaps with intense pain and discomfort. The etiology is not known, but including unrelenting, occult prostate infection or inflammation, perhaps due to the response to infection or a dysregulated immune response or a true autoimmune disease may be the reason [53].

23.3.4 Other genitourinary malignancies

Bladder cancer and renal malignancies (renal cell carcinomas and transitional cell carcinomas of the upper urinary tract) are yet another geriatric urinogenital disorder considered to be more common than in younger adults. Unfortunately, natural history, etiology, pathophysiology, and treatment and long-term treatment effects of these disorders are not studied comprehensively in geriatric adults. Transitional cell carcinoma is one of the most prevalent malignant tumors of the urinary bladder in the countries like United States; endoscopic resection being the treatment for superficial tumors. Conversely, the overall relapse rate is up to 70%, and long-term surveillance is suggested for identifying repeated disease; immunotherapy with Bacillus-Calmette-Guerin or adjuvant intravesical chemotherapy is usually employed for treatment of such recurrences. Rather, radical cystectomy and urinary diversion is the customary treatment for muscle-invasive bladder cancer; however, this major surgery may have associated risk of perioperative morbidity and mortality. But then study has also revealed that radical cystectomy with urinary diversion can be securely executed in aged patients; though, neither the long-term consequences are still assessed nor are [54–57] the effects on events of daily living, contributory activities of daily living, and overall rehabilitation status appraised. In addition, the efficacy partial cystectomy or aggressive endoscopic resection with adjuvant radiation or chemotherapy which are considered as less invasive forms of surgical therapy has also not been studied in geriatric individuals. There are also substantial instances of small, incidentally detected tumors of renal and adrenal malignancies, which are also found to be more common in elder adults and the natural history, pathophysiology, etiology of these tumors, do need additional study [58]. Since renal and adrenal tumors have been found to be chemo- and radioresistant time and again, traditional surgical therapies like radical nephrectomy, nephroureterectomy, or adrenalectomy might be employed. Moreover, new and least-invasive techniques like nephron-sparing surgery, laparoscopic surgery and cryotherapy have been employed in older adults and seem to offer reduced morbidity [59].

23.3.5 Sexual dysfunction

Sexual dysfunction is prevalent not only in young adults but their older counterparts too. But unlike other genitourinary disorders and malfunctions, sexual dysfunction should not be recognized as a normal part of aging. A population-based cross-sectional study conducted by Panser et al. on 2,115 men showed that older men (aged 70–79 years) were more apprehensive about their overall sexual function as compared to middle-aged men (aged 40–49 years) (46.6% versus 24.9%) and reported inferior actual performance in a year span [60]. They also rated upper levels of disappointment, impaired erectile function and diminished libido. Though, in a multivariate analysis, age was not an autonomous prognosticator of the outcomes. Jφnler et al. through a survey from a convenience sample of 1,680 men of diverse terrestrial regions, confirmed that the occurrence of erectile dysfunction increased with age [61]. In yet another analytical data from Massachusetts Male Aging Study, Johannes et al. reported that the basic prevalence rate for erectile dysfunction was 25.9 cases per 1,000 man-years (95%CI = 22.5–29.9) and [62] the frequency upsurged expressively with increase in age, with 12.4, 29.8 and 46.4 cases per 1,000 man-years for male who are in their 40s, 50s and 60s, respectively. The study also reported that comorbid disease, such as diabetes mellitus, heart disease and hypertension as well as lower education were the additional risk factors for erectile dysfunction; use of antacids (Hydrogen-blocker) were also found to be substantial hazard for erectile dysfunction [63]. Numerous multidimensional assessment instruments are developed for identification of the levels of sexual dysfunction and their influence on the morbidity with [64–66] suitable consistency and rationality when used with aged persons.

Similar instrument has been developed and validated for evaluation of female sexual dysfunction [67]. Some studies have recognized that sexual dysfunction in female rises with age; however, the reasons for these changes are not well understood [68–69]. In support to this, a survey data in 964 women (mean patient age 45.4 ± 16.8 years, range of 18–87 years) who were in a primary care practice reported 98.8% women expressing at least one sexual concern [70].

23.4 Nutritional consideration for elderly

The diet in aged people do not offer sufficient nutrients, required to uphold optimal health, thus results in nutrient deficits and development of degenerative diseases [71]. The geriatric patients are also more prone to developing nutritional insufficiencies, either because of little dietary intake or diminished absorption or even due to failure of conversion into active forms [72–74]. Even though energy requirement drops with increasing age, the need for protein and particular nutrients rises in the normal physiology of the body.

23.4.1 Nutritional supplements

Supplements like dietary supplements, multivitamin supplements, protein supplements and mineral supplements are in demand to satisfy the requirement in patients. European countries, particularly the United States, in the past few decades, have visualized a growing drift in use of dietary supplements for regulating their nutrient levels. An old study called Iowa Women Health Study which was conducted in 1986 disclosed that nearby 66% women (with an average age of 62 years) ingested at least one dietary supplement and the number increased to 85% in the year 2004, along with 27% women consuming four or more supplements [75]. There are many nutrition interventional studies which have sought to find the effects of diverse dosage of nutrient on the well-being of the aged people. For example, to solve the problem of sarcopenia, it is recommended to include high concentration of Leucine (Essential Amino Acids (EAAs)) in their regular routine and ingestion of whey protein supplements rich in EAAs makes it possible as it will boost muscle protein synthesis and protect against sarcopenia [76]. There are studies that suggest that folate and vitamin B6 and B12 combination to be effective in dropping serum homocysteine levels and in turn attenuates cognitive decline [77]; however, this supplementation is effective only in people having mild cognitive impairment, and it was required to be taken for chronic period in order to obtain positive results. Interestingly, osteoporosis and osteopenia cases have been decreased significantly with supplementation with different dosages of calcium and vitamin D3 [78]. Thus, the use of supplements has the objective of attaining healthy lifestyle by attenuating chronic disease risk, though, practice of supplementation should be monitored stringently since collective intake of supplement and fortified food might escalate the threat of surpassing the higher tolerable limit and in turn increase their toxicity [75].

23.4.1.1 Protein

Recommended protein levels are not obtained among geriatric individuals due to decreased daily food intake, which leads to loss of muscle mass, the disease known as sarcopenia. Studies have shown that approximately 30% of individuals with the age of 60 years or above are sarcopenic, and this number is more than 50% in people who are 80 years and older. The reduced protein turnover and failure to maintain balance between protein requirement and protein intake affects the health adversely, since lower protein levels are speculated to be responsible for chronic muscle wasting and bone health, leading to functional damage and feebleness. Therefore, aged people are suggested to consume equivalent quantity of protein throughout the day, i.e., identical quantities during breakfast, lunch and dinner [79]. Moreover, because of metabolic modifications as a normal physiological change during aging, the ability to produce muscle protein declines drastically.

23.4.1.2 Potassium

The normal range of blood potassium is 3.6–5.2 mmol/L, and hyperkalemia develops when this range exceeds the normal range which leads to extensive muscle fatigue and weakness and can cause muscle paralysis and potentially fatal problems with heart rhythm if not treated timely. Geriatric populations are predominantly at risk for high potassium levels. Low potassium levels are responsible for an augmented risk of death or hospitalization in patients with chronic kidney disease and heart failure. Studies have also shown that potassium-rich diets (fruits and vegetables) are linked with a decreased risk of hypertension, which is one of the important etiologies for renal failure. Thus, potassium-rich food is often recommended and constitutes general components of an elderly person's regular diet. Milk, a common drink, is not only rich in calcium but also supplies abundance of potassium. The geriatric patients with dental issues, high-potassium yogurt, tomatoes, boiled potatoes and bananas are malleable and easy to eat. Prunes or raisins, meat, lima beans, fish, broccoli, citrus fruits and apricots are rich sources of potassium [80].

23.4.2 Supplementary dietary botanicals for geriatrics

23.4.2.1 Cranberry and oregano for longevity promotion

Many beneficial properties like antimicrobial, antiviral, antimutagenic, antiangiogenic and antioxidative functions are exhibited by cranberry (*Vaccinium oxycoccos*) and oregano (*Origanum vulgare*). Studies have shown that oregano and cranberry (OC) extract improved lifespan, in a diet composition-dependent manner, in Mexican fruit flies (mexfly). Additionally, OC supplementation also increased longevity in middle age, but not in young age or old age. Studies have also evaluated the effect of cranberry extract alone on life- and healthspan in C. elegans and the result indicates that the cranberry extract alone is adequate to prolong lifespan, since cranberries are lofty in antioxidants and phytochemicals, like proanthocyanidins and vitamin C, which may neutralize free radicals and diminish oxidative damage and ultimately modulate signaling transduction pathways [80].

23.4.2.2 Nectarine and acai for lifespan extension

Both nectarine (*Prunus persica*) and acai (*Euterpe oleracea*) contains a variety of bioactive phytochemicals. Experiments in flies have shown increase in lifespan with nectarine supplementation. A variety of studies on experimental animals demonstrate the role of nectarine and acai in increased longevity of life and is linked with augmented lifetime reproductive output and abridged lipid oxidation. On the contrary, acai pulp supplementation endorses survival in Drosophila fed with a high-fat but not a standard diet, and the same diet composition dependent effect is also apparent in the mexfly, i.e., acai supplementation advances the survival of the mexfly fed on a high-fat and high-sugar diet. The significance of diet composition is obvious, as well, in aging intervention studies using resveratrol like pharmacological agents, i.e. experimental studies in Drosophila, mexfly and rodents like mice have revealed the longevity effects of resveratrol being dependent on the composition of diet. There are few studies which show that both nectarine and acai upholds the survival of flies with superoxide dismutase (SOD1) deficiency, since sod1 deficient flies have a short lifespan and elevated levels of oxidative damage, proposing the notion that nectarine and acai does possess antioxidant activities at the organism level. Thus, these data prove the significance of diet composition in transforming the health benefits of nutraceuticals [80].

23.4.2.3 Herbal supplements like Ginseng, Yohimbine and Icariin

A number of nutritional and herbal supplements have been employed in the treatment of ED, e.g. Ginseng, Yohimbine and Icariin. However, they lack strong experimental evidence [81]. Yohimbine, an active constituent, derived from the bark of an evergreen tree is a peripherally and central α2-blocking agent as well has a mild inhibitor of monoamine oxidase (MAOI). Studies have shown that it blocks the pre- and postsynaptic α2 receptors, and the inhibition of α 2 receptors augments the release of neurotransmitters like nitric oxide and norepinephrine in the central and peripheral nervous system and corpus cavernosum [81,82]. A study demonstrated the effective dose to be 15 mg/day (5 mg three times a day) or 15 mg 1–2 hours prior to sexual activity simultaneously with 6 g arginine glutamate (50% arginine, 50% glutamic acid) [83]. However, safety in the geriatric patients is limited due to possible side effects, for instance hypertension, tachycardia, anxiety, insomnia, hallucinations and dizziness. Another phytoconstituent, Icariin, a flavonol glycoside which is obtained from horny goat weed or Herba Epimedii has been consumed in China for increasing sexual performances since long ages; it is said to have an inhibitory effect on phosphodiester (PDE) subtypes PDE4 and PDE5, consequently upregulating the synthesis of bioactive nitric oxide and in turn exhibiting testosterone like effects [84–86]. Moreover, Ginseng is yet another well-known aphrodisiac which has found to augment erectile function, although the data obtained from few studies are still preliminary and require supplementary trials.

A recent study by Aversa Antonio aimed to assess the effects of nutraceuticals containing multiple supplemental therapeutic agents from natural sources (Virherbe®/Rekupros®) on sexual satisfaction and lower urinary tract symptoms (LUTS) in young–old men. Virherbe® and Rekupros® is developed and comprised in the Italian Health Ministry-verified pharmaceutical grade ingredients (Herbeka Srl–Agrigento, Italy). Virherbe® has a composition of a mixture of 11 supplemental facts, which is intended to improve nitric oxide production, to improve physical energy and transform sexual desire. Rekupros®, on the other hand, is a mixture having nine supplemental facts which is designed to improvise the dopaminergic and cholinergic neurotransmission, to safeguard prostate from enlargement/urinary flow alterations and to assure physiology of hormonal circadian rhythms. The study was conducted as an open-label trial, where 40 men (average age 66±13) with sexual disturbances and mild LUTS but with no cognitive/motor impairment and clinical hypogonadism were enrolled. Different parameters like sexual desire (SD; IIEF-SD domain; International Index of Erectile Function) and satisfaction (Global Assessment Question; GAQ), the capacity to perform daily activities (evaluated by 6 min walking test [6MWT]) and International Prostate Symptoms Scores (IPSS) were assessed pre and post oral administration of two capsules/day of each supplement for a period of 8 weeks. The results showed improvement in sexual desire, contentment with sex life, physical performance, and LUTS in young–old men, suggestive of potential efficacy in patients not responding to standard treatments [87].

A number of phytotherapies are employed in the treatment of BPH which includes extract of the berries of *Serenoa repens* (saw palmetto), *Pygeum africanum* (from the bark of the African plum tree), rye pollen, stinging nettle, pumpkin seed, South African star grass and quercetin. Time and again, the effects of phytotherapeutic agents imitate the actions of pharmaceuticals available in the market.

23.4.2.4 Saw Palmetto

Saw Palmetto or American dwarf palm tree (*Serenoa repens*) berry extract is considered as one of the best studied phytoconstituent for BPH management. The phytotherapy is alleged to have antiandrogenic effects, also exhibits inhibition of 5-alpha reductase types 1 and 2, prolactin growth factor, induction of proliferation, and antiestrogenic, antiedematous and anti-inflammatory effects. However, preparations have been afflicted with inadequate reliability and inaccurate statements of content. Actually, in a study of supplements for prostate disease, three out of six saw palmetto compounds tested were shown to contain less than 20% of the stated dose, and one has more than twice the stated dose in a study of commonly used supplements in prostate disease [88]. Moreover, meta-analysis studies (18 Nos.) enrolling a total of 2,900 patients who consumed saw palmetto products (together with mixture) showed a considerable improvement in overall symptom score (1.41 points), peak flow rate (1.93 mL/s) and nocturia (0.76 episodes/night) compared with placebo [89]. In yet another analysis of 14 placebo-controlled and 3 open-label trials (4,280 patients followed up for 21 days to 24 months) of a saw palmetto preparation known as Permixon® (Pierre Fabre, Castres, France) [90] demonstrated a considerable improvement in peak flow rate and decline in nocturia above placebo. Gerber and colleagues in a study [91] treated 50 men with saw palmetto 160 mg bid for 6 months who had the problem of LUTS; however, no significant changes in objective urodynamic parameters—peak urinary flow rate, post-void residual urine volume, or detrusor pressure at peak flow were observed. In a placebo controlled 6-month trial in 100 men, Willetts and colleagues [92] showed no in difference peak flow rate, or International Index of Erectile Function scores were obtained. In addition, in 2006, *The New England Journal of Medicine* published the most rigorous placebo-controlled, randomized trial of saw palmetto for BPH [93], which enrolled 225 typical BPH patients and is considered the longest (1-year) trial published till date. The study found no significant differences between active treatment and placebo for any of the outcome parameters—American

Urological Association Symptom Index (AUASI) score, maximal urinary flow rate, prostate size, residual urine volume, quality of life, or prostate-specific antigen (PSA) levels.

23.4.2.5 African plum tree

African plum tree (*Pygeum africanum* or *Prunus africanum*) bark is postulated to have inhibitory effect on various growth factors, and has anti-inflammatory, antiedematous and phytoestrogenic effects, and is thought to reduce luteinizing hormone (LH), testosterone and prolactin. However, it does not have any 5-alpha-reductase activity. It has also shown to decrease detrusor contractility and alter bladder function. In a Cochrane review (meta-analysis study) enrolling 1,500 men in 18 trials (out of 18 trials, 6 were placebo controlled) demonstrated reasonable improvement in the symptoms outcomes and flow rate, particularly nocturia [94]. Another study with a *P. africanum* preparation (Tadenan®, Debat Laboratories, Paris, France) enrolled 2,262 patients and were treated with the extract, including 12 double-blind, placebo-controlled studies. However, only a single study included patients more than 100 in number, and no study included follow-up of patients for longer than 12 weeks. Thus, since none of the trials meet the guidelines recommended by the International Consultation Conferences on BPH, these data on *P. africanum*'s efficacy cannot be considered decisive [95].

23.4.2.6 Pumpkin seed

The effect of pumpkin seeds (*Cucurbita pepo*) was studied in a randomized, placebo-controlled, 1-year trial in 476 patients with LUTS and BPH and observed significant improvement in IPSS by 6.8 points with active treatment, 1.2 points better than placebo seldom achieved with an alpha-blocker or 5-alpha-reductase inhibitor.

23.4.2.7 Rye pollen

A Cochrane review of two placebo-controlled and two direct comparative trials lasting 12–24 weeks with rye pollen extract (Cernilton) showed no improvement in urinary flow rate, residual urine, or prostate size as compared with placebo or either comparator treatment. Additionally, withdrawal due to adverse events was 4.8% for Cernilton versus 4.2% for Paraprost and 2.7% for placebo.

23.4.2.8 Stinging nettle

A 12-month double-blind, comparative trial was performed for the German stinging nettle (*Urtica dioica*) preparation Prostagutt® (Schwabe Pharma AG, Karlsruhe, Germany) in 489 patients versus finasteride. A spectacular improvement in symptom score (4.8–7.5 points) and a urinary flow rate of 2–3 mL/s were observed. Prostagutt was also found to be as effective as finasteride in a comparison, while no placebo group was included in the study [96].

23.4.2.9 South African star Grass

South African star grass (*Hypoxis rooperi*) has been studied in a randomized, placebo-controlled trials; the Harzol trial, which enrolled 200 patients randomized to 20 mg tid or placebo for 6 months, demonstrated considerable improvements compared with placebo in IPSS (7.3 points) and peak flow rate (5.2 mL/s). The other trial known as Azuprostat trial which enrolled 177 patients randomized to 65 mg/day versus placebo over 6 months demonstrated correspondingly striking, statistically considerable results (8.3 points on the IPSS, 8.8 mL/s in Qmax). Astonishingly, the improvements observed with South African star grass are superior to those achieved with nearly all 5-alpha-reductase inhibitors, alpha-blockers, or even combination therapies. A meta-analysis of four randomized, placebo-controlled trials conducted by Wilt and colleagues which included 519 men (lasting from 4 to 26 weeks) illustrated a weighted mean difference of 4.9 points in the IPSS and 3.9 mL/s in peak flow rate and were significantly different from placebo.

23.4.2.10 Quercetin

Quercetin is a bioflavonoid with documented antioxidant and anti-inflammatory properties and is said to inhibit inflammatory cytokines. It is found in foods such as red grapes, apples, tea, onions, leafy greens, wine and various berries and is implicated in the pathogenesis of CP/CPPS.29–31 In a prospective, double-blind, placebo-controlled trial by Shoskes and colleagues, the urinary component of the National Institutes of Health (NIH) Chronic Prostatitis Symptom Index (CPSI) was found to be improved by 2.7 points versus 1.5 for placebo, though it is still unclear as to whether that is a clinically significant change or not. However, this effect on urinary symptoms suggests a potential use in BPH [53].

23.4.2.11 PC-SPES and imitators

PC-SPES, a mixture of eight Chinese herbs marketed in 1996, has showed improvement and PSA reductions and thus was considered promising for prostate cancer. This supplement was standardized by chemical analysis and had batch-to-batch consistency as per the manufacturer assurance. There were many preclinical and clinical studies that were published to confirm the consensus that the formulation did decrease prostate cancer growth. Furthermore, the National Center for Complementary and Alternative Medicine and others sustained five clinical trials, some were planned, and some has already begun when complications started to get reported. Eventually, independent laboratory analysis showed that this formulation contained diethylstilbestrol, warfarin and indomethacin, after which FDA issued a warning which led to the recall of the product, and production got stopped. This instance stresses the requirement of a stringent regulated process for conduction of efficacy and safety profile studies in the polyherbal formulations [96].

23.4.3 Micronutrients and multivitamins

Supplementation en Vitamines et Mineraux Antioxydants (SU.VI.MAX) was the largest randomized trial of multivitamin and mineral supplementation in health system, which enrolled 5,141 men and 7,876 women who were followed up for a median of 7.5 years. The participants (100 Nos.) actively involved in therapy consumed a single daily capsule containing ascorbic acid 120 mg, vitamin E 30 mg, beta carotene 6 mg, selenium 100 µg and zinc 20 mg (near RDI values) showed 31% reduction in the relative risk of cancer, a 37% reduction in the relative risk of all-cause mortality, and a 48% reduction in the relative risk of prostate cancer. On the other hand, men with higher PSA values who consumed the supplement may have had an amplified risk of prostate cancer signifying that tumors may exploit certain antioxidants or nutrients from the formulation once the tumor itself has become clinically significant [97].

23.4.3.1 Zinc

Zinc levels are found to be low in the prostate tissue of patients suffering from prostate disease. Thus, its deficiency was assumed to be one of the etiologies for prostate disease. However, studies conducted at doses considerably higher than the reference daily intakes (RDI) of 11 mg/day show results that are very concerning. A health professionals follow-up study was conducted wherein 46,974 men were followed up for a long period of over 14 years showing no increased prostate cancer risk in men taking doses of up to 100 mg/day. But the relative risk of new cases of advanced prostate cancer was observed as 2.29, in male taking more than the aforementioned dose; But the relative risk of new cases of advanced prostate cancer was observed as 2.29 in male taking more than the aforementioned dose; while it was 2.37 in males taking supplemental zinc for not less than 10 years. In 2007, a trial was published, which showed that men and women taking 80 mg of zinc per day had substantial escalations in hospital admissions for genitourinary complications [98].

23.4.3.2 Selenium

The areas of the United States having the highest levels of selenium in the soil has shown to reduce the risk of cancer and in turn has encouraged many studies of selenium supplements as a preventive therapy for cancer, which also includes a randomized, controlled trial in basal and squamous cell carcinoma patients in areas having low levels of selenium in soil like Arizona.

23.4.3.3 Vitamin E

Vitamin E has been considered as a preventive therapy for numerous diseases and has facilitated the still-ongoing Selenium and Vitamin E Cancer Prevention Trial (SELECT). Nonetheless, no cardiovascular risk reduction has been obtained from multiple trials; on the contrary, the HOPE TOO trial in fact, showed an augmented risk of heart failure in addition to no attenuated cancer risk [99–100]. Additionally, high doses of vitamin E were found to significantly raise the risk of a second primary cancer or relapse in head and neck cancer patients and similarly to increase all-cause mortality expressively in patients who undertook radiation therapy [101]. Nevertheless, vitamin E obviously has a treatment prospective, which depends on the dosage or form, e.g., gamma tocopherol (major form in the diet), is more effective than alpha tocopherol (synthetic form usually found in dietary supplements) in controlling human prostate cancer cell line growth, but then again, controlled trials are still lacking in humans. Recently revealed natural form of vitamin E, vitamin E phosphate, is being verified in a small preliminary trial for determining its impact on the prostate cancer [102].

23.4.3.4 Vitamin D

Trial like Androgen-Independent Prostate Cancer Study of Calcitriol Enhancing Taxotere (ASCENT) were conducted in patients with androgen independent cancer to study vitamin D and to find if high-dose calcitriol rises the proportion of those who have a better-than 50% reduction in PSA with docetaxel or not. Study has shown that vitamin D intake is aberrantly low in prostate cancer patients, however, [103] supplementation of vitamin D should be based on need, and levels should be monitored with a simple test of 25-hydroxy vitamin D test. 32 ng/mL serum level is considered normal, however, few current indications, based on a summary of past clinical trials suggest a value of 35–40 ng/mL (90–100 nmol/L) as optimal [104]. Moreover, use of vitamin D supplementation at a dose of 400 IU/day (the usual level in multivitamins) is possibly not sufficient to correct deficiency; 800 IU or more per day also require several months to normalize blood levels of vitamin D. Thus, it is judicious to check serum levels of vitamin D in prostate cancer patients' and recommend supplements if suitable, calcium supplements, and weight-bearing exercise before prescribing bisphosphonates.

23.4.3.5 Low fat

An earlier study has shown that fat-restricted diet could slow prostate cancer growth, after which urologist have been advising patients to consume low-fat diet, but the results of primary prevention trials of low-fat diets in hormone-sensitive cancers have not been compelling. In another study by Women's Health Initiative, 20,000 women who were on a low-fat diet for 8 years neither showed any reduced risk of breast cancer nor any effect on cardiovascular disease, colorectal cancer, or the global index. In a Memorial Sloan-Kettering trial which enrolled 1,300 men illustrated no significant effect of a low-fat, high fruit and vegetable consumption diet on PSA slope or the incidence of prostate cancer over 4 years. In yet another Ornish trial [105], small reduction in PSA and in fact a significant attenuation in high-density lipoprotein (HDL) in prostate cancer patients who consumed a no-fat diet, high-dose supplements and lifestyle changes.

23.5 Conclusion

The hastened decline in the health status and well-being in geriatric population is alarming and needs quick intervention, one of the reasons being the inability to maintain proper nutritional status. The amplified dependence on medicine also affects the health by antagonistic interactions with certain nutrients. Moreover, social and economic factors, metabolic changes occurring as a part of normal physiology of aging, and the increased risk of disease have a rigorous effect on the nutritional status in significant ways. However, most of the age-related diseases can be prevented by appropriate nutritional interventions as well as intake of nutrients and antioxidant-rich food. The accurate nutritional modifications encompass a prospective to elevate the health standards of the elder population worldwide. Thus, exceptional stress must be given to the health status of elderly population for the preservation of well-being and decline in the occurrence of chronic diseases and related complications.

References

1. Amarya S, Singh K, Sabharwal M. Changes during aging and their association with malnutrition. *J Nutr Gerontol Geriatr*. 2015; 6: 78–84.
2. *World Population Ageing, Department of Economic and Social Affairs* 2015; United Nation, New York.
3. Jin K. Modern biological theories of aging. *Aging Dis*. 2010; 1: 72.
4. Rattan SIS, Sejersen H, Fernandes RA, Luo W. Stress-mediated hormetic modulation of aging, wound healing, and angiogenesis in human cells. *Ann N Y Acad Sci*. 2007; 1119:112–121.
5. Gussow, JD, Thomas PR. *The Nutrition Debate: Sorting Out Some Answers*. Palo Alto, CA: Bull Publishing, 1986. Chapter 6, Nutritional supplements: To pill or not to pill, is that the question? pp 268–341.
6. Gray GE, Paganini-Hill A, Ross RK, Henderson BE. Vitamin supplement use in a Southern California retirement community. *J Am Diet Assoc*. 1986; 86:800–802.
7. Sobal J, Muncie Jr HL, Baker AS. Use of nutritional supplements in a retirement community. *Gerontologist*. 1986; 26:187–191.
8. Worsley A. Health, wellbeing and dietary supplementation. *Recent Adv Clin Nutr*. 1986; 2: 43–56.
9. McGandy RB, Russell RM, Hartz SC et. al. Nutritional status survey of healthy noninstitutionalized elderly: energy and nutrient intakes from three-day diet records and nutrient supplements. *Nutr Res*. 1986; 6: 785–798.

10. Kirsch A, and Bidlack WR. Nutrition and the elderly: Vitamin status and efficacy of supplementation. *Nutrition.* 1987; 3: 305–314.
11. Ranno BS, Wardlaw GM, Geiger CJ. What characterizes elderly women who overuse vitamin and mineral supplements? J. *Am Diet Assoc.* 1988; 88: 347–348.
12. Burgio KL, Matthews KA, Engel BT. Prevalence, incidence and correlates of urinary incontinence in healthy, middle-aged women. *J Urol.* 1991; 146:1255–1259.
13. Malmsten UG, Milsom I, Molander U, Norlen LJ. Urinary incontinence and lower urinary tract symptoms: an epidemiological study of men aged 45 to 99 years. *J Urol.* 1997;158: 1733–1737.
14. Brown JS, Seeley DG, Fong J, Black DM, Ensrud KE, Grady D. Urinary incontinence in older women: who is at risk? Study of Osteoporotic Fractures Research Group. *ObstetGynecol* 1996; 87 (5 Pt 1):715–721.
15. Diokno AC, Brock BM, Herzog AR, Bromberg J. Medical correlates of urinary incontinence in the elderly. *Urology* 1990; 36:129–138.
16. Dugan E, Cohen SJ, Bland DR, et al. The association of depressive symptoms and urinary incontinence among older adults. *J Am Geriatr Soc.* 2000;48 (4):413–416.
17. Noelker LS. Incontinence in elderly cared for by family. *Gerontologist* 1987; 27:194–200.
18. Coward RT, Horne C, Peek CW. Predicting nursing home admissions among incontinent older adults: a comparison of residential differences across six years. *Gerontologist* 1995; 35: 732–743.
19. Jirovec MM, Wells TJ. Urinary incontinence in nursing home residents with dementia: the mobility-cognition paradigm. *Appl Nurs Res.* 1990; 3:112–117.
20. Chiang L, Ouslander J, Schnelle J, Reuben DB. Dually incontinent nursing home residents: Clinical characteristics and treatment differences. *J Am Geriatr Soc.* 2000; 48:673–676.
21. Palmer MH, German PS, Ouslander JG. Risk factors for urinary incontinence one year after nursing home admission. *Res Nurs Health.* 1991;14: 405–412.
22. Abrutyn E, Mossey J, Berlin JA, et al. Does asymptomatic bacteriuria predict mortality and does antimicrobial treatment reduce mortality inelderly ambulatory women? *Ann Intern Med.* 1994;120 (10):827–833.
23. Nordenstam GR, Brandberg CA, Oden AS, et al. Bacteriuria and mortality in an elderly population. *N Engl J Med.* 1986;314(18):1152–1156.
24. Nicolle LE, Henderson E, Bjornson J, McIntyre M, Harding GK, MacDonell JA. The association of bacteriuria with resident characteristics and survival in elderly institutionalized men. *Ann Intern Med.* 1987;106: 682–686.
25. Monane M, Gurwitz JH, Lipsitz LA, Glynn RJ, Choodnovskiy I, Avorn J. Epidemiologic and diagnostic aspects of bacteriuria: a longitudinal study in older women. *J Am Geriatr Soc.* 1995; 43(3):618–622.
26. Nicolle LE, Mayhew WJ, Bryan L. Prospective randomized comparison of therapy and no therapy for asymptomatic bacteriuria in institutionalized elderly women. *Am J Med.* 1987; 83:27–33.
27. Ouslander JG, Schapira M, Schnelle JF, et al. Does eradicating bacteriuria affect the severity of chronic urinary incontinence in nursing homeresidents? *Ann Intern Med.* 1995; 122: 749–754.
28. Raz R, Gennesin Y, Wasser J, et al. Recurrent urinary tract infections in postmenopausal women. *Clin Infect Dis.* 2000; 30(1):152–156.
29. Griebling TL, Nygaard IE. The role of estrogen replacement therapy in the management of urinary incontinence and urinary tract infection inpostmenopausal women. *Endocrinol Metab Clin North Am.* 1997; 26: 347–360.
30. Dignam R, Ahmed M, Denman S, et al. The effect of cranberry juice on UTI rates in a long term care facility. *J Am Geriatr Soc.* 1997; 45:S53.
31. Avorn J, Monane M, Gurwitz JH, Glynn RJ, Choodnovskiy I, Lipsitz LA. Reduction of bacteriuria and pyuria after ingestion of cranberry juice. *JAMA* 1994; 271(10):751–754.

32. Kontiokari T, Sundqvist K, Nuutinen M, Pokka T, Koskela M, Uhari M. Randomised trial of cranberry-lingonberry juice and Lactobacillus GG drink for the prevention of urinary tract infections in women. *BMJ* 2001; 322(7302): 1571.

33. Haidinger G, Temml C, Schatzl G, et al. Risk factors for lower urinary tract symptoms in elderly men. For the Prostate Study Group of the Austrian Society of Urology. *Eur Urol.* 2000; 37(4): 413–420.

34. Krogh J, Jensen JS, Iversen HG, Andersen JT. Age as a prognostic variable in patients undergoing transurethral prostatectomy. *Scand J Urol Nephrol.* 1993; 27:225–229.

35. Epstein RS, Lydick E, deLabry L, Vokonas PS. Age-related differences in risk factors for prostatectomy for benign prostatic hyperplasia: the VA Normative Aging Study. *Urology* 1991; 38 (1 Suppl): 9–12.

36. Cooper KL, McKiernan JM, Kaplan SA. Alpha-adrenoceptor antagonists in the treatment of benign prostatic hyperplasia. *Drugs.* 1999; 57:9–17.

37. Medina JJ, Parra RO, Moore RG. Benign prostatic hyperplasia (the aging prostate). *Med Clin North Am.* 1999; 83:1213–1229.

38. Lee M, Sharifi R. Benign prostatic hyperplasia: Diagnosis and treatment guideline. *Ann Pharmacother.* 1997;31: 481–486.

39. Breslin DS, Muecke EC, Reckler JM, Fracchia JA. Changing trends in the management of prostatic disease in a single private practice: A 5-yearfollowup. *J Urol.* 1993; 150:347–350.

40. Holtgrewe HL. Economic issues and the management of benign prostatic hyperplasia. *Urology* 1995; 46: 23–25.

41. Wilt TJ, Ishani A, Rutks I, MacDonald R. Phytotherapy for benign prostatic hyperplasia. *Public Health Nutr.* 2000; 3:459–472.

42. Lowe FC, Ku JC. Phytotherapy in treatment of benign prostatic hyperplasia: A critical review. *Urology* 1996; 48:12–20.

43. Wenninger K, Heiman JR, Rothman I, Berghuis JP, Berger RE. Sickness impact of chronic nonbacterial prostatitis and its correlates. *J Urol.* 1996; 155(3):965–968.

44. Muller A, Mulhall JP. Sexual dysfunction in the patient with prostatitis. *Curr Urol Rep.* 2006; 7: 307–312.

45. Krieger JN, Nyberg L Jr, Nickel CN. NIH Consensus definition and classification of prostatitis. *JAMA* 1999; 281:236–237.

46. Gionchetti P, Rizzello F, Campieri M. Probiotics in gastroenterology. *Curr Opin Gastroenterol.* 2002; 18: 235–239.

47. Heczko PB, Strus M, Kochan P. Critical evaluation of probiotic activity of lactic acid bacteria and their effects. *J Physiol Pharmacol.* 2006; 57(suppl 9): 5–12.

48. Reid G, Bruce AW. Probiotics to prevent urinary tract infections: The rationale and evidence. *World J Urol.* 2006; 24:28–32.

49. Falagas ME, Betsi GI, Tokas T, et al. Probiotics for prevention of recurrent urinary tract infections in women: a review of the evidence from microbiological and clinical studies. *Drugs.* 2006; 66:1253–1261.

50. Fair WR, Couch J, Wehner N. Prostatic antibacterial factor. *Ident Signific Urol.* 1976; 7:169–177.

51. Evliyaoglu Y, Kumbur H. Seminal plasma zinc analysis and bacteriological cultures in chronic staphylococcal prostatitis. *Int Urol Nephrol.* 1995; 27: 341–345.

52. Aston JL, Lodolce AE, Shapiro NL. Interaction between warfarin and cranberry juice. *Pharmacotherapy* 2006; 26: 1314–1319.

53. Nickel JC, Shoskes D, Roehrborn CG, Moyad M. Nutraceuticals in Prostate Disease: The Urologist's Role. *Rev Urol.* 2008; 10(3):192–206.

54. Rosario DJ, Becker M, Anderson JB. The changing pattern of mortality and morbidity from radical cystectomy. *BJU Int.* 2000; 85:427–430.

55. Game X, Soulie M, Seguin P, et al. Radical cystectomy in patients older than 75 years: Assessment of morbidity and mortality. *Eur Urol.* 2001; 39(5): 525–529.

56. Soulie M, Straub M, Game X, et al. A multicenter study of the morbidity of radical cystectomy in select elderly patients with bladder cancer. *J Urol.* 2002; 167(3): 1325–1328.
57. Saika T, Suyama B, Murata T, et al. Orthotopic neobladder reconstruction in elderly bladder cancer patients. *Int J Urol.* 2001; 8(10):533–538.
58. Doherty JG, Rufer A, Bartholomew P, Beaumont DM. The presentation, treatment and outcome of renal cell carcinoma in old age. *Age Ageing.* 1999; 28:359–362.
59. Hsu TH, Gill IS, Fazeli-Matin S, et al. Radical nephrectomy and nephroureterectomy in the octogenarian and nonagenarian: comparison oflaparoscopic and open approaches. *Urology* 1999;53: 1121–1125.
60. Panser LA, Rhodes T, Girman CJ, et al. Sexual function of men ages 40 to 79 years: The Olmsted County Study of Urinary Symptoms and HealthStatus Among Men. *J Am Geriatr Soc.* 1995; 43(10):1107–1111.
61. Jφnler M, Moon T, Brannan W, tone NN, Heisey D, Bruskewitz RC. The effect of age, ethnicity and geographical location on impotence and quality of life. *Br J Urol.* 1995; 75(5): 651–655.
62. Johannes CB, Araujo AB, Feldman HA, Derby CA, Kleinman KP, McKinlay JB. Incidence of erectile dysfunction in men 40 to 69 years old: longitudinal results from the Massachusetts male aging study. *J Urol.* 2000; 163(2):460–463.
63. Helgason AR, Adolfsson J, Dickman P, Arver S, Fredrikson M, Steineck G. Factors associated with waning sexual function among elderly men and prostate cancer patients. *J Urol.* 1997;158(1) :155–159.
64. Rosen RC, Riley A, Wagner G, Osterloh IH, Kirkpatrick J, Mishra A. The International Index of Erectile Function (IIEF): a multidimensional scale for assessment of erectile dysfunction. *Urology* 1997;49(6): 822–830.
65. Cappelleri JC, Siegel RL, Osterloh IH, Rosen RC. Relationship between patient self-assessment of erectile function and the erectile function domain of the international index of erectile function. *Urology* 2000; 56:477–481.
66. Glick HA, McCarron TJ, Althof SE, Corty EW, Willke RJ. Construction of scales for the Center for Marital and Sexual Health (CMASH) Sexual Functioning Questionnaire. *J Sex Marital Ther.* 1997; 23(2): 103–117.
67. Rosen R, Brown C, Heiman J, et al. The Female Sexual Function Index (FSFI): A multidimensional self-report instrument for the assessment of female sexual function. *J Sex Marital Ther.* 2000; 26(2): 191–208.
68. Purifoy FE, Grodsky A, Giambra LM. The relationship of sexual daydreaming to sexual activity, sexual drive, and sexual attitudes for womenacross the life-span. *Arch Sex Behav.* 1992; 21: 369–385.
69. Berman JR, Berman L, Goldstein I. Female sexual dysfunction: incidence, pathophysiology, evaluation, and treatment options. *Urology* 1999; 54: 385–391.
70. Nusbaum MR, Gamble G, Skinner B, Heiman J. The high prevalence of sexual concerns among women seeking routine gynecological care. *J Fam Pract.* 2000; 49: 229–232.
71. Mocchegiani E, Romeo J, Malavolta M, et al. Zinc: Dietary intake and impact of supplementation on immune function in elderly. *Age* 2013; 35: 839–60.
72. Bauer J, Biolo G, Cederholm T, et al. Evidence-based recommendations for optimal dietary protein intake in older people: A position paper from the PROT-AGE Study Group. *J Am Med Dir Assoc.* 2013; 14: 542–59.
73. Breen L, Stokes KA, Churchward-Venne TA, et al. Two weeks of reduced activity decreases leg lean mass and induces "anabolic resistance" of myofibrillar protein synthesis in healthy elderly. *J Clin Endocrinol Metab.* 2013; 98: 2604–12.
74. Araujo J R, Martel F, Borges N, Araujo JM, Keating E. Folates and aging: Role in mild cognitive impairment, dementia and depression. *Ageing Res Rev.* 2015; 22: 9–19.
75. Mursu J, Robien K, Harnack LJ, Park K, Jacobs DR. Dietary supplements and mortality rate in older women: The Iowa Women's Health Study. *Arch Intern Med.* 2011; 171: 1625–33.

76. Arnarson A, Geirsdottir OG, Ramel A, Briem K, Jonsson PV, Thorsdottir I. Effects of whey proteins and carbohydrates on the efficacy of resistance training in elderly people: Double blind, randomised controlled trial. *Eur J Clin Nutr.* 2013; 67: 1–6.

77. de Jager CA, Oulhaj A, Jacoby R, Refsum H, Smith AD. Cognitive and clinical outcomes of homocysteine_lowering B_vitamin treatment in mild cognitive impairment: A randomized controlled trial. *Int J Geriatr Psychiatry.* 2012; 27: 592–600.

78. Salovaara K, Tuppurainen M, Karkkainen M et al. Effect of vitamin D3 and calcium on fracture risk in 65-to 71-year_old women: A population-based 3-year randomized, controlled trial- the OSTPRE-FPS. *J Bone Miner Res.* 2010; 25: 1487–95.

79. Masson L. Omega-3 and omega-6 fatty acids in human health. In: Prakash D., Sharma G., editors. *Phytochemicals of Nutraceutical Importance.* CABI International Publishers; Wallingford: 2014. pp. 116–131.

80. Gupta C and Prakash D. Nutraceuticals for geriatrics. *J Tradit Complement Med.* 2015; 5(1): 5–14.

81. Albersen M, Orabi H, and Lue TF. Evaluation and treatment of erectile dysfunction in the aging male: a mini-review. *Gerontology.* 2012; 58(1): 3–14.

82. Hedner T, Edgar B, Edvinsson L, Hedner J, Persson B, Pettersson A. Yohimbine pharmacokinetics and interaction with the sympathetic nervous system in normal volunteers. *Eur J Clin Pharmacol.* 1992; 43(6): 651–656.

83. Lebret T, Hervé J-M, Gorny P, Worcel M, Botto H. Efficacy and safety of a novel combination of L-arginine glutamate and yohimbine hydrochloride: A new oral therapy for erectile dysfunction. *European Urology.* 2002; 41(6): 608–613.

84. Ning H, Xin Z-C, Lin G, Banie K, Lue TF, Lin C-S. Effects of icariin on phosphodiesterase-5 activity in vitro and cyclic guanosine monophosphate level in cavernous smooth muscle cells. *Urology* 2006; 68(6): 1350–1354.

85. Xu H-B, Huang Z-Q. Icariin enhances endothelial nitricoxide synthase expression on human endothelial cells in vitro. *Vasc Pharmacol.* 2007; 47(1): 18–24.

86. Zhang Z-B, Yang Q-T. The testosterone mimetic properties of icariin. *Asian J Androl.* 2006; 8(5): 601–605.

87. Perri A, Ilacqua A, Valenti M, Aversa A. Effects of nutraceuticals on sexual satisfaction and lower urinary tract symptoms in a cohort of young–old men. *Phytother Res.* 2018; 32(2):284–289.

88. Feifer AH, Fleshner NE, Klotz L. Analytical accuracy and reliability of commonly used nutritional supplements in prostate disease. *J Urol.* 2002; 168:150–154.

89. Wilt TJ, Ishani A, Stark G, MacDonald R, Lau J, Mulrow C. Saw palmetto extracts for treatment of benign prostatic hyperplasia: a systematic review. *JAMA.* 1998; 280(18):1604–1609.

90. Boyle P, Robertson C, Lowe F, Roehrborn C. Updated meta-analysis of clinical trials of Serenoa repens extract in the treatment of symptomatic benign prostatic hyperplasia. *BJU Int.* 2004; 93(6): 751–756.

91. Gerber GS, Zagaja GP, Bales GT, Chodak GW, Contreras BA. Saw palmetto (Serenoa repens) in men with lower urinary tract symptoms: effects on urodynamic parameters and voiding symptoms. *Urology* 1998; 51(6):1003–1007.

92. Willetts KE, Clements MS, Champion S, Ehsman S, Eden JA. Serenoa repens extract for benign prostate hyperplasia: a randomized controlled trial. *BJU Int.* 2003; 92(3): 267–270.

93. Bent S, Kane C, Shinohara K, et al. Saw palmetto for benign prostatic hyperplasia. *N Engl J Med.* 2006; 354(6): 557–566.

94. Ishani A, MacDonald R, Nelson D, Rutks I, Wilt TJ. Pygeum africanum for the treatment of patients with benign prostatic hyperplasia: A systematic review and quantitative meta-analysis. *Am J Med.* 2000; 109: 654–664.

95. Andro MC, Riffaud JP. Pygeum Africa num extract or the treatment of patients with benign prostatic hyperplasia: a review of 25 years of published experience. *Ther Res.* 1995; 56: 796–817.

96. Sokeland J, Albrecht J. Combination of Sabal and Urtica extract vs. finasteride in benign prostatic hyperplasia (Aiken stages I to II). Comparison of therapeutic effectiveness in a one year double-blind study. *Urologe A.* 1997; 36: 327–333.

97. Meyer F, Galan P, Douville P, et al. Antioxidant vitamin and mineral supplementation and prostate cancer prevention in the SU.VI.MAX trial. *Int J Cancer.* 2005; 116(2): 182–186.

98. Johnson AR, Munoz A, Gottlieb JL, Jarrard DF. High dose zinc increases hospital admissions due to genitourinary complications. *J Urol.* 2007; 177(2): 639–643.

99. Moyad MA. Selenium and vitamin E supplements for prostate cancer: Evidence or embellishment? *Urology.* 2002; 59 (4 suppl 1): 9–19.

100. Lonn E, Bosch J, Yusuf S, et al. Effects of longterm vitamin E supplementation on cardiovascular events and cancer: a randomized controlled trial. *JAMA.* 2005; 293(11): 1338–1347.

101. Bairati I, Meyer F, Jobin E, et al. Antioxidant vitamins supplementation and mortality: a randomized trial in head and neck cancer patients. *Int J Cancer.* 2006; 119(9): 2221–2224.

102. Moyad MA, Robinson LE. Cholesterol, cholesterol lowering agents/statins, and urologic disease: part IV—is vitamin E phosphate or another unique type of this vitamin the last chance for these supplements? *Urol Nurs.* 2006; 26: 415–418.

103. Wilcox A, Carnes ML, Moon TD, et al. Androgen deprivation in veterans with prostate cancer: implications for skeletal health. *Ann Pharmacother.* 2006; 40(12): 2107–2114.

104. Bischoff-Ferrari HA, Giovannucci E, Willett WC, Dietrich T, Dawson-Hughes B. Estimation of optimal serum concentrations of 25-hydroxyvitamin D for multiple health outcomes. *Am J Clin Nutr.* 2006; 84(5): 18–28.

105. Ornish D, Weidner G, Fair WR, et al. Intensive lifestyle changes may affect the progression of prostate cancer. *J Urol.* 2005; 174(3): 1065–1069.

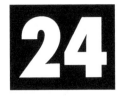

Nutrient Supplements in the Treatment of Mental Disorders in the Aging Population

Ofosua Adi-Dako
University of Ghana

Doris Kumadoh
Centre for Plant Medicine Research

Mansa Fredua-Agyeman
University of Ghana

Mary Ann Archer
Centre for Plant Medicine Research

Francis Bentil
University of Ghana

Manuela Okaijah
University of Ghana

Contents

DOI: 10.1201/9781003110866-24

24.1 General introduction

The World Health Organization (WHO) anticipates an increase in growth of the global aging population, about 60 years of age and above by the year 2050. By this time, forecast for the aged population of about 80 years and above is expected to be 400 million individuals.

Even though pharmacotherapy for instance has generally advanced and prolonged life expectancy, it is also associated with some risks in the elderly in this regard. For instance, facilitation of aging also presents with the complex issues of the management of polypharmacy required for long-term treatment of disease for such populations. Moreover, physiological and cognitive changes with age also expose the elderly to the vulnerability of adverse effects from such drugs (Singh and Bajorek, 2014) that could impact their mental health as well.

Recent reports show the continued rise in the incidence of stress-related vulnerabilities, mood and psychiatric disorder. This has heightened the research interest in preventive and therapeutic strategies to improve the mental health of the elderly. The role nutrition plays in mental health is becoming increasingly evident. Emerging findings suggest a strong correlation between a diet deficient in required nutrients and mood disorders such as anxiety, depression and neuropsychiatric conditions (Adan et al., 2019).

The elderly are susceptible to nutritional vulnerability due to physiological changes and social and economic factors they encounter later on in life. Notably, such changes are known to negatively impact their mental health. Subsequent depression and anxiety could cause the aged to lose interest in eating. With such reduced food intake, their mental health becomes further aggravated (Harbottle, 2019).

The constitution of the brain and its function depends on important nutrients such as vitamins, minerals, lipids and amino acids. In effect, the quality and type of food taken eventually affect brain function, mental health cognitive performance and the mood of an individual. Moreover, the type of dietary intake influences the production of gut microbiome, gut hormones, neuropeptides and neurotransmitters (Adan et al., 2019). Evidence from numerous systematic reviews and meta-analysis demonstrates a relationship between nutrition and mental health.

Reports from recent studies involving 33 meta-analyses of placebo-controlled randomized controlled trials and analysis of data from 10,951 participants provide strong evidence of the need of some select vital nutrients and dietary supplements in the mental health of the aging population. Studies in this regard have demonstrated how PUFAs, e.g., eicosapentaenoic acid, have complemented treatment in depression and attention-deficit/hyperactivity disorder. Folate-based supplements, high dose methyl folate and N-acetylcysteine have played beneficial roles as adjunctive treatments in mood disorders, depression and schizophrenia. (Firth et al., 2019)

Consequently, more attention should be given to the study and evaluation of the import and significance of nutritional supplements and nutrients such as polyunsaturated fatty acids (PUFAs), vitamins, minerals, antioxidants, amino acids and pre/probiotics supplements that can impact the mental health of the aged population.

Hence, this chapter, divided into four areas of nutritional interest in the elderly, seeks to demonstrate how nutritional interventions with nutraceuticals, such as polyunsaturated fatty acids (PUFAs), vitamins, minerals, antioxidants, amino acids and pre/probiotic supplements are critical for the mental well-being of the elderly.

24.2 Probiotics, prebiotic supplements and aging population

24.2.1 Gut microbiota, the basis of probiotic and prebiotic supplements

The human gut microbiota is a complex community with a behavior that has been linked to an organ in the human body and a metabolizing capacity indispensable and comparable to the liver. The human gut microbiota has been estimated to contain more than 10^{14} microorganisms, which exceeds the number of cells in the human body by a factor of 10 and contains 100 times many genes as the human genome.

The gut microbiota has been demonstrated to play essential roles in the regulation of metabolic, endocrine and immune functions and are important in human health and diseases. For instance, they contribute toward human nutrition by synthesizing and secreting vitamins, which are absorbed as nutrients by humans. They are important in the metabolism and absorption of xenobiotics including drugs. They have protective functions against various infections as they ensure colonization resistance of the gut. They ferment parts of the diet, which are not digested in the upper part of the digestive system. The good members of the microbiota are saccharolytic and produce short-chain fatty acids (SCFAs), lactate, pyruvate, ethanol, succinate and gases such as H_2, CO_2, CH_4 and H_2S as products of carbohydrate fermentation. The SCFAs contribute to the energy requirement of the host and play a key role in neuro-immunoendocrine regulation. There is now growing evidence that the microbiota has a great influence on key brain processes, which has led to a microbiota-gut-brain axis concept (Cryan and Dinan, 2012, Erny et al., 2015).

There are reports of shifts in the composition of intestinal microbiota with age. For instance, Odamaki et al. (2016) reported higher *Bifidobacterium* in infants, noting increasing proportions of *Bacterioides*, *Eubacterium* and *Clostridiaceae* as one progresses in age. Yatsunenko et al. (2012) also reported decreasing numbers of *Bifidobacterium* as one ages. A significant decrease in the relative proportions of Bacteroidetes and Firmicutes in older population in relation to adults has also been reported (Mariat et al., 2009). Elderly patients have also been reported to exhibit high levels of *E. coli* and *Bacteroidetes* (Mariat et al., 2009). There is also reported decreased species diversity with age. This together with the changes in the physiology of the elderly, for instance, decreased intestinal motility and changes in diet and malnutrition caused by lack of teeth, swallowing difficulties with old age, and a consequent increase in bacterial protein fermentation instead of saccharolytic fermentation leads to high amounts of toxic metabolites such as ammonia, phenolic compounds and amines. These toxic metabolites are often linked to diseases and infections in the elderly. For instance, small bowel bacterial overgrowth, a condition characterized by an abnormal increase in bacteria in the small intestine with associated nutrient malabsorption is often common in elderly people (Mitsui et al., 2006). There is a decreased apoptosis in the colon in old age with resultant colon cancer; inflammation, nutrient malabsorption, declined immune function and infectious diarrhea, among others.

24.2.2 Probiotics and prebiotics

Probiotics are live microorganisms that, when administered in adequate amounts, confer a health effect on the host (Hill et al., 2014). They are bacteria related to those found naturally in the human gut, particularly those supposedly found in the gut of breastfed infants because they are known to be significant in contributing toward the health effects of the microbiota. Prebiotics are selectively fermented dietary ingredients that result in specific changes, in the composition and/or activity of the gastrointestinal microbiota, consequently conferring benefit(s) upon host health. Thus the use of probiotics and prebiotics are aimed toward a healthy microbiota. Probiotics are usually good (nonpathogenic) members of the gut microbiota, which play significant role toward health and produce SCFAs as the end product of fermentation. They are usually limited to members of the lactic acid bacteria (LAB) group (chiefly the members of *Lactobacillus*) and Bifidobacteria. They are typically included in yoghurt, cheese, fermented milk products, fruit juices and other beverages. Others are available as freeze-dried supplements placed into capsules, made into tablets or sold as powder form.

The use of prebiotics is meant to selectively stimulate the growth and or activity of specific members of the colonic microbiota by providing a specific substrate for their growth and metabolism (Gibson and Roberfroid, 1995). The selective growth of those members (mostly the *Bifidobacterium* and the lactic acid group (LAB)) would cause an enhanced beneficial effect on a dysbiosed microbiota. Some of these beneficial effects include the change of the gut microbiota toward a healthier composition, improvement of intestinal functions such as prevention of constipation, treatment of diarrhea, prevention of intestinal infection and managing lactose intolerance. There is also better modulation of the immune system, reduction in risk of colon cancer, type 2 diabetes, intestinal inflammation, obesity and metabolic syndrome (Roberfroid et al., 2010). The enhanced effects are thought to be brought about by the fermentation of the prebiotics by the microbiota to produce SCFAs. Fructo-oligosaccharides (FOS), galacto-oligosaccharides (GOS) and trans-galacto-oligosaccarides (TOS) are the most commonly used prebiotics. Probiotics and prebiotics are commonly used in combination and referred to as synbiotic.

24.2.3 Probiotics and prebiotics in the elderly: Clinical evidence

As noted earlier, aging is associated with a decreased immune function, several metabolic and inflammatory disorders, diabetes, obesity, cancer, bowel diseases and increased risk of infections including *Clostridium difficile* infections (Lakshminarayanan et al., 2014). Probiotic/prebiotic interventions can improve age-related disorders (attributed to microbiota dysbiosis) by introducing specific strains with health promoting potentials and or substrates, which can increase the amount of beneficial microorganisms and thereby reduce the risk of age-related disorders. For instance, supplementation with the prebiotic xylooligosaccharides (XOSs) in patients who were more than 65 years old was shown to significantly increase the population of bifidobacteria, increase fecal moisture content and decrease fecal pH, thus generally improving intestinal health (Chung Y.C. et al., 2007). A galactooligosaccharide (GOS) mixture supplementation in the elderly (65–80 years) also led to significant increases in Bacteroides and Bifidobacteria which correlated with increased lactic acid in feces, higher IL-10, IL-8, natural killer cell activity and C-reactive protein (Vulevic et al., 2015). Also, Cicero et al. (2020) demonstrated that treatment of elderly patients with probiotics *Lactobacillus acidophilus* PBS066, *Lactobacillus reuteri* PBS072 with prebiotics resulted in statistically significant improvement in waist circumference, fasting plasma insulin, total cholesterol, high-density lipoprotein cholesterol, low-density lipoprotein cholesterol, triglycerides, high-sensitivity C-reactive protein and tumor necrosis factor alpha serum levels. Thus the synbiotic reduced blood lipids, fasting plasma glucose, waist circumference, visceral adiposity, the prevalence of metabolic syndrome, cardiovascular risk factors and insulin resistance in old patients. The consumption of *Lactobacillus rhamnosus* and prebiotic Promitor™ Soluble Corn Fiber in elderly patients aged between 60 and 80 years promoted innate immunity by increasing natural killer (NK) cell activity. The synbiotic also reduced total cholesterol and LDL-cholesterol and decreased proinflammatory cytokine IL-6 (Costabile et al., 2017). Also an increased Bifidobacteria, Actinobacteria and Firmicutes with increased butyrate production and decreased pro-inflammatory cytokine TNF- α have been reported in elderly patients consuming probiotic *Bifidobacterium longum* and inulin-based prebiotic (Macfarlane et al., 2013). Valentini et al. (2015) also reported increased Bifidobacteria, folate, vitamin B12 and reduction in homocysteine concentration with probiotic VSL#3 supplementation in the elderly.

24.2.4 Probiotics and prebiotics in mental health

The microbiota is known to play a significant role in the gut-brain axis. It has been reported that the brain and the gut can bidirectionally communicate through neurotransmitters, immunomodulation, the enteric nervous systems and SCFAs (Burokas et al., 2015). This is important for maintaining the brain functions and gut homeostasis. Parkinson's disease, Alzheimer's disease, other neurological disorders, mood disorders, severe cognitive impairment and anxiety are result of the disturbance to the bidirectional relationship. Furthermore, dysbiosis of the gut microbiota brought about by diet, drugs, infections and so on have been linked to the pathogenesis of gut-brain disorders (Rogers et al., 2016). Germ-free animals (GF) compared to conventional mice showed that the microbiota is essential for normal intrinsic and extrinsic nerve function and gut-brain signaling (McVey Neufeld et al., 2015). Other studies have also suggested that the development, function and disorders of the central nervous system and enteric nervous system is through the interaction and activation of Toll-like receptors 2 and 4 (TLR2 and TLR4) and that there is a period during life where the gut microbiota composition is very vital and any disturbance during that period could cause life-long effects of the development and function of the CNS and ENS (Heiss and Olofsson, 2019). The microbiota is known to produce glutamate and gamma-aminobutyric acid (GABA; by the conversion of glutamate), key inhibitory neurotransmitter in the nervous system (Strandwitz et al., 2019) and this has been demonstrated with probiotics, with some probiotics shown to produce GABA and serotonin (Siragusa et al., 2007, Barrett et al., 2012). Also, hydroxytryptamine (5-HT), a neurotransmitter, can be produced by the gut microbiota from tryptophan. SCFAs including acetate, propionate and butyrate produced by the microbiota can also induce immune cells.

Alzheimer's disease-related dementia, characterized by deterioration in memory, thinking and cognitive ability, is a common disease in older population. It is associated with the over production and deposition of amyloid-ß peptide which can be influenced by the gut microbiota and associated metabolites. Alzheimer's disease patients have been demonstrated to have an altered gut microbiota, suggesting the role of the microbiota in the pathogenesis of the disease. Older patients with Alzheimer's disease dementia showed lower amounts of butyrate producing bacteria and their stool samples induced lower P-glycoprotein expression levels *in vitro* than samples from older patients without dementia (Haran et al., 2019). Probiotic and selenium co-supplementation for 12 weeks improved cognitive functions and metabolic abnormality in patients with Alzheimer's disease (Tamtaji et al., 2019a).

Parkinson's disease, an important neurodegenerative disorder which affects 2%–3% of the population above 65 years, is characterized by rigidity, slowness of movement, resting tremor, depression, cognitive disturbances, depression, altered autonomic functions, etc. Also nausea, altered bowel habits (mainly constipation), dysphagia, hypersalivation are some of the gastrointestinal symptoms that characterize the disease. Parkinson's disease is associated with the accumulation of α-synuclein in the central and peripheral nervous systems (Han et al., 2020). The disease has also been linked with altered gut microbiota. For instance, Unger et al. (2016) demonstrated lower levels of SCFAs in Parkinson's disease patients relative to controls. Also, lower levels of butyrate producing fecal bacteria (*Blautia, Coprococcus* and *Roseburia*) and an abundance of mucosal *Ralstonia* have been reported in Parkinson's disease patients relative to controls (Keshavarzian et al., 2015). Supplementation with probiotics has shown improved motor function in Parkinson's disease patients (Tamtaji et al., 2019b). Also a couple of studies have demonstrated improvement of gastrointestinal function in Parkinson's disease patients including reduction in constipation, reduction of pain and bloating, improved stool consistency after consumption of probiotics or prebiotics (Barichella et al., 2016, Georgescu et al., 2016, Cassani et al., 2011).

The elderly population is also affected by depression, anxiety and stress. These disorders have also been linked to altered gut microbiota. For example, lower levels of *Bifidobacterium, Faecalibacterium* and *Ruminococcus* and higher levels of *Anaerostipes, Clostridium* and *Kebsiella* have been observed in patients with depression (Cheung et al., 2019). Administration of *Lactobacillus plantarum* PS128 showed reduction of anxiety and depression-like behaviors in mice (Liu et al., 2016). Also, administration of *Lactobacillus helveticus* NS8,

Lactobacillus rhamnosus (JB-1) and *Bifidobacterium longum* NCC3001 individually has shown evidence of reduction in anxiety, depression or cognitive function (Bravo et al., 2011, Bercik et al., 2010).

In summary, there is increasing evidence of the effects of probiotics and prebiotics on mental health. Some probiotics and prebiotics have been shown to improve cognitive and metabolic functions in patients with Alzheimer's disease, improve overall CNS function including depression, anxiety and stress, and improve quality of life of elderly patients prone to neurodegenerative diseases.

24.3 The role of antioxidants and amino acids in the mental health of the elderly

24.3.1 The importance of antioxidants in our diet

At all times, several chemical reactions continuously occur within our cells. The reduction-oxidation (redox), a common form of reaction plays a crucial role in maintaining cellular functions, including metabolic cycles and detoxification of harmful substances. As a result of these metabolic activities, reactive oxygen species (ROS) are produced as by-products. These toxic molecules produced in the body interact with DNA, lipids, and proteins to cause damage, leading to an alteration in cellular function. In a healthy cell, the balance of these ROS is maintained by endogenous substances known as antioxidants which serve to neutralize the ROS produced (Fraunberger et al., 2016).

24.3.2 Classification of antioxidants

Antioxidants can be classified into two broad classes: endogenous and exogenous. Within the body, the antioxidants consist of antioxidant enzyme defenses and additional spontaneously synthesized antioxidant compounds such as melatonin and glutathione (A primary endogenous antioxidant) (Fraunberger et al., 2016). The enzymes include Copper-zinc-SOD, and Manganese SOD catalyze the dismutation reaction of superoxide to H_2O_2 to decrease its reduction potential, Glutathione peroxidase which reduces lipid hydroperoxides to alcohols and H_2O_2 to water, Glutathione reductase (GR) maintains glutathione levels. Glutathione-S-transferase detoxifies xenobiotics. Catalase (CAT) reduces H_2O_2 to water and oxygen, and Peroxiredoxins reduce H_2O_2 to water (Ighodaro and Akinloye, 2018).

Antioxidants can be supplied by a diet outside the body with a wide range of natural and synthetic compounds (exogenous) contained in complex mixtures (such as chocolate or olive oil) or extracted to be used as a supplement (Bouayed and Bohn, 2010). They include tocopherols, resveratrol, vitamin A and vitamin C (Singh, Kesharwani and Keservani, 2017). Working together with endogenous antioxidants, these exogenous antioxidants enhance the efficiency of antioxidant gene regulation, allowing for a more enhanced and efficient defense against detrimental redox modulations (Fraunberger et al., 2016).

24.3.3 Oxidative stress, antioxidants and brain health

According to Cobley et al. (2018), the brain has several biochemical and physiological characteristics that make it vulnerable to oxidative stress. These characteristics include the following:

- **High oxygen utilization**: The brain accounts for a small proportion of body weight compared to the rest of the body. However, as it uses a high supply of available oxygen (up to 20%), toxic by-products such as hydrogen peroxide and superoxide are eventually created and begin to cause damage.
- **Presence of redox-active metals**: There is approximately 60 mg of nonheme iron naturally bound to ferritin and hemosiderin in the average adult brain. The movement of iron into the brain in a regular, healthy brain is regulated by transferrin and its associated receptors. However, if brain damage occurs, particularly in areas with a high content of iron (substantia nigra, caudate nucleus, putamen and globus pallidus), iron is released from ferritin or diffuses via microvasculature damage. This catalytic iron, once inside the brain, causes extensive amounts of damage due to the CSF's negligible iron-binding strength.
- **High calcium influx across neuronal membranes**: In the presence of reactive species such as hydrogen peroxide, an increase in intracellular calcium ions may be triggered by disruptions in mitochondrial and endoplasmic reticulum activity, specifically their calcium sequestration capacity. This causes mitochondria to increase the development of reactive species and cause more damage.
- **Autoxidizable neurotransmitters**: Catecholamine neurotransmitters (dopamine, epinephrine and norepinephrine) can react with oxygen to produce superoxide and quinones/semiquinones that readily bind to sulfhydryl side chains and deplete the already low cerebral GSH reserves.
- **Low antioxidant defenses**: There are lower concentrations of antioxidant defenses across the brain compared to the rest of the body. The only substantial antioxidant enzyme in the brain is catalase, which is very limited in its ability to detoxify H_2O_2 since it is localized microperoxisomes.

24.3.4 Restoration of levels of antioxidants

Our endogenous supply of antioxidants starts to decline while our body works to maintain its redox status, effectively reducing our ability to combat excessive amounts of reactive species. We may consume food or supplements containing natural or synthetic compounds that are either transformed directly into the endogenous antioxidant or help in its replenishment to supplement our antioxidant defenses (Fraunberger et al., 2016). Lipoic acid and

N-acetylcysteine or its amide are two representative examples (Fernandes et al., 2016). N-acetylcysteine, occurring in abundance in high protein foods, is the nutraceutical form of the amino acid cysteine and functions as a precursor of glutathione (Fernandes et al., 2016). Once NAC or NACA reaches the cell, it is absorbed into the cytosol, where the release of cysteine, the limiting reagent in the formation of GSH, is hydrolyzed (Bavarsad Shahripour, Harrigan and Alexandrov, 2014). Glutamine and cysteine are combined into γ-glutamylcysteine using γ-glutamylcysteine synthetase, where glutathione is produced by further glutamine addition (Fraunberger et al., 2016).

In mixed psychiatric samples, N-acetylcysteine (at doses of 2,000 mg/day or higher) is indicated as potentially useful for reducing depressive symptoms and increasing functional recovery. Also, by using N-acetylcysteine as an adjunctive therapy, substantial decreases in overall schizophrenia symptoms have been noted (Fernandes et al., 2016). Additionally, N-acetylcysteine has been shown to increase dopamine release in animal models (Dean, Giorlando and Berk, 2011), suggesting some promise as an adjunct when used in patients with Parkinson's disease. N-acetylcysteine may help treat schizophrenia, bipolar disorder and depression by reducing oxidative stress and reducing glutamatergic dysfunction (Dean, Giorlando and Berk, 2011).

Lipoic acid in its reduced form, dihydrolipoic acid can help restore endogenous antioxidants including vitamin C, vitamin E and GSH, which otherwise decline with age by serving as a reducing agent (Shay et al., 2009). By battling against free radicals, acting as a cofactor in several enzyme complexes, promoting the reduction of lipid peroxidation, and regenerating damaged tissues, lipoic acid can play a critical role in the treatment of various nervous system disorders. Lipoic acid can inhibit neuron damage caused by ROS produced in all neurodegenerative diseases due to its strong antioxidant effect (Cekici and Emre BakArhan, 2018). In several neurotraumatic models, it is believed to be a therapeutic agent due to its neuroprotective effects (Ekiz et al., 2017). Chronic administration of lipoic acid improves cognitive function and memory by increasing total antioxidant ability, decreasing peripheral oxidative damage, and reducing hippocampal neurodegeneration (Hagen et al., 2002). In a review study by Cekici and Emre BakArhan (2018), it was found to have important effects on psychiatric conditions which included schizophrenia, dementia, stroke, Alzheimer's and traumatic brain injury, thus necessitating its use as an adjunct in these conditions.

24.3.5 Amino acid supplementation in the mental health of the elderly.

According to the World Health Organization, about 22% of the global population is above the age of 60 (2018). The rapid growth in the aging population has a subsequent effect on the rates of mental health disorders such as depression and dementia. The typical approach to the treatment of these mental disorders is the administration of prescription drugs such as fluoxetine. Most of these drugs are associated with undesirable side effects which can lead to patient noncompliance, which plays a crucial role in worsening of symptoms, morbidity, comorbidity and mortality (Keyloun et al., 2017). To combat the issue of patient noncompliance, there has been an increased emphasis on the use of nutritional supplementation as a preventive or adjunctive treatment or curative measure in the management of mental health disorders.

Amino acids are the building blocks of proteins. There are 20 amino acids which are considered essential, and these play a role in maintaining the integrity and function of brain cells, aid in neuron regeneration and organization. Supplements containing amino acids have been found to reduce symptoms as they are converted to neurotransmitters which in turn alleviate mental health problems (Glenn, Madero and Bott, 2019).

Serine: Serine is made from another amino acid (glycine) and is a major component of phosphatidylserine. Due to the important role of phosphatidylserine in brain signaling, the nutrient can improve memory. In people with mild symptoms of Alzheimer's disease, diet supplementation with phosphatidylserine improved memory and cognitive abilities. However, it does appear that these effects wear off after supplementation stops. It may be important to continue taking phosphatidylserine to reduce symptoms of Alzheimer's. The D-isomer of serine has also been shown to be effective in improving the negative symptoms of schizophrenia via its action at the NMDA receptor (MacKay et al., 2019).

Tryptophan: Tryptophan is an essential amino acid readily available in nearly all protein containing foods. Aside from its role in protein formation, tryptophan can be converted to metabolites such as serotonin and kynurenine. Serotonin has an effect on mood and cognition hence tryptophan would be helpful in treating disorders associated with these (Jenkins et al., 2016).

Tyrosine: Tyrosine is a catecholamine precursor that can reach the brain upon oral administration. In the aging brain, dietary supplements that contain tyrosine can aid in improvement of cognitive functioning as it can correct age-related dopamine alterations.

N-acetylcysteine: N-acetylcysteine is a sulphur containing amino acid and occurs in abundance in high-protein foods as cysteine. It functions as a precursor of glutathione, a primary endogenous antioxidant. In mixed psychiatric samples, N-acetylcysteine (at doses of 2,000 mg/day or higher) is indicated as potentially useful for reducing depressive symptoms and increasing functional recovery. In addition, by using N-acetylcysteine as an adjunctive therapy, substantial decreases in overall schizophrenia symptoms have been noted (Fernandes et al., 2016). Moreover, N-acetylcysteine has been shown to increase dopamine release in animal models, suggesting some promise as an adjunct when used in patients with Parkinson's disease. N-acetylcysteine may help treat schizophrenia, bipolar disorder and depression by reducing oxidative stress and reducing glutamatergic dysfunction.

Furthermore, dietary deficiencies in protein and amino acids have been linked to dementia in the aging population. Appropriate levels of protein intake enhance memory function, support brain function and reduce the susceptibility to cognitive impairment in the elderly. The mechanism by which dietary protein intake influences brain function coupled with the effects of essential amino acid administration in dietary protein deficiencies was studied by Sato et al. Aged mice were fed a low protein diet for 2 months. The mice exhibited abnormal behavior, learning and memory disorders. There were decreased levels of neurotransmitters, e.g., gamma-aminobutyric acid, glutamate, serotonin, dopamine, norepinephrine, etc. However, on administration of the essential amino acids, phenylalanine, tryptophan, histidine, leucine, valine, isoleucine and lysine, which are a source of neurotransmitters, replacement of normal levels of glutamate was achieved. Glutamate is essential for optimal memory and learning abilities. Further studies in this area are expected to provide more information about the relation between amino acids and levels of neurotransmitters in the brain. Dietary amino acids play a significant role in supporting normal brain function (Sato et al., 2020)

The incidence and rate of Alzheimer's disease and related dementia is on the rise with the growth of the aging population. Hence, considerable attention is being focused on preventive methods such as dietary intake to improve these disease conditions. Nutritional interventions such as protein and amino acid intake plays a significant role in the management of risk factors that result in cognitive decline in the elderly. Some studies have linked the consumption of protein and amino acids, to cognition, and therefore investigations into the underlying mechanisms, and associated risk factors in this regard would provide useful information for dietary amino acid consumption for the elderly who can be susceptible to cognitive decline, for their improved mental health (Glenn et al., 2019).

Dementia and cognitive decline in the elderly are disease conditions of heightened concern as they are associated with high morbidity and mortality. The N-methyl-D-aspartate (NMDA) receptor plays an essential role in memory, learning and cognition, Some gene expressions are linked to the modulation of the N-methyl-D-aspartate receptor function which in turn influence the incidence of Alzheimer's disease and mild cognitive impairment. An enzyme, D-amino acid oxidase degrades D-amino acids, such as D-serine. Recent reports indicate that aging is related to a decline in D-serine concentrations. In effect D-serine treatment reduces neuron death, suggesting a neuroprotective function of D-Serine against neural cell death. Lin et al. hypothesized that the level of D-amino acid oxidase and associated amino acids, e.g. L-serine,

D-serine glycine, L-glutamate, D-glutamate, L-alanine and D-alanine, in the peripheral blood could be associated with senile cognitive deterioration (Lin et al., 2017).

24.4 The role of vitamins and minerals as nutrient supplements (nutraceuticals) in the treatment of mental disorders in the aging population

24.4.1 The basis for the use vitamins and minerals in mental health

The aged may be a word used to classify the elderly or those advanced in aged typically 65 years and above (https://www.encyclopedia.com/medicine/encyclopedias-almanacs-transcripts-and-maps/aging-and-aged) (2020). Adults above the age of 70 years normally encounter varied health conditions such as stroke, cardiovascular diseases, obesity and cancer. In order to maintain a general level of well-being the elderly normally take nutritional supplements. It is generally believed that natural supplements are safer; however, their use should be evaluated against other psychotic medications especially in the aged to prevent unnecessary overload of the relatively weak body system in geriatrics (Adan et al., 2019; Nguyen et al., 2020).

It has been noticed that essential vitamins and minerals as well as omega-3 fatty acids are normally not available in the right quantities deficient in people having mental disorders. Several studies have been done and show that providing these daily supplements of important nutrients may help to significantly lower the symptoms exhibited by patients with mental disorders (Lakhan and Karen, 2008).

Among the ten most common health conditions suffered by the elderly, cognitive and mental health disorders as well as malnutrition feature in addition to chronic health diseases, physical injuries and sensory impairment (Lakhan and Karen, 2008).

Vitamins are micronutrient organic compounds normally available in foods and needed for proper metabolic functions of the human body (Brown and Roffman, 2014). Vitamins function as coenzymes and antioxidants to prevent damage in the brain (Conner et al., 2017). The body is normally unable to produce sufficient quantities needed for all the metabolic functions served by them. Vitamins may be grouped as fat soluble and water-soluble (IMFNB, 1998). The fat-soluble vitamins are A, D, E and K (Csapó and Csilla, 2017).

The water-soluble vitamins are Vitamin B and Vitamin C, a group of water-soluble micronutrients, which play an important role in cognition and brain function (Parletta, Milte and Meyer, 2013).

Vitamin deficiencies have been shown in several studies to contribute significantly to mental disorders like schizophrenia (Brown and Roffman, 2014).

Studies have shown that deficiency of vitamins weaken cognizance of aged (Gaudio et al., 2016; Giannunzio et al., 2018), for instance, deficiency of vitamin B12 results in depression, mania and psychosis (Smith, Warren and Refsum, 2018), vitamin B1 deficiency results in numbness, weakness of central nervous system and beriberi (Black, 2008), deficiency of vitamin B9 (folic acid) results in depression and impairment of neurodevelopment in children (Enderami, Zarghami and Darvishi-Khezri, 2018), vitamin B3 (niacin) deficiency results in dementia (Hegyi, Schwartz and Hegyi, 2004), and deficiency of vitamin D was not reported for neuropsychiatric disorders despite several trials of vitamin D in the populace (Mohammadpour et al., 2018). Findings by Ricardo and Inês Canelas da (2019) on the correlation between vitamin D deficiency and first-episode psychosis showed no significant difference in vitamin D levels between the first-episode psychosis (FEP) and multiepisode psychosis (MEP) samples; even in countries with a significant exposure to sunlight, both the first-episode psychosis (FEP) and multiepisode psychosis (MEP) groups exhibited low levels of vitamin D; and vitamin D levels were inversely correlated with general psychopathology in first-episode psychosis (FEP). The study concluded that, there is evidence demonstrating that there are low levels of vitamin D in psychotic disorders beginning in the early stages and that vitamin D could have a pathophysiological role in psychosis. Vitamin D is involved in several brain processes, including neurodevelopment, neurotrophic activities, growth factor regulation and neuroprotective (Wrzosek et al., 2013).

The findings from research on the relation of a healthy diet rich in essential vitamins (especially diets rich in fruits and vegetables) to the management of mental disorders increases, the role of vitamin supplementation in effective treatment of mental disorders as well as maintaining a good mental health in the aged is evolving (Mann and Truswell, 2012; Fresan et al., 2019; Moreno-Agostino et al., 2019). A synthesis and appraisal of all meta-analyses of randomized controlled trials (RCTs) which had been reported involving the efficacy and safety of nutrient supplements in serious and normal and severe mental disorders was done. Results from this study indicate good safety profiles and lack of indication of contraindications with antipsychotic drugs and adverse effects (Firth et al., 2019).

24.4.2 The use of vitamins in depression

Depression is a mental disorder which can occur in childhood, adolescence and adulthood with symptoms including; loss of appetite, increased sadness and anxiety (NIMH, 2000). Nutrient supplements including vitamins are used in the treatment of mental disorder such as depression. A study conducted by Young (Young, 2007) on folate/vitamin B12 in randomized controlled trials showed that patients treated with 0.8 mg of folic acid/day or 0.4 mg of vitamin B12/day had reduced depression symptoms. Vitamin D was found to significantly reduce depressive symptoms in patients with clinical depression (Vellekkatt and Menon, 2019). Firth and colleagues (2019) used a double-blind randomized controlled trial on oral supplements, showed significant positive effects were observed at doses of 1,500–7,143 IU/day on 828 depression patients. Vitamins play roles in management of mental disorders in aging population, and vitamins A, C and E play roles in regulation of oxidative stress, cognitive decline and neurodegeneration (McGrattan et al., 2019). Deficiency of vitamin B complex results in cognitive decline in the aging population, while intake of vitamin B complex improves cognitive function. Studies on vitamins B complex for management of depression and anxiety showed some benefit for oxidative stress but no significant effect on depression or anxiety (Young et al., 2019). Deficiency of vitamin D has been observed in populations suffering from depressive disorders. A study conducted by de Koning and colleagues (de Koning et al., 2019) in a randomized controlled trial with vitamin D supplementation at a dose of 1,200 IU/day for 12 months had no effect on depressive symptoms and physical functioning in older persons with relatively low vitamin D status, clinically relevant depressive symptoms and poor physical function. However, another recent review indicated contradictory information between vitamin D for treatment of depressive symptoms (Hoffmann et al., 2019).

24.4.3 Vitamins use in bipolar disorders

Bipolar disorder occurs in the aged due to deficiency of nutrient supplements, clinically diagnosed bipolar disorder are normally a combination of manic and depressive episode (Rihmer, Gonda and Rihmer, 2006). A double-blind, placebo-controlled study showed that a single 3 g dose of vitamin C decreases manic symptoms in comparison to placebo (Naylor and Smith, 1981).

24.4.4 The use of minerals and vitamins in schizophrenia

Schizophrenia is a mental disorder that disrupts a person's normal perception of reality. Symptoms such as hallucinations, paranoia, delusions and speech/thinking impairments are presented during adolescence (Castle et al., 1991). Vitamins play roles in oxidation or reduction reaction. Deficiency of vitamin B12 was observed in the serum of patients with schizophrenia in a Dutch population; where a cross-sectional study was evaluated in 61 Dutch patients, the result was compared to healthy controls, but there was no significant different in folate and vitamin B6 levels between the groups (Kemperman et al., 2006). A similar study was reported among Dutch population with a lower plasma level of folate in 35 schizophrenia patients (Muntjewerff et al., 2003). A randomized multicenter control trials evaluated the role of vitamin supplementation in 140 schizophrenia patients who had been randomly assigned on a stable antipsychotic dose to either treatment for 16 weeks with folic acid for 2 mg/day and vitamin B12 for 400 mcg/day or placebo (Roffman et al., 2013) the result showed a significant improvement in folate+B12 group. Vitamin D deficiency early in life may also contribute to schizophrenia risk in adulthood.

McGrath and colleagues (2018) reported the association between neonatal vitamin D status and risk of schizophrenia in a large Danish cohort. The results showed that those in the lowest quantities (<20.4 noml/L) had an increased risk of schizophrenia comparable to those in higher quintiles. A meta-analysis study conducted by Belvederi Murri and colleagues showed that patients with schizophrenia had consistently lower vitamin D levels compared to healthy controls (Belvederi Murri et al., 2013).

Antioxidants such as vitamins C and E provide protection against cell damage during reactivity of oxygen containing molecules. Several studies that were conducted on vitamin C and E have proven positive and negative to the management of schizophrenia in patients. Bentsen and colleagues (Bentsen et al., 2013) evaluated vitamin C (364 mg/day) and vitamin E (1,000 mg/day) to patients with schizophrenia on antipsychotic medication. The result showed that among patients with low blood cell, the vitamin supplementation actually impaired recovery from acute psychosis compared to placebo. D'Souza and colleagues (2003) reported significantly lower plasma levels of vitamins E and C in schizophrenia patients in India when compared to the control.

A review by Brown and colleagues (Hannah and Roffman, 2015) proposed that patients with schizophrenia have lower serum concentrations of certain vitamins compared to healthy individuals. Vitamin supplementation may play a role in the treatment of schizophrenia within certain subgroups of patients. Further studies, including larger, randomized controlled trials are needed to fully elucidate the role of vitamin supplementation in the treatment of schizophrenia especially in the elderly.

Minerals play vital roles in the treatment of mental disorder, minerals such dietary magnesium, copper and zinc act as cofactors of enzymes that prevent damage from oxidative stress (Weiser et al., 1994). Magnesium is involved in multiple metabolic pathways, so normal function of the nervous system and release of neurotransmitters are dependent on magnesium (Jahnen-Dechent and Ketteler, 2012). Deficiency of magnesium in the diet could result in depression in the aging population. Eby and colleagues (Eby, Eby and Murck, 2011) reported that low magnesium level in the serum of patients could cause depression, the result from their study showed that about 50% of patients had a higher rate of depression in the lowest quartile of observation. Addition of magnesium to the diet of the patient significantly resulted in the management of depression (Tarleton and Littenberg, 2015)

Zinc plays a role in the central nervous system and function as enzymes that preserve brain zinc homeostasis (Gower-Winter and Levenson, 2012; Ranjbar et al., 2013). Clinical studies have shown that lower levels of serum zinc in the serum of patients could cause major depression (McLoughlin and

Hodge, 1990). Lower serum zinc levels have been linked with depressive symptoms. A study conducted by Maserejian and colleagues (2012) showed that low dietary zinc intake was positively associated with depression symptoms in females and patients with adequate levels of zinc responded better to SSRI anti-depressant treatment compare to those with lower levels of zinc. Schefft and colleagues (2017) in a randomized controlled trial on the evaluation of mineral supplement (zinc/magnesium) for management of depression indicated zinc was administered at 25 mg/day (elemental) as an adjunctive treatment for depression and had adequate significant effects on depressive symptoms.

Comparative studies have shown that 26 medication-free schizophrenics were found to have significantly low serum iron (Weiser et al., 1994). In addition a study in Israel where both the cerebrospinal fluid and the serum of people with schizophrenia were tested was indicative of low magnesium levels in the patients (Levine et al., 1996).

24.5 The roles of polyunsaturated fatty acids (PUFAs) as nutrients supplement in the treatment of mental disorders in aging population

24.5.1 Overview of the use of polyunsaturated fatty acids (PUFAs) as nutrients supplements

Nutrients promote good health of humans; many studies suggest that there is a considerable link between quality of diet and mental disorders, and quality of diet seems to be a factor that affects the evolution of mental disorders (Lange, 2018). Supplements are substances that can be obtained from food or manufactured synthetically, and examples include polyunsaturated fatty acids, vitamins, minerals, amino acids and pre/probiotics (Joseph et al., 2019). The primary purpose of supplements is to supply additional nutrient adequate to attain recommended nutrients levels due to insufficient level obtained from diet and provide nutrients in a form that can easily be absorbed by the human body (Joseph et al., 2019).

Nutrient supplements are used widely by the population in different countries. Polyunsaturated fatty acids are a nutrient supplement whose intake contributes to the proper function, growth and development of the human brain especially in mental disorders. Lipids, particularly omega-3 fatty acids, play a pivotal role in psychiatric disorders in addition to lessening coronary artery diseases and increasing blood flow in humans (Ji-Hyuk, 2013). Omega-3 fatty acids also play an important role in the development, function and aging of the brain. Dietary deficiency of omega-3 fatty acid in humans may result in psychiatric disorders including depression, bipolar disorder, schizophrenia, dementia, attention-deficit/hyperactivity disorder and autism

(Klaus, 2020). Neuronal membrane fluidity and functioning of some important receptors are normally maintained by eicosapentaenoic (EPA) and docosahexaenoic acid (DHA). Essential fatty acids such as linoleic acid (LA) and α-linolenic acid (ALA) are the two main groups which omega-6 and omega-3 polyunsaturated fatty acids are derived from (Tapiero et al., 2002). Omega-3 polyunsaturated fatty acids are derived from α-linolenic acid (ALA) through series of mechanism including; desaturation, elongation and β-oxidation (Simopoulos, 1999). Human obtained polyunsaturated fatty acids from their diet when metabolized in the body. Moriguchi and colleagues (Moriguchi, Greiner and Salem, 2000) have suggested that absence of omega-3 polyunsaturated fatty acids could hinder the learning and memory of experimental animals after a study.

24.5.2 Types of PUFAs and their sources

Several PUFAs contain double bonds on the carbon chain, among them are omega-3 which comes as a result of the location of the double bond between the third and fourth carbon chains, and omega-6 PUFAs between the sixth and seventh carbon chains. These two PUFAs (n-3 and n-6 PUFAs) have been widely studied. They perform pharmacological, neurological and mental health roles. Their sources have been summarized in Table 24.1.

24.5.3 Relation of PUFA to mental disorders

Polyunsaturated fatty acids are important for the growth and development of the central nervous system in the stages of human development. Adequate dietary supply of PUFAs is important for normal brain growth and development (Kris-Etherton, Grieger and Etherton, 2014; Luxwolda et al., 2014). PUFA deficiency has been suggested to be associated with psychiatry disorders such as autism spectrum disorder, depression (Kris-Etherton, Grieger and Etherton, 2014), bipolar disorder (Noaghiul and Hibbeln, 2003), schizophrenia (Peet and

Table 24.1 Omega-3 and Omega-6 Polyunsaturated Fatty Acids and Their Sources

PUFAs	Source	Biological Relevant Omega-3
Omega-3 (n-3)	Fish and meat from seals, whales, sea birds and fur-bearing animals (Anne and Hanna, 2019 Shellfish, seeds, plant oil, nuts. Fish oil (Abdelhamid, 2018)	Docosahexanoic acid (DHA) Eicosapentanoic acid (EPA) Alpha-linolenic acid (ALA)
Omega-6 (n-6)	Plant oils, (Abdelhamid, 2018) fish	linoleic acid (LA), Gamma-linolenic acid (GLA) Arachidonic acid (AA)

Horrobin, 2002), dementia syndrome (Burckhardt et al., 2016; Parletta and Nivonsenga, 2016) and attention-deficit/hyperactivity disorders (Parletta and Nivonsenga, 2016).

24.5.4 The role of PUFAs in depression

Patients with deficient omega-3PUFAs (eicosapentanoic acid and docosahexa-noic acid) in their cell plasma and dietary intake may suffer from depressive disorder. Depression may be aggravated by factors such as smoking, economic status, marital status, family history (Schaakxs, 2017) and obesity (Weich et al., 2002).

Several epidemiological and biological studies have suggested a link between omega-3PUFAs and depression (Anne and Hanna, 2019). Depression in the elderly is allied with a higher mortality rate. It occurs more in elderly people with about 50% of elderly patients having depression with dementia and 20% of patients with Alzheimer disorders in a study (Olin et al., 2002). Some studies show that rise in depression could be due to a decrease in polyunsaturated fatty acids (Sonnenberg et al., 2008) and changes in diet intake. Depression can be treated if proper attention is paid to it with additional changes to diet and inclusion of PUFA supplements (Luber et al., 2001; Krishnan et al., 2002). PUFAs (eicosapentanoic acid) have been reported as an adjunct therapy for treatment of depression (Mischoulon, 2007). Rondanelli and colleagues reported that the supplementation of PUFAs (long chain omega-3 polyun-saturated fatty acids) in elderly female patients decreased the incidence of depression, increased phospholipid fatty acids profile and improved health-related quality of life (Rodanelli, Giacosa and Opizzi, 2011). Pharmacological efficacy of omega-3PUFAs has been evaluated for treatment and manage-ment of depression (Ling, Huan and Su, 2010). Clinical studies have been done on the efficacy (Su, 2015) of omega-3PUFAs. Pottala and colleagues have suggested that a 1% increase in omega-3PUFAs reduced the vulnerabil-ity of developing depression by 28% (Pottala et al., 2012), which corresponds to the results of Von Schacky (Von Schacky, 2014) on remote assessment in nonpsychiatric conditions. Antidepressant effects of dietary intake of eicosa-pentaenoic acid (EPA) and docosahexaenoic acid (DHA) have been reported (Yang, Kim and Je, 2018), although the correlation between both PUFAs var-ies in efficacy in the management depression (Su et al., 2018; Reeves et al., 2017). A cross-sectional study by Choda and colleagues in Japanese people showed that in randomized placebo-controlled trials, omega-3PUFAs had successful positive effects on depression management confirming the role omega-3PUFAs plays in controlling depression. Nazia and colleagues (Nazia et al., 2018) also reported significant role n-3 play in controlling depression. A study conducted on 70 patients already diagnosed with depression and taking antidepressant treatment for 12 weeks. The patients were divided into two groups; intervention groups were advised to take 300 mg eicosapentae-noic acid and 200 mg docosahexanoic acid; meanwhile, the control group

500 mg corn oil capsule once daily with a meal. The result showed that omega-3PUFAs significantly decreased depression in patients as compared to control group.

24.5.5 The role of PUFAs in schizophrenia

The central nervous system plays a pivotal role in brain function; polyunsaturated fatty acids including arachidonic acid (AA) and docosahexaenoic acid (DHA) in the red blood cell membranes aid the CNS to perform its function and coordinate some important activities in the brain. Deficiency of these PUFAs and changes in dietary intake of PUFAs could result in mental disorders such as schizophrenia. Symptoms of schizophrenia include hallucination, delusion, poor speech, flattened mood, disorganized thinking and behaviors (Horrobin, 1998). Jamilian and colleagues reported the randomized placebo-controlled clinical trials on omega-3PUFAs supplementation in the treatment of schizophrenia, the results showed significant reduction in schizophrenia (Jamilian, Solhi and Jamilian, 2014). Similar evidence was reported by Pawelczyk and colleagues (Pawelczyk et al., 2016) where randomized placebo-controlled trial was lasted for six months in schizophrenia patients, and the results indicated significant reduction in the symptoms of schizophrenia patients subjected omega-3PUFAs comparable to the control group. Remote assessment of Omega-3PUFAs in schizophrenia patients indicated that replacement could result in reduction in oxidative stress (Pawelczyk et al., 2016, Pawelczyk et al., 2017). Qiao and colleagues (Qiao et al., 2018) reported mild stables reduction in schizophrenia symptoms after 12 weeks of trials foe 360 mg/day dose for DHA and 540 mg/day dose for EPA. Decrease in schizophrenia symptom was observed in Robinso and colleagues' investigation where 740 mg/day for EPA and 400 mg/day for DHA were administered for sixteen weeks (Robinson et al., 2019).

24.5.6 The role of PUFAs in attention-deficit/ hyperactivity disorders (ADHD)

Diet helps human to grow and maintain life processes, but deficiency of dietary intake of omega-3PUFAs in the developmental stages of human could have negative effects on brain development and function (Tessi et al., 2017; Bondi et al., 2014). Deficiency of n-3PUFAs in the development of infants may result in attention deficit hyperactivity disorder (Tessi et al., 2017; Montgomery et al., 2013). Several studies have been conducted on PUFAs in the management of ADHD have been indicative of positive effects of dietary supplementation (Checa-Ros et al., 2018; Long and Benton, 2013; Widenhom-Muller et al., 2014) meanwhile other reported negative effects of dietary supplementation and others also resolved that the presently obtainable evidence is unconvincing (Perera and Jeewandara, 2012; Hawkey and Nigg, 2014; Korugs and Kiliaan, 2016). Bos and colleagues (Bos et al., 2015) reported a significant decrease in symptoms of ADHD in individuals with ADHD and normally developing children at a dose administration of 0.65 g/day (EPA) and 0.65 g/day (DHA).

24.5.7 The role of PUFAs in dementia syndrome

Dementia syndrome occurs as a result of progressive decline in cognitive function owing to injury or disease in the brain beyond what might be expected from normal aging. Some of the areas particularly affected by dementia include memory, attention, judgment, language and problem solving. As humans age, cognitive function decline and so this is very common in the aged (https://www.alz.co.uk/research/ statistics). Decline in cognitive function was reported as a result of deficient intake of omega-3PUFAs (Mohajeri, Twesch and Weber, 2015) docosahexaenoic acid (DHA) plays a vital role in brain function, the quantities of docosahexanoic acid in membrane phospholipids of the brain in human triggers the brain to function and coordinates signals thus reducing decline in cognitive function. Approximately 25% of the DHA is found in the human cerebral cortex, and its level decreases due to aging and 50% of PUFAs in the CNS (Hessandri et al., 2004; Bazan et al., 2011). The degree of decline in cognitive function and deficiency in omega-3PUFAs could be detected in membranes of erythrocytes (Heude et al., 2003). Alzheimer disease is the most common cause of dementia in aging population. Studies suggest that there is a link between omega-3PUFAs and cognitive function in Alzheimer's disease (Ajith, 2018; Lukaschek et al., 2016).

24.5.8 The role of PUFAs in bipolar disorder

Bipolar disorder is a mental illness which is a combination of depressive and manic episodes that causes up-normal swings in mood, energy, activity levels and the inability to carry out day-to-day tasks. This condition is made up of different types including; bipolar-I disorder, dipolar-II disorder, and cyclothymia. Bipolar disorder typically develops in late adolescence or early adulthood.

Studies indicated that about 5% of the full spectrum of bipolar disorder was diagnosed in both men and women (Ferrari et al., 2016; Gum et al., 2009) which are based on the manifestation of at least one manic (bipolar disorder-I) or hypomanic and depressive episode (bipolar-II). Patients suffering from bipolar disorder are more disposed to other health diseases comparable to healthy persons. Proper brain function is determined by the fatty acids balance, the quantity of fatty acids in the brain relates to an average range of 60%–70% of the dry weight. The amount of docosahexaenoic acid measured in the plasma membranes of erythrocytes in bipolar disorder patients is lower compared to the docosahexaenoic acid in control patients (McNamara and Welge, 2013). Symptoms of bipolar disorder have been summarized in Table 24.2.

Table 24.2 Summary of Symptoms of Bipolar Disorders

Symptoms of a Manic Episode	Symptoms of a Depressive Episode
Increased energy, activity and restlessness	Lasting sad, anxious or empty mood
Extreme irritability	Feelings of hopelessness or pessimism
Distractibility, can't concentrate well	Feelings of guilt, worthlessness or helplessness
Little sleep needed	Loss of interest or pleasure in activities once enjoyed, including sex
Poor judgment	Decreased energy, a feeling of fatigue
Spending sprees	Restlessness or irritability
Increased sexual drive	Sleeping too much or can't sleep
Abuse of drugs, particularly cocaine, alcohol and sleeping medications	Change in appetite and/or unintended weight loss or gain
Provocative, intrusive or aggressive behavior	Difficulty concentrating, remembering, making decisions

Source: Yaday et al. (2018).

Studies showed that bipolar disorder patients have reduction in concentration of polyunsaturated fatty acids. Polyunsaturated fatty acids plays beneficial roles in recovery of bipolar disorder patients; meanwhile, the absence of polyunsaturated fatty acids in the diet of person could result in developing mental disorders (Riveros and Retana, 2018; Morris et al., 2017). Evan and colleagues (Evan et al., 2014) reported the association between polyunsaturated fatty acids in bipolar disorder patient and healthy person, the result indicated that bipolar disorder patients have decreased intake of polyunsaturated fatty acids (eicosapentaenoic acid (n-3), docosahexaenoic acid (n-3), arachidonic acid (n-6), and docosapentaenoic acid) and higher intake of saturated fats.

However, in an attempt to provide elucidation regarding the relationship between polyunsaturated fatty acids bio status and bipolar disorder, a meta-analysis was investigated by McNamara and Welge (McNamara and Welge, 2013) in comparing erythrocyte membrane polyunsaturated fatty acids composition in patients with bipolar disorder and healthy controls, the result showed that patients with bipolar-I disorder exhibited healthy erythrocyte docosahexaenoic acid deficits. There were no significant differences including linoleic acid or arachidonic acid and it was concluded that bipolar-I is associated with healthy erythrocyte docosahexaenoic acid deficits. Pomponi and colleagues (Pomponi et al., 2013) reported increased arachidonic acid and eicosapentaenoic acid and decreased docosahexaenoic acid in bipolar disorder patients. The omega-3 polyunsaturated fatty acids have been reported in preclinical and clinical trials to be an effective adjunctive for management of unipolar and bipolar disorder (Vincent et al., 2011). Gracious and colleagues (Gracious et al., 2010) reported significant improvement of overall symptom severity compared with placebo by using α linoleic acid at a dose of 0.5 g/day in psychotropic medication children and adolescent with bipolar I and bipolar II disorders for sixteen weeks.

24.6 Conclusion and future considerations

Clinical evidence derived from the evaluation of the studies demonstrates a strong relationship between vital nutrients such as PUFAs, vitamins, minerals, probiotics and prebiotic supplements and the mental health of the aged. Firth et al. (2019) attested to the safety of such nutrients with no associated adverse effects with psychiatric medications (Adi-Dako et al., 2018). The aforementioned nutraceuticals have been useful as preventive strategies or as adjunctive treatment in mental disorders, e.g. depression and schizophrenia (Firth et al., 2019).

Further randomized controlled trials could be conducted to elucidate the mechanisms of action to provide further information on the importance of these dietary supplements.

The findings provided indicate the remarkable role these nutrients play in preventive and adjunctive treatment of mental disorders and is a basis for the need for formulation considerations for such nutrients to improve mental health. Consequently, for the effectiveness of prevention and therapeutic efficacy, there is a critical need for patient-centered pharmaceutical formulation of such nutrients as dietary supplements which are well suited and tailored for the needs of the elderly. The evolving formulation needs of the elderly should be consistently evaluated and addressed. Nutrient dosage form and development addresses pertinent issues such as accuracy and frequency of dosing, preservation and stability of the efficacy of the active nutraceutical ingredients is essential (Kumadoh et al., 2020), together with the associated appropriate storage conditions. These formulation characteristics are crucial for patient-centered formulation and the convenience and compliance of the elderly for optimal preventive and treatment outcomes. The aging population also usually have a myriad of prescribed medications usually for other chronic ailments, and adjunctive treatment with nutrient supplements, should be formulated for the convenience and improved compliance of the aged. Nutrient supplements also have the additional benefits of alleviating any adverse effects in the management of polypharmacy in the treatment of chronic disease and co-morbidities in the aged.

Strides necessary for optimized geriatric mental health, would involve the use of established doses, patient-centered safe, efficacious and stable nutraceutical formulations (Kumadoh et al., 2020), with appropriate excipients for optimal bioavailability. (Kumadoh et al., 2015). The continued dissemination of evidence of efficacy of nutrient supplements could be made to clinicians and other health professionals to enhance mental health delivery services (Firth et al., 2019). Considerable attention should be given to the emerging fields of nutrition for mental health as it holds great promise in the identification of the essential nutrients for the prevention and treatment of geriatric mental health disorders. The role of patient-centered formulation design, development and delivery cannot be overemphasized (Adan et al., 2019).

References

Abdelhamid, A.S., Martin, N., Bridges, C., Brainard, J.S. et al. (2018). Polyunsaturated fatty acids for the primary and secondary prevention of cardiovascular disease. *Cochrane Database Syst Rev*. **7**:CD012345.

Adan, R.A.H. et al. (2019). Nutritional psychiatry: Towards improving mental health by what you eat. *Eur Neuropsychopharmacol*. **29**(12): 1321–1332.

Adi-Dako, O. et al. (2018). Subchronic toxicity studies of cocoa pod husk pectin intended as a pharmaceutical excipient in Sprague Dawley rats.

Ajith, T.A. (2018). A recent update on the effects of omega-3 fatty acids in Alzheimer's disease. *Curr Clin Pharmacol*. **13**:252–260.

Alessandri, J.M., Guesnet, P., Vancassel, S. et al. (2004). Polyunsaturated fatty acids in the central nervous system: Evolution of concepts and nutritional implications throughout life. *Reprod Nutr Dev*. **44**:509–538.

Alzheimer's Disease International. 2020, Dementia statistics. Available online: https://www.alz.co.uk/research/ statistics (accessed on 4 May 2020).

Arne, R., Hanna, L. (2019). The emerging role of omega-3 fatty acids as a therapeutic option in neuropsychiatric disorders. *Ther Adv Psychopharmacol*. **9**:1–18.

Barichella, M., et al. (2016). Probiotics and prebiotic fiber for constipation associated with Parkinson disease: An RCT. *Neurology* **87**(12): 1274–1280.

Barrett, E., et al. (2012). Gamma-aminobutyric acid production by culturable bacteria from the human intestine. *J Appl Microbiol*. **113**(2): 411–417.

Bavarsad Shahripour, R., Harrigan, M.R., Alexandrov, A.V. (2014). N-acetylcysteine (NAC) in neurological disorders: Mechanisms of action and therapeutic opportunities. *Brain Behavior*. **4**(2):108–122. doi:10.1002/brb3.208.

Bazan, N.G., Molina, M.F., Gordon, W.C. (2011). Docosahexaenoic acid signalolipidomics in nutrition: Significance in aging, neuroinflammation, macular degeneration, Alzheimer's, and other neurodegenerative diseases. *Annu Rev Nutr*. **31**:321–351.

Belvederi Murri, M., Respino, M., Masotti, M. et al. (2013). Vitamin D and psychosis: Mini meta-analysis. *Schizophrenia Res*. **150**(1):235–239.

Bentsen, H., Osnes, K., Refsum, H., Solberg, D.K., Bohmer, T. (2013). A randomized placebo-controlled trial of an omega-3 fatty acid and vitamins E+C in schizophrenia. *Translat Psych*. doi:10.1038/tp.2013.110.

Bercik, P. et al. (2010). Chronic gastrointestinal inflammation induces anxiety-like behavior and alters central nervous system biochemistry in mice. *Gastroenterology* **139**(6): 2102–2112 e2101.

Black, M.M. (2008). Effects of vitamin B12 and folate deficiency on brain development in children. *Food Nutr Bull*. **29**:126–131.

Bondi, C.O., Taha, A.Y., Tock, J.L. et al. (2014). Adolescent behavior and dopamine availability are uniquely sensitive to dietary omega-3 fatty acid deficiency. *Biol Psychiat*. **75**:38–46.

Bos, D.J., Oranje, B., Veerhoek, E.S. et al. (2015). Reduced symptoms of inattention after dietary omega-3 fatty acid supplementation in boys with and without attention deficit/hyperactivity disorder. *Neuropsychopharmacology*. **40**:2298–2306.

Bouayed, J., Bohn, T. (2010). Exogenous antioxidants – Double-edged swords in cellular redox state: Health beneficial effects at physiologic doses versus deleterious effects at high doses. *Oxidat Med Cell Longev*. **3**(4):228–237. doi:10.4161/oxim.3.4.12858.

Bravo, J.A., et al. (2011). Ingestion of lactobacillus strain regulates emotional behavior and central GABA receptor expression in a mouse via the vagus nerve. *Proc Natl Acad Sci U S A* **108**(38): 16050–16055.

Brown, H.E., Roffman, J.L. (2014). Vitamin supplementation in the treatment of schizophrenia. *CNS Drugs*. **28**(7):611–622.

Burckhardt, M., Herke, M., Wustmann, T., Watzke, S., Langer, G., Fink, A. (2016). Omega-3 fatty acids for the treatment of dementia. *Cochrane Database of Syst Rev*. **4**:CD009002

Burokas, A. et al. (2015). Microbiota regulation of the Mammalian gut-brain axis. *Adv Appl Microbiol.* **91**: 1–62.

Cassani, E. et al. (2011). Use of probiotics for the treatment of constipation in Parkinson's disease patients. *Minerva Gastroenterol Dietol.* **57**(2): 117–121.

Castle, E., Wessely, S., Der G., Murray, R.M. (1991). The incidence of operationally defined schizophrenia in Camberwell. *Br J Psychiat.* **159**:790–794.

Cekici, H., Emre BakArhan, Y. (2018). Potential therapeutic agent in psychiatric and neurological diseases: Alpha lipoic acid. *Acta Psychopathologica.* **04**(02). doi:10.4172/2469-6676.100165.

Checa-Ros, A., Haro-Garcia, A., Seiquer, I. et al. (2018). Early monitoring of fatty acid profile in children with attention deficit and/or hyperactivity disorder under treatment with omega-3 polyunsaturated fatty acids. *Minerva Pediatr.* Epub ahead of print 7 November 2018. doi:10.23736/S0026-4946.18.04975-7.

Cheung, S. G. et al. (2019). Systematic review of gut microbiota and major depression. *Front Psychiat* **10**:34.

Chung Y.C. et al. (2007). Dietary intake of xylooligosaccharides improves the intestinal microbiota, fecal moisture, and pH value in the elderly. *Nutr Res* **27**: 756–761.

Cicero, A.F.G. et al. (2020). Impact of a short-term synbiotic supplementation on metabolic syndrome and systemic inflammation in elderly patients: A randomized placebo-controlled clinical trial. *Eur J Nutr.* **60**: 655–663.

Cobley, J.N., Fiorello, M.L., Bailey, D.M. (2018). 13 Reasons why the brain is susceptible to oxidative stress. *Redox Biol.* Elsevier B.V. **15**(February):490–503. doi:10.1016/j.redox.2018.01.008.

Conner, T.S., Brookie, K.L., Carr, A.C. et al. (2017). Let them eat fruit! The effect of fruit and vegetable consumption on psychological well-being in young adults: A randomized controlled trial. *PLoS One* **12**: e0171206.

Costabile, A., et al. (2017). Effects of soluble corn fiber alone or in synbiotic combination with lactobacillus rhamnosus GG and the pilus-deficient derivative GG-PB12 on fecal microbiota, metabolism, and markers of immune function: A randomized, double-blind, placebo-controlled, crossover study in healthy elderly (Saimes Study). *Front Immunol* **8**:1443.

Cryan, J. F. and T. G. Dinan (2012). Mind-altering microorganisms: the impact of the gut microbiota on brain and behaviour. *Nat Rev Neurosci.* **13**(10):701–712.

Csapó, János, A., Cilla, J.P. (2017). The role of vitamins in the diet of the elderly I. Fat-soluble vitamins. Acta Universitatis Sapientiae, Alimentaria.

Dean, O., Giorlando, F., Berk, M. (2011). N-acetylcysteine in psychiatry: Current therapeutic evidence and potential mechanisms of action. *J Psychiat Neurosci.* **36**(2):78–86. doi:10.1503/jpn.100057.

de Koning, E.J., Lips, P., Penninx, B.W.J.H., Elders, P.J.M. et al. (2019). Vitamin D supplementation for the prevention of depression and poor physical function in older persons: The D-Vitaal study, a randomized clinical trial. *Am J Clin Nutr.* **110**(5):1119–1130.

D'Souza, B., D'Souza, V. (2003). Oxidative injury and antioxidant vitamins E and C in Schizophrenia. *Ind J Clin Biochem IJCB.* **18**(1):87–90.

Eby, G.A., Eby, K.L., Murck, H. (2011). Magnesium and major depression. Magnesium in the central nervous system, pp. 313–330.

Ekiz, A. et al. (2017). Functional and structural changes of the urinary bladder following spinal cord injury; treatment with alpha lipoic acid. *Neurourol Urodynamics.* **36**(4):1061–1068. doi:10.1002/nau.23083.

Enderami, A., Zarghami, M., Darvishi-Khezri, H. (2018). The effects and potential mechanisms of folic acid on cognitive function: A comprehensive review. *Neurol Sci.* **2018**(39):1667–1675.

Erny, D., et al. (2015). Host microbiota constantly control maturation and function of microglia in the CNS. *Nat Neurosci* **18**(7): 965–977.

Evans, S.J., Ringrose, R.N., Harrington, G.J., Mancuso, P. et al. (2014). Dietary intake and plasma metabolomics analysis of polyunsaturated fatty acids in bipolar subjects reveal dysregulation of linoleic acid metabolism. *J Psychiatr.* **57**:58–64.

Eyles, D.W., Trzaskowski, M., Vinkhuyzen, A.A. et al. (2018). The association between neonatal vitamin D status and risk of schizophrenia. *Sci Rep.* **8**(1):1–8.

Fernandes, B.S. et al. (2016). N-acetylcysteine in depressive symptoms and functionality: A systematic review and meta-analysis. *J Clin Psychiat.* **77**(4):e457–e466. doi:10.4088/JCP.15r09984.

Ferrari, A.J., Stockings, E., Khoo, J.P. et al. (2016). The prevalence and burden of bipolar disorder: Findings from the Global Burden of Disease Study 2013. *Bipolar Disord.* **18**(5):440–450.

Firth, J. et al. (2019). The efficacy and safety of nutrient supplements in the treatment of mental disorders: A meta-review of meta-analyses of randomized controlled trials. *World Psychiatry.* **18**(3): 308–324.

Fraunberger, E.A. et al. (2016). Redox modulations, antioxidants, and neuropsychiatric disorders. *Oxidative Med Cell Longev.* **2016**. doi:10.1155/2016/4729192.

Fresan, U., Bes-Rastrollo, M., Segovia-Siapco, G. et al. (2019). Does the mind diet decrease depression risk? A comparison with mediterranean diet in the SUN cohort. *Eur J Nutr.* **58**:1271–1282.

Gaudio, S., Wiemerslage, L., Brooks, S.J., Schioth, H.B. (2016). A systematic review of resting-state functional-MRI studies in anorexia nervosa: Evidence for functional connectivity impairment in cognitive control and visuospatial and body-signal integration. *Neurosci Biobehav.* **71**:578–589.

Georgescu, D., et al. (2016). Nonmotor gastrointestinal disorders in older patients with Parkinson's disease: is there hope? *Clin Interv Aging.* **11**: 1601–1608.

Giannunzio, V, Degortes, D, Tenconi, E et al. 2018, Decision-making impair- ment in anorexia nervosa: new insights into the role of age and decision-making style. *Eur Eat Disord.* **26**, pp.302–314.

Gibson, G.R., Roberfroid, M.B. (1995). Dietary modulation of the human colonic microbiota: introducing the concept of prebiotics. *J Nutr.* **125**(6):1401–1412.

Glenn, J.M., Madero, E.N., Bott, N.T. (2019). Dietary protein and amino acid intake : Links to the maintenance of cognitive health. *Nutr Jr.* **11**(6):1315.

Gower-Winter, S.D., Levenson, C.W. (2012). Zinc in the central nervous system: From molecules to behavior. *Biofactor.* **38**(3):186–193.

Gracious, B.L., Chirieac, M.C., Costescu, S., Finucane, T.L. et al. (2010). Randomized, placebo-controlled trial of flax oil in pediatric bipolar disorder. *Bipolar Disord.* **12**:142–154.

Gum, A., King-Kallimanis, B., Kohn, R. (2009). Prevalence of mood, anxiety, and substance-abuse disorders for older Americans in the national comorbidity survey-replication. *Am J Geriat Psychiatry.* **17**:769–813.

Hagen, T.M. et al. (2002). Feeding acetyl-L-carnitine and lipoic acid to old rats significantly improves metabolic function while decreasing oxidative stress. *Proc Nat Acad Sci U S A.* **99**(4):1870–1875. doi:10.1073/pnas.261708898.

Han, D., et al. (2020). Proteostasis of alpha-Synuclein and Its Role in the Pathogenesis of Parkinson's Disease. *Front Cell Neurosci* **14**:45.

Hannah, E., Brown, J., Roffman L. (2015). Vitamin supplementation in the treatment of schizophrenia. *CNS Drugs E mBio* **10**(3).

Harbottle, L. (2019). The effect of nutrition on older people's mental health. *Br J Community Nurs.* **24**(Sup7):S12–s16.

Hawkey, E., Nigg, J.T. (2014). Omega-3 fatty acid and ADHD: Blood level analysis and meta-analytic extension of supplementation trials. *Clin Psychol Rev.* **34**:496–505.

Hegyi, J., Schwartz, R.A., Hegyi, V. (2004). Pellagra: Dermatitis, dementia, and diarrhea. *Int J Dermatol.* **43**:1–5.

Heiss, N.C., Olofsson, E.L. (2019). The role of the gut microbiota in development, function and disorders of the central nervous system and the enteric nervous system. *J Neuroendocrinol*. **31**:e12684.

Heude, B., Ducimetière, P., Berr, C. (2003) Cognitive decline and fatty acid composition of erythrocyte membranes – The EVA Study. *Am J Clin Nutr*. **77**:803–808.

Hill, C., et al. (2014). Expert consensus document. The International Scientific Association for Probiotics and Prebiotics consensus statement on the scope and appropriate use of the term probiotic. *Nat Rev Gastroenterol Hepatol*. **11**(8):506–514.

Hoffmann, K., Emons, B., Brunnhuber, S., Karaca, S., Juckel, G. (2019). The role of dietary supplements in depression and anxiety – A narrative review. *Pharmacopsychiatry*. **52**:261–79.

Horrobin, D.F. (1998). The membrane phospholipid hypothesis as a biochemical basis for the neurodevelopmental concept of schizophrenia. *Schizophr Res*. **30**:193–208.

https://www.encyclopedia.com/medicine/encyclopedias-almanacs-transcripts-and-maps/aging-and-aged, 2020 (Date visited 01/12/2020)

Ighodaro, O.M., Akinloye, O.A. (2018). First line defence antioxidants-superoxide dismutase (SOD), catalase (CAT) and glutathione peroxidase (GPX): Their fundamental role in the entire antioxidant defence grid. *Alex J Med*. **54**(4):287–293. doi:10.1016/j.ajme.2017.09.001.

Institute of Medicine. Food and Nutrition Board, IMFNB. (1998). *Dietary Reference Intakes: Thiamin, Riboflavin, Niacin, Vitamin B6, Folate, Vitamin B12, Pantothenic Acid, Biotin, and Choline*. Washington, DC: National Academy Press.

Jahnen-Dechent, W., Ketteler, M. (2012). Magnesium basics. *Clin Kidney J*. **5**:i3–i14.

Jamilian, H., Solhi, H., Jamilian, M. (2014). Randomized, placebo-controlled clinical trial of omega-3 as supplemental treatment in schizophrenia. *Glob J Health Sci*. **6**:103–108.

Jenkins, T. A. et al. (2016). Influence of tryptophan and serotonin on mood and cognition with a possible role of the gut-brain axis', *Nutr Jr*. **8**(1):56.

Ji-Hyuk, L. (2013). Polyunsaturated fatty acids in children. *Pediat Gastroenterol Hepatol Nutr*. **16**(3):153–161.

Joseph, F., Scott, B.T., Kelly, A. et al. (2019). The efficacy and safety of nutrient supplements in the treatment of mental disorders: a meta-review of meta-analyses of randomized controlled trials. *World Psychiatry*. **18**:308–324.

Kemperman, R.F., Veurink, M., van der Wal, T. et al. (2006). Low essential fatty acid and B-vitamin status in a subgroup of patients with schizophrenia and its response to dietary supplementation. *Prostagland Leukotr Essent Fatty Acids*. **74**(2):75–85.

Keshavarzian, A., et al. (2015). Colonic bacterial composition in Parkinson's disease. *Mov Disord*. **30**(10):1351–1360.

Keyloun, K. et al. (2017). Adherence and persistance across antidepressant therapeutic classes: a retrospective claims analysis among insured us patients with major depressive disorder. *CNS Drugs*. **31**:421–32.

Klaus, W.L. (2020). Omega-3 fatty acids and mental health. *Glob Health J*. **4**(1). doi:10.1007/s40263-017-0417-0.

Konigs, A., Kiliaan, A.J. (2016). Critical appraisal of omega-3 fatty acids in attention-deficit/hyperactivity disorder treatment. *Neuropsychiatr Dis Treat*. **12**:1869–1882.

Kris-Etherton, P.M., Grieger, J.A., Etherton, T.D. (2009). Dietary reference intakes for DHA and EPA. *Prostaglandins Leukot Essent Fatty Acids*. **81**:99–104.

Krishnan, K.R., Delong, M., Kraemer, H. et al. (2002). Comorbidity of depression with other medical diseases in the elderly. *Biol Psychiat*. **52**:559–588.

Kumadoh, D., et al. (2015). Development of oral capsules from Enterica herbal decoction-a traditional remedy for typhoid fever in Ghana.

Kumadoh, D., et al. (2020). Determination of shelf life of four herbal medicinal products using high-performance liquid chromatography analyses of markers and the Systat Sigmaplot software. *J Appl Pharmac Sci*. **10**(06):072–080.

Lakhan, S.E., Karen, F.V. (2008). Nutritional therapies for mental disorders. *Nutr J.* **7**(2). doi:10.1186/1475-2891-7-2.

Lakshminarayanan, B., et al. (2014). Compositional dynamics of the human intestinal microbiota with aging: implications for health. *J Nutr Health Aging.* **18**(9):773–786.

Lange, K.W. (2018). Diet, exercise, and mental disorders – Public health challenges of the future. *Mov Nutr Health Dis.* **2**:3959.

Levine, J., Rapoport, A., Mashiah, M., Dolev, E. (1996). Serum and cerebrospinal levels of calcium and magnesium in acute versus remitted schizophrenic patients. *Neuropsychobiology.* **33**(4):169–172.

Lin, C.-H., Yang, H.-T., Chiu, C.-C., Lane, H.-Y.J.S.R. 2017. Blood levels of D-amino acid oxidase vs. *Amino Acids Ref Cognit Aging.* **7**, 1–10.

Lin, P.Y., Huang, S.Y., Su, K.P. (2010). A meta-analytic review of polyunsaturated fatty acid compositions in patients with depression. *Biol Psychiatry.* **68**(2):140–7.

Liu, Y.W., et al. (2016). Psychotropic effects of Lactobacillus plantarum PS128 in early life-stressed and naive adult mice. *Brain Res* **1631**:1–12.

Long, S.J., Benton, D. (2013). A double-blind trial of the effect of docosahexaenoic acid and vitamin and mineral supplementation on aggression, impulsivity, and stress. *Hum Psychopharmacol.* **28**:238–247.

Luber, M.P., Meyers, B.S., Williams-Russo, P.G. et al. (2001). Depression and service utilization in elderly primary care patients. *Am J Geriatr Psychiat.* **9**:169–176.

Lukaschek, K, Von Schacky, C, Kruse, J et al. (2016). Cognitive impairment is associated with a low omega-3 index in the elderly: Results from the KORA-age study. *Dement Geriatr Cogn Disord.* **42**:236–245.

Luxwolda, M.F., Kuipers, R.S., Boersma, E.R. et al. (2014). DHA status is positively related to motor development in breastfed African and Dutch infants. *Nutr Neurosci.* **17**:97–103.

Macfarlane, S., et al. (2013). Synbiotic consumption changes the metabolism and composition of the gut microbiota in older people and modifies inflammatory processes: A randomised, double-blind, placebo-controlled crossover study. *Aliment Pharmacol Ther.* **38**(7):804–816.

MacKay, M.-A. B. et al. (2019). d-serine: Potential therapeutic agent and/or biomarker in schizophrenia and depression? *Front Psychiatry,* **10**:25.

Mann, J., Truswell, A.S. (2012). *Essentials of Human Nutrition.* 4th ed. New York: Oxford University Press, 2012.

María, E., Riveros and Mauricio, A. (2018). Retama, are polyunsaturated fatty acids implicated in histaminergic dysregulation in bipolar disorder? A hypothesis, *Front Physiol.* **9**: Article 693.

Mariat, D., et al. (2009). The Firmicutes/Bacteroidetes ratio of the human microbiota changes with age. *BMC Microbiol* **9**:123.

Maserejian, N.N., Hall, S.A., McKinlay, J.B. (2012). Low dietary or supplemental zinc is associated with depression symptoms among women, but not men, in a population-based epidemiological survey. *J Affect Disord.* **136**(3):781–788.

McGrattan, A.M., McEvoy, C.T., McGuinness, B., McKinley, M.C., Woodside, J.V. 2019, Effect of dietary interventions in mild cognitive impairment: A systematic review. *Br J Nutr.* **120**(12):1388–1405.

McLoughlin, I.J., Hodge, J.S. (1990). Zinc in depressive disorder. *Acta Psychiatr Scand.* **82**(6):451–453.

McNamara, R.K., Welge, J.A. (2016). Meta-analysis of erythrocyte polyunsaturated fatty acid biostatus in bipolar disorder. *Bipolar Disord.* **18**:300–306.

McVey Neufeld, K.A., et al. (2015). The gut microbiome restores intrinsic and extrinsic nerve function in germ-free mice accompanied by changes in calbindin. *Neurogastroenterol Motil.* **27**(5):627–636.

Mischoulon, D. (2007). Update and critique of natural remedies as antidepressant treatments. *Psychiatr Clin North Am.* **30**:51–68.

Mitsui, T., et al. (2006). Small bowel bacterial overgrowth is not seen in healthy adults but is in disabled older adults. *Hepatogastroenterology.* **53**(67):82–85.

Mohajeri, M.H., Troesch, B., Weber, P. (2015). Inadequate supply of vitamins and DHA in the elderly: Implications for brain aging and Alzheimer-type dementia. *Nutrition.* **31**:261–275

Mohammadpour, N., Jazayeri, S., Tehrani-Doost, M. et al. (2018). Effect of vitamin D supplementation as adjunctive therapy to methylphenidate on ADHD symptoms: A randomized, double blind, placebo-controlled trial. *Nutr Neurosci.* **21**:202–209

Montgomery, P., Burton, J.R., Sewell, R.P. et al. (2013). Low blood long chain omega-3 fatty acids in UK children are associated with poor cognitive performance and behavior: a cross-sectional analysis from the DOLAB study. *PLoS One.* **8**:e66697.

Moreno-Agostino, D., Caballero, F.F., Martin-Maria, N., Tyro- volas, S., et al. (2019). Mediterranean diet and wellbeing: evidence from a nationwide survey. *Psychol Health.* **34**:321–335.

Moriguchi, T., Greiner, R.S., Salem, N. Jr. (2000). Behavioral deficits associated with dietary induction of decreased brain docosahexaenoic acid concentration. *Jn Neurochem.* **75**:2563–2573.

Morris, G., Walder, K., McGee, S.L., et al. (2017). A model of the mitochondrial basis of bipolar disorder. *Neurosci Biobehav.* **74**:1–20.

Muntjewerff, J.W., van der Put, N., Eskes, T. et al. (2003). Homocysteine metabolism and B-vitamins in schizophrenic patients: low plasma folate as a possible independent risk factor for schizophrenia. *Psychiat Res.* **121**(1):1–9.

National Institute of Mental Health: Depression. *National Institute of Mental Health, National Institutes of Health* 2000. US Department of Health and Human Services, Bethesda (MD). Reprinted 2002.

Naylor, G.J., Smith, A.H. (1981). Vanadium: A possible aetiological factor in manic depressive illness. *Psychol Med.* **11**:249–256.

Nazia, Y., Hammad, H., Zaheer, A., Kausar, S., Kouser, S. (2018). Role of omega-3 polyunsaturated fatty acid in the management of major depressive disorder. *Int J Med Res Health Sci.* **7**(11):178–185.

Noaghiul, S., Hibbeln, J.R. (2003). Cross-national comparisons of seafood consumption and rates of bipolar disorders. *Am J Psychiatry.* **160**:2222–2227.

Nguyen, S., Lavretsky, H. (2020). Emerging complementary and integrative therapies for geriatric mental health. *Curr Treat Opt Psychiat.* **7**(1):1–24.

Odamaki, T., et al. (2016). Age-related changes in gut microbiota composition from newborn to centenarian: a cross-sectional study. *BMC Microbiol.* **16**:90.

Olin, J.T., Schneider, L.S., Katz, I.R., Meyers, B.S. et al. 2002, Provisional diagnostic criteria for depression of Alzheimer disease. *Am J Geriatr Psychiatry.* **10**:125–128.

Parletta, N., Niyonsenga, T., Duff, J. (2016). Omega-3 and omega-6 polyunsaturated fatty acid levels and correlations with symptoms in children with attention deficit hyperactivity disorder, autistic spectrum disorder and typically developing controls. *PLoS One.* **11**:e0156432.

Pawelczyk, T., Grancow-Grabka, M., Kotlicka-Antczak, M. et al. (2016). A randomized controlled study of the efficacy of six-month supplementation with concentrated fish oil rich in omega-3 polyunsaturated fatty acids in first episode schizophrenia. *J Psychiatr Res.* **73**:34–44.

Pawelczyk, T., Grancow-Grabka, M., Trafalska, E. et al. (2017). Oxidative stress reduction related to the efficacy of n-3 polyunsaturated fatty acids in first episode schizophrenia: Secondary outcome analysis of the OFFER randomized trial. *Prostaglandins Leukot Essent Fatty Acids.* **121**:7–13.

Peet, M., Horrobin, D.F. (2002). A dose-ranging exploratory study of the effects of ethyl-eicosapentaenoate in patients with persistent schizophrenic symptoms. *Jn Psychiatr Res.* **36**:7–18.

Perera, H., Jeewandara, K.C., Seneviratne, S., Guruge, C. (2012). Combined ω -3 and ω-6 supplementation in children with attention-deficit hyperactivity disorder (ADHD) refractory to methylphenidate treatment. *J Child Neurol.* **27**:747–753.

Pomponi, M. et al. (2013). Plasma levels of n-3 fatty acids in bipolar patients: Deficit restricted to DHA. *J Psychiatr.* **47**:337–342.

Pottala, J.V., Talley, J.A., Churchill, S.W. et al. (2012). Red blood cell fatty acids are associated with depression in a case-control study of adolescents. *Prostagland Leukot Essent Fatty Acids.* **86**:161–165.

Qiao, Y., Mei, Y., Han, H. et al. (2018). Effects of omega-3 in the treatment of violent schizophrenia patients. *Schizophr Res.* **195**:283–285.

Ranjbar, E., Kasaei, M.S., Mohammad-Shirazi, M., Nasrollahzadeh, J., Rashidkhani, B., Shams, J. et al. (2013). Effects of zinc supplementation in patients with major depression: A randomized clinical trial. *Iran J Psych.* **8**(2):73.

Reeves, J.L., Otahal, P., Magnussen, C.G. et al. (2017). DHA mediates the protective effect of fish consumption on new episodes of depression among women. *Br J Nutr.* **118**:743–749.

Ricardo, C., Inês Canelas da, S. (2019). Symptomatic Correlates of Vitamin D Deficiency in First-Episode Psychosis, *Psychiat J.* **2019**:7. Article ID 7839287.

Rihmer, Z, Gonda, X and Rihmer, A 2006, Creativity and mental illness. *Psychiatr Hung.* **21**, no.4:288–294

Roberfroid, M., et al. (2010). Prebiotic effects: metabolic and health benefits. *Br J Nutr* **104 Suppl 2**: S1–63.

Robinson, D.G., Schooler, N.R., Rosenheck, R.A., Lin, H. et al. (2019). Predictors of hospitalization of individuals with first-episode psychosis: Data from a 2-year follow-up of the raise-ETP. *Psychiatr Serv.* **7**:569–577.

Roffman, J.L., Lamberti, J.S., Achtyes, E. et al. (2013). Randomized multicenter investigation of folate plus vitamin B12 supplementation in schizophrenia. *JAMA Psychiatry.* **70**(5):481–489.

Rogers, G. B., et al. (2016). From gut dysbiosis to altered brain function and mental illness: mechanisms and pathways. *Mol Psychiatry* **21**(6):738–748.

Rondanelli, M., Giacosa, A., Opizzi, A. et al. (2011). Long chain omega 3 polyunsaturated fatty acids supplementation in the treatment of elderly depression: Effects on depressive symptoms, on phospholipids fatty acids profile and on health-related quality of life. *J Nut Health Aging.* **15**(1):37.

Sato, H., Tsukamoto-Yasui, M., Takado, Y., Kawasaki, N., Matsunaga, K., Ueno, S., Kanda, M., Nishimura, M., Karakawa, S., Isokawa, M.J.F.I.N. (2020). Protein deficiency-induced behavioral abnormalities and neurotransmitter loss in aged mice are ameliorated by essential amino acids. **7**:23.

Schaakxs, R. et al. (2017). Risk factors for depression: Differential across age? *Am J Geriat Psychiat.* **25**(9):966–977.

Schefft, C., Kilarski, L.L., Bschor, T. et al. (2017). Efficacy of adding nutritional supplements in unipolar depression: A systematic review and meta-analysis. *Eur Neuropsychopharmacol.* **27**:1090–109.

Shay, K.P. et al. (2009). Alpha-lipoic acid as a dietary supplement: Molecular mechanisms and therapeutic potential. *Biochimica et Biophysica Acta Gen Sub.* **1790**(10):1149–1160. doi: 10.1016/j.bbagen.2009.07.026.

Simopoulos, A.P. (1999). Essential fatty acids in health and chronic disease. *Am Jn Clin Nutr.* **70**:560–569.

Singh, P., Kesharwani, R.K., Keservani, R.K. (2017). Antioxidants and vitamins: Roles in cellular function and metabolism. Roles in cellular function and metabolism. *Sust Energ Enhanc Hum Func Activ*:385–407. doi:10.1016/B978-0-12-805413-0.00024-7.

Singh, S., B. Bajorek (2014). Defining 'elderly' in clinical practice guidelines for pharmacotherapy. *Pharma Prac.* **12**(4):489–489.

Siragusa, S., et al. (2007). Synthesis of gamma-aminobutyric acid by lactic acid bacteria isolated from a variety of Italian cheeses. *Appl Environ Microbiol.* **73**(22):7283–7290.

Smith, A.D., Warren, M.J., Refsum, H. (2018). Vitamin B12. *Adv Food Nutr Res.* **83**:215–279.

Sonnenberg, C.M., Deeg, D.J., Comijs, H.C., Van Tilburg, W., Beekman, A.T. (2008). Trends in antidepressant use in the older population: Results from the LASA-study over a period of 10 years. *J Affect Disor.* **111**:299–305.

Strandwitz, P., et al. (2019). GABA-modulating bacteria of the human gut microbiota. *Nat Microbiol.* **4**(3):396–403.

Su, K.P. (2015). Personalized medicine with Omega-3 fatty acids for depression in children and pregnant women and depression associated with inflammation. *J Clin Psychiatry.* **76**(11):e1476–e1477.

Su, K.P., Yang, H.T., Chang, J.P. et al. (2018). Eicosapentaenoic and docosahexaenoic acids have different effects on peripheral phospholipase A2 gene expressions in acute depressed patients. *Prog Neuropsychopharmacol Biol Psychiatry.* **80**:227–233.

Tamtaji, O.R., et al. (2019). Probiotic and selenium co-supplementation, and the effects on clinical, metabolic and genetic status in Alzheimer's disease: A randomized, double-blind, controlled trial. *Clin Nutr* **38**(6):2569–2575.

Tamtaji, O.R., et al. (2019). Clinical and metabolic response to probiotic administration in people with Parkinson's disease: A randomized, double-blind, placebo-controlled trial. *Clin Nutr.* **38**(3):1031–1035.

Tapiero, H., Ba, G.N., Couvreur, P., Tew, K.D. (2002). Polyunsaturated fatty acids (PUFA) and eicosanoids in human health and pathologies. *Biomed Pharmacother.* **56**:215–222.

Tarleton, E.K., Littenberg, B. (2015). Magnesium intake and depression in adults. *J Am Board Fam Med.* **28**(2):249–256.

Tesei, A., Crippa, A., Ceccarelli, S.B. et al. (2017). The potential relevance of docosahexaenoic acid and eicosapentaenoic acid to the etiopathogenesis of childhood neuropsychiatric disorders. *Eur Child Adolesc Psychiatry.* **26**:1011–1030.

Unger, M.M., et al. (2016). Short chain fatty acids and gut microbiota differ between patients with Parkinson's disease and age-matched controls. *Parkinsonism Relat Disord* **32**:66–72.

Valentini, L., et al. (2015). Impact of personalized diet and probiotic supplementation on inflammation, nutritional parameters and intestinal microbiota – The RISTOMED project: Randomized controlled trial in healthy older people. *Clin Nutr* **34**(4): 593–602.

Vellekkatt, F., Menon, V. (2019). Efficacy of vitamin D supplementation in major depression: a meta-analysis of randomized controlled trials. *J Postgrad Med.* **65**:74–80

Vicent, B.M., Gabriel, R.F., Gabriela, D.C. et al. (2011). Therapeutic use of omega-3 fatty acids in bipolar disorder. *Expert Rev Neurother.* **11**(7):1029–1047.

Von Schacky, C. (2014). Omega-3 index and cardiovascular health. *Nutrients.* **6**:799–814.

Vulevic, J., et al. (2015). Influence of galacto-oligosaccharide mixture (B-GOS) on gut microbiota, immune parameters and metabonomics in elderly persons. *Br J Nutr* **114**(4): 586–595.

Weich, S. et al. (2002). Mental health and the built environment: A cross-sectional survey of individual and contextual risk factors for depression. *Br J Psychiat.* **180**(5):428–433.

Weiser, M., Levkowitch, Y., Neuman, M., Yehuda, S. (1994). Decrease of serum iron in acutely psychotic schizophrenic patients. *Int J Neurosci.* **78**(1):49–52.

Widenhorn-Müller, K., Schwanda, S., Scholz, E., Spitzer, M. (2014). Effect of supplementation with long-chain ω-3 polyunsaturated fatty acids on behavior and cognition in children with attention deficit/hyperactivity disorder (ADHD): A randomized placebo-controlled intervention trial. Prostaglandins Leukort. *Essent Fat Acids.* **91**:49–60.

World Health Organisation. (2018). https://www.who.int/news-room/fact-sheets/detail/mental-health-of-older-adults

Wrzosek, M., Lukaszkiewicz, J., Wrzosek, M. et al. (2013). Vitamin D and the central nervous system. *Pharmacol Rep.* **65**(2):271–278.

Yadav, J., Sharma, S.K., Singh, L., Singh, T. (2013). Bipolar disorder in adults. *Int Res J Pharm.* **4**, no.6:34–38

Yang, Y., Kim, Y., Je, Y. (2018). Fish consumption and risk of depression: Epidemiological evidence from prospective studies. *Asia Pac Psychiatry*. **10**:e12335.

Yatsunenko, T., et al. (2012). Human gut microbiome viewed across age and geography. *Nature*. **486**(7402): 222–227.

Young, L.M., Pipingas, A., White, D.J., Gauci, S., Scholey, A. (2019). A systematic review and meta-analysis of B vitamin supplementation on depressive symptoms, anxiety, and stress: Effects on healthy and 'at-risk' individuals. *Nutrients*. **11**(9):2232.

Young, S.N. (2007). Folate and depression–a neglected problem. *J Psychiatry Neurosci*. **32**, no. 2:80–82.

Safety and Efficacy Determination in Antiaging Nutraceuticals

Vaibhav Changediya
Parul University

Contents

25.1 Aging

Structural and functional changes take place due to complex biological phenomena over time in a living organism which is called aging. There is a quite interesting relationship between diet and aging. The aging phenomenon can be slowed down by consumption of antioxidants and decreased caloric intake.

DOI: 10.1201/9781003110866-25

Oxygen plays many important roles in the body [1]. First and foremost, it is required to maintain life. However, the reactive oxygen species (ROS) produced by oxygen is injurious to health and one of the key factors responsible for aging. Healthy food and dietary antioxidants are important to increase quality of life and slow down the aging process. The microelements such as manganese, zinc, selenium, iron and dietary antioxidants such as probiotics, vitamin A, vitamin C, vitamin D and vitamin E are slowing down the aging process because of their ability to decrease the amount of ROS in cells, which results in an increase in lifespan of organisms. The objective of this chapter is to highlight the significance of antiaging nutraceuticals and to discuss safety and efficacy of antiaging nutraceuticals [2,3].

Aging is characterized by physiological changes in cells and tissues that result in increased risk of disease and death. It depends on both internal and external factors. Internal factors are naturally occurring processes that take place within the cell. External factors include ultraviolet irradiation hormonal imbalances, nutritional deficiencies, chronic sun exposure, etc. We can decrease skin aging by adopting proper prevention measures including a balanced diet, skin care and antioxidant-enriched supplements. By adopting these methods, we can reduce the harmful effects of free radicals [1]. The impact of nutrition on the aging process has been a matter of interest not only in the case of animal research but in humans as well (Figure 25.1).

25.2 Signs of aging

The signs of aging are wrinkles around the eyes, brows and regions of the neck. There is a decline in maximal heart rate due to a decrease in oxygen use capacity, and approximately more than 10,000 neurons of the brain become not functioning properly, vision becomes dim, and the maximal capacity of the kidney and liver to filter waste material decreases [4].

25.3 Theories of aging

Based on common assumptions, the following theories have been postulated to describe the phenomenon of aging.

25.4 Free radical theory

Free radicals are highly reactive, uncharged species having an unpaired valence electron. These free radicals are required in various metabolic processes, including in the synthesis of hormones protection of the body from infection and for production of energy which is released from food. The free radicals are required in particular amounts in all these conditions. The excess production

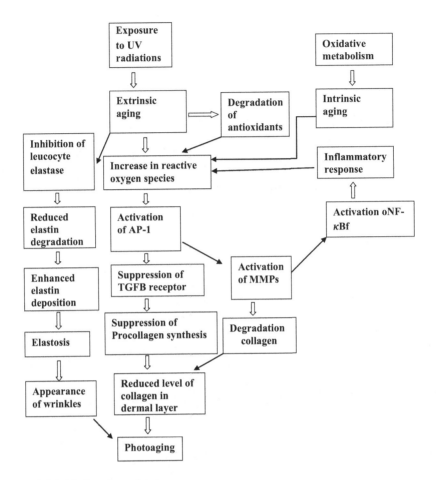

Figure 25.1 *Mechanism of aging.*

of free radicals is responsible for specific damage to the body including DNA, elastin and collagen [5]. Damage occurs due to free radical takes or pulls an electron likely from a neighboring molecule, to pair its unpaired electron and convert the molecule to a free radical. The oxidative damage occurs to macromolecules like DNA and proteins is undergoes accumulation but is not significant enough to cause aging. Oxygen plays many significant roles in the body. Not only is it required for life, but it is also involved in the production of many potentially harmful compounds. The DNA molecule undergoes genetic mutations by free radical attacks resulting in synthesis of dysfunctional protein. This mutation may be repair by DNA-repairing enzymes. Free radicals are generated during energy production, i.e., ATP. The mitochondria lose their efficiency for ATP production during the aging process, The several scientific studies proves that mitochondrial DNA is more prone to mutation than core DNA [5]. A decrease in consumption of calories results in slowing the aging phenomenon and promotes lifespan in rats, spiders, flies, fish, etc. [2]. Older rodents are generally involved in these kinds of studies in which they are given a special diet full of vitamins and minerals [6,7,8].

25.5 Stochastic theory

The stochastic theory is also called the wear-and-tear theory and was proposed by August Weismann [9]. According to Weisman, an excess of fat, certain injuries and infections, and excessive irradiation with UV light are the main causes of aging. This theory was later modified by Hart and Setlow (1974) who proposed that aging is due to DNA damage and mutation in proteins.

25.6 Mitochondrial decline theory

According to this theory, cytochrome c oxidase, an enzyme that plays a vital role in the mitochondrial electron transport chain (ETC), continuously decreases over time in both vertebrates and invertebrates [10]. Therefore, there are close connections between MDTA and FRTA. Improving the antioxidant defense system also increases the functional decline of mitochondria and at the same time also decreases the amount of free radicals.

25.7 Theory of ubiquitin proteasomal system decline

According to this theory, misfolding and aggregation of proteins are the reasons behind aging. It is a complex consisting of 20S core chamber and two 19S caps attached to it from each end [11]. This causes an accumulation of misfolded proteins leading to the development of several neurodegenerative diseases such as Alzheimer's and Parkinson's [12–14].

25.8 Immunologic theory

A wide range of foreign molecules are detected and destroyed by the immune system to preserve the healthy cells. It is reported that a characteristic of the immune system to resist infectious diseases reduces over time, therefore increasing the risk of death in the elderly [7].

25.9 Nutraceuticals

Nutraceuticals is a broad term including all types of food with health or medical effect. In the world, regulations on functional food and nutraceuticals are developed along with the development of new products. As the name suggests, "nutra" means food and "ceutical" refers to the medicinal product properties. According to the definition by the Foundation for Innovation in Medicine (FIM), nutraceuticals are "food or food ingredients providing medical and health benefits, including prevention and treatment of diseases" [15].

This nomenclature is not aligned across legal regulations in different countries. A large number of substances including vitamins, carotenoids, flavonoids, minerals, etc. have *in vitro* or *in vivo* clinically important antioxidant properties. There is great interest in antiaging substances obtained from food which have beneficial effects on digestive and immune systems and modulate inflammatory and degenerative processes in the body, and the most popular components are antioxidants, especially coenzyme Q10, phytoestrogens, probiotics and omega-3 fatty acids.

25.10 Nutraceuticals for deficiency

The National Institutes of Health (NIH) recommends that if you do not eat a variety of nutritious foods, then "some supplements might help you get adequate amounts of essential nutrients" [16]. They further state, before recommending to follow the food guide, that "supplements can't take the place of the variety of foods that are important to a healthy diet". Indeed, a general belief exists that supplementation is only useful in periods of deficiency and, historically, there is no denying this observation. Vitamins C or D can prevent scurvy and rickets, respectively and these are classic examples of the utility of nutrition to prevent disease.

25.11 Why are nutraceuticals needed?

Humans require food to survive, and our evolutionary history is filled with agricultural advancements that have resulted in the stable production of food free from harmful pathogens. For example, whole grains such as wheat and rice contain three layers: bran, endosperm and germ. The bran layer provides physiological benefits ranging from improving digestion, regulation of cholesterol and glucose absorption. The germ layer consists of phytochemicals, B vitamins and vitamin E, whereas the endosperm consists primarily of carbohydrates and proteins. While fortification has become the solution to maintain the nutritional value of wheat, other products that undergo similar processing may not be as fortunate. Moreover, highly processed and foods of convenience, which make up nearly half of our daily total caloric intake, further deteriorate quality of the food supply [17]. Couple processing with the drastic alterations in the diversity of our food supply that has favored, instead of more nutritional varieties, cultivars resistant to fluctuations in growing conditions and that better survive.

According to the definition by the Foundation for Innovation in Medicine (FIM), the nutraceuticals are "food or food ingredients providing medical and health benefits, including prevention and/or treatment of diseases" [18].

According to the above definition, all foods or food supplements can be defined as nutraceuticals. 'Health benefits' refer to long-term health improvement or decreasing the risk of development of chronic diseases. Nutraceuticals differ from functional foods as they are used in prevention and treatment of illnesses and they include supplements as well, while functional food is in the form of regular food [3]. Nutraceuticals is a broad term including all types of food with health or medical effect. It is closely connected to medical claim term, which is a sensitive matter in the field of regulations of functional foods. The meaning of nutraceuticals is in many aspects very close to the term 'healthy food' [19,20].

25.12 Important nutrients for slowing the aging process

The term antiaging medicine deserves to redefine aging as a goal or target for biomedical and scientific investigation, challenging the way aging has been understood up to now [21]. Diet plays a significant role in the treatment of different diseases, and the proper choice of nutrients can help in prevention of illness and enhance the quality of life. Epidemiological surveys suggest a strong connection between the intake of specific dietary elements (e.g., antioxidants) and a decrease in the risk of cancer, coronary heart diseases or cataract [22,23]. The intake of food supplements significantly corrects the deficiency in folic acid, vitamins E and B12, and iron. Persons who regularly consume dietary supplements have the intake of calcium above the average. Also, a significant correlation is observed in regular intake of food supplements and respecting dietary recommendations [25].

A large group of substances including vitamins, carotenoids, flavonoids and minerals have exhibited clinically significant *in vitro* and *in vivo* antioxidant characteristics. Apart from this, carotenoids and flavonoids also show significant antioxidant characteristics. All those natural compounds found in various foods, vegetables and beverages can be utilized as significant sources of antioxidants [24]. Flavonols, flavones, anthocyanins, catechins and proanthocyanidins are the most common classes of flavonoids, whereas dietary carotenoids include carotene, cryptoxanthin, lutein, zeaxanthin and lycopene. Carotenoids and flavonoids are secondary metabolites synthesized by plants, mostly after various stresses (mechanical, chemical, UV radiation, environmental and microbiologic stresses). Reactive oxygen species in plants induces a series of reactions leading to the production of carotenoids and polyphenolic compounds that protect plants from injury. Beta-carotene is a pigment of plant which the body can convert into vitamin A; it serves as an antioxidant and strengthens the body system [26,27]. Rich sources of beta-carotene are yellow and orange fruits and vegetables and green vegetables with dark green leaves. Vitamin A (retinol) induces the cells to divide freely in the process of cellular differentiation. Vitamin A prevents penetration of microorganisms that cause disease, by keeping cell membranes, stimulating immunity, and it is needed for bone, protein and growth hormone formation. Vitamin A is playing a significant role for good vision and potentially important for prevention of eye diseases like glaucoma and cataract, which are predominantly seen in older age.

Vitamin C is a water-soluble vitamin, which acts as a strong antioxidant. One of the most important functions of vitamin C is protection of low-density lipoprotein (LDL) cholesterol from oxidative damage [28]. The main food sources of vitamin C are broccoli, red paprika, pomegranate, acerola, citrus fruit, strawberry, tomatoes and green vegetables in general. Vitamin E is an antioxidant protecting cellular membranes and other lipid-soluble body parts like LDL cholesterol. The protection of LDL cholesterol from oxidation can decrease the rate of heart diseases such as coronary disease. It is recommended to take a natural form of vitamin E, d-α-tocopherols [29,30] (Table 25.1).

Apart from the potential advantages of these nutraceuticals, they suffer from poor aqueous solubility, stability, etc. [31]. To overcome these challenges, various solvent systems, complexation techniques and different colloidal systems (vesicles, microemulsion, liposomes, etc.) are used. Among these, the colloidal systems have exhibited greater solubilization efficiency toward hydrophobic molecules [32]. Therefore, in recent years, researchers are focusing their interest on colloidal delivery systems.

There is a growing overlap between conventional food (including beverages) and food supplements, including energy bars and teas or liquids. What could be considered a functional food under a given set of circumstances may be named a dietary supplement, medical food, food for special dietary use or nutraceutical under different circumstances, depending on its ingredients (active components) and the claims reported on its label (Borchers AT, Keen CL, Gerswin). The term nutraceutical was originally coined by Stephen DeFelice, who defined nutraceuticals as "food or part of a food that provides medical or health benefits, including the prevention and treatment of a disease". This concept has been proposed as a modern approach to food science, and the area of possible use has been defined as beyond the diet, but before the drugs. Nutraceuticals are continuously developed and have quickly spread worldwide. Food supplements, as per their micronutrient content, can be used to improve the health of individuals in need.

From our point of view, it is imperative to have more information on safety and efficacy based on clinical studies rather than only in vitro studies. The first step in assessing the action of nutraceuticals is to distinguish them from the other food-derived products, particularly food supplements, which are not always included in daily dietary habits in the presence of a specific need. This exercise may require: (i) appropriate target identification; (ii) safety assessment; (iii) a clear understanding of the mechanism of action; (iv) efficacy assessment substantiated by clinical studies; (v) an evaluation of possible unwanted side effects; and (vi) an evaluation of possible interactions with

Table 25.1 Classification of Nutraceuticals with their Sources and Potential Benefits

Sr. No.	Chemical Constituents	Structures	Food Source	Potential Benefits	Drawbacks
1	Polyphenolic compounds Resveratrol (RSV)		Grapes, peanuts, berries	Antioxidant, anticancer, reduce cholesterol, anti-inflammatory	Poor water solubility, high metabolic rate
2	Curcumin (Cur)		Turmeric root	Antioxidant, anticancer, anti-inflammatory, improves liver functions	Poor water solubility, chemical instability, low absorption, rapid metabolism
3	Quercetin (QT)		Apples, onion, grapes, dark cherries, red wine, etc.	Antioxidant, anticancer, controls diabetes and hypertension	Poor water solubility, high metabolic rate, inactive metabolic product
4	Genistein		Soya beans, legumes	Antioxidant, reduces breast and prostate cancers	Poor water solubility and intestinal permeability
5	Daidzein		Soya beans, legumes	Antioxidant and anti-inflammatory	Poor water solubility and hence poor absorption

(Continued)

Table 25.1 (Continued) Classification of Nutraceuticals with their Sources and Potential Benefits

Sr. No.	Chemical Constituents	Structures	Food Source	Potential Benefits	Drawbacks
6	Carotenoids Lycopene		Tomatoes, pink grapefruit, guava, papaya, watermelon.	Antioxidant, protect against formation of cancer mainly prostate, bladder, cervical, leukemia	Poor solubility, dose-associated toxicity, nonspecificity, small half lifetime
7	Lutin		Corn, egg yolk, spinach	Anticancer (colon), protects the eyes against muscular degeneration	Poor water solubility, chemical instability, nonspecificity
8	β-Carotene		Carrots	Antioxidant, anticancer, protects cornea against UV light	Poor solubility
9	α-Carotene		Corn avocado	Protect eyes from muscular degeneration and cataracts	Poor water solubility
10	Isothiocyanate sulforaphane		Cauliflower, broccoli, cabbage,	Anticancer	Poor water solubility
11	Benzylisothiocyanate (BITC)		Cauliflower, broccoli, cabbage,	Anticancer, antibacterial	Poor water solubility

(Continued)

Table 25.1 (Continued) Classification of Nutraceuticals with their Sources and Potential Benefits

Sr. No.	Chemical Constituents	Structures	Food Source	Potential Benefits	Drawbacks
12	Alkaloids Quinine (QN)		Cinchona	Antimalarial	Poor water solubility
13	Morphine		Opium poppy	Antidepressant, pain killer	Poor water solubility
14	Noncarotenoids Saponin		Legumes (chicks, peas, all pulse crop)	Reduced cholesterol level in blood	Poor water solubility
15	Terpineol		Pine oil, petit grain oil.	Anticancer	Poor water solubility

(Continued)

Table 25.1 (Continued) Classification of Nutraceuticals with their Sources and Potential Benefits

Sr. No.	Chemical Constituents	Structures	Food Source	Potential Benefits	Drawbacks
16	Perillyl alcohol		Cherries and mints	Anticancer	Poor water solubility
17	Capsaicin		Capsicum (hot peppers)	Anticancer activity against liver, colonic and bladder cancer	Poor water solubility, uncontrolled dose-associated toxicity
18	Piperin		Black pepper, jalapeno peppers	Help in digestion	Poor water solubility
19	Omega-3 fatty acids		Flaxseed oil, fish oil, soybean, spinach	Maintenance of brain function, reduces cholesterol level	Poor oxidative stability and water solubility

(Continued)

Table 25.1 (Continued) Classification of Nutraceuticals with their Sources and Potential Benefits

Sr. No.	Chemical Constituents	Structures	Food Source	Potential Benefits	Drawbacks
20	Vitamins vitamin A		Sweet potatoes, fish liver, lettuce, dark leafy greens etc.	Antioxidant, essential for growth of healthy vision, skin and mucous membranes, may aid in the prevention and treatment of certain cancers and in the treatment of certain skin disorders	Light sensitive and poor water solubility
21	Vitamin E		Almonds, spinach, sunflower seed, palm oil, etc.	Antioxidant, helps to form blood cells, boosts immune system.	Poor water solubility, short half lifetime
22	Vitamin K		Green leafy vegetables, green leafy lettuce	Essential for blood clotting	Poor water solubility and hence poor absorption

other products (e.g. food, food supplements and drugs). Therefore, it is important to clearly identify their specificity in view of their possible use and utility in the pharmaceutical arena.

25.13 State of the art and future trend

The first step in food regulation in was established in 1997 with the Green Paper on Food Law, which outlined the need for new and improved legislation in the field white paper on Food Safety 2000 [33]. These papers led to the General Food Law Regulation [Regulation EC No. 178/2002 of the European Parliament and of the Council 2002], which established the principle and foresaw the creation of an independent organization called the European Food Safety Authority (EFSA) with the specific task of giving scientific advice based upon scientific assessment of the beneficial health effects and associated risks related to food intake [Regulation EC No. 178/2002]. The risk assessment and risk evaluation can also be included as a part of the EFSA mandate from a European Member State or stakeholder [34]. This step should then be followed by a specific action from local national authorities, who take the suggestions on board and propose appropriate legislation and regulation in the field. The mission of the EFSA is to "provide the basis for the assurance of a high level of protection of human health and consumer interest with respect to food".

Nevertheless, while nutraceuticals should always have specific added health value for the prevention or treatment of pathological conditions, food supplements may not be required to have this characteristic [35]. Notwithstanding the differences existing between them that were outlined previously, Article 2 of Directive 2002/46/ EC (Directive 2002/46/EC of the European Parliament and of the Council 2002) defines only food supplements as "foodstuffs, the purpose of which is to supplement the normal diet and which are concentrated sources of nutrients or other substances with a nutritional or physiological effect, alone or in combination, marketed in dose form, namely, forms such as capsules, pastilles, tablets, pills and other similar forms, sachets of powder, ampoules of liquids, drop dispensing bottles, and other similar forms of liquids and powders designed to be taken in measured small unit quantities", [36] without mentioning nutraceuticals [Directive 2002/46/]. Food supplements can contain substances with a physiological effect other than nutritional value and so can nutraceuticals, according to our view. A product must be available in a concentrated form and should be taken in the proper pharmaceutical form to fall under Directive 2002/46/EC.

Nutraceuticals can be marketed with the same pharmaceutical form of food supplements. We instead propose a different classification approach for these products to differentiate them from food supplements (Directive 2002/46/). The current European Directive 2002/46/EC on food supplements mainly focuses inter alia on vitamins and minerals as supplements and foresees that maximum amounts of vitamins and minerals must consider the upper safe levels established by scientific risk assessment considering different consumer groups and the intake of vitamins and minerals derived from other dietary sources. Prior to 2002, food supplements were subjected to national regulations, which set the legislation framework and risk assessment management. Regarding food supplements, the European Responsible Nutrition Alliance (ERNA) suggested a risk management model for determining maximum risk levels for different nutrient intakes based on the population safety index in 2004. In 2006, ERNA contributed to the establishment of guidelines for nutrition and health claim regulations, suggesting these guidelines as a tool for companies to provide correct communication about the many health benefits of vitamins, minerals, omega 3 fatty acids, etc. [37].

The key aspect here is that food supplements and nutraceuticals are both considered to be derived foodstuffs, which means that, in many cases, the precautionary principle valid for food is applied to food supplements, and the term nutraceutical is used for products available on the market without proper assessment of their beneficial health effects, except in cases specifically provided in the food supplement legislation itself. It would hence be advisable that the European Commission or authorities in charge explore the possibility of including nutraceuticals in their Directives or Regulations by defining a new category that differentiates them from food supplements and pharmaceuticals. In particular, no effective, shared regulatory system exists in the USA regarding medical or health claims for nutraceuticals, even though these products have entered mainstream science and medicine and the consumer marketplace. This lack of rules negatively influences the market for these products, can generate confusion among consumers, and eventually, can lead to possible misuse [38].

Nutraceuticals that demonstrate specific pharmacological activities can claim beneficial health effects for pathological conditions, and if they are considered vegetal supplements (in cases of vegetal origin), they can be covered by legislation for food supplements. An EFSA positive opinion would be necessary to assess and recognize their potential use and hence market the nutraceutical as a pharma-food, demonstrating the large difference that exists between nutraceuticals and food supplements. Regulation EC 1924/2006 on nutrition and health claims made on food was issued to harmonize the laws and different legislations among Member States to guarantee safety and efficacy and to simultaneously protect the internal market by providing proper, understandable information to consumers [Regulation EC No. 1924/200] [39]. In accordance with this Regulation, any health or nutritional claims on food must be approved from EFSA before marketing. Health claims are generally related to nutritional profiles, the overall nutritional composition of a foodstuff and the presence of nutrients that have been scientifically recognized as having a beneficial effect on health. National regulations often apply in the absence of specific shared international rules concerning recommendations or any endorsements by national medical associations. Nutraceuticals are generally reported to have good safety profile with few unwanted side effects and high bioavailability [40]. Their application area ranges from metabolic syndrome and inflammation control to Alzheimer's disease [4,22–27]. It must, however, be noted again that current European legislation does not mention the term nutraceutical [41].

Nutraceutical Research and Education Act specifically dedicated to the review and approval of nutraceuticals and the development of programs stimulating clinical research in this field with the aim of substantiating all health claims with clinical data [48]. The realization of these actions and proper worldwide availability of information could: (i) be beneficial for individuals; and (ii) be beneficial for research in this area; and (iii) realize a proactive approach toward preventing, rather than curing, pathological conditions, many of which may arise from improper diet and lifestyle (e.g. metabolic syndrome). This outcome is, however, not always easy to achieve in populations and remains to be completed. Efficacy, together with safety, is to be considered of utmost importance for nutraceuticals. European Council Regulation (EC) No. 178/2002 on food introduced a precautionary principle in the risk management process in 2002 [42,43]. Risk analysis in authorization procedures and claims approval may also be relevant for nutraceuticals, food supplements and functional foods [15]. When possible harmful health effects are identified, affecting the health of humans, the environment, plants and animals [44].

The first step of safety assessment was established in 1997 with Regulation EC No. 258/97 of the European Parliament and of the Council on novel foods and novel food ingredients. Both recognized the need to have a safety assessment through a shared procedure before placing food supplement on the market. In November 2015, Regulation EU 2015/2283 of the European Parliament and of the Council on novel foods revised the rules to define and place novel foods on the market within the European Union [45,46].

Nutraceuticals are still not mentioned in the 2015 Regulation, notwithstanding their potential medicinal use to prevent/cure some pathological conditions. It may be feasible to apply current legislation for pharmaceutical regarding efficacy, safety and health effect assessment to nutraceuticals with the same restrictions [47]. Another possible approach could be to start by reconsidering Directive 1999/21/EC, which defines processed or formulated products that are intended for the dietary management of individuals with disrupted metabolism, or in special physiological conditions, and must be prescribed by a medical doctor and used under their supervision as PARNUTS [Commission Directive 1999/21] [49,50]. PARNUTS legislation could be adopted to draw a possible scheme for nutraceutical validation with the aim of clearly distinguishing them from food supplements and/or from functional foods intended for particular nutritional or clinical uses. According to Directive 89/398/EEC, PARNUTS should have a special composition for their claimed nutritional/medical purposes and should be clearly different from foodstuffs for dietary use [28]. These products should be addressed to individuals who do not qualify for pharmacological treatment and who could benefit from alternative treatment given their proven efficacy. In this case, the possible target population could be quite wide considering the growing impact on health due to improper lifestyles, particularly metabolic syndrome, which includes different pathological health conditions, such as hypertriglyceridemia, hypertension, hypercholesterolemia, type II diabetes and obesity [34,35].

25.14 The need for scientific rationale

The proper starting point for nutraceutical concept assessment should begin with a sharp difference between nutraceuticals and food supplements. Food supplements have been already defined as previously reported. Regarding nutraceuticals, we propose the following definition: (i) for food of vegetal origin, a nutraceutical is the phytocomplex and (ii) for food of animal origin, a nutraceutical is the pool of secondary metabolites. Both are concentrated and administered in the proper pharmaceutical form. They are capable of providing beneficial health effects, including the prevention and/or the treatment of a disease [51,52].

Table 25.2 collects some of the most common definitions of these products together with other food-derived products. Many of them belong to the food supplement category, which also includes herbal products; these food supplements are often miscategorized with nutraceuticals.

Table 25.2 Some of the Most Common Definitions of These Products Together with Other Food-Derived Products

Food supplement (United States Government Office, 1994)	A product (other than tobacco) in the form of a capsule, powder, soft gel or gel cap intended to supplement the diet to enhance health that bears or contains one or more of the following dietary ingredients: a vitamin, mineral, amino acid, or other botanical or dietary substance.	United States Food and Drug Administration (FDA). Dietary Supplement Health and Education Act (DSHEA). U.S. Department of Health and Human Services. 1994. United States. Public Law 103–417, available at FDA Website: http://www.fda.gov.
Food supplement (EU, 2002)	Food product whose purpose is to supplement the normal diet and which consists of a concentrated source of nutrients or other substances with nutritional effects or physiological, single or in combination, marketed in dosed formulations, such as capsules, tablets, tablets or pills, designed to be taken in small individual quantities measured.	EU Directive 2002/46/EC

(Continued)

Phytochemical (Bloch and Thomson, 1995)	Substances found in edible fruit and vegetables that can be ingested daily (in quantities of grams) by humans and that exhibit a potential to favorably modulate human metabolism to prevent cancer and other diseases (isoflavones, resveratrol, garlic allyl sulphides, tomato lycopene, onion quercetin, etc.).	Bloch A, Thomson CA. Position of The American Dietetic Association (phytochemical and functional foods). J Am Diet Assoc 1995; 95: 493–496.
Nutraceuticals (De Felice, 1995)	Food or part of food that provides medical or health benefits, including the prevention and/or treatment of a disease.	DeFelice SL. The nutraceutical revolution: its impact on food industry R&D. Trends Food Sci Technol 1995; 6: 59–61.
Nutraceuticals (Zeisel, 1999; DSHEA, 1994)	A diet supplement that delivers a concentrated form of a biologically active component of food in a nonfood matrix to enhance health.	Zeisel SH. Regulation of "Nutraceuticals". Science. 1999: 285; 1853–5. Food and Drug Administration, FDA, Dietary Supplement Health and Education Act of 1994 (DSHEA), United States.
Nutraceuticals (Brower, 1998)	Any substance that is a food or a part of a food and is able to induce medical and health benefits, including the prevention and treatment of disease.	Brower V. Nat Biotechnol 1998; 16: 728.
Nutraceuticals (Merriam Webster Dictionary, 2015)	A foodstuff (as a fortified food or dietary supplement) that provides health benefits in addition to its basic nutritional.	Merriam Webster Online Dictionary. 2015. Merriam Webster Inc., P.O. Box 281, Springfield, MA 01102, United States.
Nutraceuticals (ENA, 2016)	Nutritional products that provide health and medical benefits, including the prevention and treatment of disease.	European Nutraceutical Association (ENA). 2016. Science behind Nutraceuticals. In E. N. Association (Ed.), (Vol. 2016). 594 Basel, Switzerland.
Functional food (Zeisel, 1999)	Nutrient consumed as part of a normal diet but delivering one or more active ingredients (that have physiological effects and may enhance health) within the food matrix.	Zeisel SH. Regulation of "Nutraceuticals". Science 1999: 285; 1853–5. Food and Drug Administration, FDA, Dietary Supplement Health and Education Act of 1994 (DSHEA), United States.
Functional food (Diplock et al., 1999)	Product which is shown in a satisfactory manner that, in addition to adequate nutritional effects, induces beneficial effects on one or more target functions of the organism, significantly improving the health status and welfare or reducing the risk of disease.	Diplock A, Aggett P, Ashwell M, Bornet F, Fern E, Roberfroid M. The European Commission concerted action on functional foods science in Europe (FUFOSE). Scientific concepts of functional foods in Europe. Consensus document. Br J Nutr 1999; 81: S1–S27.
Functional food (Hardy, 2000)	Any food or ingredient that has a positive impact on an individual's health, physical performance, or state of mind, in addition to its nutritive value.	Hardy G. Nutraceuticals and functional foods: introduction and meaning. Nutrition 2000; 16: 688–689.

(*Continued*)

Table 25.2 (Continued) Some of the Most Common Definitions of These Products Together with Other Food-Derived Products

Food for medical use (EU, 1999)	Complete nutritional food with a formulation of nutrients standards, which may constitute the sole source nutrition for the person to whom it is addressed. Or alternatively: complete nutritional food with a formulation of nutrient adapted to a specific disease, disorder or medical condition, which may constitute the only source of nutrition for the person to whom it is addressed. Or alternatively, nutritionally incomplete food with a formulation standard nutrient or adapted for a specific disease, disorder or medical condition, which it is not suitable to be used as the only source of nutrition.	EU Directive 1999/21/ EC.

The first step to assess therapeutic efficacy should be based on positive evidence from clinical data [53]. This step should include the contribution of different professionals and different expertise, ranging from food chemistry and food safety to structure–activity studies, with the aim of assessing the mechanism of action, nutritional aspects, pharmacology, pharmacokinetics and pharmacodynamics of each nutraceutical. The utmost importance of the clinical aspects of any study concerning nutraceuticals as pharma-foods (e.g., in vivo clinical trials) or any possible interactions between food and/or drugs assumed together with nutraceuticals is not to be underestimated [9,37]. Medical doctor involvement in these studies is a crucial step for proper evaluation of both safety and efficacy assessment [54,55].

Figure 25.2 indicates the differences between food supplements and nutraceuticals, signifying the efficacy/safety requirements for these products. Figure 25.2 outlines a proposed scheme that describes the necessary steps to consider when identifying and developing a new nutraceutical. It should be noted that the necessary time to develop a new nutraceutical is reduced compared to time required to develop a new drug, considering the natural origin of the constituents of a nutraceutical. Priority steps are indicated. The first step of utmost importance is the identification of the heath condition to specific legislation on efficacy, safety, production and use in therapy to be authorized and marketed. The dose and mechanism of action must be identified in detail, as must possible undesired side effects and pharmacokinetics depending on the dose and method of administration. Once a medicinal product is placed on the market, its benefit/risk ratio continues to be assessed throughout its entire lifespan. The adoption of nutraceuticals in daily diets may help prevent the onset of pathological conditions [56].

The starting point for identifying and testing a nutraceutical should be making a proper therapeutic hypothesis, such that the hypothesis is reproducible

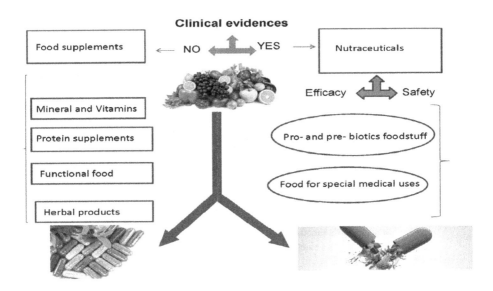

Figure 25.2 *Differences between food supplements and nutraceuticals.*

and supportive in the modulation of a target capable of producing a beneficial health address, followed by an assessment of safety and efficacy with clinical trials and a complete and accurate study/assessment of the mechanism of action. The absence of unwanted side effects and efficacy are crucial steps prior to submitting an application to EFSA in Europe (or to the equivalent authority in other countries) for a health claim to be authorized and advertised on the product label before advertising the product or putting it on the market. The admitted claims are generally indicated as helps to develop or stimulate a beneficial effect, and they often refer to substances or pre- or probiotics, not to a phytocomplex itself, as promoting a beneficial health effect [57,58] (Figure 25.3).

All the above-mentioned food-derived products are considered generally safe, but regulatory criteria are different in different countries; for example, in Japan, functional foods are defined according to their use of natural ingredients, whereas in the United States, they can also contain ingredients produced with biotechnology. One possible source of confusing information could be administration of the pharmaceutical form – pills, tablets and capsules – which can be the same for food supplements and nutraceuticals. However, nutraceuticals should have proven clinical efficacy, beneficial health effects, greater bioavailability and safety beyond their nutritional value. The lack of a common legislation is huge challenge for nutraceutical globalization because the existence of different regulations can generate confusion and also give a somewhat dissimilar definition of products that are present in different countries. Active substances, which can either be extracted from plants as phytocomplexes or can be of animal origin, can create a very promising nutraceutical toolbox that

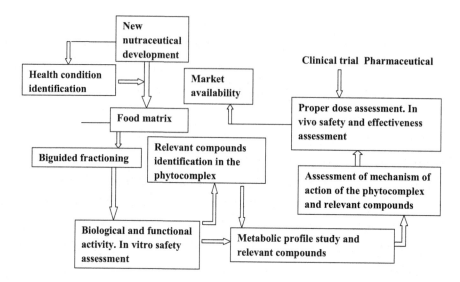

Figure 25.3 *A proposal for regulatory framework for nutraceuticals.*

is useful for promoting health, preventing disease, or offering general medicinal properties, given their proven clinical efficacy when they are concentrated and administered in a suitable pharmaceutical form [4]. This category encompasses food supplements, vitamin- and/or mineral-based formulations, herbal supplements and animal origin products [59].

The main focus on food supplement legislation has thus far addressed their safety and labelling, whereas less emphasis has been given to product claims and intended use of these supplements than for pharmaceuticals. This last aspect is accomplished through good manufacturing practice regulations, which should also be enforced. The terms nutraceuticals and food supplements are commonly used without differentiating between them [40,41]. A clear and common regulation system allowing the identification and classification of these products at an international level that clearly indicates quality, efficacy, mechanism of action and safety could benefit potential consumers as well as the industry also. Obtaining health claims approval could also represent a growing challenge for stakeholders because nutraceuticals are currently in a grey area between pharmaceuticals and medicinal food [60].

25.15 Safety and efficacy

The agency generally depends on evidence gathered from clinical investigations approved by the manufacturers of the products, along with reports of adverse events in actual use. For several reasons, the FDA's data is not sufficient when it comes to antiaging investigation [61]. Some investigation, such as lifestyle changes that have not been proved to affect aging processes, lies outside of the FDA's regulatory purview because they constitute the practice of medicine rather than the use of a drug or medical device. The practice of medicine is regulated by state law, through a combination of state medical board oversight and private suits for malpractice. Those physicians who practice in a manner that is unsafe or ineffective can face disciplinary action. But a state medical board infrequently warns physicians for illegal practice. The threat of potential malpractice suits also does not seem to determine the proliferation of antiaging services. Another obstacle to effective FDA regulation of antiaging products is the Dietary Supplement Health and Education Act (DSHEA) implemented in 1994, which allows certain antiaging products to be marketed as "dietary supplements" without safety or efficacy data. The definition of a dietary supplement in this law and legislation is extremely broad; virtually any antiaging product would qualify as a dietary supplement as long as it did not make a claim to treat a specific disease. Prior to the DSHEA, a product that claimed, for example, to "provide you with Improved skin texture, Increased Sex drive, Increased Energy level, Increased muscle mass, Decreased Cholesterol, Improved Cognitive Thinking Skills, Improved Immune System, and Improved Bone Density" (Hormonal Anti-aging Center, 2003) would have been regulated as a drug because it proved to affect the structure or function of the body (Federal Food, Drug, and Cosmetic Act, 1994). Since the DSHEA, however, products for which such assumptions are made and which are sold as dietary supplements are not subject to FDA regulation as drugs. Moreover, the DSHEA has reversed the traditional process for increasing safety and efficacy. It is mandatory for the manufacturer of a new drug or medical device to establish safety and efficacy before marketing. The agency can take action to restrict its sale or remove it from the market in case a dietary supplement is unsafe [62]. Finally, manufacturers of dietary supplements are not required to disclose information about adverse events to the FDA. The FDA recently has launched guidelines for dietary supplement manufacturers required to verify that their products contain the ingredients listed on the label (FDA, 2003), but still they are lacking safety and efficacy data [63].

Even in the case of drugs and devices that are subject to full FDA legislation, the agency faces a number of difficulties in ensuring safety and efficacy. Is symptomatic relief sufficient, in which case manufacturers might be allowed to make antiaging assumptions for products such as anti-inflammatory drugs? Indeed, what counts as a symptom of aging, and what qualifies as symptomatic relief? How should the FDA deal with the quality of many symptoms? Even if the FDA imposed severe restrictions on antiaging assumptions, this would not prevent practitioners from prescribing drugs that are unproven for antiaging uses, such as human growth hormone. The Federal Food, Drug, and Cosmetic Act does not restrict physicians from prescribing products for off-label indications. The manufacturer of a drug or device must notify the FDA of adverse event reports stemming from off-label use (U.S. Department of Health and Human Services, 2001), but adverse events in general are significantly under reported [64].

25.16 Safety and efficacy determination of antiaging nutraceuticals

Conventional food (including beverages) and food supplements show growing overlap between them, including energy bars and teas or liquids. This overlap becomes even wider when we consider functional foods and nutraceuticals. The term nutraceutical was originally coined by Stephen DeFelice as a combination of the words nutrient and pharmaceutical. WHO defined nutraceuticals as "food or part of a food that provides medical or health benefits, including the prevention and treatment of a disease" [48]. This concept has been proposed as a modern approach to food science, and the area of possible use has been defined as beyond the diet, but before the drugs [3,4]. The definition of nutraceuticals and a legitimate assessment of their potential in medicine are still contradictory being shared and accepted worldwide [5]. The nutraceutical definition often overlaps and the rationale behind the use of these products is becoming more and more important in their distinction. Nutraceuticals are growing and developed at tremendous rate and have rapidly spread worldwide [8]. Existing contradictory information in the field of nutraceutical is generating confusion about the possible effective use of these products, which are available on the market and in pharmacies. Food supplements, as per their micronutrient content, can be used to improve the health of individuals in need. In general, many of the health claims that are currently associated with food supplements, pro- and prebiotics, herbal products and functional foods may not properly be substantiated by scientific data on their safety, efficacy and effect on health and/or pathological conditions [65,66].

The claims are mainly unsubstantiated due to a lack of studies on possible mechanisms of action and a lack of in vivo research confirming the claimed beneficial health effects on specific pathological conditions. Another significant aspect is that the data reported in the literature mainly come from in vitro studies which are focused on single food constituents (micronutrients). Safety is of prime importance, as there is also the chance of contamination by inorganic and organic origins in these products [10,11]. Moreover, the ingredients themselves may cause health problems, and proper information on possible unwanted side effects should be provided on the label. From our point of view, it is imperative to have more information on safety and efficacy based on clinical studies rather than only in vitro studies, and it is also important for better understanding of the mechanism of action and bioavailability of these products. The first step in assessing the action of nutraceuticals is to distinguish them from the other food derived products, particularly food supplements, which are not always included in daily dietary habits in the presence of a specific need [12]. This exercise may require: (i) appropriate identification of target; (ii) safety evaluation; (iii) an understanding of the mechanism of action; (iv) efficacy assessment by clinical studies; (v) an evaluation of possible unwanted side effects; and (vi) an evaluation of possible interactions with other products (e.g., food, food supplements and drugs).

We think that a different strategy is needed for nutraceutical concept assessment and their use, and the existing assessment protocol for pharmaceutical products may be considered as a initiating point. Solving the discrepancies between the different accepted definitions of nutraceuticals and their regulatory requirements will be a significant challenge. An outline of the lack of shared regulations regarding nutraceuticals as pharma foods is needed [13]; Nutraceuticals are considered to be in the green area after diet, but before drugs. Therefore, it is important to clearly identify their specificity in term of their possible use and application in the pharmaceutical area.

The efficacy of each test product was objectively evaluated by measuring the evaluation parameters (i.e., SELS, TEWL, EC) at the test sites prior to the initial application of the test product and 15 minutes after the initial application. Evaluation parameters were then measured after7, 14, 28, and 56 days of test product use [67].

25.17 Surface evaluation of living skin (SELS)

SELS was measured by a Visioscan Instrument which uses a specially designed camera and halogen lamps to obtain images that permit the user to characterize the topography of the skin surface [68].

25.18 Tran epidermal water loss (TEWL)

TEWL represents the level of water that constantly transpires through the skin. In this study, TEWL was used as an indicator of skin barrier protection [6]. TEWL was measured with a computerized evaporimeter in a quiet area, apart from the general traffic and activity of the test center. Readings were obtained by placing the probe lightly in contact with the skin [69].

25.19 Electroconductivity (EC)

EC was measured with a Nova Dermal Phase Meter. The DPM measures skin impedance, an indicator of the retained water content of the skin. Qualified subjects reported to the test facility and were examined by a trained technician. Faces were devoid of topical treatments. Subjects equilibrated to the ambient environment for 30 minutes before baseline measurements of surface evaluation of living skin (SELS), transepidermal water loss (TEWL) and electroconductivity (EC). SELS uses an optical system in a special camera that measures four parameters related with skin surface topography: roughness, scaling, smoothing, and wrinkling. This method provides analysis of living skin directly; indirect methods (e.g., profilometric) require replicas and pictorial representations of skin topography. However, when using SELS, the four skin parameters are mutually interdependent [5]. Subjects were instructed to apply the day cream test product to the face and neck every morning. After the use of a facial cleanser, subjects patted their skin dry and applied enough of the test product to form a thin layer on the skin. The test product was then massaged into the skin. The night cream test product was applied to the face every evening, and the eye cream was applied above and below the eyes every morning and evening. The day lip cream was applied in and around the lips twice in the morning and twice in the afternoon, and the night lip cream was applied in and around the lips once at night [70].

One of the aging theories connects aging with excessive formation of free radicals, and its balance can be re-established by adequate intake of anti-oxidants. A large group of substances have clinically significant antioxidant characteristics. Diet plays an important role in the treatment of many diseases, and the right choice of nutrients can help in disease prevention and improve the quality of life. Regular intake of antioxidant-rich foods (fruit, vegetables, and whole-wheat grains) has a favorable health impact, which can slow down or delay the aging process of the skin [71].

References

1. Lee J, Koo N, Min DB. Reactive oxygen species, aging and antioxidative nutraceuticals. *Compr Rev Food Sci Food Saf.* 2006; 3:21–33.
2. Schagen SK, Zampeli VA, Makrantonaki E et al. Discovering the link between nutrition and skin aging. *Dermato-Endocrinology.* 2012; 4 (3):298–307.
3. Vranešić-Bender D. The role of nutraceuticals in anti-aging medicine. *Acta Clin Croat.* 2010; 49:537–544.
4. Kwak NS, Jukes DJ. Functional foods. Part 2: The impact on current regulatory terminology. *Food Control.* 2001; 12:109–117.
5. Patel P, Singh SK. The aging gut and the role of prebiotics, probiotics, and synbiotics: A review. *J Clin Gerontol Geriatr.* 2014; 5(1):3–6.
6. Agarwal V. An ayurvedic insight to ageing with its preventive measures. *Int J Res Ayurveda Pharm.* 2013; 4:31–33.
7. Wickens AP. Ageing and the free radical theory. *Respir Physiol.* 2001; 128:380–381.
8. George AJ, Ritter MA. Thymic involution with ageing: Obsolescence or good housekeeping? *Immunol Today.* 1996; 17(6):267–272.
9. Xu Q, Parks CG et al. Multivitamin use and telomere length in women. *Am J Clin Nutr* 2009; 89:1857–1863.
10. Lueckenotte AG. Theories of ageing. In: Gerontologic nursing, 2nd edn. Holly Evans Madison Publisher, 2000; pp 21–24.
11. Rath SK, Shinde A. Review of antioxidant activity of Rasayana herbs ayurveda. *Int J Ayurvedic Herb Med* 2012; 2(1):202–217.
12. Peng C, Wang X, Chen J et al. Biology of ageing and role of dietary antioxidant. *Bio Med Res Int.* 2014:1–13.
13. Benzi G, Pastoris O, Marzatico F et al. The mitochondrial electron transfer alteration as a factor involved in the brain aging. *Neurobiol Aging.* 1992; 13:361–368.
14. Thrower JS, Hoffman L, Rechsteiner M et al. Recognition of the poly ubiquitin proteolytic signal. *EMBO J.* 2000; 19:94–102.
15. NIH. Dietary Supplements: What You Need to Know, Available at: https://ods.od.nih.gov/HealthInformation/DS_WhatYouNeedToKnow.aspx.

16. American Academy of Pediatrics, Committee on Genetics. Folic acid for the prevention of neural tube defects. *Pediatrics*, 1999; 104: 325–327.
17. M. Hegedus, B. Pedersen and B. O. Eggum. The influence of milling on the nutritive value of flour from cereal grains. 7. Vitamins and tyrptophan. *Qual. Plant. – Plant Foods Hum. Nutr.* 1985; 35: 175–180.
18. M. de Lourdes Samaniego-Vaesken, E. Alonso-Aperte and G. Varela-Moreiras. Vitamin food fortification today. *Food Nutr. Res.* 2012; 56: 54–59.
19. M. Nardocci et al. Consumption of ultra-processed foods and obesity in Canada. *Can. J. Public Health.* 2019;110: 4–14.
20. R. L. Bailey, J. J. Gahche, P. E. Miller, P. R. Thomas and J. T. Dwyer. Why US adults use dietary supplements. *JAMA Intern. Med.* 2013; 173: 355–361.
21. Morganti P. The photoprotective activity of nutraceuticals. *Clin Dermatol* 2009;27:166–74.
22. Food and Nutrition Board, Institute of Medicine. Dietary reference intakes. Washington (DC): National AcademyPress, 2002.
23. Therond P, Bonnefont-Rousselot D, Davit-Spraul A, Conti M, Legrand A. Biomarkers of oxidative stress: An analytical approach. *Curr Opin Clin Nutr Metab Care.* 2000; 3:373–84.
24. Mykyty CE. Anti-aging medicine: A patient/practitioner movement to redefine aging. *Soc Sci Med.* 2006; 62:643–53.
25. Sebastian RS, Cleveland LE, Goldman JD, Moshfegh AJ. Older adults who use vitamin/mineral supplements differ from nonusers in nutrient intake adequacy and dietary attitudes. *J Am Diet Assoc.* 2007; 107:1322–32.
26. Hercberg S, Czernichow S, Galan P. Tell me what your blood beta-carotene level is, I will tell you what your health risk is! The viewpoint of the SUVIMAX researchers. *Ann Nutr Metab.* 2009; 54: 310–2.
27. Sommerburg O, Keunen JEE, Bird AC, van Kujik JGM. Fruits and vegetables that are sources for lutein and zeaxanthin: The macular pigments in human eyes. *Br J Ophthalmol.* 1998; 83:907–10.
28. Balz F. Antioxidant vitamins and heart disease. Presented at the 60th Annual Biology Colloquium, Oregon State University, Corvallis, Oregon, February 25, 1999.
29. Prahl S, Kueper T, Biernoth T, Wöhrmann Y, Münster A, Fürstenau M, et al. Aging skin is functionally anaerobic: Importance of coenzyme Q10 for antiaging skin care. *Biofactors* 2008; 32: 245–55.
30. Micke O, Schomburg L, Buentzel J, Kisters K, Muecke R. Selenium in oncology: From chemistry to clinics. *Molecules* 2009; 14:3975–88.
31. Messina MJ. Legumes and soybeans: Overview of their nutritional profiles and health effects. *Am J Clin Nutr.* 1999;70:439–450.
32. Craig WJ. Phytochemicals: Guardians of our health. *J Am Diet Assoc.* 1997; 97(10 Suppl 2):199–204.
33. White paper on Food Safety. 2000. Available at http://ec.europa. eu/dgs/health_food-safety/library/pub/pub06_en.pdf (last accessed 31 March 2020).
34. Regulation EC No 178/2002 of the European Parliament and of the Council of 28 January 2002 laying down the general principles and requirements of food law, establishing the European Food Safety Authority and laying down procedures in matters of food safety. Available at http://eur-lex.europa.eu/. (last accessed March 2020).
35. Directive 2004/27/EC of the European Parliament and of the Council of 31 March 2004 amending Directive 2001/83/EC on the Community code relating to medicinal products for human use. Available at http://eurlex.europa.eu (last accessed March 2020).
36. Directive 2002/46/EC of the European Parliament and of the Council of 10 June 2002 on the approximation of the laws of the Member States relating to food supplements. Available at Feur-lex.europa.eu.
37. ERNA. European Responsible Nutrition Alliance. Vitamin and mineral supplements: A risk management model. Brussels. Belgium. Available at www.erna.org: ERNA, 2004 (last accessed March 2020).

38. ERNA. European Responsible Nutrition Alliance. 2006. Available at https://ec.europa. eu/food/sites/food/files/safety/docs/labelling (last accessed 31 March 2020).

39. Regulation EC No 1924/2006 of the European Parliament and of the Council of 30 December 2006 on nutrition and health claims made on foods. 2006. Available at https://eur-lex.europa.eu (last accessed March 2020).

40. Augustin MA, Sanguansri L. Challenges and solutions to incorporation of nutraceuticals in foods. *Annu Rev Food Sci Technol.* 2015; 6: 463–77.

41. Abuajah CA, Ogbonna A, Osuji C. Functional components and medicinal properties of food: A review. *J Food Sci Technol.* 2015; 52: 2522–9.

42. Dadhania VP, Trivedi PP, Vikram A, Tripathi DN. Nutraceuticals against neurodegeneration: A mechanistic insight. *Curr Neuropharmacol.* 2016; 14: 627–40.

43. Olaiya CO, Soetan KO, Esan AM. The role of nutraceuticals, functional foods and value added food products in the prevention and treatment of chronic diseases. *Afr J Food Sci.* 2016; 10: 185–93.

44. Yang N, Kaarunya Sampathkumar K, Joachim Loo SC. Recent advances in complementary and replacement therapy with nutraceuticals in combating gastrointestinal illnesses. *Clin Nutr.* 2016; 36: 968–79.

45. Wildman R, Keller M. Nutraceuticals and functional foods. In: Handbook of Nutraceuticals and Functional Foods, 2nd edn, ed Wildman REC. Boca Raton: CRC press, 2016.

46. Santini A, Tenore GC, Novellino E. Nutraceuticals: A paradigm of proactive medicine. *Eur J Pharm Sci.* 2017; 96: 56–61.

47. Directive of the Council 89/389/EEC. Foodstuff intended for particular nutritional use. 1989. Available at https://eur-lex.europa.eu (last accessed March 2020).

48. De Felice S. FIM Rationale and Proposed Guidelines for the Nutraceutical Research & Education Act – NREA. FIM's 10th Nutraceutical Conference November 10–11, 2002. The Waldorf-Astoria, New York City, USA. http://www.fimdefelice.org/ archives/arc. researchact.html (last accessed March 2020).

49. Regulation EC No 258/97 of the European parliament and of the council of 27 January 1991 concerning novel foods and novel food ingredients. Available at https://eur-lex. europa.eu (last accessed March 2020).

50. Commission Regulation EC No 1852/2001 of 20 September 2001 laying down detailed rules for making certain information available to the public and for the protection of information submitted pursuant to European Parliament and Council Regulation (EC) No 258/97. *Off J Eur Communities.* 2001; L253/ 17–8.

51. Regulation EU 2015/2283 of the European Parliament and of the Council of 25 November 2015 on novel foods, amending Regulation (EU) No 1169/2011 of the European Parliament and of the Council and repealing Regulation (EC) No 258/97 of the European Parliament and of the Council and Commission Regulation (EC) No 1852/2001. *Off J Eur Union.* 2015; L327/1–22.

52. Commission Directive 1999/21/EC. On dietary foods for special medical purposes. *Off J Eur Communities.* 1999; L91/29.

53. O'Neill S, O'Driscoll L. Metabolic syndrome: A closer look at the growing epidemic and its associated pathologies. *Obes Rev.* 2015; 16: 1–12.

54. Dragsbæk K, Neergaard JS, Laursen JM, Hansen HB, Christiansen H, Beck-Nielsen H, et al. Metabolic syndrome and subsequent risk of type 2 diabetes and cardiovascular disease ineilderly women: Challenging the current definition. *Medicine.* 2016; 95: 48–52.

55. Rautiainen S, Manson JE, Lichtenstein AH, Sesso HD. Dietary supplements and disease prevention – a global overview. *Nat Rev Endocrinol.* 2016; 1: 407–20.

56. McCarville JL, Caminero A, Verdu EF. Novel perspectives on therapeutic modulation of the gut microbiota. *Ther Adv Gastroenterol.* 2016;9:580–93.

57. Commission Regulation (EU) No 1047/2012 of 8 November 2012 amending Regulation (EC) No 1924/2006 with regard to the list of nutrition claims. *Off J Eur Union.* 2012; L 310/36.

58. Bagchi D. *Nutraceutical and Functional Food Regulations in the United States and Around the World*. Boston, MA: Academic Press. 2008; 115–364.

59. Voinea L, Popescu DV, Negrea MT. Good practices in educating and informing the new generation of consumers on organic foodstuffs. *Amfiteatru Economic*. 2015;17:488–506.

60. Nally JD. *Good Manufacturing Practices for Pharmaceuticals*, 6th edn. New Vernon, NJ: CRC Press, 2016.

61. Kessler, DA. The regulation of investigational drugs. *N Engl J Med*. 1989;320:281–288.

62. Wolfe, SM. (2003). Statement on medical malpractice. The Health Research Group, Public Citizen. Retrieved on March 19, 2003, from http://www. citizen.org/publications/release.cfm.

63. Ahmad, S. Adverse drug event monitoring at the Food and Drug Administration: Your report can make a difference. *J Gen Int Med*. 2003;18:57–60.

64. Washington Legal Foundation v. Friedman, 13 F. Supp.2d 51 (D.D.C. 1998).

65. Sercombe L, Veerati T, Moheimani F, et al. Advances and challenges of liposome assisted drug delivery. *Front Pharmacol*. 2015;6:286.

66. Agarwal S, Kumari PVK. Advances in Novasome technology – A review. *Int J Appl Pharm*. 2013;5:1–4.

67. Pinsky MA, inventor. Materials and methods for delivering antioxidants into the skin. US Patent, filed 2010.

68. Singh A, Malviya R, Sharma PK. Novasome – A breakthrough in pharmaceutical technology: A review article. *Adv Biol Res*. 2011;5:184–189.

69. BFischer TW, Wigger-Alberti W, Elsner P. Direct and non-direct measurement techniques for analysis of skin surface topography. *Skin Pharmacol Appl Skin Physiol*. 1999;12(1–2):1–11.

70. Seitz JC, Spencer TS. The use of capacitive evaporimetry to measure the effects of topical ingredients on transepidermal water loss (TEWL) [Abstract]. *Clin Res*. 1982;30:608A.

71. Leveque JL, de Rigal J. Impedance methods for studying skinmoisturization. *J Soc Cosmet Chem*. 1983;34(8):419–428.

Index

Note: **Bold** page numbers refer to tables and *italic* page numbers refer to figures.

liver 69–70
  skeletal muscles 70–71, *71*
outcomes
  energy intake variations 80–81
  reduced dietary variety 81–83, **83**
  taste and smell, with aging
    processes 81
physical activity 76–77
recovery
  dietary supplements 85, *85*
  functional food 84
  medical foods 84–85
  nutraceuticals 85–88
regulation 73
  coenzyme 74–75, *75*
  cycle *74*
  intake changes 73
  micronutrients 75–76
sympathetic nervous system 78
temperature 78
epidermal growth factor (EGF) 433
epigallocatechin-3-gallate (EGCG)
  149–150
epigallocatechingallate (EGCG) 122,
  390–391, 455
epigenetics 34, 290
  in age-related diseases 383–385
  aging
    cellular, animal and insect models
     385–388
    DNA modification 381–382
    histone modifications 382–383
    noncoding RNA 383
  alteration 380, 410
  nutrition 388–389
    flavonoids 389–390
    isoflavonoids 392
    isothiocyanates 392–393
    polyphenol catechins 390–391
    short-chain fatty acids 393
    stillbenoids 391–392
esophageal motility 431
Eugenia Jambolana 598
European Food Safety Authority (EFSA) 16
European Medicines Agency (EMA) 16
European Union (EU) 578–579
excipient food 424
eyelids 242, *243*
eyes 227
  etymological derivations and synonyms
    227–228
  ocular immunity 240, *241,* 242
  predominance of *Mahabhoota* 228
  Tridosha and ocular health 228–229

fats metabolism 78
fat-soluble vitamins 453–454
Federal Food, Drug and Cosmetic Act
  (FD&C Act) 16
Feinberg, A.P. 383
de Felice, S.L. 146, 170, 216, 593
fenugreek 598
fermented functional foods 7–9
FFs *see* functional foods (FFs)
Ficus benghalensis 177
Firth, J. 663, 671
fisetin 507–508
flavonoids 6, 94–96, 219, 389, 417–418
  apigenin 390
  beneficial properties 116–119, *119*
  beneficial role *124*
  curcumin 389–390
  effects 119–121
  epigenetics 389–390
  oro-dental challenges 484
  quercetin 390
  structure and classification **117–118**
  United States nursing homes 524
fluorosis 611
folate 87, 268
Food and Agriculture Organization
  (FAO) 2
food disorders 267
Food Safety and Standards Authority
  (FSSA) 17
Food Standards Australia and New Zealand
  (FSANZ) 16
food with functional claims (FFC) 14, 17
foot massage 255
form sense 231
frailty 413
Franceshi 207
free radical theory 233
Freund, A. 500
fucoidan 5
functional dyspepsia 443–444
functional foods (FFs)
  classification 3, **3**
  definition 1
  energy metabolism 84
  fermented 7–9
  formulation approaches 10, 14, **15**
  marine foods 3–5, **5**
  market 1–2, 14, 16
  metabolic syndrome 600
  non-dairy milk beverage 7–9, **8**
  phytochemicals **9,** 9–10, **11–13**
  prebiotics 6
  probiotics 6–7, **7**

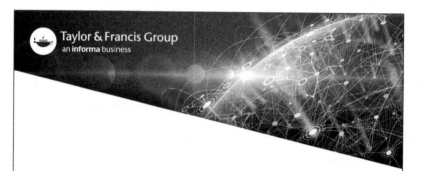

Taylor & Francis eBooks

www.taylorfrancis.com

A single destination for eBooks from Taylor & Francis with increased functionality and an improved user experience to meet the needs of our customers.

90,000+ eBooks of award-winning academic content in Humanities, Social Science, Science, Technology, Engineering, and Medical written by a global network of editors and authors.

TAYLOR & FRANCIS EBOOKS OFFERS:

A streamlined experience for our library customers

A single point of discovery for all of our eBook content

Improved search and discovery of content at both book and chapter level

REQUEST A FREE TRIAL
support@taylorfrancis.com

Printed in the United States
by Baker & Taylor Publisher Services